Advances in Corneal Research

Selected Transactions of the
World Congress on the Cornea IV

Advances in Corneal Research

Selected Transactions of the
World Congress on the Cornea IV

Edited by

Jonathan H. Lass

*Case Western Reserve University
and University Hospitals of Cleveland
Cleveland, Ohio*

Springer Science+Business Media, LLC

Library of Congress Cataloging-in-Publication Data

World Congress on the Cornea (4th : 1996 : Orlando, Fla.)
   Advances in corneal research : selected transactions of the World
Congress on the Cornea IV / edited by Jonathan H. Lass.
       p.   cm.
   "Proceedings of the World Congress on the Cornea IV, held April
17-19, 1996, in Orlando, Florida"--T.p. verso.
   Includes bibliographical references and index.
   ISBN 978-1-4613-7460-2   ISBN 978-1-4615-5389-2 (eBook)
   DOI 10.1007/978-1-4615-5389-2
   1. Cornea--Surgery--Congresses. 2. Cornea--Diseases--Congresses.
3. Cornea--Pathophysiology--Congresses.   I. Title.
   [DNLM: 1. Corneal Diseases--congresses.   2. Corneal
Transplantation--congresses. 3. Corneal Stroma--congresses.
4. Refractive Errors--surgery--congresses. 5. Contact Lenses-
-congresses. 6. Keratitis--congresses.   WW 220 W927c 1997]
RE336.W6   1996
617.7'19--DC21
DNLM/DLC
for Library of Congress   97-42705
                                                                 CIP

Proceedings of the World Congress on the Cornea IV, held April 17–19, 1996, in Orlando, Florida

ISBN 978-1-4613-7460-2

© 1997 Springer Science+Business Media New York
Originally published by Plenum Press,New York in 1997
Softcover reprint of the hardcover 1st edition 1997

10 9 8 7 6 5 4 3 2 1

PREFACE

These Proceedings of the Fourth International Congress on the Cornea continue a tradition of summarizing the state-of-the art basic and clinical research in cornea and external diseases since the first Congress was held in 1964. Reflecting the emerging importance of refractive surgery, two of the twelve sessions of the Congress were devoted to refractive surgery; this is reflected in an emphasis in these Proceedings. In addition, an entire session was devoted to the molecular and cellular biology of the cornea with important new information on the role of growth factors and cytokine modulation of corneal wound healing. Within these Proceedings an international group of expert researchers and practitioners provide the latest insights into the tear film and ocular surface, corneal transplantation and eyebanking, the corneal stroma and endothelium, contact lenses, microbial and nonmicrobial keratitis, keratoconus, and world corneal health.

Notable subjects covered include the latest understanding of the barrier function of the ocular surface epithelium, corneal hydration control, the molecular mechanisms controlling gene expression in corneal wound healing, stromal–epithelial interactions in the cornea, the immunology of blepharitis, the effect of contact lenses on the conjunctiva, morphologic and functional evaluation of the human corneal endothelium, long-term follow-up of penetrating keratoplasty in keratoconus, the Tampa trephine penetrating keratoplasty, and the refractive results of the Nidek EC-5000 excimer laser. In addition to the papers included in these Proceedings, there is a complete listing of all the abstracts of the 179 papers and 103 posters presented at the Fourth Congress.

Our objective in this book is to provide a comprehensive survey of the advances in cornea, external disease, and refractive surgery in the past 10 years since the last Congress was held in 1987. With the participation of an international group of leading experts, this book will allow the reader to appreciate the scope of knowledge in these fields throughout the world and hopefully will stimulate further advances to be reported at the Fifth International Congress on the Cornea 10 years from now.

Jonathan H. Lass
Cleveland, Ohio

ACKNOWLEDGMENTS

This volume contains 48 papers and abstracts presented at the Fourth International Congress on the Cornea held in Orlando, Florida, from April 17 to April 19, 1996. Over 500 participants from 32 countries gathered to define the current state of clinical progress in our subspecialty since the Third International Congress held in 1987 in Washington, D.C. Prior congresses, held in Washington in 1964 and 1976, have been stimuli for progress in the pursuit against world corneal blindness. Since its founding by Dr. John Harry King, the Castroviejo Society has been the major sponsor of these congresses, including this Fourth Congress. The Castroviejo Society was named in honor of Ramon Castroviejo, who is remembered as one of the seminal leaders in the field of corneal transplantation. Further support of this congress was provided by the Contact Lens Association of Ophthalmologists (CLAO) under its President, Dr. Donald Doughman; the Eye Bank Association of America (EBAA) under its President, Dr. William Reinhart; the International Society of Refractive Surgery (ISRS) under its President, Dr. Richard Lindstrom; the Ocular Microbiology and Immunology Group (OMIG) under its President, Dr. Gilbert Smolin; and Tissue Banks International (TBI) under its Executive Director, Mr. Frederick Griffith.

The Fourth Congress was pleased to honor leaders in the field over the past 30 years since the First Congress. These leaders included Drs. James Aquavella, Jose Barraquer, Jules Baum, S. Arthur Boruchoff, Stuart Brown, Jorge Buxton, Douglas Coster, Tadeu Cvintal, Richard Forster, Claes Dohlman, Merrill Grayson, Barrie Jones, Herbert Katzin, Herbert Kaufman, Peter Laibson, Howard Leibowitz, Michael Lemp, Enrique Malbran, Sr., A. Edward Maumenee, Saiichi Mishima, Madan Mohan, Akira Nakajima, Guillermo Pico, Sr., Frank Polack, Martin Reim, Daniel Taylor, Richard Troutman, and Alberto Urrets-Zavalia.

Special thanks are due to my codirectors, Drs. Shigeru Kinoshita and David Schanzlin, for their tireless effort in the organization and direction of this Congress; to the Planning Committee, including Drs. James Aquavella, Jules Baum, Peter Donshik, Gary Foulks, James McCulley, and Ronald Smith, for their assistance in the design and planning of the Congress; and to the moderators of the 12 sessions listed below, who invited the participants for their sessions and selected the free papers and posters. These individuals included:

Contact Lenses	Peter Donshik, M.D.
	Jan Kok, M.D.
Corneal Transplantation and Eye Banking	Matthias Böhnke, M.D.
	Roger Meyer, M.D.
	Gullapalli Rao, M.D.

Corneal Stroma and Endothelium	William Bourne, M.D.
	Mitsuru Sawa, M.D.
Keratoconus	Jay Krachmer, M.D.
	Yves Pouliquen, M.D.
Microbial Keratitis–Non-Viral	Joseph Frucht-Pery, M.D.
	Thomas Liesegang, M.D.
Microbial Keratitis–Viral	David Easty, M.D.
	Y. Jerold Gordon, M.D.
Molecular and Cellular Biology, Genetics	Timo Tervo, M.D.
	Steven Wilson, M.D.
Non-Microbial Keratitis and Immunology	C. Stephen Foster, M.D.
	Peter Watson, M.D.
Ocular Surface, Lids, Tears	Anthony Bron, M.D.
	William Mathers, M.D.
	Teruo Nishida, M.D.
Refractive Surgery	Rubens Belfort, M.D.
	Joseph Colin, M.D.
	John Marshall, Ph.D.
	Jeffery Robin, M.D.
	Theo Seiler, M.D.
	George Waring, M.D.
World Corneal Health	Chandler Dawson, M.D.
	Hugh Taylor, M.D.

Finally, thanks go to Susan Krister and Educational Meeting Management for their assistance in the organization of the meeting, Connie Koran for editorial services, and profound gratitude and appreciation to the following major corporate sponsors whose support made the Fourth Congress and this book possible: Vistakon, Alcon, Allergan, Chiron Vision, KeraVision, Storz, and the Japanese sponsors (Alcon Japan Limited, Bausch & Lomb Japan, CIBA Vision, HOYA Corporation, Inami Ophthalmic Instruments, JCR Pharmaceuticals, Johnson & Johnson Vision Products, Matsumoto Medical Instruments, Otsuka Pharmaceutical, Rohto Pharmaceutical, San Contact Lens Company, Santen Pharmaceutical, and Senju Pharmaceutical).

CONTENTS

Session I. Ocular Surface, Lids, Tears

Session II. Corneal Transplantation and Eye Banking

Session III. Corneal Stroma and Endothelium

Sessions IV and XII. Refractive Surgery

Session V. Molecular Biology, Cellular Biology, and Genetics

Session VI. Contact Lenses

Session VII. Microbial Keratitis — Viral

Session VIII. Keratoconus

Session IX. Non-Microbial Keratitis and Immunology

Session X. World Corneal Health

Session XI. Microbial Keratitis — Non-Viral

Session I

Ocular Surface, Lids, Tears

THE EVOLUTION OF LID MARGIN CHANGES IN BLEPHARITIS

A. J. Bron and J. M. Tiffany

Nuffield Laboratory of Ophthalmology
University of Oxford
Oxford, United Kingdom

ABSTRACT

Anterior blepharitis affects the lash-bearing region of the lids. It may be seborrhoeic or non-seborrhoeic and is associated with an increased prevalence of lid commensals. Colonization with *S. aureus*, although not necessarily associated with blepharitis, increases the risk and may be accompanied by lid crusting, collarettes, styes, and folliculitis. Enhanced cell-mediated immunity to *S. aureus* may provide a partial explanation for the folliculitis. *S. aureus* carriage is very high in atopes, while ulcerative blepharitis is associated with *Candida* superinfection. There is a strong link between anterior blepharitis and skin diseases such as seborrhoeic dermatitis, acne rosacea, atopy, and psoriasis.

Posterior blepharitis is usually due to obstructive meibomian gland disease resulting from hyperkeratinization of the meibomian ducts, or from cicatricial events. The latter may dominate the picture in cicatrizing disorders such as trachoma. Posterior blepharitis is strongly associated with skin disorders; focal blepharitis occurs with seborrhoeic dermatitis and diffuse blepharitis with atopy and acne rosacea. Meibomian seborrhoea may be a hypersecretory disorder, although an obstructive element may explain the excess of expressible lipid; a hyposecretory form of meibomian gland disease is also a theoretical possibility. In both anterior and posterior blepharitis, constitutional features of meibomian lid composition, together with the action of lipid commensals on such lipids, may determine some features of the diseases.

INTRODUCTION

This paper reviews the evolution of lid changes in anterior and posterior marginal blepharitis. The diagnostic term "blepharitis" is not used with great accuracy. In an English study of ophthalmic diagnosis in general practice,[1] use of the term by General Practitioners had a low specificity (0.23) and a low positive predictive value (26%). Even among ophthalmologists, differentiation of anterior from posterior changes is often not attempted and many papers use the word as a portmanteau term which does not distinguish the two. It is important for ophthalmologists to make this distinction, since although anterior and posterior blepharitis frequently occur together, they can occur independently and may have different etiologies.

ANTERIOR BLEPHARITIS

McCulley et al.[2] provided a classification of chronic blepharitis based on morphological and microbiological features in which anterior blepharitis was described as staphylococcal, seborrhoeic, and mixed, while posterior blepharitis was described as Meibomian seborrhoea and primary or secondary meibomitis (Fig. 1).

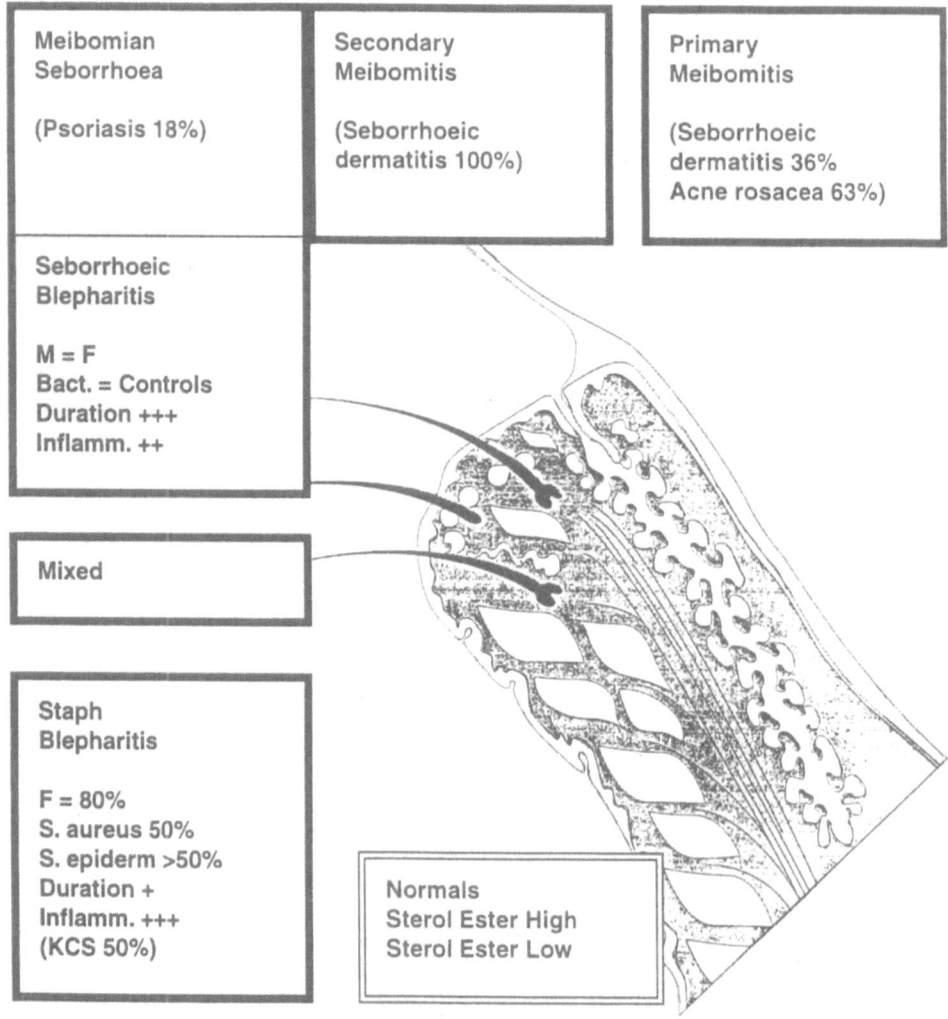

Figure 1. Classification of chronic blepharitis (McCulley et al., 1982).

Table 1. Frequency of skin disorder in chronic blepharitis (McCulley et al., 1982)

Skin disorder	None	SEB	SEBR	Rosacea	Atopy	Psoriasis
Staph bleph	64	9	9	0	9	–
SEB. bleph	0	100	0	0	11	–
SEB. bleph + Meib.Seb	0	82	0	0	9	18
SEB. bleph + 2° Meib.	0	100	6	12	0	12
Primary meibomitis	0	36	0	63	0	–
Normals	80	0	10	0	0	–
"Other"	50	0	0	0	9	–

n = 90

Controls 33

Seb.d. = seborrhoeic dermatitis; sebr. = seborrhoea

Associations with Skin Disease

McCulley et al.[2] noted strong dermatological associations with both anterior and posterior forms of chronic blepharitis; an exception was the Staphylococcal form of anterior blepharitis, where the association was weak. In staphylococcal blepharitis there was an association with seborrhoeic dermatitis, seborrhoea, or atopy in 9% of each of these disorders; in 64% of this group there was no association with skin disease (Table 1).

In the seborrhoeic form of anterior blepharitis, or in seborrhoeic blepharitis occurring with meibomian seborrhoea or focal meibomitis, there was an association with seborrhoeic dermatitis in 82–100% of patients, suggesting that the skin disease was in some way causal. Seborrheic dermatitis did not occur in their normal controls. Psoriasis was also associated with some forms of blepharitis.

Huber-Spitzy et al.[3] also examined the relationship between skin disorders and blepharitis in a series of 407 patients with chronic blepharitis, classified more simply into seborrhoeic, squamous, and ulcerative (Table 2). Seventy-two percent were associated with the same triplet of skin diseases identified by McCulley[2] (seborrhoeic dermatitis, 33%; acne rosacea, 27%; and atopic dermatitis, 12%). In 28% there was no such association. Seborrhoeic blepharitis was almost equally distributed between those with seborrhoeic dermatitis and acne rosacea, while squamous blepharitis occurred chiefly with seborrhoeic dermatitis. Apart from a few patients with acne rosacea, ulcerative blepharitis was confined almost entirely to patients with atopic dermatitis. Although these authors are in general agreement, there are differences in their findings which may be population dependent.

These dermatological associations might be expected to impose certain age, sex, and behavioral constraints on these populations with chronic blepharitis. In a further study, Huber-Spitzy et al.[4] found that blepharitis presented in relative youth in atopic dermatitis (age 19–31 years) and its activity might either wax and wane with the activity of the der-

Table 2. Frequency of skin disorder in chronic blepharitis (Huber-Spitzy, 1991)

	SEB. D.	Rosacea	Atopy	Total
Seborrhoeic bleph.	21	24	0.7	46
Squamous bleph.	12	2.7	0.5	15
Ulcerative bleph.	0	0.5	10	11

n = 407

Seb. d. = seborrhoeic dermatitis

matitis (as noted by Hogan[5]) or behave independently. Patients with seborrhoeic dermatitis were more likely to be young men presenting in their second and third decades. Those with acne rosacea presented in their seventh and eighth decade in this series and women were affected twice as often as men. It should be said, however, that in the series of McCulley et al.,[2] no particular age-or sex-specific relationship was discerned between the blepharitis groups except that 80% of the staphylococcal blepharitis group were women (compared to 56% males and 44% females overall), and were of a younger age, averaging 42 years compared to the average for all groups of 50 ± 18.9 (range 6–86 years). The time from onset of lid symptoms to presentation was shortest in the staphylococcal group (1.7 years) and in the primary meibomitis group (2.4 years) compared to an average of 8.1 to 11.64 years for other groups.

Bacterial Factors in Anterior Blepharitis

Staphylococci have been considered to have a causative role in blepharitis for several decades, since the original observations of Thygeson.[6,7] Several groups have indicated the means by which bacteria might contribute to both forms of blepharitis, either directly by infection or indirectly, through their actions on lipids[8] or by immune mechanisms.[9]

The Role of Lipids

Shine and McCulley[10,11] and Shine et al.[12] have indicated that in normal subjects, meibomian lipid composition may differ constitutionally, one group having very low levels of cholesterol esters and esters of unsaturated fatty acids (normal/cholesterol absent: N[CA]) and the other group, high levels of these fractions (normal/cholesterol present: N[CP]). Patients with each form of chronic blepharitis resemble this latter group and it was proposed that they are vulnerable to the actions of esterases and lipases produced by bacterial colonizing the lids, such as *S. aureus*, and commensal organisms, such as coagulase-negative staphylococci and *Propionobacterium acnes* (CoNS and *P. acnes*).[13]

Furthermore, Shine et al.[12] have shown *in vitro*, that the growth of *S. aureus* may be stimulated by the presence of cholesterol and it is relevant that the group of normals whose meibomian lipid is cholesterol-rich (N[CP]), show twice as many Staphylococcal strains on their lid margins as the cholesterol-poor group (N[CA]). It has been suggested on the basis of the above that constitutional meibomian lipid composition may influence the evolution of chronic blepharitis in two ways:

1. Esterases produced by normal lid commensals and colonizing *S. aureus* release fatty acids and cholesterol in that group of subjects whose secretions are rich in lipid esters. Released fatty acids could act as a general irritant in any form of blepharitis and could be the source of soaps responsible for "meibomian foam."
2. Cholesterol released from cholesterol esters will act as a stimulus to *S. aureus* growth and increase the risk of colonization, infection, and immunization.

The Role of Staphylococci in Anterior Blepharitis

Since a proportion of normal lids are culture-positive for *S. aureus*, it appears that colonization alone may not give rise to disease, but the increased frequency of colonization and the increased numbers of *S. aureus* found in association with anterior blepharitis suggests a causative role, which has been accepted for many years.

Table 3. Frequency of positive culture
for *S. aureus* from the lid margin

	Percent
Normals[15, 16]	8
	6
Mixed blepharitis[14]	11
Staph. blepharitis[16]	40
Blepharitis in atopy[4]	76
Retinoid toxicity[17]	79

Table 3 gives the frequency of positive culture for *S. aureus* in patients with blepharitis in different series. There are many such reports, using differing culture techniques in different populations; the data in the table are given simply for comparison. Groden et al.[14] found no difference in frequency of *S. aureus* in the lids of normal subjects (15%, compared to 11% in blepharitis), but the blepharitis was not broken down into categories and the study was not prospective. This study was of interest, however, in showing an increased degree of bacterial lid colonization, with a wide range of organisms, in "blepharitis" patients compared to normals. Positive cultures for *S. aureus* (using various techniques) have been found in 6–15% of normal lids in various studies[14–16] and were found in 40% of the Staphylococcal blepharitis patients reported by Dougherty and McCulley,[16] 76% of patients with blepharitis associated with atopic dermatitis (whether or not accompanied by ulcerative or squamous blepharitis)[3] and 79% of the blepharitis associated with retinoid toxicity.[17]

"Staphylococcal blepharitis," as defined by McCulley, is characterized clinically by the presence of lid crusting and collarettes and could include other features such as folliculitis and styes. McCulley et al.[2] and Dougherty and McCulley[16] found that although almost 100% of patients in their Staphylococcal group were culture-positive for CoNS (almost universal for normal lids), the proportion of *S. aureus*-positive patients was 40%, compared to a frequency of 8% in their controls. This implies that although the clinical phenotype is correlated statistically with the occurrence of *S. aureus* in the group, it is an imperfect marker in the individual case, perhaps because a single culture result does not describe the bacterial history of the lids but alternatively because the phenotype can be generated in other ways. Thus it is recognized that positive cultures for bacterial pathogens in an individual vary over time.[18,19] By the same token, since a proportion of normal lids are culture-positive for *S. aureus*, it is apparent that colonization alone is not sufficient to give the clinical disease. There would be an advantage in defining anterior blepharitis on the basis of clinical morphology alone (e.g., seborrhoeic and non-seborrhoeic), while refining the diagnosis for an individual patient on the basis of further information on their microbial and allergic status.

Two mechanisms of staphylococcal damage have been proposed, one infective and involving the release of exotoxins, and the other allergic and involving cell-mediated immunity.

Mondino et al.[20] developed a model of blepharitis by immunizing rabbits with Staphylococcal cell wall antigen. Ficker et al. found that 40% of patients with mixed forms of chronic blepharitis showed enhanced cell-mediated immunity (CMI) to the A-protein of *S. aureus*.[21] This far exceeded the percentage who were culture-positive for *S. aureus*, suggesting that if CMI has a role, it is to provide the immune environment for inflammatory lid reactions during periods of *S. aureus* recolonization. In this view, eradication of *S. aureus* from the lids by antimicrobial therapy would reduce the opportunity of stimulating CMI-based reactions by colonizing *S. aureus*.[22] (In the study by Ficker et al.,[21] it should be noted that the frequency of positive culture for *S. aureus* varied with technique: 22.5% of 80 subjects assessed by the scrub technique, and 9.5% of the total group of 116, by lash culture.)

It must be accepted, however, that neither a positive culture nor an enhanced CMI status itself is a confirmation that a given blepharitis is caused by a staphylococcal mechanism.

Other Infective Mechanisms

In the atopic patients studied by Huber-Spitzy et al.,[4] 76% of cases were culture-positive for *S. aureus*, regardless of whether they had squamous or ulcerative blepharitis. However, a positive culture for *Candida sp.* occurred only in the ulcerative blepharitis group. This suggests a special role for *Candida* in this group of patients. It was attributed to the frequent use of corticosteroids in atopes and treated effectively by antimycotics.

POSTERIOR BLEPHARITIS

The salient features of posterior blepharitis is meibomian gland dysfunction (MGD), a term adopted by Jester et al.[23] The term is synonymous with the terms "meibomianitis"

Table 4. Classification of meibomian gland diseases

1. Reduced number:	Congenital deficiency[24]
2. Replacement:	Dystichiasis[25]
	Metaplastic
3. Hyposecretory*	Secondary
4. Meibomian gland dysfunction[2,25,28]	
focal or diffuse[29]	Obstructive/cicatricial
primary, or secondary to:	
local disease	
anterior blepharitis;	
conjunctivitis e.g., *trachoma*; *pemphigoid*; *atopy*	
chemical burns[30]	
systemic disease	
seb. dermatitis[27]	*anhydrotic ect. dyspl*
acne rosacea[27]	*ectrodactyly syndrome*[31,32]
atopy[27]	*turner syndrome*
ichthyosis[25]	*fungal*[4]
psoriasis[29]	*toxic:*
	13-CIS ret. acid[33-35]
	polychlorinated biphenols[35-37]
other	epinephrine[23] (rabbit)
internal hordeolum	
chalazion	
concretions	
5. Hypersecretory**	
meibomian seborrhoea[38-40]	
6. Neoplastic	
7. Suppurative	

*Hypothetical: Evidence is not yet available for primary hyposecretion.
**Although there is evidence for an accumulation of meibomian oils within the glands, there is none yet for overproduction, as opposed to excessive release on expression.

and "meibomitis" (see above). Clinically there are inflammatory signs on the lid margin associated with the disease, but inflammatory cells are sparse within the gland itself. A general list of causes of meibomian gland disease is provided in Table 4 (refs.[24-40]). Excellent methods are now available to assess meibomian gland status and its impact on the ocular surface. These include: measurement of casual oil levels on the lid margin and its delivery rate by meibometry,[41,42] grading the clinical features of oil gland disease,[29] grading expressibility and quality of the meibomian oil,[28] and measuring gland drop-out by meibography.[28,43] The thickness of the preocular oil layer of the tear film can be gauged by interferometry[44-50] and the evaporative water loss can be measured by evaporimetry.[51-53] The contribution of oil gland deficiency and of aqueous tear deficiency to ocular surface disease are discussed in the NEI/Industry report on dry eyes.[54]

The meibomian glands are richly-innervated holocrine glands, related to the sebaceous glands in structure and function. The delivery of meibomian lipid onto the lid margin results from a secretory process and is supplemented by lid action. There is evidence that the absence of muscular lid action during sleep encourages nocturnal accumulation, which is discharged upon waking.[41,55]

Norn has suggested, on the basis of staining with Sudan Red dye, that only 45% of the meibomian glands are functional at a given time.[56] Expression of clear lid oil is taken as a feature of normal lid function. Norn has shown that the proportion of glands from which oil can be expressed decreases with age, without apparently decreasing the thickness of the preocular oil film (Fig. 2).[56] He suggested that excretion might decrease with age. This would explain the paradoxical finding that casual oil levels on the lid margin rise with age.[57]

Classification of Meibomian Gland Dysfunction

Three major types of meibomian gland dysfunction may be considered (Table 5) and are discussed below.

Hypersecretory MGD (Meibomian Seborrhoea). Meibomian seborrhoea is characterized by the release of large volumes of lid oil at the lid margin by expression over the

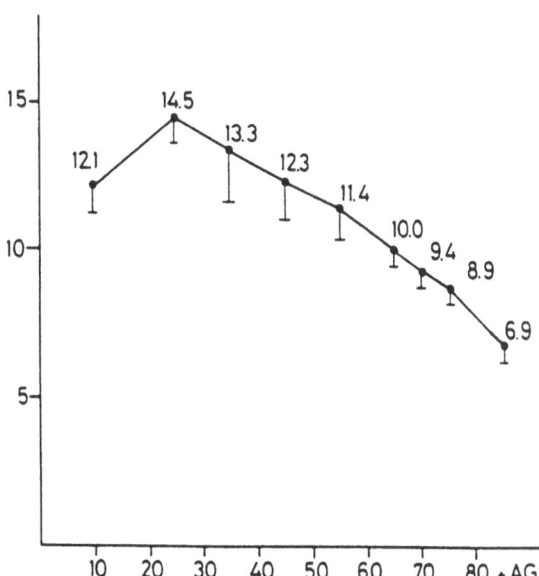

Figure 2. Expressibility of secretion from meibomian glands. Dependence on age. Abscissa: age; ordinate: average number of expressible glands. Bars: SEM. (From Norn, 1987 with permission).

Table 5. Models of meibomian gland disease

Type	Meibography	Delivery	Expression
Hypersecretory[1]	no drop-out	high	non-viscous: high volume
Obstructive	drop out	low	viscous: low volume
Hyposecretory[2]	no drop-out	low	low volume

[1]A hypersecretory state is mooted to exist in association with seborrhoeic dermatitis and to be equivalent to seborrhoea. It does not exclude coexistent obstructive disease, which could be responsible for a damming back of secretion, which would be expressed in increased quantity. This could mimic a hypersecretory state.
[2]A hyposecretory state not secondary to obstruction, is at present theoretical.

tarsal plate. It is assumed to be due to a hypersecretory state of the meibomian glands, paralleling that encountered in the sebaceous glands in cystic acne. It is reported to be associated with seborrhoeic dermatitis in 100% of cases,[2] but is also encountered in acne rosacea. However, it is recognized by some authors that the clinical features of the disease could result from a damming back of secretions in the presence of partial obstruction, in which case it could be an early stage of obstructive disease. It should be possible to distinguish true hypersecretion from partial obstruction using meibometry, and by directly demonstrating an increased delivery. This approach is currently under study in our department.

Hyposecretory MGD. There is evidence from studies of retinoid toxicity in animals, such as the Syrian hamster, that meibomian gland toxicity in this condition is due in part to a loss of acinar tissue in the absence of duct hyperkeratinization.[34] This is in keeping with the sebaceous atrophy that is the therapeutic goal of treatment when these drugs are used in the treatment of cystic acne.[58] At present there would be difficulty in distinguishing a hyposecretory form of MGD from obstructive MGD, although it might be suggested by a reduced delivery rate in the absence of gland drop-out and it is possible that meibography could quantify loss of gland volume. In experimental and human retinoid toxicity the meibomian gland changes are associated with ductal keratinization and obstructive signs.

Obstructive MGD. Obstructive meibomian gland disease is the most common form of meibomian gland disease (MGD). As with anterior blepharitis, this is strongly associated with skin disease, although it is also encountered in patients who do not volunteer any skin complaint.

McCulley et al.[2] identified two forms of meibomitis corresponding to obstructive MGD:

- Primary meibomitis was described as a diffuse form with extensive plugging of the glands, associated in 36% of cases with seborrhoeic dermatitis and in 63% of cases with acne rosacea.
- Secondary meibomitis was described as a "spotty" or focal disorder associated with seborrhoeic dermatitis (100%) or to a lesser extent with rosacea or psoriasis. (Our preference is to use the term "primary" to mean that there is no known associated local or systemic disease, and the term "secondary" when there are known lid or systemic factors; this differs from McCulley's usage.)

A question that arises is whether focal MGD gives rise to the diffuse form. This may be the case, but has not been shown. Although there may be a diffuse form with limited morphological disturbance to the gland orifices (i.e., absence of pouting or plugging), as noted above, expressibility of lid oil decreases with age[59] and there is room for confusing the effects of age with those of MGD itself. Thus, the clinician could encounter diffuse reduction of oil expressibility as an age phenomenon. It is possible that gland drop-out could be a useful differentiating feature.

Obstructive MGD is commonly encountered in cicatricial disorders of the conjunctiva but the frequency is poorly documented because serious secondary changes such as trichiasis, entropion, and ectropion overwhelm the clinical picture.[60,61] It is of interest that the frequency of meibomian plugging is increased in patients with conjunctivitis[59] and several observers have noted a relation between giant papillary conjunctivitis due to contact lens wear and the occurrence of meibomian gland disease.[62,63] Although attention usually has been focused on the role of MGD in causing contact lens intolerance and GPC, it is an attractive alternative to consider that the conjunctivitis initiates the MGD by causing periductular fibrosis.

The sequence of events in obstructive MGD is suggested by the findings in animal models:

- In a genetically determined model of hyperkeratinization, the "Rhino mouse," there is ductal obstruction by keratinizing cells and extravagant cystic change in the ducts and acinar tissue.[64]
- Daily topical application of epinephrine to rabbit eyes induces a severe obstructive meibomian gland disease, characterized by ductal occlusion and cystic expansion of the glands.[23,65]
- A similar condition has been induced in rabbit and primate eyes with systemic polychlorinated biphenols and mimics the changes encountered in human toxicity.[36,37]
- The effects of experimental occlusion of the meibomian orifices have been studied by Mishima and Maurice[66] and recently by Gilbard[67] and have demonstrated an increase in tear osmolarity followed by ocular surface changes including Bengal Rose staining and loss of conjunctival glycogen. This model best explains the clinical features that occur in meibomian keratoconjunctivitis.[26]

Histological studies of the meibomian glands from patients with MGD support the concept of duct obstruction due to hyperkeratinization.[68]

Some morphological features of obstructive MGD are shown in Fig. 3 and grading is described elsewhere.[29] We hypothesize that they are accounted for by a combination of obstructive and cicatricial events, as follows:

Obstructive

- The key event is hyperkeratinization of the meibomian duct lining leading to duct obliteration by the lining epithelium and shed keratinized cells. In the normal gland, shed cells are not usually found free within the duct. Increased keratin content has been measured in the expressed secretions from MGD patients.[69]
- There is some extrusion of shed cells which appear at the duct orifice as pouting or plugging of the gland orifice.
- Damming back of secretions leads to cystic dilatation of the ducts and acinar tissue.
- Ultimately there is a disuse atrophy of the acini due to persistent obstruction.

Other events in MGD suggest that additional processes are involved in its evolution which may be termed cicatricial. These include the following events which usually occur in a patchy fashion:

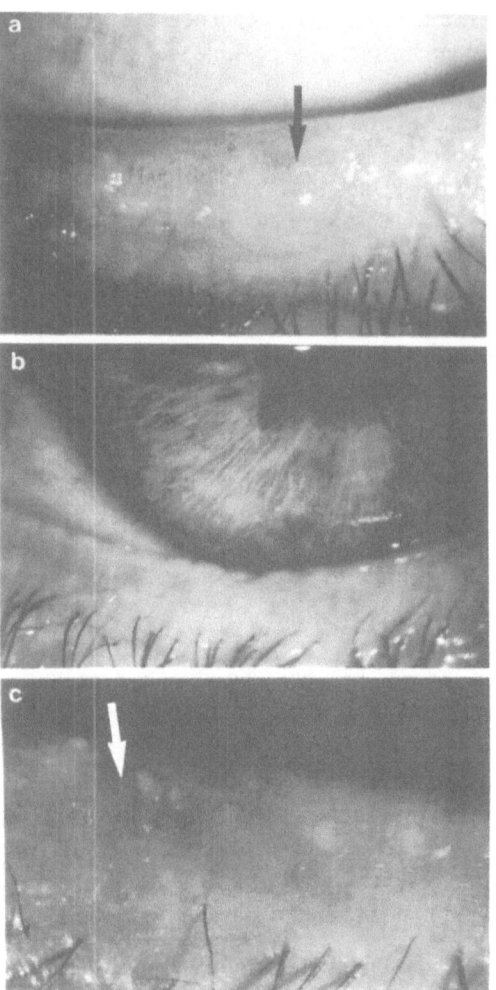

Figure 3. Clinical features of obstructive meibomian gland disease: a) expression of cloudy meibomian oil (arrow); b) focal mucosal absorption; c) plugged and opacified meibomian orifices which have been dragged proximally (upper left) by the cicatricial changes of trachoma. A focus of mucosal absorption (arrow) is also seen on the posterior lid margin.

Cicatricial

- The meibomian ducts, which normally run in the plane of the lid within the tarsal plate, become visible at the lid margin, due to a process of elongation, distortion, and exposure under a thinned mucus membrane. In the early stages lid oil can be expressed from such ducts.
- The orifices move behind the mucocutaneous junction.[29,56] This is an important event functionally, since the associated glands cannot deliver their oil to the pre-ocular tear film effectively from this position although oil could be floated to the surface of the tear film.
- The mucous membrane of the lid margin may be thin and/or the mucocutaneous junction may migrate proximally onto the tarsal plate. This is encountered particularly in cicatrizing conjunctival disease (Fig. 4). A ridging of the mucocutaneous junction may precede these events. Focal absorption of the meibomian orifices and periductal tissue at the lid margin, called "dimpling" by Cher, may be seen.[70]

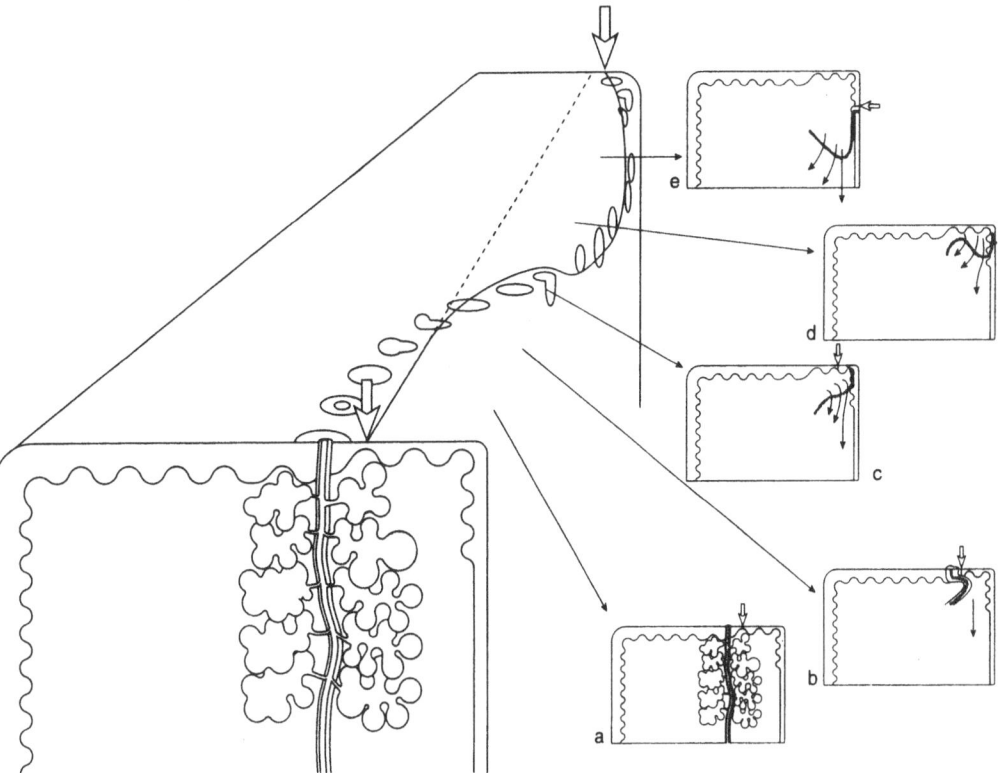

Figure 4. Schematic representation of the evolution of obstructive meibomian gland disease. a) Section thorough normal lid. b) Early gland obstruction with pounting of an orifice or plugging of a duct and early cicatricial changes. The elongated duct is visible through thin conjunctiva; the mucocutaneous junction (↓) is drawn proximally. c–e) Progressive cicatricial change draws the mucocutaneous junction orifices and ductules proximally. Their relationship varies according to lid location. The dotted line represents the original position of the mucocutaneous junction in the normal lid.

These various events are most reasonably interpreted as due to a process of absorption and cicatrization within the submucosa which drags the ductular apparatus proximally and renders it visible. The early marginal changes are seen in the absence of overt tarsal scarring.

In cicatricial conjunctivitis such as that due to trachoma, the lid is thickened by scarring and it is of interest that in trachoma the tarsal plate has been found to be of normal thickness while the thickening is accounted for by vertical collagenous bands.[71] Such a process would explain the ductular findings described here.

From the above, it can be seen that ductal plugging or pouting is the clinical sign of hyperkeratinization, while ductal exposure and retroplacement of the orifices are the clinical signs of submucosal scarring.

Lipid Factors in Posterior Blepharitis

Causative factors in the evolution of MGD include changes in meibomian lipid composition referred to earlier.[16] Meibomian gland disease is not an infective condition; expressed secretions usually show fewer positive cultures than those for the lid margins themselves. Any role that bacteria may have is probably indirect. It has been noted already that bacteria are generally more plentiful and strains more varied on lids with all forms of blepharitis. It is likely that the products of lipolysis contribute to the symptoms of MGD.

Some studies have raised the question of whether chemical changes in meibomian lipids (such as an increase in fatty acid or fatty alcohol chain length or saturation, or a decrease in branching) could initiate obstruction by raising lipid viscosity at normal lid temperature. Such evidence is not yet available, but it is of interest that the lipids of chalazion have a higher melting point than normal meibomian lipids.[72]

Posterior Blepharitis and Ocular Surface Disease

Posterior blepharitis in its mildest form may be asymptomatic. It is assumed that symptoms may arise from the effects of inflammatory mediators. However, although vasodilatation occurs on the lid margins, there are limited periglandular inflammatory signs in the absence of the granulomatous changes of chalazia. It is possible that duct and gland distention are a cause of symptoms, which could explain the relief afforded by lid massage.

Mathers and co-workers[28,73] have shown in patients with chronic blepharitis that meibomian gland drop out and decreased quality and quantity of expressed meibomian secretions correlates with increased tear evaporation and osmolarity. There was not a significant correlation with the Schirmer test. In a related study by Shimazaki et al.,[74] the presence of MGD correlated with an increased Schirmer test and it was inferred that hyperosmolarity in this group of patients was a reflex stimulus to tear production.

McCulley and Sciallis described a condition of meibomian keratoconjunctivitis (MKC) as an important cause of symptoms in severe, chronic blepharitis.[26] Signs of obstructive MGD were associated with conjunctival injection, punctate keratitis, and superficial punctate keratitis (SPK). In all cases, MKC was associated with some form of skin disease such as seborrhoea sicca (11.5%), acne rosacea (34.6%), or seborrhoeic dermatitis on its own (38.5%) or in combination with atopy (15.4%). The SPK was thought to differ from that associated with anterior blepharitis. On the basis of a prominent interference pattern on the surface of the tear film it was concluded at that time that the punctate keratitis was not due to a quantitative deficiency of tear lipid. Presumably some other qualitative factor was thought to be responsible. The findings of Mathers et al. suggest that a quantitative loss is likely to be important.[28,73]

Combined Anterior Blepharitis and MGD

Combined disease is not uncommon and is encountered in seborrhoeic blepharitis[2] and also as a specific complication of systemic retinoid therapy.[17] This is an intriguing association, since the hyperkeratinization of the anterior blepharitis occurs here despite the anti-keratinizing action of the retinoids. Possibly the frequent finding of a positive culture for S. aureus is of relevance.

Although in our experience combined anterior and posterior blepharitis occurs particularly in atopic blepharitis, Huber-Spitzy et al. recorded it in only 14% of their patients with atopy.[3,4]

CONCLUSIONS

It has been apparent on reviewing the literature that there is a relative paucity of information about the progression of the two major forms of blepharitis. This is partly because symptomatic blepharitis tends to be treated once it is diagnosed. Nonetheless, it has been possible to draw a number of inferences about its evolution.

The definition of chronic marginal blepharitis can be simplified by confining description to clinical phenotypes and elaborating the clinical diagnosis with other information relating to microbial and other features (Table 6).

Anterior blepharitis may be termed seborrhoeic or non-seborrhoeic on the basis of clinical features and is associated with an increased prevalence of normal lid commensals. There may or may not be colonization with *S. aureus*. The condition runs a remittent course influenced by the presence and activity of associated skin disease which may determine some aspects of the timing of presentation and severity of disease. The presence of *S. aureus* introduces a risk for marginal lid ulceration, styes, and folliculitis. Enhanced CMI to *S. aureus* may be partly responsible for the folliculitis. *S. aureus* carriage is very high in atopes, while marginal ulcers are almost entirely associated with *Candida* superinfection. Ulcerative changes lead to lid margin absorption and deformity.

Posterior blepharitis is usually due to obstructive meibomian gland disease, resulting from hyperkeratinization and blockade of the gland ductules. There is also an important cicatricial element and the relationship between these two components is not certain. However, the cicatricial element may dominate the picture in cicatrizing conjunctival disorders. Posterior blepharitis is strongly associated with skin disease, seborrhoeic dermatitis being associated with focal changes and atopy and acne rosacea with diffuse changes. Posterior blepharitis is not associated with infection of the glands, but the bacteria are more profusely present on the lids in this as in other chronic blepharitis. The lytic enzyme produced by these commensals may play a role in the pathogenesis and symptoms. Symptoms may be due to changes in the lids themselves, but extensive MGD may cause symptomatic, evaporative dry eye.

Meibomian seborrhoea may be a distinct disease in its own right, mimicking the features of sebaceous hypersecretion. Its association with seborrhoeic dermatitis makes this likely. However, it has yet to be excluded that it represents a form of partial obstruction with damming back of secretions. A hyposecretory MGD is currently a theoretical possibility for which the only candidate is retinoid-induced blepharitis.

There is still a great deal to be learned about the evolution of chronic blepharitis. Excellent methods are now available to study the components of each of the major forms of the disease. In those disorders where the etiological factors are known, such as the dermatoses, cicatrizing conjunctival disease and radiation damage to the ocular surface, there

Table 6. Classification of chronic blepharitis

Anterior	
Seborrhoeic (squamous)	(*S. aureus* +/-)
Non-seborrhoeic*	(*S. aureus* +/-)
with: crusting, collarettes, ulceration, folliculitis, enhanced CMI	
Posterior	
Obstructive MGD	focal; diffuse: primary; secondary
Hypersecretory	(meibomian seborrhoea)
Hyposecretory	(existence unproven)
Other features which may be associated with blepharitis: chalazia,	
concretions, conjunctivitis, ocular surface disease, dry eye.	

*A positive culture for *S. aureus*, in the presence of the clinical features listed below, entitles the diagnosis of staphyloccoal blepharitis.

is now the opportunity to carry out longitudinal studies which will clarify their mechanism.

REFERENCES

1. J.H. Sheldrick, Vernon, S.A., and Wilson, A., Study of diagnostic accord between general practitioners and an ophthalmologist. *Br. Med. J.* 304:1096 (1992).
2. J.P. McCulley, Dougherty, J.M., and Deneau, D.G., Classification of chronic blepharitis *Ophthalmology* 89:1173 (1982).
3. V. Huber-Spitzy, Baumgartner, I., Buhler-Sommeregger, K, et al., Blepharitis - a diagnostic and therapeutic challenge. A report on 407 consecutive cases. *Graefes Arch. Klin. Exp. Ophthalmol.* 229:224 (1991).
4. V. Huber Spitzy, Buhler-Sommeregger K, Arocker-Mettinger E., et al., Ulcerative blepharitis in atopic patients - is Candida species the causative agent. *Br. J. Ophthalmol.* 76:272 (1992).
5. M.J. Hogan, Atopic keratoconjunctivitis. *Trans. Am. Ophthalmol. Soc.* 50;265 (1952).
6. P. Thygeson, Etiology and treatment of blepharitis. A study in military personnel. *Arch. Ophthalmol.* 36:445 (1946).
7. P. Thygeson, The etiology and treatment of blepharitis: a study in miliary personnel. *Milit. Surg.* 98:191 (1946).
8. J.P. McCulley,. Meibomian secretions in chronic blepharitis. *Proceedings of the World Congress on the Cornea IV,* Orlando. In press. (1997).
9. D.V. Seal, Immunology of staphylococcal blepharitis. *Proceedings of the World Congress on the Cornea IV, Orlando.* In press (1997).
10. W.E. Shine and McCulley, J.P., The role of cholesterol in chronic blepharitis. *Invest. Ophthalmol. Vis. Sci.* 32:2272 (1991).
11. W.E. Shine and McCulley, J.P., Role of wax ester fatty alcohols in chronic blepharitis. *Invest. Ophthalmol. Vis. Sci.* 34:3515 (1993).
12. W.E. Shine, Silvany, R., and McCulley, J.P., Relation of cholesterol-stimulated *Staphylococcus aureus* growth to chronic blepharitis. *Invest. Ophthalmol. Vis. Sci.* 34:2291 (1993).
13. J.M. Dougherty and McCulley, J.P., Bacterial lipases and chronic blepharitis. *Invest. Ophthalmol. Vis. Sci.* 27:486 (1986).
14. L.R. Groden, Murphy, B., Rodnite, J., and Genvert, G.I., Lid flora in blepharitis. *Cornea* 10:50 (1991).
15. D. Badiani, Bron, A.J., Elkington, A., et al., The use of a novel transport method for the quantification of the external eye. *Microb. Ecol. Health Dis.* 1:57 (1988).
16. J.M. Dougherty, and McCulley, J.P., Comparative bacteriology of chronic blepharitis. *Br. J. Ophthalmol.* 68:524 (1984).
17. H.J. Blackman, Peck, G.L., Olsen, T.G., and Bergsman, D.R., Blepharo-conjunctivitis: a side effect of 13-cis-retinoic acid therapy for dermatologic diseases. *Ophthalmology* 86:753 (1979).
18. J. Nolan, Evaluation of conjunctival and nasal bacterial cultures before intraocular operations. *Br. J. Ophthalmol.* 51:483 (1967).
19. M.R. Allansmith, Anderson, R.P., and Butterworth, M., The meaning of preoperative cultures in ophthalmology. *Trans Am. Acad. Ophthalmol. Otolaryngol.* 73:683 (1969).
20. B.J. Mondino, Caster, A.L., and Dethlefs, B., A rabbit model of staphylococcal blepharitis. *Arch. Ophthalmol.* 105:409 (1987).
21. L. Ficker, Ramakrishnan, M., Seal, D.V., and Menday, P., Role of cell-mediated immunity to staphylococci in blepharitis. *Am. J. Ophthalmol.* 111:473 (1991).
22. D.V. Seal, Wright, P., Ficker, L., et al., Placebo controlled trial of fusidic acid gel and oxytetracycline for recurrent blepharitis and rosacea. *Br. J. Ophthalmol.* 79:42 (1995).
23. J.V. Jester, Nicolaides, N., and Smith, R.E., Meibomian gland studies: histologic and ultrastructural investigations. *Invest. Ophthalmol. Vis. Sci.* 20:537 (1981).
24. A.J. Bron, Tiffany, J.M., Kaura, R., and Mengher, L.S., Disorders of tear lipids and mucous glycoproteins. In *External Eye Disease*, D.L. Easty, and Smolin, G., eds., Butterworths, London (1985).
25. A.J. Bron, and Mengher, L.S., Congenital deficiency of meibomian glands. *Br. J. Ophthalmol.* 71:312 (1987).
26. J.P. McCulley, and Sciallis, G.F., Meibomian keratoconjunctivitis. *Am. J. Ophthalmol.* 84:788 (1977).
27. J.P. McCulley. Meibomitis. In *The Cornea*, H.E. Kaufman, Barron, B.A., McDonald, M.B., and Waltman, S.R., eds., Churchill Livingstone, New York (1988).

28. W.D. Mathers, Shields, W.J., Sachdev, M.S., et al. Meibomian gland dysfunction in chronic blepharitis. *Cornea* 10:277 (1991).

29. A.J. Bron, Benjamin, L., and Snibson, G.R., Meibomian gland disease. Classification and grading of lid changes. *Eye* 5:395 (1991).

30. F.J. Holly, and Lemp, M.A. Tear physiology and dry eyes. *Surv. Ophthalmol.* 22:69 (1977).

31. J.L. Baum, and Bull, M.J., Ocular manifestations of the ectrodactyly, ectodermal dysplasia, cleft-lip and palate syndrome. *Am. J. Ophthalmol.* 78:211 (1974).

32. B.J. Mondino, Bath, P.E., Foos, R.Y., et al. Absent meibomian glands in the ectrodactyly ectodermal dysplasia, cleft lip-palate syndrome. *Am. J. Ophthalmol.* 97:496 (1984).

33. F.T. Fraunfelder, LaBraico, J.M., and Meyer, S.M., Adverse ocular reactions possibly associated with isotretinoin. *Am. J. Ophthalmol.* 100:534 (1985).

34. R.W. Lambert, and Smith, R.E., Effects of 13-cis-retinoic acid on the hamster meibomian gland. *J. Invest. Dermatol.* 92:321 (1989).

35. H. Ikui, Sugi, K., and Uga S., Ocular signs of chronic chlorobiphenyl poisoning (Yusho). *Fukuoka Acta Med.* 60:432 (1969).

36. Y. Ohnishi, Ikui, S., Kurimoto, S., and Kawashima, K., Further ophthalmic studies of patients with chronic chlorobiphenyls poisoning. *Fukuoka Acta Med.* 66:640 (1975).

37. Y. Ohnishi, and Kohno, T., Polychlorinated biphenyls poisoning in monkey eye. *Invest. Ophthalmol. Vis. Sci.* 18:981 (1979).

38. H.W. Cowper, Meibomian seborrhoea. *Am. J. Ophthalmol.* 5:25 (1922).

39. S.R. Gifford, The etiology of chronic meibomitis. *Am. J. Ophthalmol.* 4:566 (1921).

40. S.R. Gifford, Meibomian glands in chronic blepharo-conjunctivitis. *Am. J. Ophthalmol.* 4:489 (1921).

41. C.K.S. Chew, Jansweijer, C., Tiffany, J.M., et al., An instrument for quantifying meibomian lipid on the lid margin: the Meibometer. *Curr. Eye Res.* 12:247 (1993).

42. A.J. Bron, Control of meibomian secretion and its role in ocular surface disease. (The Castroviejo Lecture), American Academy of Ophthalmology (1993).

43. J.B. Robin, Jester, J.V., Nobe, J., et al., In vivo transillumination biomicroscopy and photography of meibomian gland dysfunction. A clinical study. *Ophthalmology* 92:1423 (1985).

44. M.S. Norn, Semiquantitative interference study of fatty layer of precorneal film. *Acta Ophthalmol.* 57:766 (1979).

45. H. Hamano, Hori, M., Kawabe, H., et al., Bio-differential interference microscopic observations on anterior segment of eye. First communication: Observations of precorneal tear film. *J. Jpn. Contact Lens Soc.* 21:229 (1979).

46. J-P. Guillon, Tear film structure and contact lenses. In *The Preocular Tear Film in Health, Disease, and Contact Lens Wear*, F.J. Holly, ed., Dry Eye Institute, Lubbock, Texas (1986).

47. T. Olsen, Reflectometry of the precorneal film. *Acta Ophthalmol.* 63:432 (1985).

48. D.R. Korb, Baron, D.F., Herman, J.P., et al., Tear film lipid layer thickness as a function of blinking. *Cornea* 13:354 (1994).

49. M.G. Doane, Abnormalities of the structure of the superficial lipid layer on the in vivo dry-eye tear film. In *Lacrimal Gland, Tear Film, and Dry Eye Syndromes. Basic Science and Clinical Relevance*, D.A. Sullivan, ed., Plenum, New York (1994).

50. J.M. Tiffany, Chew, C.K.S., Bron, A.J., and Quinlan, M., Availability of meibomian oil and thickness of the oil layer on the precorneal tear film. *Invest. Ophthalmol. Vis. Sci.* 34:821 (1993).

51. M. Rolando, and Refojo, M.F., Tear evaporimeter for measuring water evaporation rate from the tear film under controlled conditions in humans. *Exp. Eye Res.* 36:25 (1983).

52. K. Tsubota, and Yamada, M., Tear evaporation from the ocular surface. *Invest. Ophthalmol. Vis. Sci.* 33:2942 (1992).

53. W.D. Mathers, Ocular evaporation in meibomian gland dysfunction and dry eye. *Ophthalmology* 100:347 (1993).

54. Report of the National Eye Institute/Industry Workshop on Clinical Trials in Dry Eyes. *CLAO J.* 21:221 (1995).

55. A.J. Bron, Reflections on the tears. A discourse on the classification, diagnosis and management of dry eye. The Doyne Lecture. *Eye* In Press (1997).

56. M. Norn, Meibomian orifices and Marx's line studied by triple staining. *Acta Ophthalmol.* 63:698 (1985).

57. C.K.S. Chew, Hykin, P.G., Jansweijer, C., et al., The casual level of meibomian lipids in humans. *Curr. Eye Res.* 12:255 (1993).

58. M. Landthaler, Kummermehr, J., Wagner, A., and Plewig, G., Inhibitory effects of 13-cis-retinoic acid in human sebaceous glands. *Arch. Dermatol. Res.* 269:297 (1980).

59. M. Norn, Expressibility of meibomian secretion. Relation to age, lipid precorneal film, scales, foam, hair, and pigmentation. *Acta Ophthalmol.* 65:137 (1987).

60. P. Wright. Cicatrizing conjunctivitis. The Doyne Lecture. *Trans. Ophthalmol. Soc. U.K.* 105:1 (1986).

61. W. Bernauer, Broadway, D.C., and Wright P., Chronic progressive conjunctival cicatrisation. *Eye* 7:371 (1993).

62. N.F. Martin, Rubinfeld, R.S., Malley, J.D., and Manzitti, V., Giant papillary conjunctivitis and meibomian gland dysfunction blepharitis. *CLAO J.* 18:165 (1992).

63. W.D. Mathers, and Billborough, M., Meibomian gland function and giant papillary conjunctivitis. *Am. J. Ophthalmol.* 114:188 (1992).

64. J.V. Jester, Rajagopalan, S., and Rodrigues, M., Meibomian gland changes in the rhino (hr^rh/hr^rh) mouse. *Invest. Ophthalmol. Vis. Sci.* 29:1190 (1988).

65. J.V. Jester, Nicolaides, N., Kiss-Palvolgyi, I., and Smith, R.E., Meibomian gland dysfunction. II. The role of keratinization in a rabbit model of MGD. *Invest. Ophthalmol. Vis. Sci.* 30:936 (1989).

66. S. Mishima, and Maurice, D.M., The oily layer of the tear film and evaporation from the corneal surface. *Exp. Eye Res.* 1:39 (1961).

67. J.P. Gilbard, Rossi, S.R., and Heyda, K.G., Tear film and ocular surface changes after closure of the meibomian gland orifices in the rabbit. *Ophthalmology* 96:1180 (1989).

68. V.J. Gutgesell, Stern, G.A., and Hood, C.I., Histopathology of meibomian gland dysfunction. *Am. J. Ophthalmol.* 94:383 (1982).

69. B.L. Ong, Hodson, S.A., Wigham, T., et al., Evidence for keratin proteins in normal and abnormal human meibomian fluids. *Curr. Eye Res.* 10:1113 (1991).

70. I. Cher, The simple meibomian dimple. *Proceedings of the World Congress on the Cornea IV, Orlando.* In press (1997).

71. A.A. Al-Rajhi, Hidayat, A., Nasr, A., and Al-Faran, M., The histopathology and the mechanism of entropion in patients with trachoma. *Ophthalmology* 100:1293 (1993).

72. J.M. Tiffany, and Dart, J.K.G., Normal and abnormal functions of Meibomian secretion. Proc. Vith. Congr. Eur. Soc. Ophthalmol. *Roy. Soc. Med. Intl. Congr. Symp. Ser.* 40:1061 (1981).

73. W.D. Mathers, Lane, J.A., and Zimmerman, M.B., Tear film changes associated with normal aging. *Cornea* 15:229 (1996).

74. J. Shimazaki, Sataka, M., and Tsubota, K., Ocular surface changes and discomfort in patients with meibomian gland dysfunction. *Arch. Ophthalmol.* 113:1266 (1995).

IMMUNOLOGY AND THERAPY OF MARGINAL ULCERATION AS A COMPLICATION OF CHRONIC BLEPHARITIS DUE TO *S. aureus*

David Seal[1] and Linda Ficker[2]

[1]Tennent Institute of Ophthalmology
Western Infirmary
Glasgow Scotland, United Kingdom
[2]Moorfields Eye Hospital
City Road
London, United Kingdom

ABSTRACT

Two immunological hypotheses have been proposed for the marginal keratitis (MK) complications of blepharitis due to *S. aureus* related to the increased presence of Langerhan cells, Cl complement, and IgM antibody in the peripheral cornea.

The first hypothesis suggests that recurrent MK has an etiological mechanism similar to that of peripheral corneal ulcers associated with collagen vascular diseases, in which immune complexes are considered important. The immune complexes deposit in the peripheral cornea; these deposits are formed by *S. aureus* cell wall antigen from lids and IgM antibody, activate Cl and its cascade to C5a, which is potent chemotactically for neutrophils.

The second hypothesis proposes that MK is due to a cell-mediated immune (CMI) reaction expressed as delayed-type hypersensitivity. This hypothesis is supported by the presence of Langerhan cells peripherally in which cell wall antigens, especially protein A, would be processed. They secrete cytokines which act chemotactically for mononuclear cells including CD4 Thl lymphocytes.

Both hypotheses would expect satisfactory treatment with topical steroids for the inflammatory, non-infectious etiology. The CMI theory better explains unilateral MK from local conjunctival-enhanced CMI as well as the observed occurrence of MK with systemic enhancement to *S. aureus* cell wall protein A. This could be treated by staphlylococcal desensitization.

Advances in Corneal Research, edited by Lass
Plenum Press, New York, 1997

INTRODUCTION

Marginal keratitis and ulceration present as a recurring problem in patients with chronic blepharitis due to *S. aureus*. These features, described by Thygeson[1] and by Hogan in 1946 and 1962, respectively,[2] continue to occur today.

Mondino has investigated extensively the condition in a rabbit model[3,4] and has shown an association with production of antibody and delayed hypersensitivity (DH), due to cell mediated immunity (CMI) to *S. aureus,* as well as to coagulase-negative staphylococci;[5] the latter does not occur in the human.[6] About 40% of chronic blepharitics have enhanced DH to *S. aureus*, which is not expected in the normal population.[6]

Two distinct hypotheses have emerged to explain the immunogenesis of occurrence of repeated marginal ulceration (Figure 1), secondary to *S. aureus* blepharitis. These are discussed below.

IMMUNE COMPLEX HYPOTHESIS

It has been suggested that toxins of *S. aureus* cause punctate epithelial breakdown that allows staphylococcal antigens to penetrate the stroma to complex with IgM found in the peripheral cornea.[7] This in turn activates the Cl component of complement found there, with a resulting cascade to C5a which acts chemotactically for polymorphonuclear leucocytes (PMNs) and causes release of cytokines. This in turn could result in marginal ulceration of similar etiology to immune complex disease associated with rheumatoid factor (IgM) to self IgG. Previous exposure to *S. aureus* antigens from chronic ulcerative blepharitis leads to increase in IgM present in the peripheral cornea and hence to a cycle of chronicity of marginal ulcer associated with chronic blepharitis. Steroids would be expected to inhibit the activity of macrophages, although not necessarily reducing macrophage activation by cytokines, and to inhibit cytokine release with additional suppression of PMN activity.

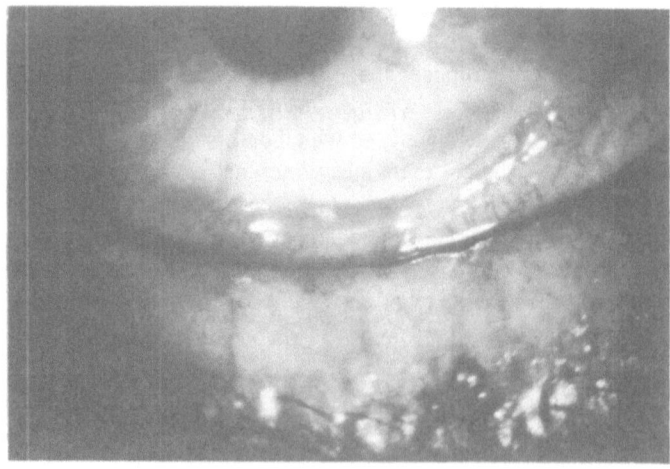

Figure 1. Marginal ulcer with severe blepharitis.

CELL MEDIATED IMMUNE HYPOTHESIS

A hypothesis of cell-mediated immune reaction in MK has been proposed in humans, based on investigative work.[6] Recurrent episodes of chronic blepharitis due to *S. aureus* leads to local conjunctival enhancement of CMI, expressed as DH, to cell wall antigens of *S. aureus*, especially protein A. This may also occur in an individual who has developed systemic enhancement from previous exposure to *S. aureus* infection or colonization at other sites.

S. aureus repeatedly colonizes the lids of both normals (approximately 10%) and atopes[8] (approximately 50%) from other sites of human carriage, as well as causing chronic folliculitis in patients with blepharitis. Cell wall antigens from *S. aureus*, especially protein A with/without ribitol teichoic acid, dissipate through the tear film and corneal epithelium into the peripheral cornea, aided by blinking. In the peripheral cornea, these antigens are processed by Langerhan cells (LC), which lie between the epithelial cells with a dendritic morphology.

LC are only found in the peripheral cornea, and are the only corneal cells to express the MHC class II antigens without prior inducement by cytokines.[9] Irritation to the central cornea, however, such as with herpetic infection can result in centripetal migration of these cells.

LC have receptors for the F_c portion of the antibody molecule. This may be relevant for endocytosing *S. aureus* protein A, as it also binds to the F_c receptor so that cross-linking may take place mediated by antibody molecules in a non-specific manner. These cells express the major histocompatibility class (MHC) II receptor and also take up antigen by pinocytosis. Upon exposure to antigen, the LC or other antigen processing cells (APC) undergo functional maturation and gain ability to present the antigen to CD4 T helper cells attracted to the area by cytokine production. This includes "memory" lymphocyte cells, primed from previous *S. aureus* exposure. The APCs take up antigens intra-cellularly and express them on the cell surface as antigenic peptides bound to MHC molecules; during antigen processing partial degradation takes place to oligopeptides with unfolding of the secondary structure.[9]

Corneal epithelial cells can produce IL-1, so activating macrophages, which then express MHC class II molecules and become APCs.[9] They will then process antigenic peptides (i.e., protein A) in a binary complex with MHC class II similarly to LCs. Macrophages can process particulate antigens including whole bacteria such as staphylococci, but can more effectively process soluble antigens viz. protein A, internalized in endocytic vesicles.

The CD4 T helper cell (Th) is responsible for most DH reactions. The Th1 subtype mediates DH, not given by the "2" subtype, based on an array of cytokines produced by T cell clones[10,11] Th1 produces IL-2 and interferon(IFN)-gamma, responsible in part for the induration response of the DH reaction. Th1 and 2 cross-regulate each other's activities via cytokine production by one inhibiting production by the other viz. IFN-gamma inhibits the effect of IL-4 on B lymphocytes - this may be the mechanism for in-vivo observation of a strong DH response with weak antibody production and vice versa so that preferential 'up-regulating' of the Th1 response down-regulates the Th2 response.

In extra-ocular sites, Th2 lymphocytes play a key role in immediate hypersensitivity reactions, producing IL4 and IL5 secretion by B cells and expression of IgE receptors, and producing IL-4, which induces mast cell proliferation.[9] Th2 cells are found in the conjunctiva of patients with vernal disease in children. This explains why patients with severe allergic keratoconjunctivitis as adults have very high IgE antibodies, associated with IL-5 induction of eosinophils, have lids colonized by *S aureus* but lack DH to *S. aureus* protein A.[8]

The activated CD4 Th cell secretes IFN-gamma at the site of antigen entry, inducing class II expression on non-professional APC, which activates them. The recognition of the MHC-peptide complex of the APC by a T cell receptor initiates an intra-cellular signal transduction pathway within the cell.[9] The molecules that are then produced increase binding of Th cells to APC and are called adhesion molecules (ADM). This includes the 55 kd monomeric transmembrane glycoprotein belonging to the Ig gene superfamily and for CD8 two 34 kd alpha chain molecules.

The cell-cell interaction (APC and Th lymphocyte) combination of CD3-TCR, recognizing the MHC/oligopeptide antigen expressed, and the complex of CD4 and CD5 receptors activates p59 and p56 tyrosine kinases by dephosphorylation as an "activity cascade." This in turn induces synthesis of IL-2 and its receptor expression to give proliferation of selected antigenic specificity resulting in the inflammatory DH reaction. The activity of these tyrosine kinases, and the activity cascade, is blocked by the drug cyclosporin which acts on calcineurin blocking T cell activation. Fucidin has a similar action, which may explain its beneficial effect for treating the blepharitis of rosacea, usually associated with both *S. aureus* colonization of the lids and systemic enhanced DH to it, with a topical preparation (Fucithalmic).

T lymphocytes exert their local effector function by secreting cytokines in tissue for direct interaction with target cells.[10,11] IFN-gamma induces expression of MHC class II molecules by keratinocytes, epithelial cells, endothelial cells, and fibroblasts, which can all vary in their capacity to serve as APCs. They can all process and present immunogenic peptides complexed with MHC class II molecules. However, they differ in capacity to produce co-stimulatory signals and do not stimulate resting T cells which require IL-2 to become activated.[9]

The cellular response is regulated by expression of ADMs on inflammatory cells and vascular endothelium, which in turn is controlled by cytokines that can also act as chemotactic factors for PMNs. These ADMs cause an adhesion cascade of PMNs and lymphocytes via the nearby limbal vascular endothelium, when they bind to it and then migrate to the site of activated lymphocytes in the peripheral cornea. Memory Th lymphocytes will also migrate to this site if the patient has previously-induced systemic enhancement to *S. aureus* cell wall antigens. The expression of integrins (B_1, B_2, B_3) attracts these activated Th cells to the inflammatory site. The expression of B_1 is up-regulated on the surface of activated memory cells which binds to the counter receptor on vascular endothelium (VLA-4, member of Ig superfamily) resulting in extravasation to the site (peripheral cornea) of the processed antigen (protein A). The expression of ICAM- 1 -B_2 integrin is needed for neutrophils which may be more relevant for the immune complex hypothesis.

New vessels have their origins at the perilimbal plexus of conjunctiva venules and capillaries. Such corneal neovascularization can occur at any level and must be considered in any immuno-pathological hypothesis since immunological privilege may be compromised.

HUMAN STUDIES

One hundred sixteen patients with chronic blepharitis of mixed etiology, some of whom had suffered from marginal keratitis and ulceration, were tested intradermally in the forearm for DH to *S. aureus* antigens, including killed *S. aureus*, killed CNS, and purified protein A (Sigma Laboratories).[6] A DH reaction was recorded in 40% of subjects after 48

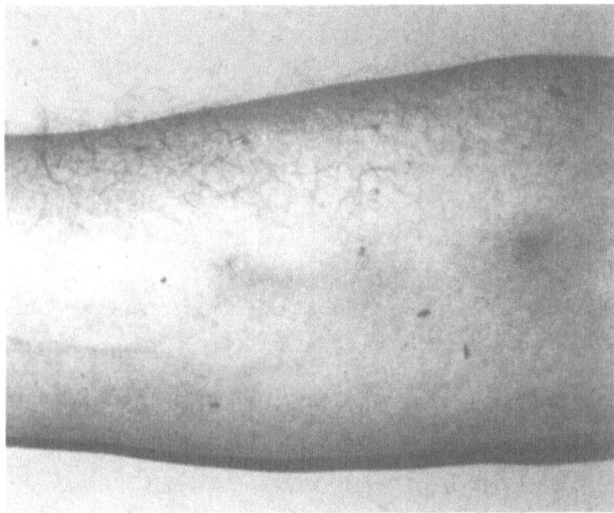

Figure 2. Arm (right) of blepharitic injected intra-dermally with killed CNS, saline, and killed *S. aureus* (right, enhanced reaction; others, no reaction).

hours for *S. aureus*, and a very enhanced reaction for protein A, but not for CNS (Figures 2 and 3). This suggested that ribitol teichoic acid of the staphylococcal cell wall did not play a role in the human and that protein A of the *S. aureus* cell wall was prolific at inducing DH. This situation is very different from that in the rabbit, in which it is possible to produce DH to CNS, but not subsequent blepharitic disease in the lids or a phlyctenular response in the cornea, and in which animal the role of protein A appeared minimal.[3–5] This would not be the first time that the rabbit has been shown to differ from the human, not only immunologically[12] but also for the pathogenesis of virulent bacteria for the human viz. *Streptococcus pyogenes* to which the rabbit is relatively inately resistant.

DRUG THERAPY

An understanding of the pathogenetic mechanism involved in marginal ulceration and keratitis, secondary to chronic blepharitis due to *S. aureus*, is essential if new treatment modalities are to be developed to suppress it. The role of the immune complex hypothesis versus the cell mediated immune hypothesis needs to be finally resolved. If the immune complex hypothesis becomes more germane to the clinical situation, then drug therapy targeted at inhibiting immune complex formation will be required.

Steroids continue to be used as an effective anti-inflammatory drug, although it is not clear for which of the two hypotheses considered above they are suppressing cytokine release and inhibition of cellular activity;[11] they are expected to reduce the inflammatory effects consequent to both of them. While providing effective treatment in the short term, they are of no long term benefit, and have no prophylactic role, which reflects our lack of full understanding of this common condition.

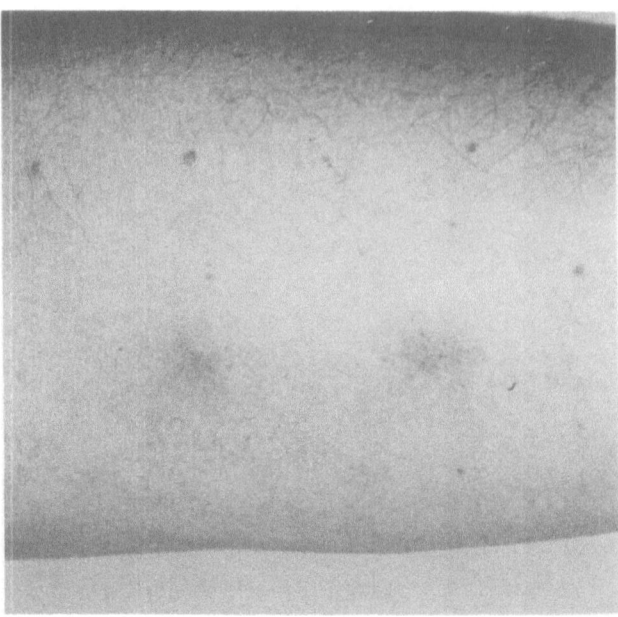

Figure 3. Arm (left) of blepharitic injected intra-dermally with *S. aureus* protein A (left, enhanced reaction) and thiomersal (right, control).

New drug therapy related to the CMI theory includes further investigation of the role of fusidic acid in the effective treatment of the blepharitis of rosacea, working on its cyclosporin-like activity as described. Additionally, new drugs could include diamidine therapy, with pentamidine, propamidine (Brolene, UK) or hexamidine (Desmodine, France), based not only on their anti-staphylococcal antibiotic effect but on the multi-factorial intra-cellular effect of the diamidine molecule.[14] This binds non-intercalatively to DNA, and modifies cellular function including inhibition of enzymes,[15] that could include inhibition of enzymes required for antigen degradation and processing with MHC class II molecules similarly to chloroquine, which is thought to act by increasing cellular pH.

Other possible approaches include desensitization with production of blocking antibody (IgM and IgG) to protein A. This should suppress the presence of the antigen in tissue and, if the DH hypothesis is correct, should not only lead to a general reduction in DH, which was recorded by Mudd[16] some years ago, but also to a reduction in the recurrence and severity of the marginal disease; it will be important to induce a Th2, and not a Th1, response. However, if the immune complex hypothesis is correct, then the patient may become worse and not better, because there will be increased IgM in the peripheral cornea which will give more complexes, not less, resulting in a greater degree of inflammation. Thygeson[17] had experimented with a toxoid vaccine, probably contaminated with protein A, to induce anti-toxin antibodies and had claimed some success. This field is fertile for pursuit.

ACKNOWLEDGMENTS

We are very grateful to Dr. John Hay for advice and comment.

REFERENCES

1. P. Thygeson, Marginal corneal infiltrates. *Trans. Amer. Acad. Ophthalmol.* 51:198 (1946).
2. M.J. Hogan, Daiz-Bonnet, V., Okumoto, M., and Kimura SJ., Experimental staphylococcic keratitis. *Invest. Ophthalmol.* 1:267 (1962).
3. B.J. Mondino, and Kowalski, R.P., Phlyctenulae and catarrhal infiltrates. Occurrence in rabbits immunized with staphylococal cell walls. *Arch. Ophthalmol.* 100:1968 (1982).
4. B.J. Mondino, Caster, A.L., and Dethlefs, B., A rabbit model of staphylococcal blepharitis. *Arch. Ophthalmol.* 105:409 (1987).
5. B.J. Mondino, and Adamu, S., Ocular immune response to *Staphylococcus epidermidis*. In, *The Cornea. Transactions of the World Congress on the Cornea III,* D.H. Cavanagh, ed., Raven Press, New York, (1988).
6. L. Ficker, Ramakrishnan, M., Seal, D.V., and Wright, P., Role of cell-mediated immunity to Staphylococci in blepharitis. *Amer. J. Ophthalmol.* 111:473 (1991).
7. B.J. Mondino, Inflammatory diseases of the peripheral cornea. *Ophthalmol.* 95:463 (1988).
8. S.J. Tuft, Ramakrishnan, M., Seal, D.V., and Kemeny, D.M., Role of *Staphylococcus aureus* in chronic allergic conjunctivitis. *Ophthalmol.* 99:180 (1992).
9. R.L. Hendricks, and Tang, Q., Cellular immunity. Chapter 6. In: *Ocular Infection and Immunity*, J.S. Pepose, Holland, G.N., and Wilhelmus, K.R. eds., MosbyYear Book Inc., St. Louis (1996).
10. S.W. Cousins, Chemical mediators of ocular inflammation. Chapter 5. In: *Ocular Infection and Immunity,* J.S. Pepose, Holland, O.N., and Wilhelmus, K.R.,eds., Mosby-Year Book Inc., St. Louis (1996).
11. Rosenbaum J., Towards cytokine insight in sight. *Brit. J. Ophthalmol.* 79:970 (1995).
12. R.E. Langman, *The immune system. Evolutionary principles. Guide to Our Understanding of This Complex Biological Defense System.* Academic Press, London (1989).
13. D.V. Seal, Wright, P., Ficker, L., et al., Placebo controlled trial of fusidic acid gel and oxytetracycline for recurrent blepharitis and rosacea. *Brit. J. Ophthalmol.* 79:42 (1995).
14. J. Hay, Kirkness, C.M., Seal, D.V., and Wright, P., Drug resistance and acanthamoeba keratitis: the quest for alternative anti-protozoal chemotherapy. *Eye* 8:555 (1994).
15. M.A. Anion, Bennett, N.D., Cairns, D., and Hay, J., Selective effects of pentamidine on cytosolic and granule-associated enzyme release from zymosan-activated human neutrophilic granulocytes. *J. Pharm. Pharmacol.* 46:394 (1994).
16. S. Mudd, Taubler, J.B., and Baker, A.G., Delayed-type hypersensitivity to *Staphylococcus aureus* in human subjects. *J. Reticulo. Endothel. Soc.* 8:493 (1970).
17. P. Thygeson, Treatment of staphylococcic blepharo-conjunctivitis with staphylococcus toxoid. *Arch. Ophthalmol.* 26:430 (1941).

3

MEIBOMIAN MARGINAL DIMPLES

Clinical Indicants of Reactive Pathogenic Processes

Ivan Cher

Department of Ophthalmology
University of New South Wales
Sydney, Australia

ABSTRACT

Lipids in meibomian secretion have been incriminated as inducers of some eyelid disorders. Consideration of eyelid dimples provides additional clinical evidence for this hypothesis. We need to draw attention to focal dimples and related indentations in eyelid margins; to demonstrate their intra-tarsal and marginal associations, as well as their relationship to meibomian duct-gland complexes (DGC); and to identify possible inducer agents and mechanisms. Patients with lesions of this type were sought and recruited from private and hospital clinics. The subject lesions were photographed revealing no signs of infection or neoplasia. Affected lid margins were inert and free of surface inflammation. On the other hand, a disordered DGC was found beneath each indentation, which in turn coincided with the relevant meibomian orifice. It was demonstrable that the dimpling process extended, in some cases, to notches, serrations and grooves. Associated intra-tarsal disorders found, were comedonic accumulation of meibum, linear granuloma, calcification and atrophic "drop-out" of DGC. Among marginal associations of dimpling were adjacent focal trichiasis and zones of lash deviation. Aberrant meibomian lashes were also encountered with dimples and, in individual cases, some combinations of these findings also occurred. From these appearances it was concluded that the indentations arose from post-inflammatory contracture along the DGC axis, aggravated in some by loss of submarginal bulk ("drop-out"). Strangulation by fibrosis may contribute to "drop-out." In aggregate, the findings support the view that there exist autotoxic pro-inflammatory and pro-metaplastic inducers derivable from meibum irrespective of bacterial liberation of free fatty acids. The constraint of comedo and granuloma to spindle shape suggests that pathogenesis can occur without breaching the walls of the DGC.

Advances in Corneal Research, edited by Lass
Plenum Press, New York, 1997

INTRODUCTION

In chronic meibomian gland disease, thickening, irregularity, and disturbance of normal contour of the lid margin occur.[1,2,3] However, in a thorough listing of meibomian lid lesions, marginal indentation, either focal or diffuse, does not feature.[2] One mention of atrophic dimple has been found in the literature.[4]

The possibility of irritation of eyelid tissues by meibomian secretion ("meibum"[5]) is acknowledged in seborrhoeic meibomitis[3] and in pathogenesis of chalazia.[3] Additional clinical evidence for such a significant mechanism would be valuable.

In spite of lack of emphasis in the current literature, indentations in the eyelid margins, particularly in the simplest form of the meibomian dimple, appear to support the belief that several different reactive eyelid lesions and irregularities arise because of retention of meibum.

The goals of the study reported here are to draw attention to these focal dimples and other related indentations of the eyelid margin; to demonstrate the intra-tarsal and marginal associations, as well as their relationship to meibomian duct-gland complexes (DGC); and to identify possible inducer agents and mechanisms.

PATIENTS AND METHODS

This paper reviews indentations of the margin and posterior lid edge. Clinical evidence is marshaled and conclusions drawn from exemplary cases. This is not a population study and does not establish the prevalence of the lesions demonstrated.

Patients for this study were recruited from routine private and hospital practices. Lesions of this type were sought, evaluated, and photographed, using both routine camera and slit-lamp photography. All clinical photographs were originally in 35mm Kodachrome, reproduced in half-tone for this study. In some of the illustrative cases presented here, ideally presentable matching photographs of both the tarsal and the marginal aspects of the lesion being studied, were not attained. One example of infra-red transillumination meibography is also included in this paper. For this, Kodak black and white high-speed infra-red film was used.[6]

FINDINGS

Various marginal indentations and their associations are now illustrated by the figures that follow. In all cases the patient was free of symptoms, unless there was also present irritation from eroding meibomian concretion or eyelash deformation disturbing the cornea. The simplest (and presumably earliest) marginal indentation coincides with a meibomian orifice in association with a disturbed DGC. If the indentation does not reach the posterior lid edge, then the term "dimple" is appropriate.

In **Figure 1** there is an example of a dimple. **Figure 2** shows light glowing underneath a dimple, transmitted to the margin from a hyperlucent comedo-like accumulation of meibomian secretion within the affected gland ("Fibre-optic sign").[2] **Figure 3** displays a stage in which the dimple extends posteriorly to form a notch. Lateral extensions of the indentation process will also be demonstrated **(Figures 19 & 20)**.

A granuloma associated with a meibomian dimple, not causing a notch is demonstrated by **Figure 4**. The linear or spindle shape is worthy of note. (The darker linear streak in line with the granuloma is the shadow of the everting rod.)

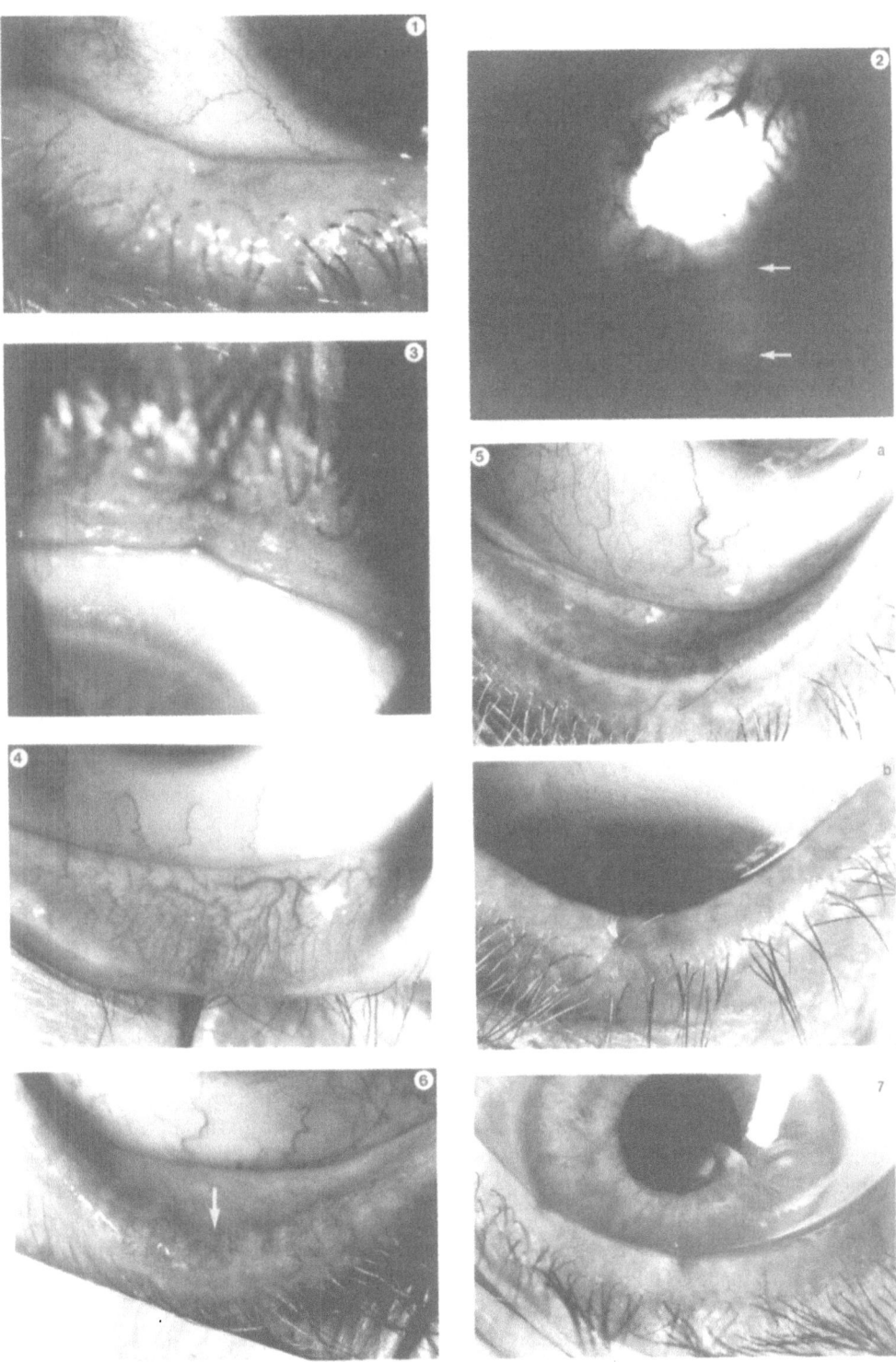

Figures 1–7.

Figures 5a & 5b show intra-tarsal inflammation with calcification underlying two dimples, and metaplasia within one of the glands (aberrant lash).

In **Figure 6** there is ubiquitous meibomian dysfunction. Loss of a meibomian DGC ("drop-out")[6] is indicated by the arrow, being recognizable clinically without infra-red meibography.

Figure 7 shows a notch associated with "drop-out" of DGC, while **Figure 8** demonstrates this type of "drop-out" atrophy of DGC portrayed by infra-red transillumination photography. **Figure 8** is not a photograph of the same case demonstrated in **Figure 7**.

In **Figure 9a** the notch is associated with an adjacent zone of lashes deviating towards the nose, The view of the tarso-conjunctiva in this case also demonstrates loss of the relevant DGC **(Figure 9b)**, indicated by an arrow.

Figure 10 shows lash-line distortion, actual trichiasis being associated with the notch. **Figure 11a** displays an eyelash which is part of a focus of trichiasis. This lash has grown posteriorly through the back surface of the dimple to lie under the tarsal conjunctiva. This is the rare condition known as Cilium incarnatum internum, digitally enhanced in **Figure 11b** * **(This case is one of two illustrated in this paper showing focal congestion near the site of the dimple).**

The next two examples show that the meibomian disorder has produced not only dimples but also metaplastic aberrant eyelashes. As in **Figure 5**, the lash may arise within the dimple orifice itself **(Figure 12)**. In **Figure 13**, two aberrant lashes are growing in the neighborhood of a dimple.

An example of duplex dimple appears in **Figures 5a & 5b**. In **Figure 14** four dimples are grouped without notching the posterior lid edge. In **Figure 15** multiple indentations are present causing serration of the posterior lid edge.

Figures 16 & 17 show multiple dimples along the length of upper lids, and each upper lid is grossly hypertrophied. **Figure 18** shows the contour on slit illumination of the case in **Figure 17**.

In **Figure 19** a group of dimples appears to have fused to form a short horizontal groove and in **Figure 20** an extensive groove runs the length of the lid margin.

SUMMARY OF FINDINGS AND DISCUSSION

In the cases presented here, signs of neoplasia or infection were not found. Except for two cases, the tissues near the dimples illustrated were free of congestion. Each dimple or notch occurred precisely at the orifice of an individually disordered intra-tarsal DGC. In addition, the intra-tarsal and the marginal associations found indicate that each indrawn meibomian orifice is invariably associated with focal chronic low-grade DGC inflammation and fibrosis, evidenced also by the presence in some patients of lash deformation, i.e. there exists in these patients localized posterior blepharitis with fibrotic and metaplastic sequelae.

In some of these cases "drop-out" was recognizable clinically as well as meibographically. Multiple and fused variants of indentations were found. The photographs reproduced here indicate that longitudinal marginal grooves may be examples of extended

---

* The slide of **Figure 11a** was enhanced to disclose the extent of subconjunctival penetration by the ingrowing lash using AAdobe Photoshop@. The Kodachrome slide was scanned. Red tones were reduced using color correction curves. The adjusted image was converted to black and white and contrast increased, producing **Figure 11b**.

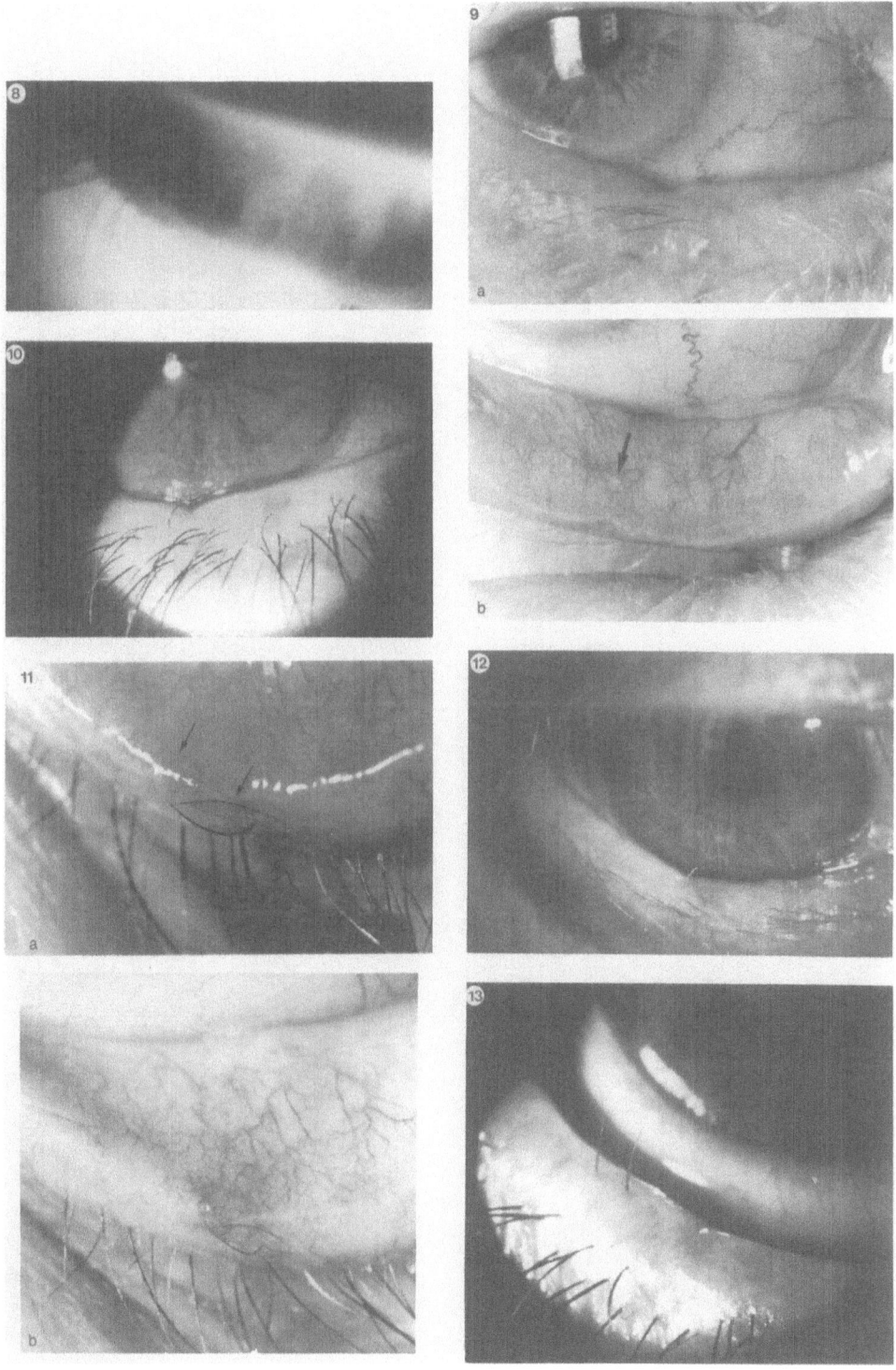

Figures 8–13.

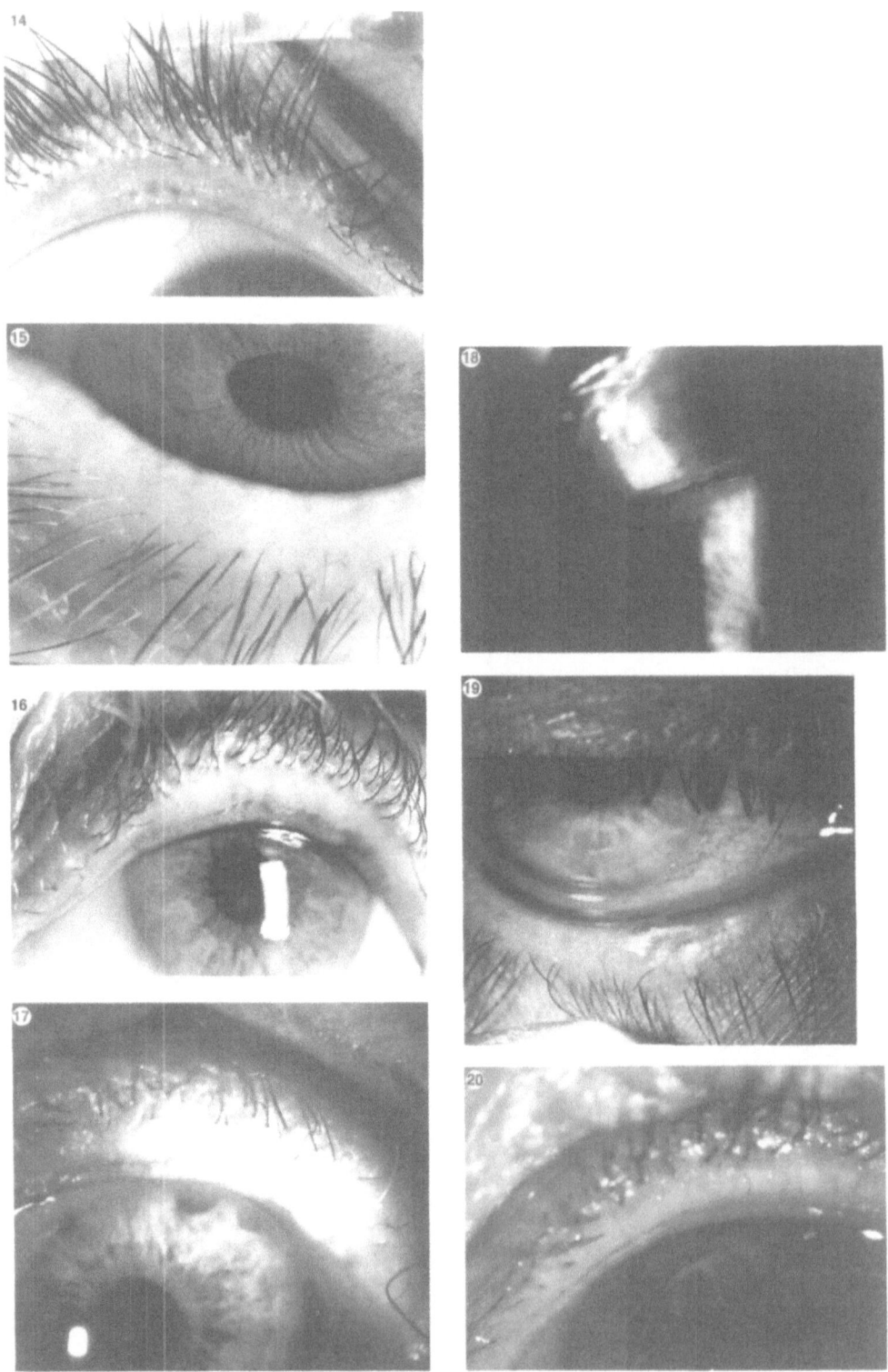

Figures 14–20.

fusion of adjacent dimples. This study revealed that it is possible for epidermal metaplasia (aberrant meibomian lash) to occur together with the dimpling process.

This study also confirmed that inflammation of the posterior lid lamella (tarso-conjunctiva) can be responsible for expanding lid thickness. (Paradoxically such chronic inflammation can also bring about loss of tissue bulk and thinning of the lid.) The cases shown in this report indicate an additional mode of altered lid dimensions, namely depressions or indentations in various forms along the lid margin. It is clear that dimpling can extend through the posterior lid edge forming a notch.

Other findings of this study are that intra-tarsal associations underlying the focal solitary marginal lesions are (1) retained meibomian secretion (Comedo) in which "fibre-optic sign" can be demonstrated; (2) another association in the tarsus, spindle-shaped granuloma; (3) localized calcification (post-inflammatory) associated with a dimple; and (4) with notches at least, evidence of "drop-out."

The observations suggest that where isolated dimples and notches occur, the marginal surface is inert (i.e., marginal blepharitis is absent). Among other findings were mesodermal cicatrization shown by trichiasis and nasal-ward diversion of lashes. This deviation was not, in every case, limited locally to the site of an indentation, but was also to be seen in several illustrations extending along the lid as an association of diffuse meibomian dysfunction. Retrograde subconjunctival ingrowth of eyelash, and epidermal metaplasia producing aberrant lashes also occurred. In individual cases, various combinations of different reactive lesions were found.

Trichiasis is well recognized and being cicatricial in nature.[3] The illustrations in this report demonstrate that dimple or notch can coexist with trichiasis and other lash disturbances. Cicatrization contributes to the indentations as it does to trichiasis.

In the case of solitary dimpling, one can invoke axial fibrous contracture of the underlying gland (compare nipple retraction in scirrhous carcinoma of breast). Anchored at fundus, the shrinking gland draws in its orifice. The linear nature of the granuloma portrayed in **Figure 4** provides an inflammatory base on which to anticipate linear shrinkage along the affected gland.

"Drop-out" occurring in association with marginal lid indentations may arise partly from other fibrous processes—for example cicatrizing a pre-existing granuloma—Chalazion scar.[7] Peri-acinar, centripetal, cicatricial strangulation may also play a role. Build-up of internal secretion pressure may be an additional cause of atrophy of the basal meibomian epithelium, in cases distinguished by enough resistant obstruction of the orifice.[8] Advance of the fibrosis can lead from dimple to trichiasis anteriorly and notch posteriorly. In the type of cases being discussed here, the intra-tarsal findings remote from the surface confirmed that the process initiating the marginal changes begins in the DGCs deeply in the tarsus. The occurrence of a dimple attended by comedo alone (without granuloma or drop-out), suggests that prolonged, mere retention of secretion in the tarsus can provoke low-grade inflammation even be it only subclinical in degree.

This study revealed that dimples or any of the tarsal or marginal findings can be present without a suggestion of microbial infection. In other meibomian diseases, absence of significant micro-organismal infection is recognized;[3] micro-organisms described not as *causative* but as *incidental*. Chalazia are generally sterile,[9] as can be even the pustular and cystic lesions of acne.[10] The literature already incriminates irritation by meibomian lipids, in development of chalazion, seborrhoeic meibomitis, some blepharitides and in conjunctivitis meibomiana.[3]

Evaluation of clinical signs in tarsus and margin associated with dimples illuminate etio-pathogenesis of meibomian disease from a new standpoint. The range of conditions described in this study epitomizes the manner in which primary meibomian dysfunction can lead on to secondary eyelid damage by inflammation and metaplasia. It also demonstrates chronic, low-grade, non-infective, meibocentric processes and invites consideration of the mechanisms for "drop-out."

The minuscule focal lesion of the lid margin, the meibomian dimple, its extensions posteriorly and sidelong and its effects on the lashes anteriorly, together with the deep and superficial associations in the eyelid provide useful clinical evidence re-calling attention to meibomian secretion as source of autotoxic pro-inflammatory and pro-metaplastic inducers of eyelid pathology, i.e. previously unemphasized clinical evidence.

CONCLUSIONS

Dimples, notches, and grooves arise from non-infective post-inflammatory fibrosis and cicatricial retraction along the axes of affected meibomian DGCs. "Drop-out" of DGC also reduces bulk under the posterior lid margin, encouraging notch formation. "Drop-out" may itself occur through resorption of granuloma, through fibrotic strangulation and through pressure atrophy of basal epithelium. The sub-surface intra-tarsal inflammation without infection suggests that liberation of free fatty acids by bacterial action upon meibomian lipids should not be invoked as inducer of the inflammation underlying dimples and their extensions.

The absence of infection, the minuscule focus, the meibocentric locus, the association with eyelash deformities, dimpling accompanying even overtly passive comedo, all support the view that (irritant material derived from) retained meibum can provoke reactive meibomian disease (RMD) in the adjacent tissues.

The anatomical constraint of comedo and granuloma into linear or spindle shape suggests that such autotoxic stimulus might provoke RMD by acting even through the intact walls of an affected DGC.

Meibomian glands are holocrine glands whose lipid cell membranes are themselves lost into the formation of meibomian secretion. It appears that chronically retained meibum can become pro-inflammatory and pro-metaplastic. A model candidate for such a meibomian inducer or mediator might, for example, be Leukotriene B4 (LTB4), a cytokine derived from arachidonic acid (a lipid substance released from phospholipid cell membranes).[11] LTB4 has been shown to cause epidermal hyperproliferation as well being a mediator of inflammation in vitro and in vivo.[11] As an inducer of hyperproliferation, it could also contribute to primary obstruction of the meibomian duct by excessive epithelial growth, followed by hyperkeratinisation, with implications for the pathogenesis of (primary) obstructive meibomian dysfunction (OMD).

REFERENCES

1. M. Grayson, *Disease of the Cornea*, 2nd Edition, The CV Mosby Company, St Louis (1983).
2. A.J. Bron, Benjamin, L., and Snibson, G.R., Meibomian Gland Disease. Classification of Lid Changes. *Eye* 5: 395 (1991).
3. W.S. Duke-Elder, and MacFaul, P.A., The Ocular Adnexa, Chapter 2, In: *System of Ophthalmology, Vol 13, Part 1*, W.S. Duke-Elder, ed., Henry Kimpton, London (1974).
4. M.R. Allansmith, The chronically red eye. *Audio-digest Ophthalmol.* 21(8):Side B (1983).
5. N. Nicolaides, Kaitaranta, J.K., Rawdah, T.N., et al., Meibomian Gland Studies. *Invest. Ophthalmol. Vis. Sci.* 20–24: 522 (1981).

6. J.B. Robin, Jester, J.V., Nobe, J., et al., *In vivo* transillumination biomicroscopy and photography of meibomian gland dysfunction: A clinical study. *Ophthalmology* 92: 1423 (1985).

7. W.D. Mathers, Shields, W.J., Sachdev, M.S., et al., Meibomian Gland Dysfunction in Chronic Blepharitis. *Cornea* 10(4): 277 (1991).

8. J. Shimazaki, Sakata, M., and Tsubota, K., Ocular surface changes and discomfort in patients with Meibomian Gland Dysfunction. *Arch. Ophthalmol.* 113: 1266 (1995).

9. K.V. Cahill, and Burns, J.A.(Discussion), Management of Benign Lid Lesions. In: *Focal Points Vol VII Module 2.* R.P. Carroll, ed., American Academy of Ophthalmology, San Francisco (1989).

10. T.B. Fitzpatrick, and Haynes, H.A., Skin Lesions of General Medical Significance. Chapter 50 In, *Harrison's Principles of Internal Medicine. 10th Edition.* R.G. Petersdorf RG, et al., eds., McGraw-Hill, Tokyo (1983).

11. J.T. Elder, Fisher, G.J., Duell, E.A., et al., Regulation of keratinocyte growth and differentiation: Interactive signal transduction pathways. Chapter 8 In, *Physiology and Molecular Biology of the Skin. Vol 1, 2nd Edition*, L.A. Goldsmith, ed., Oxford University Press, New York (1991).

4

DEVELOPING THE OPTIMAL ARTIFICIAL TEAR

Jeffrey P. Gilbard

Cornea Research Unit, Schepens Eye Research Institute
Department of Ophthalmology, Harvard Medical School
Advanced Vision Research, Inc.

ABSTRACT

Development of what has been called "the optimal artificial tear solution" was based on a two-pronged strategy. This strategy was first, to develop a profound understanding of the pathogenesis of dry-eye disease, and second, to develop a comprehensive understanding of why the eye needs a tear film. As an eye becomes dry, through either decreased tear production or increased evaporation, the tear film loses water and tear film osmolarity increases. The increase in osmolarity dehydrates the ocular surface and drives the disease process. TheraTears™, based on clinical studies, has the hypotonicity necessary to rehydrate the tear film, thwarting the disease process and permitting rehydration of the ocular surface.

As a result of a blood-tear barrier, the living cells on the surface of the eye depend upon the tear film for two life-sustaining requirements: oxygen and electrolytes. TheraTears™, based on clinical studies, has an electrolyte balance matching that seen in the normal human tear film; this electrolyte balance has been shown in pre-clinical studies to be crucial for the maintenance of normal goblet-cell density. By providing this electrolyte balance, and lowering elevated tear film osmolarity, TheraTears™, in pre-clinical studies, permits healing to proceed. TheraTears™ has specifically been shown in pre-clinical studies to restore both conjunctival goblet-cell density and corneal glycogen levels in dry-eye disease.

INTRODUCTION

In 1976 I began a research program designed to develop the first therapeutic tear solution. Our research team had a two-pronged strategy: (1) To develop a profound understanding of the pathogenesis of dry-eye disease, and (2) to develop a comprehensive understanding of why the eye needs a tear film.

Advances in Corneal Research, edited by Lass
Plenum Press, New York, 1997

There are many papers in the literature that carefully describe changes observed in the tear film and ocular surface in dry-eye disease. The limitation of these studies is that they were unable to place these observations in chronological sequence and they were unable to describe the natural history of dry-eye disease. For this reason, in 1986 we began to study rabbit models of dry-eye disease.[1-5] With these studies, performed over a four-year period, it was demonstrated that elevated tear film osmolarity was the first change measurable in a spectrum of dry-eye diseases. It was found that tear film osmolarity may increase through one of two general mechanisms: decreased tear secretion or increased tear film evaporation. Secretion may decrease through any mechanism that damages lachrymal gland tissue or any mechanism that decreases corneal sensation. Evaporation may increase through either large palpebral fissure width, occurring normally or in the context of thyroid eye disease, or through meibomian gland dysfunction, commonly resulting from chronic posterior blepharitis.[6]

Whether osmolarity increases through decreased tear production or increased tear film evaporation, the surface diseases that unfold share common features. First, increased water transport occurs across the conjunctival epithelium,[2,7] resulting from the increased osmotic gradient across the conjunctiva; this increase in water transport between conjunctival cells causes increased conjunctival cell desquamation. Occurring simultaneously with these changes is a decrease in conjunctival goblet-cell density and corneal glycogen levels. Since the attachments between corneal cells are stronger than those between conjunctival cells, the cornea is more resistant to the increase in tear film osmolarity. As a re-

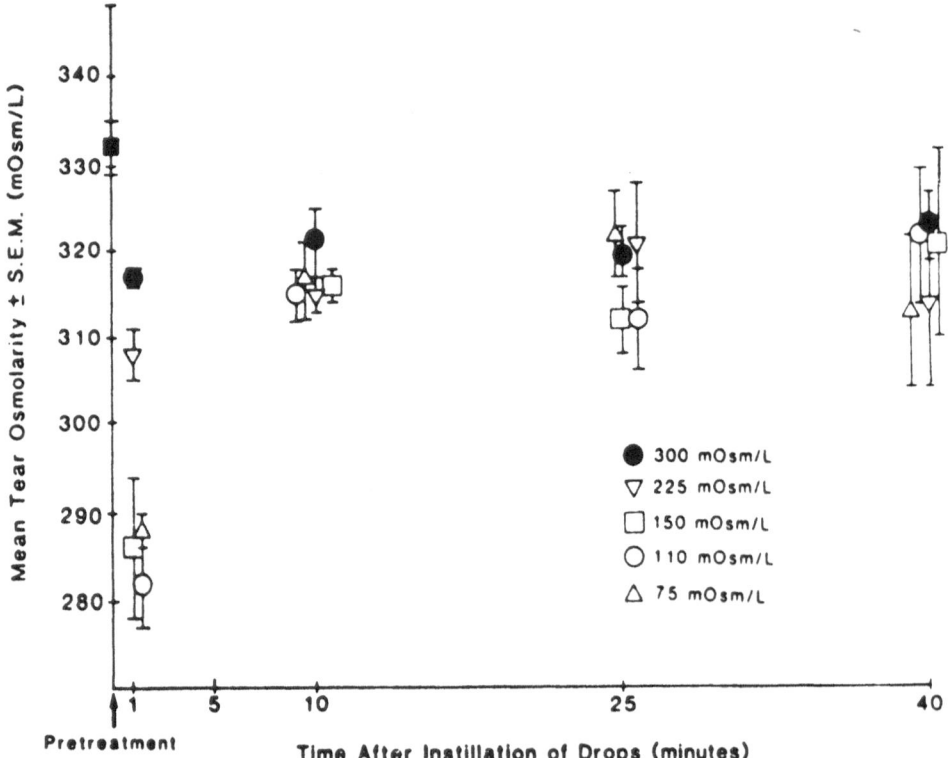

Figure 1. The effect of various hypotonic solutions and an isotonic solution on tear film osmolarity in keratoconjunctivitis sicca patients. Published courtesy of *Ophthalmology* (1885; 92: 646–650).

sult the cornea, in contrast to the conjunctiva, remains morphologically normal until much later in the disease process. Ultimately the attachments between corneal cells give way and increased movement of water between corneal cells results in increased corneal cell desquamation. As the corneal epithelium becomes more altered, cell surface glycoproteins are lost and tear film instability results. Ultimately, as the osmotic gradient continues to pull water out of the ocular surface, intercellular water, and intracellular edema are lost. Loss of intercelluar water increases ionic bonding between cells, and decreased cell shedding at this stage probably accounts for the "squamous metaplasia" described late in the disease.[8]

An artificial tear then, designed to be therapeutic, would need first to effectively lower elevated tear film osmolarity. So we did clinical studies in patients with keratoconjunctivitis sicca to determine how hypotonic an eye drop would need to be to effectively lower elevated tear film osmolarity (Figure 1).[9] As seen in Figure 1, an isotonic (300 mOsm/L) drop, while obviously wetting and lubricating the eye, does not lower elevated tear film osmolarity — does not rehydrate the tear film. In addition, at one minute after instillation, a hypotonic drop approximately two-thirds isotonic (225 mOsm/L) does not fully lower elevated tear film osmolarity. The eye drop measuring about 150 mOsm/L ultimately became the basis for the solution known as "TheraTears[TM]." A solution of this osmolarity takes tear film osmolarity from 332 mOsm/L before instillation to about 285 mOsm/L one minute after instillation. What does this accomplish? The ocular surface epithelium and the tear film are normally in an osmotic equilibrium—the osmolarity of the tear film reflects the osmolarity of the ocular surface. So when tear film osmolarity measures 332 mOsm/L the surface of the eye is 332 mOsm/L as well. At the moment tear film osmolarity drops to 285 mOsm/L, the ocular surface is still 332 mOsm/L; the eye drop has flipped the osmotic gradient and water now moves back into the ocular surface. Evidence for this fluid movement is seen at the ten minute time point. Osmolarity is up to about 316 mOsm/L, reflecting movement of water from the tear film into the ocular surface.

Additional evidence for this water movement is provided by studies in which rabbit models for keratoconjunctivitis sicca (KCS) were treated four times a day, Monday through Friday, with TheraTears[TM].[10] In these studies tear samples were taken on Monday mornings, after a weekend of no treatment. TheraTears[TM] treatment produced a reduction in tear film osmolarity that was statistically significant after 8 weeks of treatment (Figure 2). This treatment effect was not observed with treatment with control isotonic nor hypotonic (230 mOsm/L) solutions. This same effect on tear film osmolarity was observed in the single-site double-masked clinical study.[11] It is believed that this progressive and sustained lowering of tear film osmolarity reflects movement of water into the ocular surface. It is likely that the substantia propria under the conjunctival epithelium acts as a sponge and becomes cumulatively rehydrated. As its hydration status improves this loose connective tissue acts like a sustained release device, establishing a lower osmolarity for the ocular surface and the tear film in equilibrium with it. As tear film osmolarity approaches normal, the mechanism responsible for disease progression is thwarted.

It turns out, however, that for an eye drop to be therapeutic for dry eye it must do more than lower elevated tear film osmolarity. It must also perform the crucial biologic functions of the tear film. This is because average tear volume is only 7 μl while an eye drop is 30 μl. So an eye drop, once instilled in the eye, essentially replaces the components of the existing tear film.[12,13] Why, then, does the eye need a tear film? The eye needs a tear film because there is a blood tear barrier.[14] As a result the living cells on the surface of the eye have two crucial requirements that are met by the "tear supply" rather than by a blood supply: oxygen and electrolytes. Oxygen is provided by direct absorption from the

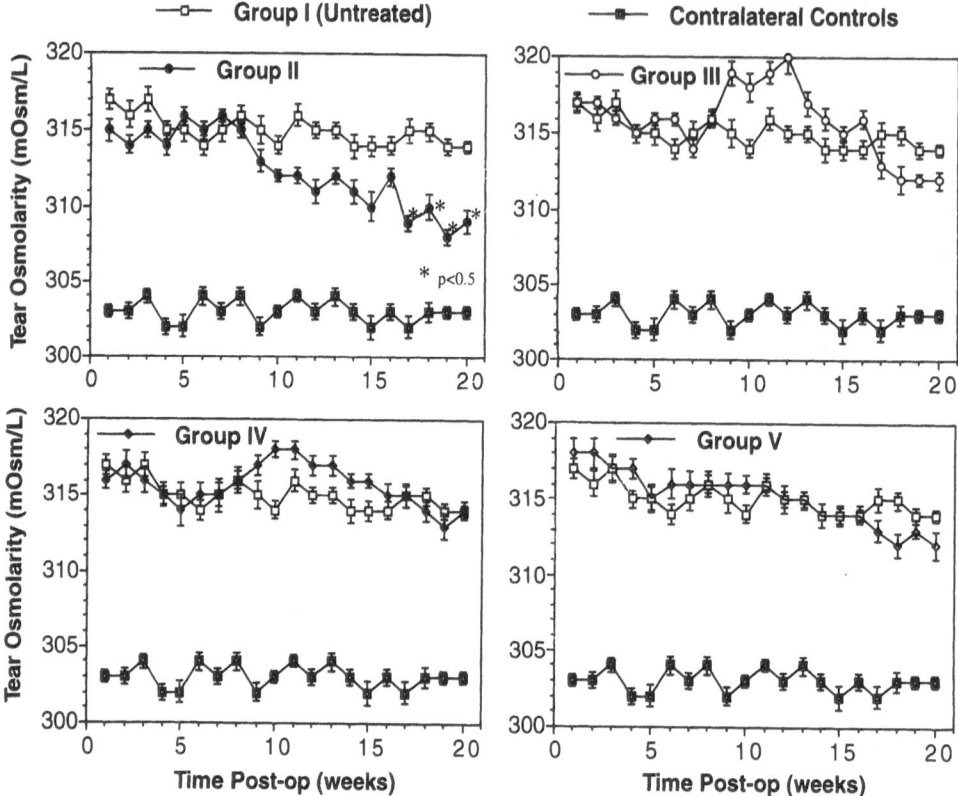

Figure 2. The effect of QID treatment with various tear solutions. Treatment with TheraTears™ (Group II, upper left) produced a statistically significant reduction in tear film osmolarity at 8 weeks. This treatment effect was not observed with the control solutions. Modified from *Ophthalmology* (1992; 99:600–604).

air, while electrolytes are provided by the tear film. We were able to measure the electrolyte composition of the human tear film in nanoliter tear samples[15] (Figures 3A-5A), and show that the electrolyte balance seen in the human tear film was crucial for the maintenance of normal conjunctival goblet-cell density[11,16] (Figures 3B-5B). This electrolyte composition (Solution 15) became the electrolyte vehicle for TheraTears.™

We hypothesized that treatment with TheraTears™ would restore conjunctival goblet cells and corneal glycogen levels in dry-eye disease. Given the evidence that goblet-cell density in normal conjunctiva takes 8 weeks to recover following injury,[1] the treatment period in this experiment was designed to last twelve weeks. Indeed, in preclinical studies, it was found that QID treatment with TheraTears™ for 12 weeks resulted in a statistically significant restoration of conjunctival goblet cells and corneal glycogen levels compared to untreated controls (Figures 6, 7). Treatment with two control unpreserved solutions, one isotonic and the other hypotonic, had no effect on goblet-cell density or corneal glycogen. Treatment with an isotonic preserved solution significantly decreased conjunctival goblet-cell density and corneal glycogen (Figures 6, 7).[10] In our single-site double-masked clinical study an analogous reduction in rose Bengal staining was observed, and subjectively patients preferred TheraTears™ over a hypotonic preserved control by a nine-to-one margin.[11]

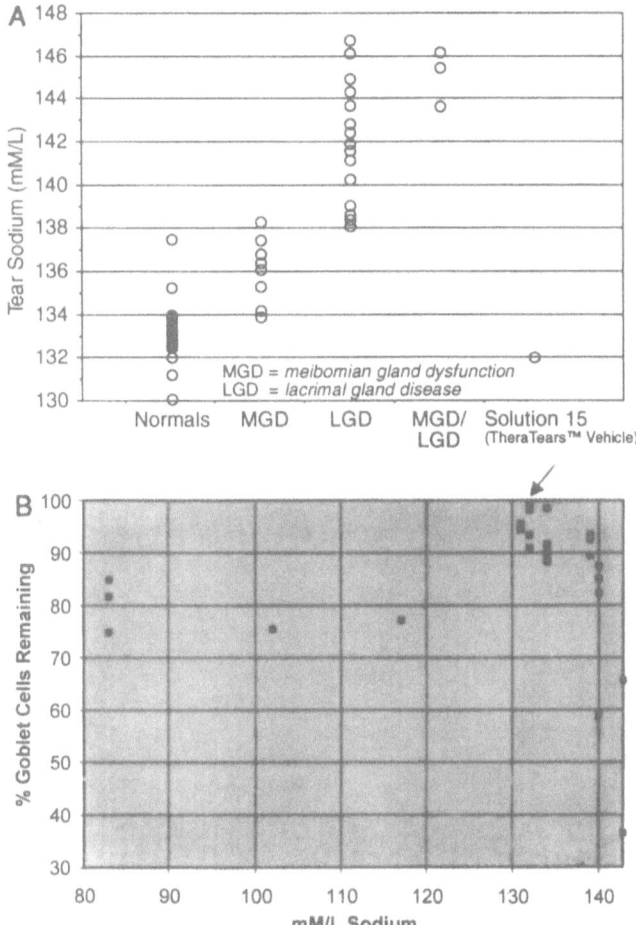

Figure 3. A. Tear sodium in healthy and dry-eye disease. TheraTears™ vehicle (Solution[15]) sodium concentration (132 mM/L) is displayed for comparison. Modified from *Int. Ophthalmol. Clin.* (1994; 34:27–36). B. Effect of sodium concentration of electrolyte-balanced solutions on conjunctival goblet-cell density after 12 hours of exposure. Arrow indicates TheraTears™ electrolyte vehicle. A sodium concentration of 132 mM/L is required for goblet cell maintenance.[16]

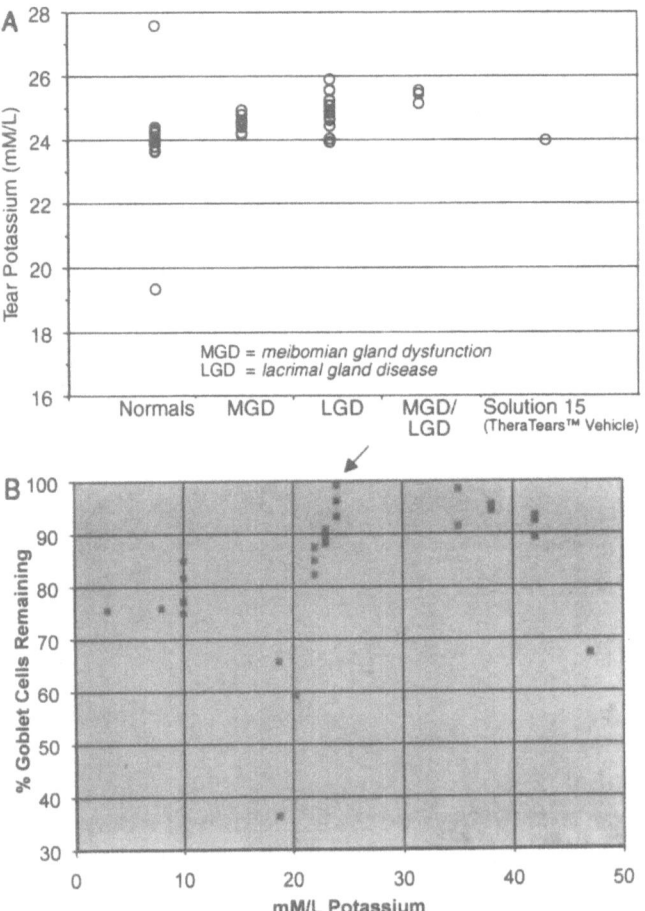

Figure 4. A. Tear potassium in health and dry-eye disease. TheraTears[TM] vehicle potassium concentration (24 mM/L) is displayed for comparison. Modified from *Int. Ophthalmol. Clin.* (1994; 34:27–36). B. Effect of potassium concentration of electrolyte-balanced solutions on conjunctival goblet-cell density after 12 hours of exposure. Arrow indicates TheraTears[TM] electrolyte vehicle. A potassium concentration of 24mM/L is required for goblet cell maintenance.[16]

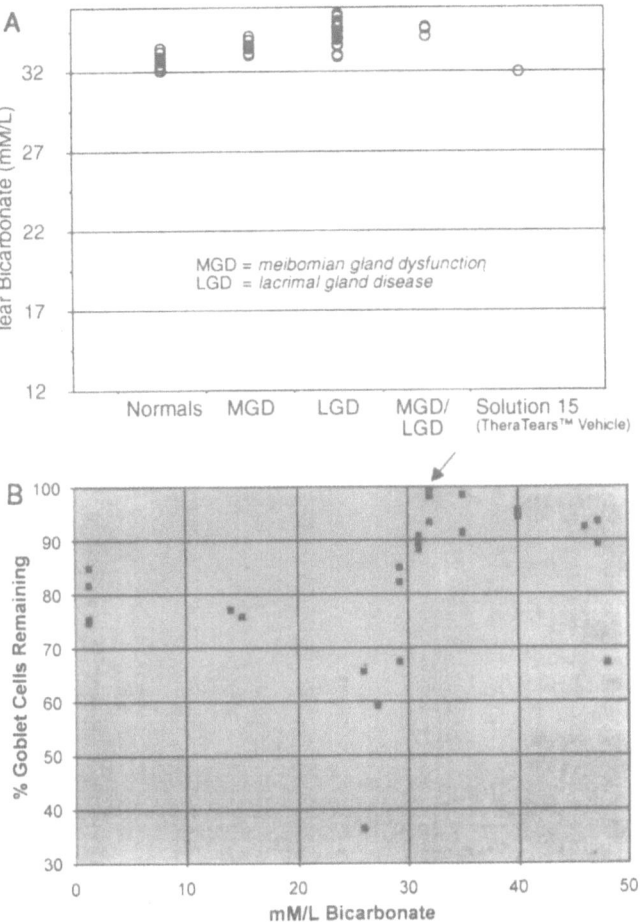

Figure 5. A. Tear bicarbonate in health and dry-eye disease. TheraTears[TM] vehicle bicarbonate concentration (32 mM/L) is displayed for comparison. Modified from *Int. Ophthalmol. Clin.* 1994; 34:27–36. B. Effect of bicarbonate concentration of electrolyte-balanced solutions on conjunctival goblet cell density after 12 hours of exposure. Arrow indicates TheraTears[TM] electrolyte vehicle. A bicarbonate concentration of 32 mM/L is required for goblet-cell maintenance.[16]

In summary, TheraTears[TM] has two mechanisms of action, one directed at the disease process, and the other directed to fulfill tear film function. First, it has the hypotonicity necessary to rehydrate the tear film so that the tear film can rehydrate the eye. And second, it has the electrolyte balance required to permit the natural healing process to proceed.

ACKNOWLEDGMENTS

The TheraTears[TM] technology described in this review has been issued U.S. Patent 4,775,531 (Inventor — Dr. Gilbard; Assignee — Schepens Eye Research Institute). Foreign patents have issued and are pending. Dr. Gilbard is President and CEO of Advanced Vision Research, Inc., the company that has brought TheraTears[TM] to market.

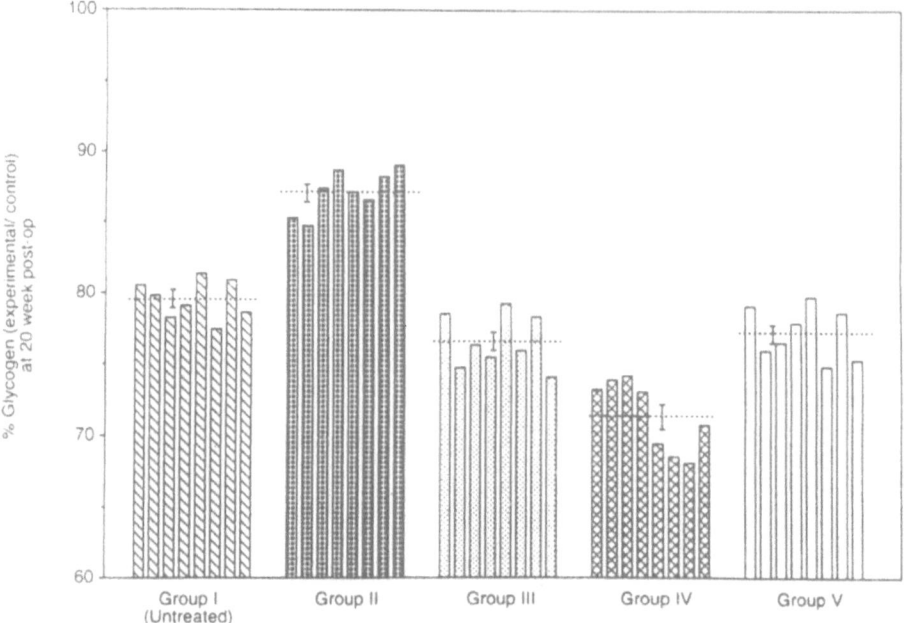

Figure 6. The effect of 12 weeks of treatment with four different artificial tear solutions on conjunctival goblet-cell density. A significant restoration of goblet-cell density was observed in Group Ii rabbits treated with TheraTears^{TM} (p<0.01). Published courtesy of *Ophthalmology* (1992; 99:600–604).

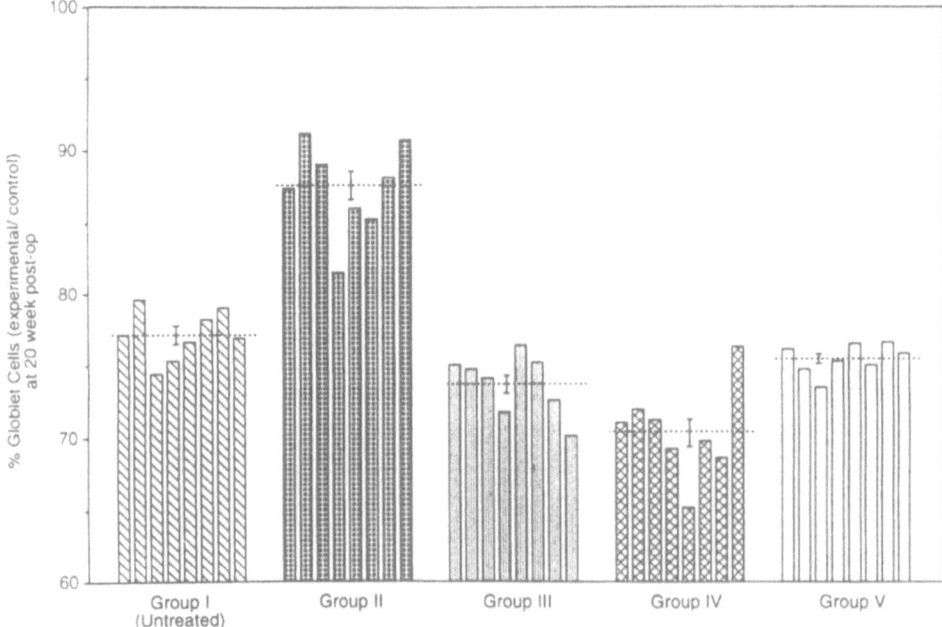

Figure 7. The effect of 12 weeks of treatment with 4 different artificial tear solutions on corneal glycogen levels. A significant restoration of corneal glycogen was observed in Group II rabbits treated with TheraTears^{TM} (p<0.01). Published courtesy of *Ophthalmology* (1992; 99:600–604).

REFERENCES

1. J.P. Gilbard, Rossi, S.R., and Gray, K.L., a new rabbit model for keratoconjunctivitis sicca. *Invest. Ophthalmol. Vis. Sci.* 28:225 (1987)

2. J.P. Gilbard, Rossi, S.R., Gray, K.L., et al., Tear film osmolarity and ocular surface disease in two rabbit models for keratoconjunctivitis sicca. *Invest. Ophthalmol. Vis. Sci* 29:374 (1988).

3. J.P. Gilbard, Rossi, S.R., and Gray Heyda, K., Tear film and ocular surface changes after closure of the meibomian gland orifices in the rabbit. *Ophthalmology* 96:1180 (1989).

4. J.P. Gilbard, Rossi, S.R., Gray, K.L., and Hanninen, L.A., Natural history of disease in a rabbit model for keratoconjunctivitis sicca. *Acta Ophthalmol.* 67(Suppl. 192):96 (1989).

5. J.P. Gilbard, and Rossi, S.R., Tear film and ocular surface changes in a rabbit model of neurotrophic keratitis. *Ophthalmology* 97:308 (1990).

6. J.P. Gilbard, Rossi, S.R., and Gray, K.L., Mechanisms for increased tear film osmolarity. In *The Cornea: Transactions of the World Congress on the Cornea III.* H.D. Cavanagh, ed., Raven Press, Ltd., New York (1988).

7. H. Sjogren: Keratoconjunctivitis sicca. In *Modern Trends in Ophthalmology*, F. Ridley and Sorsby, A., eds., Butterworth, London (1940).

8. J.P. Gilbard, Dry eye disorders. In *Principles and Practice of Ophthalmology*, D.M. Albert and Jakobiec, F.A., eds., W.B. Saunders Company, Philadelphia (1994).

9. J.P. Gilbard, and Kenyon, K.R., Tear diluents in the treatment of keratoconjunctivitis sicca. *Ophthalmology* 92:646 (1985).

10. J.P. Gilbard, and Rossi, S.R., An electrolyte-based solution that increases corneal glycogen and conjunctival goblet cell density in a rabbit model for keratoconjunctivitis sicca. *Ophthalmology* 99:600 (1992).

11. J.P. Gilbard, Rossi, S.R., and Gray Heyda, K., Ophthalmic solutions, the ocular surface, and a unique therapeutic artificial tear formulation. *Am. J. Ophthalmol.* 107:348 (1989).

12. A. Jordan, and Baum, J., Basic tear flow. Does it exist? Ophthalmology 87:920 (1980).

13. S. Mishima, Gasset, A., Klyce, S.D., and Baum, J.L., Determination of tear volume and tear flow. *Invest. Ophthalmol.* 5:264 (1966).

14. G. Raviola, Conjunctival and episcleral blood vessels are permeable to blood-borne horseradish peroxidase. *Invest. Ophthalmol. Vis. Sci.* 24:725 (1983).

15. J.P. Gilbard, Human tear film electrolyte concentrations in health and dry-eye disease. *Int. Ophthalmol. Clin.* 34:27 (1994).

16. J.P. Gilbard, Non-toxic ophthalmic preparations. US Patent 4,775,531. Oct. 4, 1988.

5

BARRIER FUNCTION OF OCULAR SURFACE EPITHELIUM

Shigeru Kinoshita, Norihiko Yokoi, and Aoi Komuro

Department of Ophthalmology
Kyoto Prefectural University of Medicine
Kyoto, Japan

ABSTRACT

This paper demonstrates three different types of corneal epithelial barrier dysfunction: mechanically and/or immunologically oriented (as in superficial punctate keratopathy); genetically regulated (as in corneal dystrophy); and biologically based (as in conjunctival epithelial invasion of the cornea). Corneal epithelial barrier function was examined by measuring fluorescein uptake using a newly-designed fluorophotometer, after instillation of 3 µl of 0.5% fluorescein. Fluorescein uptake (mean ± standard error, ng/ml) in the central cornea 30 minutes later was 21.4 ± 1.6, 81.9 ± 8.9, 269.0 ± 26.9, and 1400.9 ± 197.2 in normal controls (Grade 0), Grade 1, Grade 2, and Grade 3 superficial punctate keratopathies, respectively, showing significant progression of epithelial barrier dysfunction with severity of clinical manifestation. Among the corneal dystrophies, gelatinous drop-like dystrophy (2584.6 ± 791.7, p = 0.0001), granular dystrophy (351.6 ± 157.5, p = 0.0001) and lattice dystrophy (599.7 ± 222.0, p = 0.001), but not macular dystrophy (51.2 ± 0.3, p = 0.011), showed markedly increased fluorescein uptake in comparison to normal corneas. Extremely high fluorescein uptake in gelatinous droplike dystrophy is speculative of corneal epithelial cell membrane abnormality. The corneas covered by conjunctival epithelium, as proved by impression cytology, showed increased fluorescein uptake (472.1 ± 144.6, p = 0.0001) in comparison to normal controls.

INTRODUCTION

Corneal epithelial cells are constantly renewed by the proliferation of basal cells and terminally differentiated to superficial cells, thereby maintaining biological homeostasis.[1] The epithelial layer serves as mechanical, biological, and immunological barrier to the outer environment. For instance, the healthy epithelial barrier protects ocular inner tissues from infectious agents, inflammatory substances, water permeation, etc.[2-3] When corneal epithelial function is disturbed, epithelial staining with fluorescein is visible by biomicroscopy. Biomicroscopic observation with sodium fluorescein is, therefore, a crucial clinical tool for detecting corneal epithelial abnormality. However, very few observers recognize that this method can be used to qualitatively evaluate corneal epithelial barrier function. In other words, the investigation of corneal epithelial barrier function is essential for assessing epithelial health.

There are several ways to quantitatively measure barrier function, each using different methodologies and/or different hardware setups.[4-14] Among them, specially designed fluorophotometry using topically-applied sodium fluorescein as a tracer molecule via the corneal epithelial layer has been demonstrated to be a reliable quantitative method for clinical use.[13] The method reported here has several advantages, including shorter measurement time, smaller focal diamond area, and accurate placement of measuring area. This study, therefore, investigated corneal epithelial barrier dysfunction in various ocular surface diseases using this system, reported previously.[13] Based on the resulting data, the concept that there are at least three different types of corneal epithelial barrier dysfunction is introduced. These dysfunctions include mechanically and/or immunologically oriented, genetically regulated, and biologically based dysfunction.

SUBJECTS AND METHODS

Subjects

With fully informed consent, three different categories of corneal epithelial abnormalities, as described below, were enrolled in this study: 65 superficial punctate keratopathies, 21 corneal dystrophies, and seven scarred corneas with superficial neovascularization, for examining conjunctival epithelial invasion on the cornea.

The 65 superficial punctate keratopathy eyes were either mild dry eye conditions only or combined with drug toxicity, allergic reactions, etc. Patient ages ranged from 18–83 years (52.8 ± 2.4 years, mean ± standard error). The 21 corneal dystrophies comprised seven gelatinous droplike corneal dystrophy, six granular corneal dystrophy, six lattice corneal dystrophy, and two macular corneal dystrophy. Ages ranged from 13 to 72 years (49.4 ± 4.2 years). The seven scarred corneas with superficial neovascularization were seen in patients 21–73 years old (48.0 ± 8.7 years); their epithelial characteristics at the central corneas were examined after fluorophotometry by an impression cytological technique reported previously.[15,16] The samples were fixed with 10% buffered formalin and stained with periodic acid Schiff for the presence of goblet cells. Five samples had many goblet cells, indicating the presence of conjunctival epithelium on the cornea; two samples were corneal epithelium.

A total of 100 eyes of healthy volunteers served as controls, ages ranging from 10–79 (33.6 ± 1.9 years).

Assessment of Corneal Epithelial Barrier Function by Fluorophotometry

Corneal epithelial barrier function was evaluated on the basis of corneal fluorescein uptake. This was done as described previously, using a slit-lamp fluorophotometer (Anterior fluorometer™ FL-500; KOWA Co., Ltd.: Tokyo, Japan).[13] Briefly, the size of the measurement plane was 0.3 × 0.15 mm in horizontal-vertical section; the focal diamond was 0.66 × 0.33 mm, horizontal-vertical section from the corneal surface respectively. The largest area of the receiving system focal diamond is easily adjusted to the corneal surface while the observer views the corneal from the front, and its fluorescent light may be received directly in front. A measurement angle of 30° was selected, and measurement time was reduced to 0.2 seconds to eliminate bias introduced by blinking and eye movement. With the instrument focused on the central cornea, background intensity was measured 10 times and averaged.

In this procedure, 3 µl of a 0.5% (5 mg/ml) BSS PLUS (Alcon; Fort Worth, USA) fluorescein solution was instilled to the lower conjunctival sac of each eye with an Eppendorf micropipette, in non-contact fashion, followed by washing of the tarsal and bulbar conjunctiva with 20 ml of BSS PLUS 10 minutes later. Twenty minutes after eye washing, fluorescein intensity was measured 10 times at the central cornea, and the data were averaged. The mean value of background fluorescein was then subtracted; the counts obtained were converted into fluorescein concentrations using calibration lines incorporated in the software. Based on this fluorescein uptake concentration, corneal epithelial barrier function was evaluated.

Clinical Evaluation of Corneal Epithelial Abnormalities

After fluorophotometry, all ocular surfaces were stained with sodium fluorescein, observed biomicroscopically, and photographed. All eyes with corneal and/or conjunctival epithelial defects were excluded. For superficial punctate keratopathy and normal controls, the clinical manifestations of corneal epithelium were classified into four grades by two corneal specialists: no superficial punctate keratopathy anywhere on the cornea (Grade 0); no superficial punctate keratopathy on 8 mm diameter central cornea (Grade 1); mild superficial punctate keratopathy on 8 mm diameter central cornea, with lesions sparse in density (Grade 2); severe superficial punctate keratopathy on 8 mm diameter central corneal, with high-density lesions overlapping (Grade 3). Statistical analyses were performed using Student's t test.

RESULTS

Superficial Punctate Keratopathy in Normal Cornea

Fluorescein uptakes (mean ± standard error, ng/ml) in the central cornea from measurement at 30 minutes after fluorescein instillation (20 minutes after washing) were 21.4 ± 1.6 in Grade 0 (normal volunteers); 81.9 ± 8.9 in Grade 1; 269.0 ± 26.9 in Grade 2; and 1400.9 ± 197.2 in Grade 3. These data represent a statistically significant increase in corneal fluorescein uptake with increased severity of clinical manifestation (p = 0.0001, Grade 0 vs. Grade 1; p = 0.0001, Grade 1 vs. Grade 2; p = 0.0001, Grade 2 vs. Grade 3)(Figs. 1 and 2).

Corneal Dystrophy

Fluorescein concentration at central corneas 30 minutes later was 2584.6 ± 791.7 in gelatinous droplike corneal dystrophy, 351.6 ± 157.5 in granular corneal dystrophy, 599.7 ± 222.0 in lattice corneal dystrophy type 1, and 51.2 ± 0.3 in macular corneal dystrophy. Gelatinous droplike dystrophy (p = 0.0001), granular dystrophy (p = 0.0001), and lattice

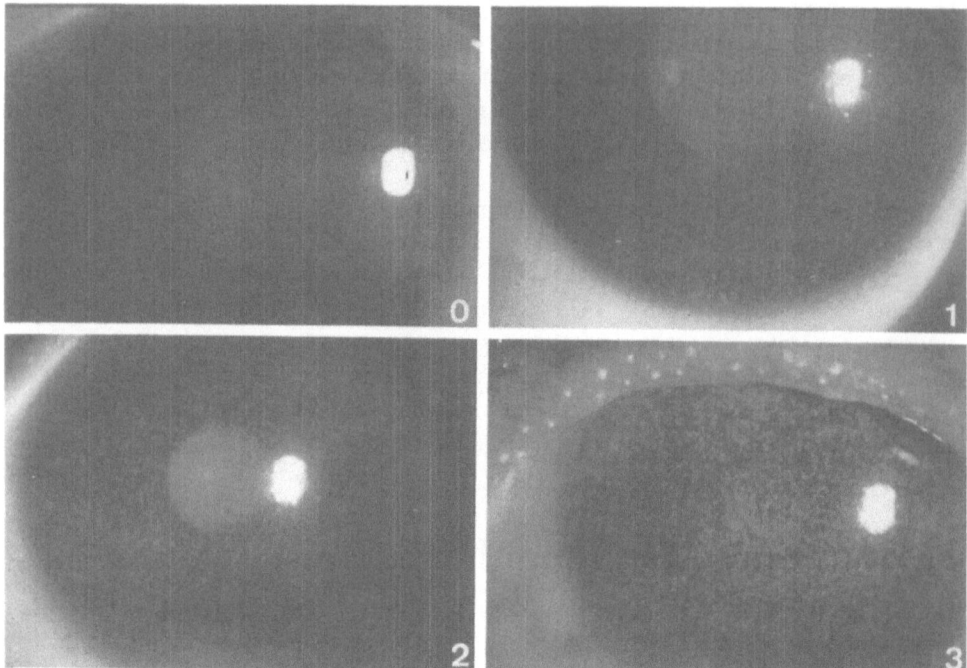

Figure 1. Representative manifestation of corneal surface stained with fluorescein in each grade: Grade 0, no superficial punctate keratopathy anywhere on cornea; Grade 1, no superficial punctate keratopathy on 8 mm diameter central cornea; Grade 2, mild superficial punctate keratopathy on 8 mm diameter central cornea; Grade 3, severe superficial punctate keratopathy on 8 mm diameter central cornea.

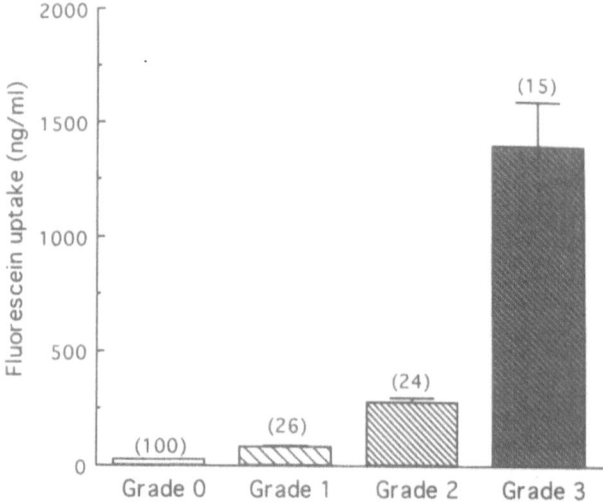

Figure 2. Fluorescein uptake in central cornea at 30 minutes after 3 μl of 0.5% fluorescein instillation in eyes with superficial punctate keratopathy and normal volunteer. There was significant increase in fluorescein uptake with grade.

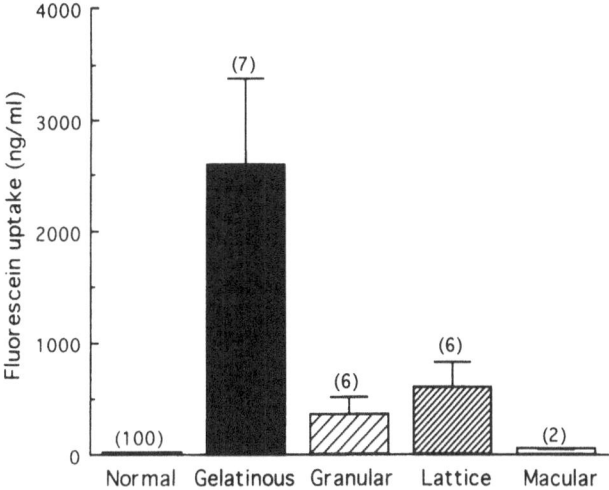

Figure 3. Fluorescein uptake in central cornea at 30 minutes after 3μl of 0.5% fluorescein instilation in eyes with corneal dystrophies: normal, normal cornea; gelatinous, gelatinous droplike corneal dystrophy; granular, granular corneal dystrophy; lattice, lattice corneal dystrophy; macular, macular corneal dystrophy. Gelatinous droplike, granular, and lattice corneal dystrophies showed statistically increased uptake.

dystrophy (p = 0.0001), but not macular dystrophy (p = 0.011), showed markedly increased fluorescein uptake in comparison to normal corneas (Fig. 3). Among these, gelatinous droplike cornea dystrophy developed extremely high fluorescein uptake, indicating excessive damage to corneal epithelial barrier function (Fig. 4).

Conjunctival Epithelial Invasion of the Cornea

Central corneas covered by conjunctival epithelium with superficial neovascularization, as confirmed by impression cytology, showed statistically increased fluorescein uptake (472.1 ± 144.6) at 30 minutes after fluorescein instillation, as compared to normal control (p = 0.0001)(Figs. 5 and 6). There was no difference (p = 0.9213) in fluorescein uptake between vascularized (20.3 ± 1.5 and normal corneas, if covering epithelium was of corneal origin.

DISCUSSION

This study clearly demonstrates that there are at least three different types of corneal epithelial barrier dysfunction: mechanical and/or immunological damage to superficial corneal epithelial cells due to dry eye condition, drug toxicity, allergic reaction, etc., as represented by superficial punctate keratopathy; corneal epithelial abnormality regulated genetically, as in corneal dystrophy; and covering cornea by an epithelial layer possessing different biological characteristics from corneal epithelium, such as conjunctival epithelium. These three types of dysfunction enable easier hydrophilic molecule permeation to corneal stroma.

Mechanical and/or immunological damage to superficial corneal epithelial cells yields various degrees of superficial punctate keratopathy due to tight junction abnormality, cell membrane abnormality, or both. Corneal epithelial barrier function is presumably

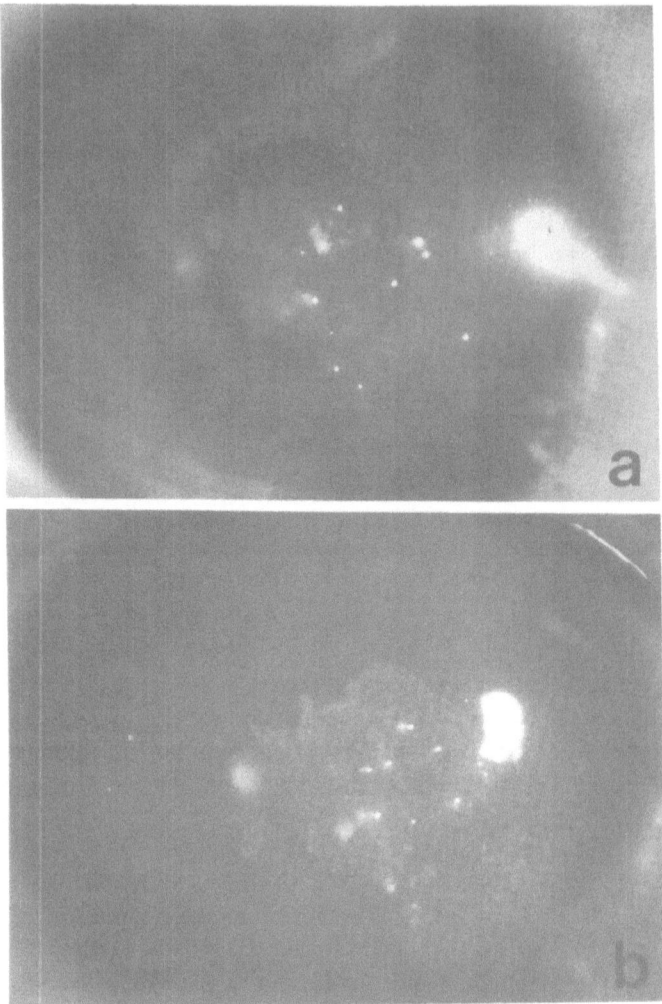

Figure 4. Corneal manifestation of gelatinous droplike corneal dystrophy: central corneal exhibited several elevated nodules with scarring (a); corneal epithelial cell layer stinaed with fluorescein was more broad than pathological area, but did not reach to the limbus (b).

damaged in such cases; in fact, corneal epithelial barrier function, as assessed by the fluorphotometry-based method, correlates well to clinical manifestations observed via biomicroscope with fluorescein dye. The present results confirmed the preliminary findings mentioned above.[13] Therefore, it is possible that the corneal fluorescein uptake value can be used as quantitative indicator for evaluating corneal epithelial barrier function. In fact, fluorescein uptake by the wounded cornea was markedly reduced over time during the wound healing process after corneal epithelial ablation, but the timing of functional and anatomic recovery[17] was not the same. Actually, functional recovery, as represented by corneal epithelial barrier function, was a few weeks behind recovery of clinical manifestation (data not shown). All these findings suggest that corneal epithelial barrier function is a sensitive indicator of corneal epithelial cell layer disturbance.

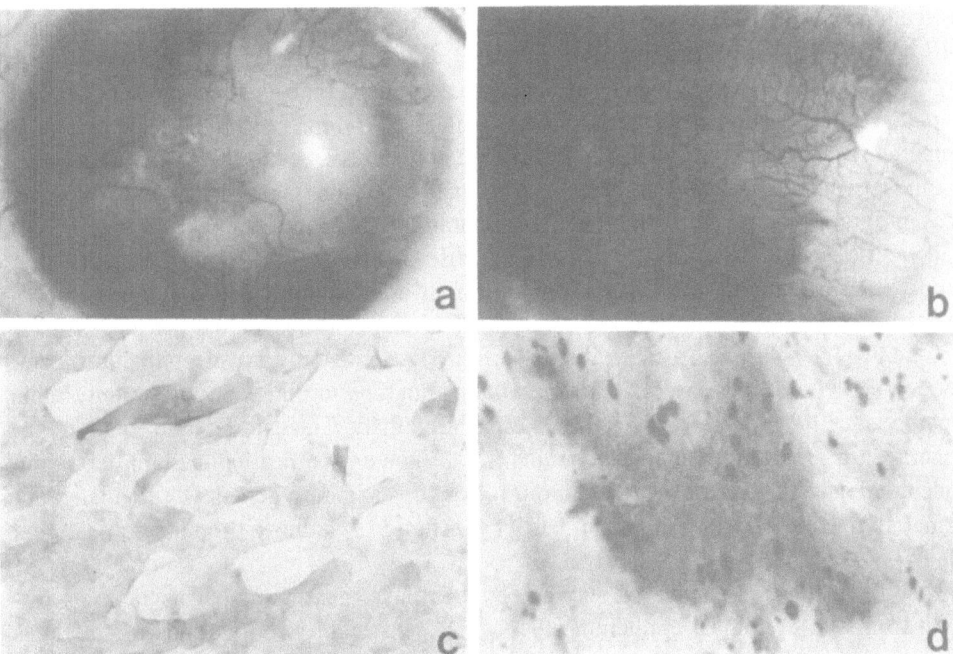

Figure 5. Scarred corneas with superficial neovascularization and their superficial epithelial cells taken by impression cytology: (1) scarred cornea with corneal epithelium; (b) scarred cornea covered by conjunctival epithelium; (c) impression cytology taken from eye (a) showing corneal epithelial cells; (d) impression cytology from eye (b) indicating many goblet cells. Although (a) and (b) show similar corneal manifestations, epithelial cell characteristics over cornea are different.

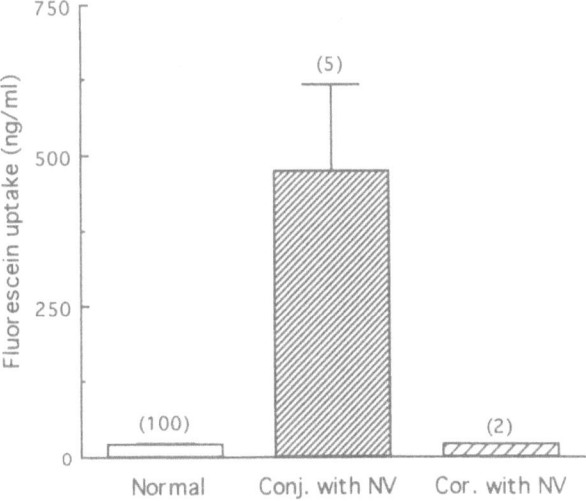

Figure 6. Fluorescein uptake at central cornea at 30 minutes after 3μl of 0.5% fluorescein instillation in eyes with scarred corneas: Conj. With NV, conjunctival epithelium covered cornea with neovascularization; Cor. With NV, corneal epithelium on cornea with neovasclarization.

To the best of the authors' knowledge, this is the first report describing the abnormal barrier function of the corneal epithelial cell layer in such corneal dystrophies as gelatinous droplike corneal dystrophy, lattice corneal dystrophy, and granular corneal dystrophy. Among these, the abnormality of the corneal epithelial barrier function in gelatinous droplike corneal dystrophy was striking (approximately 100 times more permeable than in normal corneal epithelium). Gelatinous droplike corneal dystrophy, the so-called primary familial amyloidosis of the cornea[18–19] occasionally seen in Japanese, but not in other races, progressively develops amyloid deposition in the superficial corneal stroma, but not in the corneal epithelium. However, since this disease inevitably recurs a few years after corneal transplantation,[20] and since droplike lesions are mainly extended as far as limbal tissues where corneal epithelial stem cells are present,[21] it is speculated that the primary abnormality may be of corneal epithelial origin. The data on corneal epithelial barrier function and clinical observation, shown in the photograph in Fig. 4, strongly suggest this hypothesis: cell membrane abnormality is especially likely. The data on lattice and granular corneal dystrophies may indicate similar involvement of corneal epithelium, though in moderate degree. Therefore, our laboratory is now investigating genetically regulated abnormal substances affecting epithelial barrier function in gelatinous droplike corneal dystrophy.

When the cornea is covered with an epithelial layer possessing barrier function different from that of corneal epithelium, the layer's permeability to hydrophilic molecules such as sodium fluorescein must also be different. Since normal conjunctival epithelial cells are more permeable than corneal epithelium in animals[8] and humans,[22] it is reasonable to assume that regenerated epithelium of conjunctival origin over the cornea is more permeable than corneal epithelium. In fact, results indicate that when conjunctival epithelium retains its original characteristics, showing the presence of many goblet cells, the epithelial layer is approximately 20 times more permeable than corneal epithelium. This is, therefore, an accurate and non-contact way of observing the epithelial biological characteristics, corneal or conjunctival, in vascularized cornea. Whether the barrier function changes when conjunctival epithelial cells change their biological characteristics to those of corneal epithelial cells[23] remains an unsolved question.

ACKNOWLEDGMENTS

Supported in part by a research grant from the Japanese Ministry of Education, Science and Culture of Japan, and a research fund from the Kyoto Foundation for the Promotion of Medical Science.

REFERENCES

1. I.K. Gipson, and Sagrue, S.P., Cell biology of the corneal epithelium. In, *Principles and Practice of Ophthalmology, Basic Science*, D.M. Albert, ed., W.B. Saunders, New York (1994).
2. S.D. Klyce, and Beuermann R.W., Structure and function of the cornea. In, *The Cornea*, H.E. Kaufman, Barron, B.A., McDonald, M.B., and Waltman, S.R., eds., Churchill Livingstone, New York (1988).
3. S.D. Klyce, and Crosson, C.E., Transport processes across the rabbit epithelium: a review. *Curr. Eye Res.* 4:427 (1985).
4. R.F. Brubaker, Maurice, D.M., and McLaren, J.W., Fluorometry of the anterior segment, In, *Noninvasive Diagnosis Techniques in Ophthalmology*, B.R. Masters, ed., Springer-Verlag, New York (1993).
5. R.A. Thoft, and Friend, J., Permeability of regeneratied corneal epithelium. *Exp. Eye Res.* 21:409 (1975).

6. R.A. Berkowitz, Klyce, S.D., Salisbury, J.D., and Kaufman, H.E., Fluorophotometric determination of the corneal barrier after penetrating keratoplasty. *Am. J. Ophthalmol.* 92:332 (1981).

7. E.J.F.M. de Kruijf, Boot, J.P., Laterveer, L., et al., A simple method for determination of corneal epithelial barrier in humans. *Curr. Eye Res.* 6:1327 (1987).

8. A.J.W. Huang, Tseng, S.C.G., and Kenyon, K.R., Paracellular permability of corneal and conjunctival epithelia. *Invest. Ophthalmol. Vis. Sci.* 30:684 (1989).

9. M. Gobbels, and Spitznas, M., Influence of artificial tears on corneal epithelium in dry-eye syndrome. *Graefe's Arch. Clin. Exp. Ophthalmol.* 227:139 (1989).

10. D.L. Bernal, and Ubels, J.L., Quantitative evaluation of the corneal epithelial barrier: effect of artificial tears and preservatives. *Curr. Eye Res.* 10:645 (1991).

11. Y. Want, Chen, M., and Wolosin, J.M., ZO-1 in corneal epithelium; stratal distribution and synthesis induction by outer cell removal. *Exp. Eye Res.* 57:283 (1993).

12. S-W Chang, and Hu, F-R., Changes in corneal autofluorescence and corneal barrier function with aging. *Cornea* 12:493 (1993).

13. N. Yokoi, and Kinoshita, S., Clinical evaluation of corneal epithelial barrier function with slit-lamp fluorophotometer. *Cornea* 14:485 (1995).

14. B.E. McCarey, Reaves, T., Al, S., Noninvasive measurement of corneal epithelial permeability. *Curr. Eye Res.* 14:505 (1995).

15. M. Ohji, Ohmi, G., Kiritoshi, A., and Kinoshita S.., Goblet cell density in thermal and chemical injuries. *Arch Ophthalmol.* 105:1686 (1987).

16. K. Nishida, Kinoshita, S., Ohashi, Y., et al., Ocular surface abnormalities in aniridia. *Am. J. Ophahtlmol.* 120:368 (1995).

17. M.D. McCartney, and Cantu-Crouch, D., Rabbit corneal epithelial wound repair; tight junction reformation. *Curr. Eye Res.* 11;15 (1992).

18. K. Nakaizumi. A rare case of corneal dystrophy. *Nippon Ganka Gakkai Zasshi* 18:949 (1914).

19. C.A. Miller, and Krachmer, J.H., Epithelial and stromal dystrophies. In, *The Cornea,* H.E. Kaufman, Barron, B.A., Mcdonald, M.B., and Waltman, S.R., eds., Churchill Livingstone, New York (1988).

20. S. Ohzono, Ogawa, K., Kinoshita, S., et al., Recurrence of corneal dystrophy following keratoplasty. *Rinsho Ganka (Jpn. J. Clin Ophthalmol.)* 38:1160 (1984).

21. A. Scheermer, Galvin, S., and Sun, T.T., Differentiation-related expression of a major 64K corneal keratin in vivo and in culture suggests limbal location of corneal epithelial stem cells. *J. Cell. Biol.* 103:49 (1986).

22. K. Yokoi, Yokoi, N., Komuro, A., et al., Evaluation of the barrier function of conjunctival epithelium using anterior fluorphotometer. *Rinsho Ganka (Jpn. J. Clin. Ophthalmol.)* 48:1160 (1994).

23. S. Kinoshita, Friend, J., and Thoft, R.A., Biphasic cell proliferation in transdifferentiation of conjunctival to corneal epithelium in rabbits. *Invest. Ophthalmol. Vis. Sci.* 24:1008 (1983).

6

CLINICAL ASSESSMENT OF CONJUNCTIVAL DAMAGE AND TEAR FILM STABILITY IN DRUG-INDUCED EPITHELIAL KERATOPATHY

Norihiko Yokoi, Aoi Komuro, Yoko Takehisa, and Shigeru Kinoshita

Department of Ophthalmology
Kyoto Prefectural University of Medicine
Kyoto, Japan

ABSTRACT

In this study 26 eyes of 14 patients diagnosed with drug-induced epithelial kera-topathy, 10 eyes of five patients with Sjögren's syndrome, and 10 eyes of five normal vol-unteers were examined for damages to conjunctival epithelium using sulforhodamine B (SRB) and rose bengal (RB). In both stainings the damage at the nasal and temporal bul-bar conjunctiva was scored (0 to 3) on the basis of severity; the values were totaled for the eye. In drug-induced keratopathy, precorneal tear film changes were also examined using a new tear surface observing system.

In drug-induced epithelial keratopathy, conjunctival epithelial damage was disclosed in two eyes of two patients by both SRB and RB (both score 1). In Sjögren's syndrome, prominent conjunctival epithelial damage was detected (SRB score: 5.1[mean]; RB score: 4.8 [mean]), with no staining in normal eyes. Precorneal tear instability was seen in 15 eyes of nine patients with drug-induced epithelial keratopathy (out of 18 eyes in 10 pa-tients); this finding disappeared after corneal damage resolution.

Results of this study reveal that in drug-induced epithelial keratopathy conjunctival epithelial damage is minimal, even when the corneal epithelium is severely damaged and tear/corneal surface interaction is deteriorated.

INTRODUCTION

In the clinical setting, drug-induced corneal epithelial damage is often encountered; its clinical importance is undisputed.[1] In some cases, however, it cannot be diagnosed eas-ily. In addition, drug effect alone cannot easily be isolated from the clinically manifested corneal epithelial damage, since adverse effects of eyedrops on corneal epithelium some-times overlap those of the disease. For example, dry eye, which accompanies damaged corneal epithelium, is likely to be adversely affected by eyedrops[2] because dry eye patients require frequent instillation and their already-disrupted corneal epithelium is easily subject to damage by drug and/or preservatives. Therefore, in the treatment of ocular surface epithelial diseases, including dry eye, it is important to consider possible adverse effects of eyedrops on pre-existing corneal epithelial damage.

There have been many reports regarding the toxic effect of topical eye drugs on corneal epithelium.[1-5] For example, β-blocker eyedrops often cause corneal epithelial damage[6,7] and topical anesthetics sometimes disrupt corneal epithelium.[8] Moreover, preservatives, including benzalkonium chloride, are reportedly involved in corneal epithelial damage.[1-5] In contrast, clinical information concerning adverse effect of eyedrops on conjunctival epithelium,[9] which is as likely to be compromised as corneal epithelium is not widely available.

This study employed clinically useful dyes (sulforhodamine B[10] and rose bengal[11]) to examine conjunctival epithelial involvement in drug-induced epithelial keratopathy, as compared with the Sjögren's syndrome and normal healthy eyes. Precorneal tear condition, presumably compromised in drug-induced keratopathy, was also investigated.

SUBJECTS AND METHODS

A total of 46 eyes of 24 subjects were enrolled in this study, including 10 eyes of five normal, healthy volunteers (three males, two females; age: 40–65 years, 55.2 ± 9.4 [mean ± SD]), 10 eyes of five Sjögren's syndrome patients (one male and four females; age: 46–62 years, 54.6 ± 6.0 [mean ± SD]), and 26 Eyes of 14 patients diagnosed with drug-induced epithelial keratopathy (nine males, five females; age: 36–85 years, 62.5 ± 15.4 [mean ± S.D.]). All drug-induced keratopathy patients had been exposed to frequent instillation of several types of eyedrops and/or antiglaucoma eyedrops: six eyes of three patients had been exposed to over-the-counter drugs (no precise data on eyedrops); five eyes of three patients had been exposed to a combination of several types of eyedrops, including 0.3% ofloxacin, 0.1% betamethasone, 0.5% cefmenoxime, 2% glutathione, 1% chondroitin sulphate, and 0.05% flavinadenin dinucleotide. In one patient, both eyes had been exposed to 0.1% betamethasone eyedrops with excessive instillation and four eyes of two patients had been exposed to β-blocker, including 2% carteolol or 0.5% timolol in combination with several types of eyedrops, including 0.04% dipivefrine, 0.3% floxacin, 0.1% fluorometholone, and 0.1% hyaluronate. In another patient, both eyes had been exposed to 0.05% betaxolol β_1-blocker. Characteristically, seven eyes of four patients had been exposed to a recently developed antiglaucoma drug, and prostaglandin $F_{2\alpha}$ derivative, isopropyl unoprostone, which has been commercially available in Japan since 1994, in combination with β-blocker (timolol or carteolol). Of the 14 patients with drug-induced keratopathy, 12 patients were bilaterally involved and two patients had unilateral involvement.

To evaluate conjunctival epithelial damage, sulforhodamine B (SRB) and rose bengal (RB) staining were used (0.5%, 10 µl and 1%, 2µl, respectively). It has been reported that SRB is far better for detecting conjunctival epithelial damage than is fluorescein.[10] Moreover a recent study has shown that RB can detect damage of the mucin layer covering the ocular surface epithelium.[12] These stainings were separately scored (0 to 3 points) at the nasal and temporal bulbar conjunctiva, based on damage severity, in reference to the method of van Biestelveld.[11] The scores were then totalled for the eye. For photography of sulforhodamine B staining of conjunctival epithelial damage, exciter filter (BPB-53; Fuji Photo Film Co., Ltd.; Tokyo, Japan) were mounted on the photoslit lamp (SC 1200; Kowa Co., Ltd.; Tokyo, Japan).

Precorneal tear film stability in drug-induced epithelial keratopathy was also evaluated non-invasively using a newly-developed specular reflection video-recording system, which is a modification of Doane's device[13] for observing the precorneal tear surface. Briefly, the specular reflex light from the tear surface, a circular area 2 mm in diameter, was collected through a video camera to a TV monitor. A live image of the tear surface at the central cornea was recorded and observed. As another predisposing factor, tear deficiency was evaluated in drug-induced epithelial keratopathy cases using Schirmer I test[14] after complete healing of epithelial keratopathy.

RESULTS

SRB and RB staining demonstrated no bulbar conjunctival epithelial damage in normal eyes. In Sjögren's syndrome patients, severe conjunctival epithelial damages were demonstrated using SRB and RB staining (SRB score: 5.1 ± 1.8 [mean $\pm$ S.D.]); RB score: 4.8 ± 1.5 [mean $\pm$ S.D.]). A representative case is shown in Fig. 1. In drug-induced epithelial keratopathy, minimal bulbar conjunctival epithelial damage was seen in only two eyes of two patients (both staining scores 1); the other cases exhibited no involvement of the bulbar conjunctival epithelium (Fig. 2B, C; Fig. 3B,C).

In drug-induced epithelial keratopathy, corneal epithelial damages were classified into two types based on appearance two minutes after fluorescein staining: one showed excessive fluorescein permeability[15] (17 eyes of nine patients; Fig 2A) in which fluo-

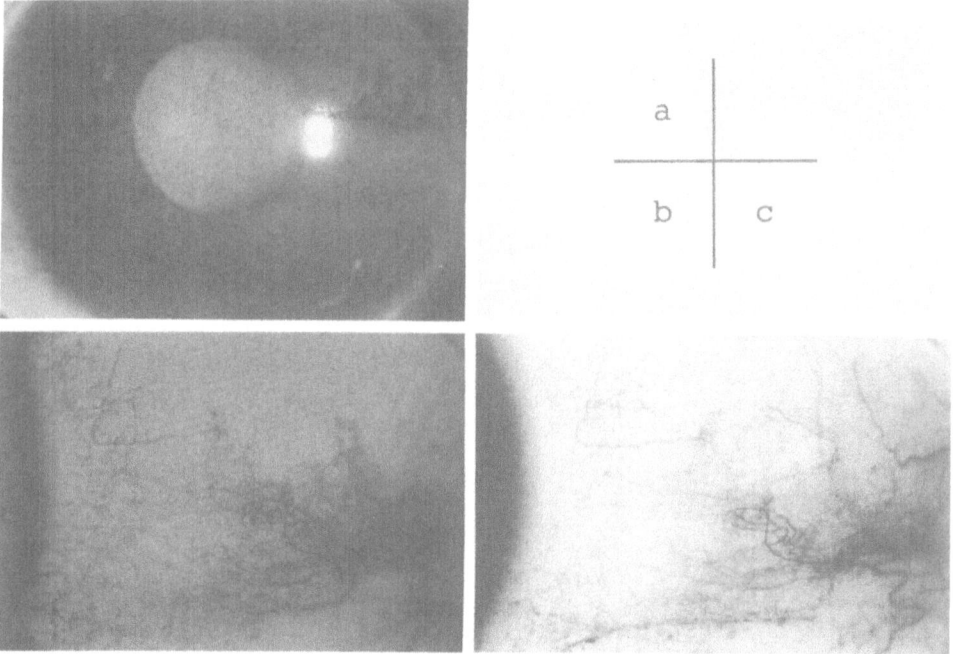

Figure 1. (Yokoi and associates) A case of Sjögren's syndrome showing minimal superficial punctate epithelial keratopathy as corneal involvement (a). Sulforhodamine B and rose bengal staining showed severe conjunctival epithelial damage (b and c, respectively). Only temporal bulbar conjunctiva is shown.

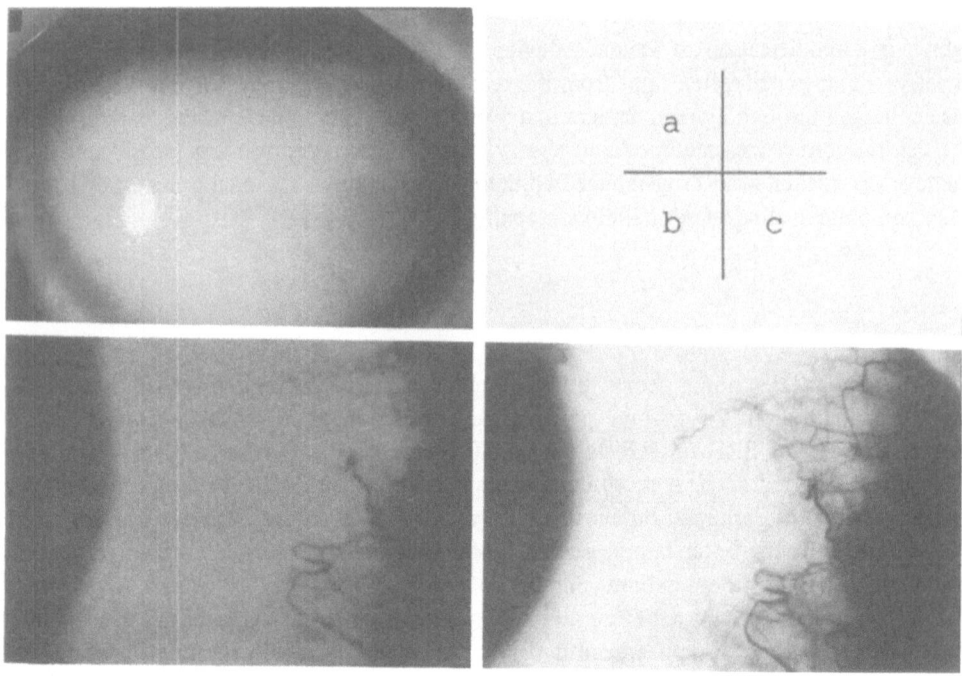

Figure 2. (Yokoi and associates) A case showing excessive fluorescein permeability as corneal involvement (a) . Sulforhodamine B and rose bengal staining showed no involvement in conjunctival epithelium (b and c, respectively). Only temporal bulbar conjunctiva is shown.

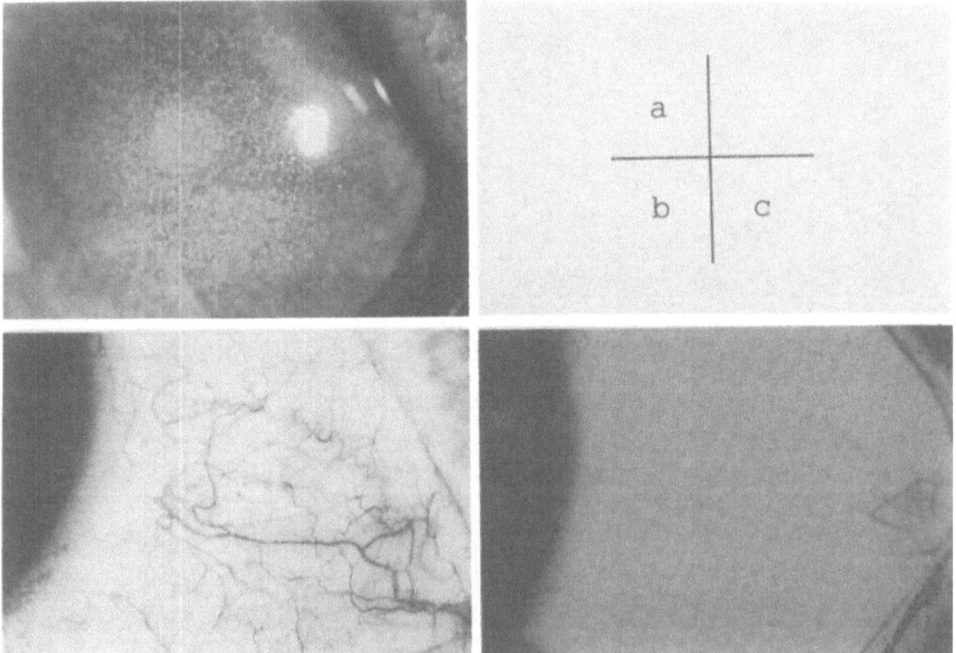

Figure 3. (Yokoi and associates) A case showing predominant superficial punctate epithelial keratopathy as corneal involvement (a). Sulforhodamine B and rose bengal staining showed no involvement in conjunctival epithelium (b and c, respectively). Only temporal bulbar conjunctiva is shown.

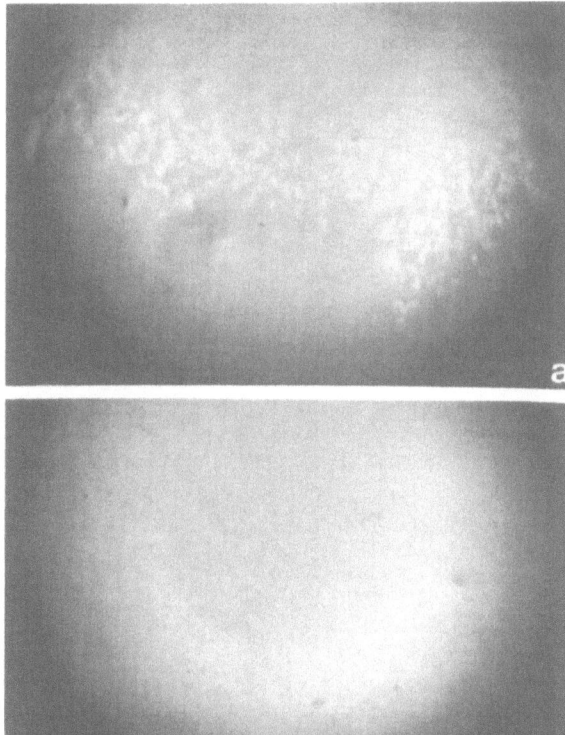

Figure 4. (Yokoi and associates) Precorneal tear film of case shown in Fig. 2, which showed very thin and spontaneous breakup of tears on corneal surface (a), indicating severely deteriorated tear/corneal surface interaction. Two weeks after stoppage of responsible drug, frequent instillation of preservative-free eye drops had improved this finding (b).

rescein dye diffusely permeated into the cornea with unclear margins (delayed staining); the other type showed prominent superficial punctate epithelial keratopathy (nine eyes of five patients; Fig 3A) in which fluorescein discretely pooled in the epithelial lesions with clear margins; this is a well-known type in clinical situations. In Sjögren's syndrome, only superficial punctate keratopathy was detected (Fig. 1A); no epithelial lesions were detected in the corneas of normal eyes.

In 15 eyes of nine patients with drug-induced epithelial keratopathy (examined cases: 18 eyes of 10 patients), observation of precorneal tear film revealed that it had become thinner and broken up spontaneously, in so-called "non-invasive breakup,"[16] indicating tear instability on the corneal surface (Figs 4A and 5A). This abnormal tear finding was completely resolved in all cases after the resolution of corneal damage (Figs. 4B and 5B). Schirmer's test indicated that tear deficiency (less than 5 mm) in eight eyes of five patients (examined cases: 26 eyes of 14 patients) of drug-induced epithelial keratopathy.

DISCUSSION

The adverse effect of eyedrops on ocular surface epithelium is mainly classified into two types, based on ocular surface effect: predominantly cytotoxic and predominantly allergenic. As regards the former, there have been many reports on corneal epithelial damage, manifested as superficial punctate keratopathy, diffuse epithelial keratopathy, and, in

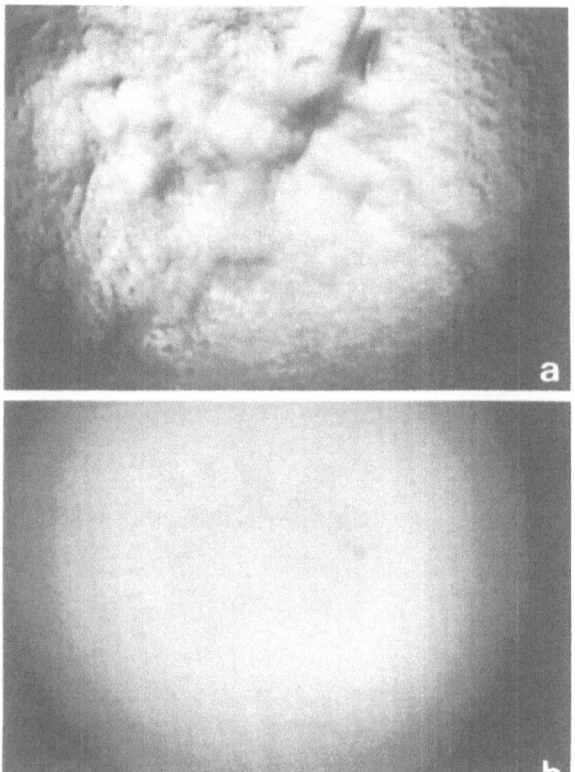

Figure 5. (Yokoi and associates) Precorneal tear film of case shown in Fig. 3, which showed spontaneous brakup of tears on corneal surface (a). Two weeks after stoppage of responsible drug, frequent instillation of preservative-free eyedrops had improved this finding (b).

severe form, epithelial defect.[17] As regards the allergenic type, allergic conjunctivitis showing conjunctival hyperemia and follicular response is often experienced. The most severe form is ocular pseudopemphigoid.[18,19] From this point of view, the drug-induced keratopathies examined in this study were caused by the former mechanism given the lack of conjunctival allergic response. As seen in the examined cases, the detection of enhanced fluorescein permeability two minutes after fluorescein staining is considered an important finding suggesting a cytotoxic mechanism of eyedrops. This is interpreted as implying deteriorated cell membrane permeability, which permits easier fluorescein permeation into cells. It has been reported that preservatives, represented by benzalkonium chloride, can, by their strong surface activity, alter the hydrophobic nature of cell membrane, which acts to inhibit the permeation of hydrophilic molecules. Since fluorescein has intermediate value of lipid/water partition coefficient (0.6), it detects disrupted cell membrane barrier function without difficulty.

Interestingly, the present study showed that in drug-induced keratopathy, bulbar conjunctival epithelium is minimally compromised, even when the corneal epithelium is severely damaged. Moreover, this findings was contrasted greatly with the high conjunctival staining scores by sulforhodamine B and rose bengal in Sjögren's syndrome. To explain this fact, the following hypothesis has been proposed: the conjunctival epithlium has far less tight a barrier function than the corneal epithelim;[20] drugs and/or preservatives mainly enter the subconjunctival space via the paracellular route. This can also explain why conjunctiva is predominantly affected in drug toxicity by the allergic mechanism.

Specular microscopic study of damaged corneal epithelium demonstrated tear instability. In view of the minimal involvement of conjunctival epithelium as observed in this study, this tear instability is induced by the disruption of corneal epithelium, which secretes mucin-like glycoprotein as demonstrated by the recent studies.[21] However, in patients using β-blocker eyedrops, goblet cell density is reportedly diminished.[7] The exact mechanism responsible for drug-induced tear abnormality will, therefore, require further examination. This tear/corneal surface disinteraction in drug-induced keratopathy could contribute to producing additional corneal epithelial damage by dry-up mechanism; in this study, as therapy, preservative-free artificial tears were instilled frequently, and the causative eyedrops stopped.

In conclusion, in drug-induced epithelial keratopathy, conjunctival epithelial damage is minimal, even when corneal epithelial damage is severe. This characteristic is quite different from that of dry eye, in which conjunctival epithelial damage is more predominant than that in the corneal epithelium. Evaluation of conjunctival epithelial damage is therefore important in differentiating drug-induced keratopathy from dry eye; even in dry eye, disproportionally damaged corneal epithelium, as opposed to conjunctival damage, may imply the contribution of drug toxicity. Moreover, in drug-induced corneal epithelial damage, precorneal tear film stability is quite deteriorated on the disrupted corneal surface. This fact may be another important aspect in treating drug-induced keratopathy.

ACKNOWLEDGMENTS

Supported in part by a research grant from Kyoto Foundation for the Promotion of Medical Science, and the intramural research fund of Kyoto Prefectural University of Medicine.

REFERENCES

1. F.M. Wilson, II., Adverse external ocular effects of topical ophthalmic medications. *Surv. Ophthalmol.* 24:57 (1979).
2. M. Gobbels, and Spitznas, M., Influence of artificial tears on corneal epithelium in dry-eye syndrome. *Graefe's Arch. Clin. Exp. Ophthalmol.* 227:139 (1989).
3. N.L. Burstein, Corneal cytotoxicity of topically applied drugs, vehicles and preservatives. *Surv. Ophthalmol.* 25:15 (1980).
4. R. Marsh, and Maurice, D.M., The influence of non-ionic detergents and other surfactants on human corneal permeability. *Exp. Eye. Res.* 11:43 (1971).
5. N.L. Burstein, Preservative alteration of corneal permeability in humans and rabbits. *Invest. Ophthalmol. Vis. Sci.* 25:1453 (1984).
6. E. Kuppens, Stolwijk, T., van Best J., and de Keizer, R., Topical timolol, corneal epithelial permeability and autofluorescence in glaucoma by fluorophotometry. *Graefes Arch. Clin. Exp. Ophthalmol.* 232;215 (1994).
7. J.M. Herreras, Pastor, J.C., Calonge, M., and Asensio, V.M., Ocular surface alteration after long-term treatment with an antiglaucomatous drug. *Ophthalmology* 99:1082 (1992).
8. M. Boljka, Kolar, G., and Vidensek J., Toxic side effects of local anaesthetics on the human cornea. *Br. J. Ophthalmol.* 78:386 (1994).
9. D. Broadway, Grierson, I., and Hitchings, R., Adverse effects of topical antiglaucomatous medications on the conjunctiva. *Br. J. Ophthalmol.* 77:590 (1993).
10. J.A. Eliason, and Maurice, D.M., Staining of the conjunctiva and conjunctival tear film. *Br. J. Ophthalmol.* 74:519 (1990).
11. O.P. van Bijsterveld, Diagnostic tests in the sicca syndrome. *Arch. Ophthalmol.* 82:10 (1969).

12. R.P.G. Feenstra, and Tseng, S.C.G., Comparison of fluorescein and rose bengal staining. *Ophthalmology* 99:605 (1992).

13. M. Doane, An instrument for *in vivo* tear film interferometry. *Optom Vis. Sci.* 66:383 (1989).

14. O. Schirmer, Studien zur physiologie und pathologie der traänenabsonderung un traänenabfuhr. *Arch. Klin. Exp. Ophthalmol.* 59:197 (1903).

15. K. Miyamoto, Inoue, Y., and Ohashi, Y., Three cases of drug-induced keratitis with remarkably increased corneal epithelial permeability. *J. Jpn. CL. Soc. 35:317 (1993).*

16. L.S. Mengher, Bron, A.J., Tonge, S.R., and Gilbert, D.J., A non-invasive instrument for clinical assessment of the pre-corneal tear film stability. *Curr. Eye Res.* 4:1 (1985).

17. I.R. Schwab, and Abbott, R.L., Toxic ulcerative keratopathy: an unrecognised problem. *Ophthalmology* 96:1187 (1989).

18. J.T. Patten, Cavanagh, H.D., and Allansmith, M.R. Induced ocular pseudopemphigoid. *Am. J. Ophthalmol.* 82:272 (1976).

19. P.M. Fiore, Jacobs, I.H., and Goldberg, D.B., Drug-induced pemphigoid. A spectrum of diseases. *Arch. Ophthalmol.* 105:1660 (1987).

20. A.J.W. Huang, Tseng, S.C.G., and Kenyon, K.R., Paracellular permeability of corneal and conjunctival epithelia. *Invest. Ophthalmol. Vis. Sci.* 30:684 (1989).

21. H. Watanabe, Fabricant, M., Tisdale, A.S., et al., Human corneal and conjunctival epithelia produce a mucin-like glycoprotein for the apical surface. *Invest. Ophthalmol. Vis. Sci.* 36:337 (1995).

7

CORNEAL EPITHELIAL REJECTION AFTER ALLOGRAFT CONJUNCTIVAL TRANSPLANTATION FOR LIMBAL PAPILLOMA

A Case Report

Francisco José de Lima Bocaccio,[1,2] Sérgio Kwitko,[1] Daniel Fridman,[1] Jussara Ribeiro Duarte,[2] Mauro Antonio Chies,[1] and Juliana Bocaccio Yaluk[1]

[1]Cornea Service, Department of Ophthalmology
Hospital de Clínicos de Poroto Alegre
Rio Grande do Sul, Brasil
[2]Cornea Service, Department of Ophthalmology
Irmandade Santa Casa de Misericordia de Porto Alegre
Rio Grande do Sul, Brasil

ABSTRACT

The authors report a case of typical corneal epithelial rejection two months after allogenic limbal-conjunctival graft for a recurrent limbal-conjunctival papilloma in a 62-year-old female patient. The HLA donor-recipient pair was haploidentical (50% identity). This observation suggests a clear conjunctival epithelial transdifferentiation onto corneal epithelium. This is the first report, to the best of the authors' knowledge, of allograft conjunctival transplantation for this disease and of corneal epithelial rejection after such a procedure. In this case, there was no rejection of the conjunctival graft, and corneal rejection was successfully treated with oral prednisone and topical 1% prednisolone.

INTRODUCTION

Extensive experimental and clinical work has demonstrated the importance of limbal basal epithelial cells, the "stem cells," for the so-called "transdifferentiation," i.e., transformation of conjunctival epithelial cells into cells biochemically and morphologically similar to the corneal epithelium. This occurs when the entire corneal epithelium is removed, and the limbal area is intact, or when a new limbal conjunctival tissues is transplanted to an affected area after removal of the entire corneal epithelia.[1–8]

Conjunctival transplantation is one of the several approaches for limbal tumor as an obstacle for its recurrence after tumor removal.[4] This paper reports a case of corneal epithelial rejection after an allograft conjunctival transplantation for a recurrent limbal papilloma.

CASE REPORT

A 65-year-old woman was sent to the Cornea Service in December, 1994 because of a recurrent limbal papilloma after simple surgical removal.

Slit lamp examination disclosed a 360° mass that clinically appeared to be a recurrent papilloma (Fig. 1). The tumor covered part of the para-central cornea, distorting central corneal curvature, leading to a decreased visual acuity(count fingers at 3 meters).

Removal of the entire mass, with a superficial keratectomy and an allograft conjunctival transplantation, was performed in April, 1995 under subconjunctival anesthesia.

Allograft conjunctival transplantation was preferred to autograft because the fellow eye presented corneal and conjunctival abnormalities secondary to staphylococcal ble-

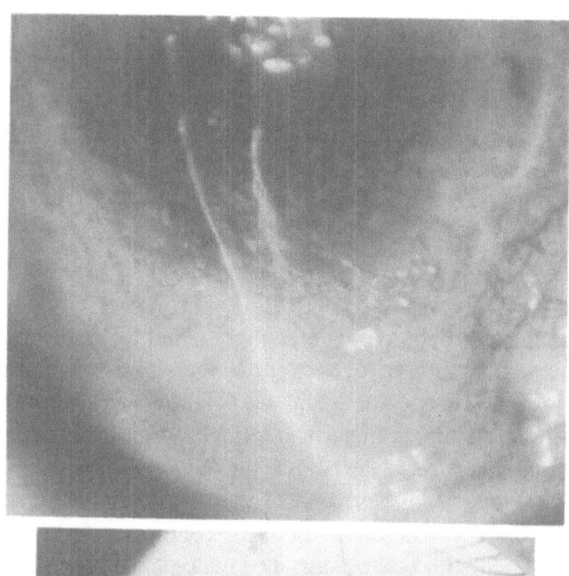
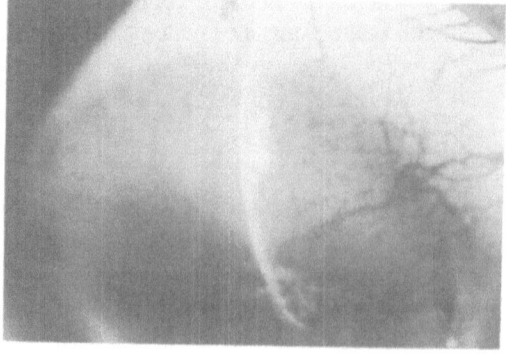

Figure 1. Recurrent papilloma: inferior aspect.

pharitis. Donor tissue was obtained from the amblyopic left eye of the patient's daughter as this donor had only one HLA Class I mismatch with the recipient. HLA typing for Class I and Ii antigens, as well as crossmatching against peripheral blood mononuclear cells were performed prior to surgery.

Conjunctival transplantation was performed according to the surgical technique described by Thoft[1] and modified by Kenyon and Tseng.[9] Two 3 x 7 mm conjunctival flaps were sutured onto recipient corneal limbus, inferiorly and superiorly, with two 10.0 nylon buried sutures at the cornea and two 8.0 vicryl® sutures at the conjunctival side, taking care to keep the limbal side of the flap facing the recipient limbus.

Both donor and recipient eyes were patched for at least 24 hours. Cycloplegic and neomycin-dexamethasone drops every eight hours, and a patch of the recipient eye were maintained until the epithelial defect healed completely. No immunosuppressive therapy was used because of HLA-matched donor. After the complete epithelial healing, the eye was kept with nonpreserved artificial tears (0.5% methylcellulose) every two hours for the next two weeks, and tapered according to the fluorescein staining.

One week postoperatively, conjunctival donor flaps were well adhered to the recipient eye, without edema and with normal vascularization and color. Complete corneal epithelium healing was already noted seven days after surgery and best-corrected visual acuity was 20/200 (Fig. 2).

Two months after surgery the patient returned complaining of blurred vision and a foreign body sensation. Slit lamp examination disclosed a typical corneal epithelial rejection line and an inferior punctate fluorescein staining (Fig. 3).

Treatment with topical 1% prednisolone every hour was indicated. As no improvement was noted with five days of treatment, oral prednisone (40 mg/day) was started. Two weeks later the rejection line disappeared and the cornea was clear. Best-corrected visual acuity was 20/30 (Fig. 4).

Five months after surgery, a recurrence of the papilloma started inferiorly (Fig. 5), so a new inferior superficial keratectomy with tumor and adjacent inferior conjunctival removal was performed with no complications. Three months later the patient presented again with a typical corneal epithelial rejection line inferiorly, and was successfully treated with topical 1% prednisolone.

One year after allograft conjunctival transplantation, the cornea was clear with no signs of tumor recurrence or other epithelial corneal rejection line and the best corrected visual acuity was still 20/30 (Fig. 6).

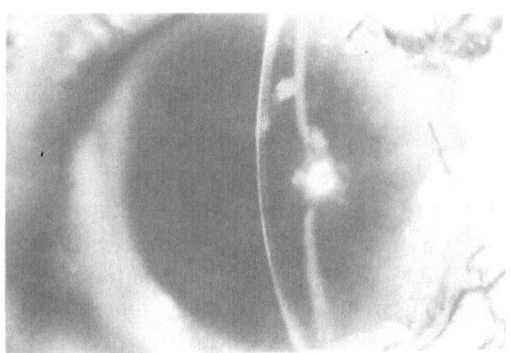

Figure 2. One week post-operatively - VA 20/200.

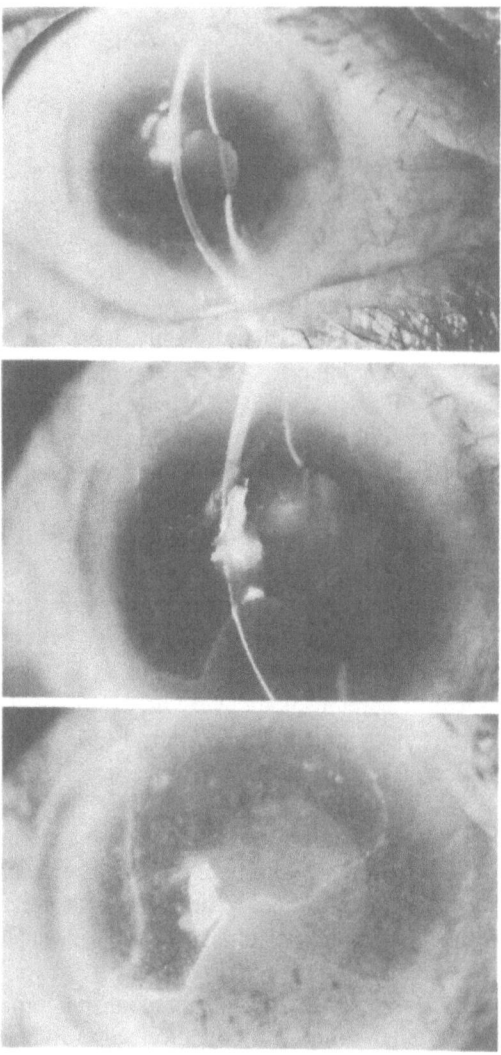

Figure 3. Corneal epithelial rejection line with inferior punctate fluorescein staining.

DISCUSSION

Autologous conjunctival transplantation to promote a normal transdifferentiation in cases of severe unilateral alkali burn was first suggested by Thoft in 1977.[1] The success of this procedure is directly related to the presence of a healthy conjunctival epithelium in the unaffected fellow eye. This procedure has been performed with success for several unilateral surface disorders, such as chemical and thermal burns, trophic ulcers, recurrent pterygia, contact lens associated keratopathy, and limbal tumors.[1,8–16]

However, when patients have bilateral surface involvement, such as in bilateral burns, Stevens-Johnson syndrome, Lyell syndrome, cicatricial pemphigoid, trachoma, aniridia, and ectodermal dysplasia, there is no healthy conjunctival epithelium in the fel-

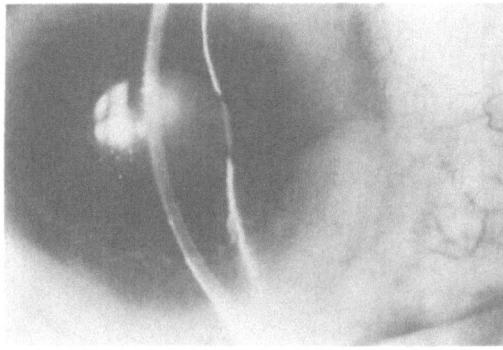

Figure 4. Two weeks after treatment of rejection.

low eye. For these cases, in 1983 Thoft suggested transplantation of corneal epithelia from fresh donor cadaver eyes, a surgical procedure called "keratoepithelioplasty."[2] Very little has been published about the results of this procedure.[2,17]

Weise et al.[18] reported encouraging results of allograft conjunctival transplantation in non-human primates. Tseng et al.,[7] Tsai et al.,[5] and Tsubota et al.[19] have also reported good results performing allograft conjunctival transplantation obtained from non-tissue-matched cadaver donor eyes, with strong systemic immunosuppression. The Cornea Service at Hospital de Clinicasde Porto Alegre recently reported encouraging preliminary results of allograft conjunctival transplantation for bilateral surface disorders, where donor conjunctiva was obtained from HLA-matched relatives, without immunosuppression.[3] More recently, Tan et al. have also shown good results of limbal transplantation from either HLA-matched relatives or cadaveric donor eyes with immunosuppression.[6]

Because the conjunctiva is a vascular tissue, allograft rejection of conjunctival flap is to be expected of non-matched donors are used without intensive immunosuppressive therapy. A rate of 29.4% of rejection episodes (5 of 17 eyes) of conjunctival flap after allograft conjunctival transplantation for bilateral ocular surface disorders has been reported previously. All of these cases had either incompatible donors or haplo-identical HLA donors for a repeated allograft conjunctival transplantation. A similar rate was reported by Tseng et al.[7] (30%), and Tsubota et al.[19] (22.2%), who obtained conjunctivas from non-tis-

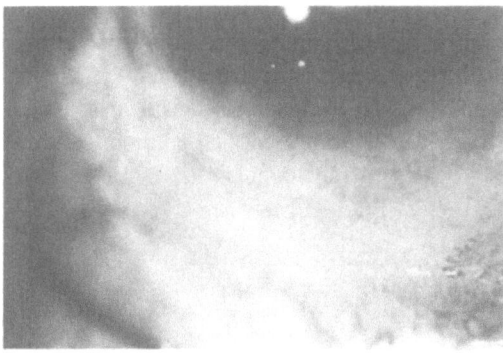

Figure 5. Recurrence of papilloma: appearance of inferior conjunctiva five months after surgery.

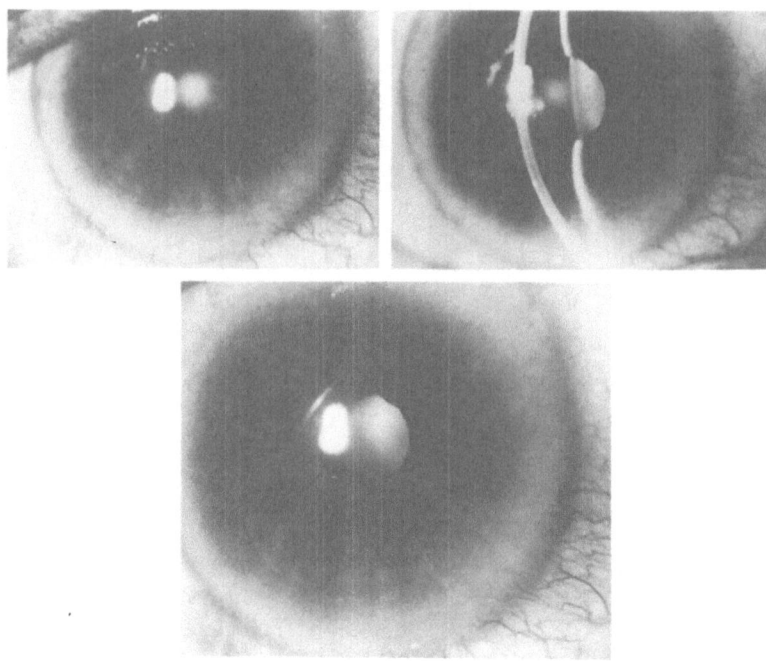

Figure 6. Slit lamp aspect: one year after surgery - VA 20/30.

sue-matched cadaver donor eyes. Thoft[14] also reported rejection of donor cadaver corneal lenticules in some cases of keratoepithelioplasty with no disturbance of corneal epithelial integrity. Tsai et al.[5] have reported no rejection in their series of 16 eyes using systemic immunosuppression for non-matched allograft limbal transplantation. Tan et al.[6] reported only one rejection (11.1%) episode in their series of nine HLA-matched allograft limbal transplantations, using systemic immunosuppression, subsequent to a *Staphylococcus aureus* keratitis.

The interesting finding of the case described herein is the development of a corneal epithelial rejection line two months after allogenic conjunctival transplantation, without disturbing the conjunctival flap, i.e., a rejection of the donor epithelial cells that were covering the recipient corneal that had transdifferentiated from donor conjunctival cells.

Pfister[4] reported a similar case of corneal epithelial rejection line 6 weeks after an allograft limbal transplantation for alkali burn from a non-matched cadaver eye that resolved with fluormetholone. However, this report seems to be the first, to the best of the author's knowledge to describe a rejection of corneal epithelium after allograft conjunctival transplantation from a live HLA-matched donor.

ACKNOWLEDGMENTS

The authors gratefully acknowledge Eduardo Vaconcellos, M.D. for referring the patient and for the first video documentation, and Diane Marinho, M.D. and Samuel Rymer, M.D. for the useful advice and discussions.

REFERENCES

1. R.A. Thoft, Conjunctival transplantation. *Arch. Ophthalmol.* 95:1425 (1977).
2. R.A. Thoft, Keratoepithelioplasty. *Am. J. Ophthalmol.* 97:1 (1984).
3. S. Kwitko, Marinho, D., Barcaro, S., et al., Allograft conjunctival transplantation for bilateral ocular surface disorders. *Ophthalmology* 102(7):1020 (1995).
4. R.R. Pfister, Corneal stem cell disease: concepts, limbal stem cells. *CLAO J.* 120(1): 64 (1994).
5. RJ-F Tsai, and Tseng, S.C.G., Human allograft limbal transplantation for corneal surface reconstruction. *Cornea* 13(5):389 (1994).
6. D.T.H. Tan, and Flicker, L.A., Limbal transplantation. *Ophthalmology* 103:29 (1996).
7. S.C.G. Tseng, Chen, J.J.Y., Huang, A.J.W., et al., Classification of conjunctival surgeries for corneal diseases based on stem cell concept. *Ophthalmol. Clin. North Am.* 3:595 (1990).
8. M.J. Carvalho, Mourac, R.C., Cunha, M., et al., Limbal autograft transplantation for severe ocular burn. *Arq. Bras. Oftalmol.* 57:167 (1994).
9. K.R. Kenyon, and Tseng, S.C.G., Limbal autograft transplantation for ocular surface disorders. *Ophthalmology* 96:709 (1989).
10. S. Kinoshita, Friend, J., and Thoft, R.A., Biphasic cell proliferation in transdifferentiation of conjunctival to corneal epithelium in rabbits. *Invest. Ophthalmol. Vis. Sci.* 24:1008 (1983).
11. M.S. Shapiro, Friend, J., and Thoft, R.A., Corneal re-epithelialization from the conjunctiva. *Invest. Ophthalmol. Vis. Sci.* 21:135 (1981).
12. S. Kinoshita, Kiorpes,T.C., Friend, J., and Thoft, R.A., Limbal epithelium in ocular surface wound healing. *Invest. Ophthalmol. Vis. Sci.* 23:73 (1982).
13. R.A. Thoft and Friend, J., Biochemical transformation of regenerating ocular surface epithelium. *Invest. Ophthalmol. Vis. Sci.* 16:14 (1977).
14. R.A. Thoft, Conjunctival surgery for corneal disease. In *The Cornea: Scientific Foundations and Clinical Practice, Third Edition,* G. Smolin and Thoft, R.A., eds., Boston, Little, Brown (1994).
15. R.J.F. Tsai, Sun, T.T., and Tseng, S.C.G., Comparison of limbal and conjunctival autograft transplantation in corneal surface reconstruction in rabbits. *Ophthalmology* 97:446 (1990).
16. T.E. Clinch, Goins, K.M., and Cobo, L.M., Treatment of contact lens-related ocular surface disorders with autologous conjunctival transplantation. *Ophthalmology* 99:534 (1992).
17. P.W. Turgeon, Nauheim, R.C., Roat, M.I., et al., Indications for keratoepithelioplasty. *Arch. Ophthalmol.* 108:233 (1990).
18. R.A. Weise, Mannis, M.J., Vastine, D.W., et al., Conjunctival transplantation. Autologous and homologous grafts. *Arch. Ophthalmol.* 103:1736 (1985).
19. K. Tsubota, Toda, I., Saito, H., et al., Reconstruction of the corneal epithelium by limbal allograft transplantation for severe ocular surface disorders. *Ophthalmology* 102:1486 (1995).

8

AUTOMATED EXTRACTION OF MORPHOLOGICAL AND MORPHOMETRIC CHARACTERISTICS OF THE CONJUNCTIVAL VASCULATURE

Christopher G. Owen,[1] Timothy J. Ellis,[2] and E. Geoffrey Woodward[1]

[1]Applied Vision Research Centre
City University
London, United Kingdom
[2]Information Engineering Centre
City University
London, United Kingdom

ABSTRACT

This report investigates a novel technique for delineating conjunctival vasculature from the scleral background. A Canny edge detector was used for accurate vessel edge detection, along with a "ravine finder" to define the axis of the vessel. A connectivity labeling algorithm was used to link adjacent pixels into strings in order to define vessel segments. This allows width measurement of numerous vessel segments, using appropriate triples of points, based on a central ravine point and two vessel boundary points. An initial investigation was conducted on 20 patients. Ages ranged from 20 to 65 years (mean=42.2, standard deviation=13.5 years). Results may indicate an increase in the number of larger vessels with age (ranging from 0.100 to 0.175 mm). Analysis shows a lognomial distribution of vessel widths. Potential applications of this technique are myriad. With further development of the connectivity algorithm individual vessels could be tracked allowing further morphometric and morphological characteristics to be quantified. This will only further the understanding of vascular "abnormality."

INTRODUCTION

Examination of the conjunctival vasculature is a useful source of information for many systemic and ocular disorders. Conjunctival and episcleral vessels consist of a multilayered intricate vascular pattern which is readily observed through its transparent mucus

Advances in Corneal Research, edited by Lass
Plenum Press, New York, 1997

membrane, and thus open to computational assessment. Unlike retinal vasculature, which is observed through transparent refractive structures such as the cornea and lens leading to altered magnification, the bulbar conjunctival blood supply is from two sources, depending upon location, both originating from the ophthalmic artery via the internal carotid. Perilimbal bulbar conjunctival vessels (4 to 6 mm from the limbus)[1] stem from the episcleral arterial circle, which originates from the long posterior ciliary artery via the major circle of the iris (the intraocular arterial circle),[2] the anterior ciliary arterial network, and anterior cilary arteries which branch from the extraocular muscular arteries. The peripheral bulbar conjunctivae (>6 mm from the limbus) is supplied via the lacrimal artery (originating from the ophthalmic artery), which branches into the palpebral arcades before crossing the fornix to become bulbar conjunctival vessels.[2,3]

Usually only bulbar conjunctival hyperemia is noted. This is often subjectively assessed using ordinal ranking classifications, which at best are made with photographic reference plates.[4] However, observers are said to overestimate the "true" width of a vessel.[5] Hence, a number of computer- assisted techniques of conjunctival hyperemia assessment have been described. Automated examination of vessel area[6,7,8] and relative redness[8] are useful in monitoring ocular effects to certain insults observed in longitudinal time sequences. Contact lens wear,[4,9,10] contact lens wearing time,[11] and *in vivo* ocular irritancy of contact lens cleaning solutions[12] all have been subjectively shown to effect conjunctival hyperemia. Other factors to be considered include the biocompatibility of ocular medications, as well as the therapeutic effectiveness of ocular medications in the treatment of conjunctivitis, episcleritis, scleritis, uveitis, and other non-infective conditions which cause hyperaemia such as acute closed angle glaucoma and carotid carvenous sinus fistula. Another use has been to evaluate the success of certain surgical treatments such as monitoring the vascular response to glaucomatous bleb surgery.[13]

Systemic conditions, such as diabetes,[14,15] hypertension,[16] sickle cell anemia,[17,18] renal failure,[19] and glaucoma,[20] are all known to effect the morphological and morphometric characteristics of the bulbar conjunctival vasculature (such effects have also been reported in retinal vasculature). Morphological vasculature changes caused by disease may go undetected if only vessel area and relative redness measurements are taken. The availability of objective, accurate, and reliable measurements holds the potential for precise quantitative assessment and monitoring of clinically relevant vessel dimensions and distributions.

The problem of extracting detailed morphometric and morphological measurements of blood vessels using digital image processing has been addressed by a number of authors in a variety of contexts.[6,21,22,23] However, the problems associated with the image measurement process are far from trivial. Using a standard photographic method for obtaining images of the conjunctiva, vessels at different depths are subject to varying levels of focus blur and contrast. In addition, since the vessels exist in a three-dimensional structure, individual vessels change in contrast and become blurred along their length as they move deeper into the conjunctiva. Also, the imaging geometry (a semi-spherical surface) and illumination source (directional flash) create a non-uniform reflectance image. Finally, the presence of the iris and eye lashes in the image introduce confusing structures.

The problem of measuring the vessels' size, shape and topology firstly requires reliable detection of the complete vessel (or at least a substantial proportion of it). The most widely adopted approach to solving this problem has been to use edge detection algorithms to identify points on the vessel boundaries and axis and then to track these points along the axis.[6,21–23] Models of the vessel cross-section, based on rectangular,[23] Gaussian,[21] or half-elliptical profiles,[22] have been used to try to achieve optimal detection of the vessel.

Effects of age on the morphometric and morphological characteristics of the bulbar conjunctival vasculature have been studied. McMonnies and Ho[24] subjectively assessed conjunctival hyperemia in non-contact lens wearers using a photographic reference scale. The results showed increasing levels of hyperemia with age, and greater vascularity in males than females. Differences in hyperemia were small and considered clinically insignificant. By inspecting digitized images, Kovalchek et al.,[25] revealed greater meandering of bulbar conjunctival postcapillaries in patients up to 40 years of age. The occurrence of bulbar conjunctival microaneurysms, ischemia, and proliferative networks was only apparent in the older age group. They also found an increase in bulbar conjunctival vessel area associated with age. It is known that bulbar conjunctival hyperemia (a 3 grade increase in subjective grade) is associated with a 0.5°C increase in surface temperature. This confirms the association between calor and rubor.[26] A study by Alió and Padron[27] showed that the absolute temperatures of the center of the cornea, limbus, sclera, and outer canthus decreases with age, perhaps indicating a reduction in vascular perfusion; this appears to contradict the above findings. However, ocular thermography is prone to experimental artefacts which are difficult to control. Using novel morphological feature detectors, this study investigated the effects of age on the conjunctival vasculature.

MATERIALS AND METHODS

Twenty individuals free from systemic and ocular abnormality were photographed. Ages ranged from 20 to 65 years (mean=42.2, standard deviation [s.d.]=13.5 years). Images of the dextro lateral conjunctivae were captured using a Nikon FS-2 photo-slit lamp with a xenon flash tube, on Ilford HP5 plus monochrome film (ASA 400). Images were taken through a Wratten 35 (purple) filter to maximize image information content.[28] The angle between observation and illumination systems was set to 30°, with the optical axis being approximately normal to the curved conjunctival surface (this has been experimentally found to minimize specular reflections from the conjunctival epithelium). Images were acquired on the maximum magnification setting of the slit lamp (x30), which corresponds to a magnification of x 3.184 at the film plane. Images were then recorded to compact disc (CD) to 3072 x 2048 pixels per 36 x 24 mm slide. Hence 1 mm in object space will be represented by 272 pixels on the CD image. A resolution of 272 pixels per mm corresponds to a pixel size of 3.7 μm per pixel. However, the photo-CD image format provides for a number of reduced resolution versions of the digital image within the same file: 1536 x 1024, 768 x 512, 384 x 256 and 192 x 128 pixels. Hence, an appropriate scaling factor (i.e., 2,4,8 or 16) must be applied to the calibration value for these images.

IMAGE ANALYSIS ALGORITHMS

The approach adopted for the measurement of the vessel widths and lengths is based on edge detection, but makes no explicit use of a vessel model. Instead, the vessels, which in the grey level images appear dark against a lighter background, are initially detected using a "ravine finder." This method identifies local minima in the grey level image and marks points appropriately. This is used to define the axis of the vessels. The edges of the vessels are detected using a standard Canny edge detector,[29] which performs Gaussian smoothing, gradient-based edge detection, non-maximum suppression of proximal edges and finally hysteresis thresholding. The Canny operator is widely used in computer vision,

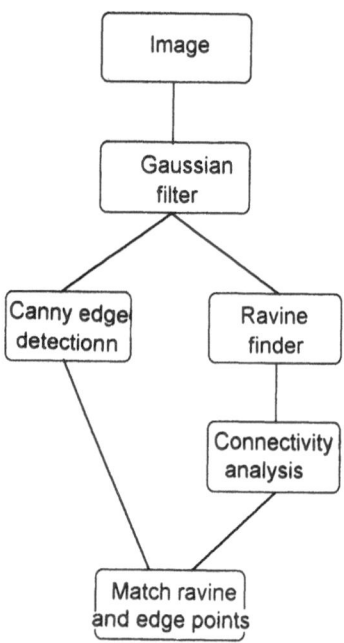

Figure 1. Flowchart of image analysis operations.

and its capability for accurate edge location and good detection performance are well known. For the present work we have used an efficient implementation of the Canny algorithm based on the work of Deriche[30] which employs recursive image filtering. Figure 1 shows a simplified flowchart of the sequence of processing steps.

The points detected by the ravine finding algorithm are processed with a connectivity labeling algorithm which links adjacent pixels into strings, defining segments of the vessels. In order to provide reliable estimates of the individual vessel widths, appropriate triples of points, based on a central ravine point and two vessel boundary points, must be detected. This is performed in the following fashion. At each ravine point the orientation of the vessel with respect to the image co-ordinate axis is estimated. This is performed by using a simple least squares filter on a small number (typically seven) of adjacent center-line ravine points (see Figure 2). Tracking perpendicularly from the center point outwards

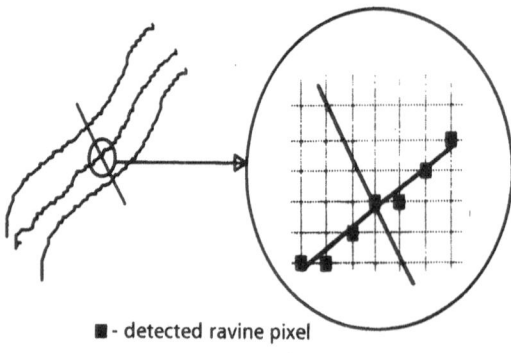

■ - detected ravine pixel

Figure 2. Determination of local orientation of ravine centre line using least squares fit to pixel data (estimated over 7 pixels). Search direction for vessel boundaries is perpendicular to the direction of this line.

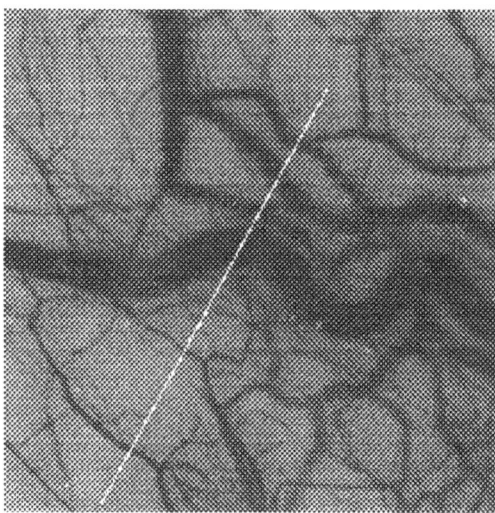

Figure 3. Sub-section of image showing the line profile used in Figures 4 and 5.

in both directions allows the detection of the blood vessel boundaries using the Canny-based edges extracted previously. Genuine blood vessels are distinguished from other noise and artifacts in the image by recognizing approximately symmetric pairs of boundary points. That is, points whose distance from the axis point to each of the boundary points is, within a threshold, equal.

IMAGE ANALYSIS RESULTS

To illustrate the operation of the vessel edge detection, Figure 3 shows a 256 x 256 portion of one of the images we have analyzed. A sequence of image points has been extracted along the profile (235 pixels) indicated by the white line drawn onto the image. Figure 4 shows a plot of the image data along the profile, superimposed on top of which are two Gaussian filtered profiles, using standard deviations of 2.1 and 4.1 pixels. One particular point to note is the smoothing of the wider filter (s.d. = 4.1 pixels) that suppresses the internal structure within the widest vessel (pixels 85–105), enabling the ravine detector to reliably detect only single local minima within the vessel.

Figure 5 shows the output from the Canny/Deriche edge detector. Typically, this output is thresholded at 1 in order to detect edges within the image. As can be seen in comparing the plots in figure 5a and 5b, although the narrower filter (s.d. = 2.1 pixels) detects more edges, some of these will be attributed to image noise, artifact and faint vessels, and their detection may complicate the vessel tracking algorithm.

The image data set was analyzed using five ranges of standard deviation for the Gaussian filtering - 1.4, 2.1, 2.8 and 4.1 and 8.0 pixels. This range, for the resolution of images used (512 x 512, taken from the 768 x 512 resolution images of the Kodak Photo-CD digitized image data sets) appeared to give an adequate representation for most vessels imaged (see Figure 3). Figure 6 shows the operation of the vessel boundary and axis detection algorithms, applied to the original grey-level image in Figure 3. The increasing smoothing operation of the Gaussian filtering is apparent over the five image sets, with an increasing sensitivity to larger vessel widths as the standard deviation of the filter increases.

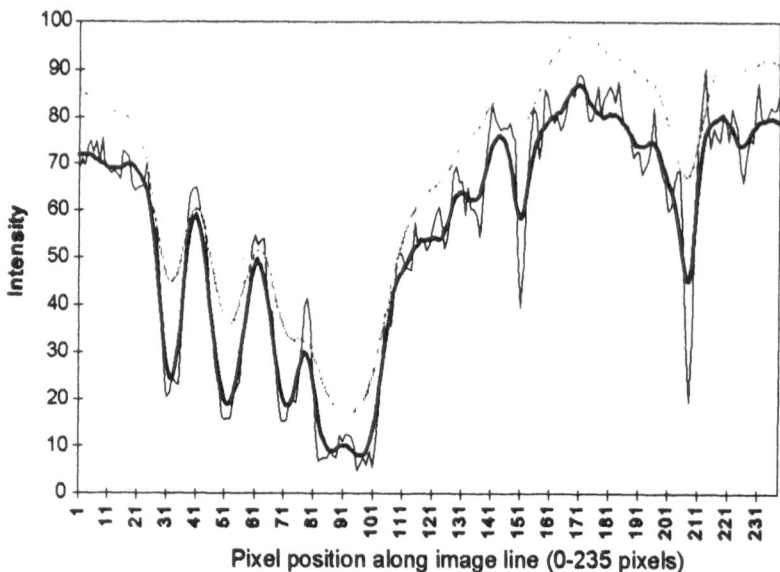

Figure 4. Grey-level pixel line profile extracted from a image shown in Figure 3 (noisy thin solid line). Other two traces show the result of Gaussian smoothing the image data, using standard deviations of 2.1 (thick solid line) and 4.1 (broken line).

Figures 7–12 show a set of images indicating the success of the algorithm in detecting the vessel boundaries. Figure 7 shows the original full size (512 x 512) image. Figure 8 shows the output vessel boundary detection using the Canny/Deriche edge detector (s.d. = 2.1). It can be seen that the vessel boundaries for many of the medium sized vessels are well detected. Figure 9 shows the results of the ravine finder, which have detected a good proportion of the vessels in the image. Figure 10 then shows the vessel axis points remaining after the connectivity labeling algorithm has determined points which are spatially adjacent in the image. These axis points are shown superimposed on the original grey level image in Figure 11. Figure 12 shows the combination of vessel boundaries and connected vessel axes. This data is then used by the vessel tracking algorithm to make measurements of vessel widths over the length of each segment.

VESSEL WIDTH RESULTS

Vessel segment widths for the 20 patients were analyzed. Vessel boundary detection with the Canny/Deriche edge detector s.d. = 2.1 visually appeared to give the best results. Hence only data from this detection filter was included. Vessel segment widths were categorized into 0.025 mm bins. Bins ranged from 0–<0.025 mm to 0.475–0.500 mm (in 0.025 mm increments). None of the vessel segments measured exceeded 0.500 mm. The number of vessel segments measured in each width range was recorded. This allowed a histogram of the number of vessels segments measured of differing widths for each patient. Initial analysis shows a lognomial distribution of vessel width data. Older patients appear to have a greater number of larger diameter vessel widths than younger patients (in the range of 0.100 to 0.175 mm). However, the peak vessel width for all age groups is the same (between 0.075 to <0.100 mm). Figure 13 shows a histogram of the number of vessels segments measured of differing widths for a patient of 65 and 24 years of age. This indicates an increased population in the larger vessels between the two ages.

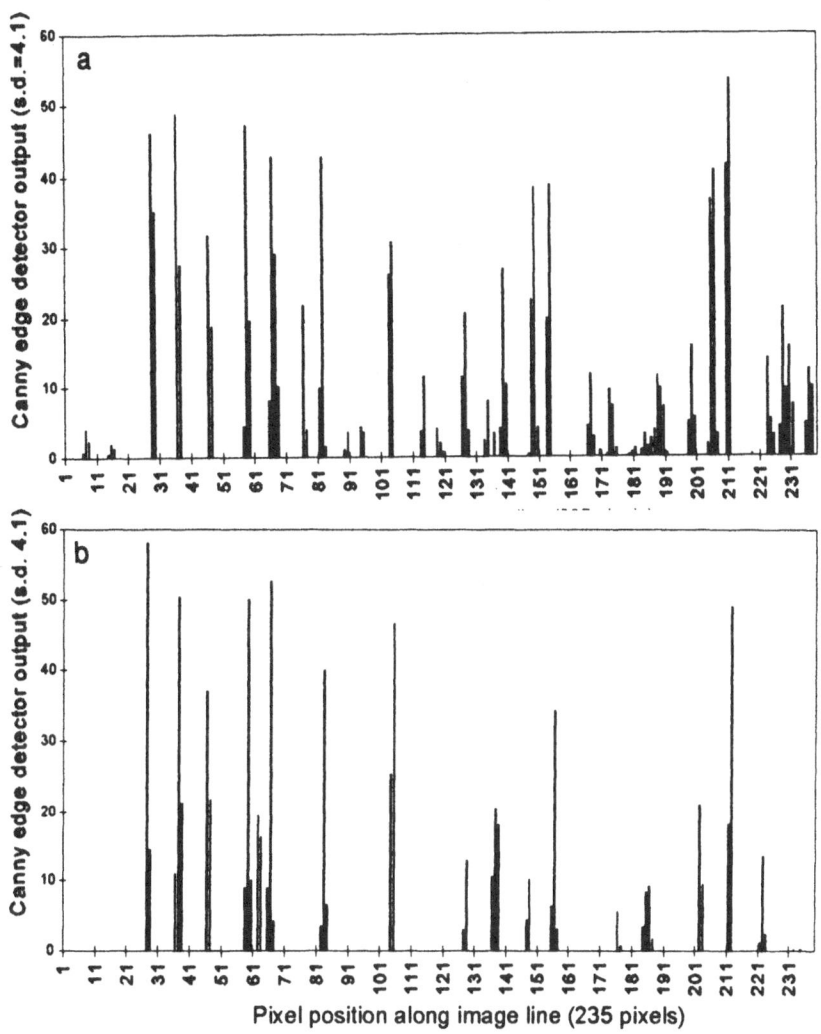

Figure 5. Output from the Canny edge detector for data in figure 2, (a) s.d. = 2.1, (b) s.d. = 4.1. Peaks in graph correspond to steepest gradient on filtered signal.

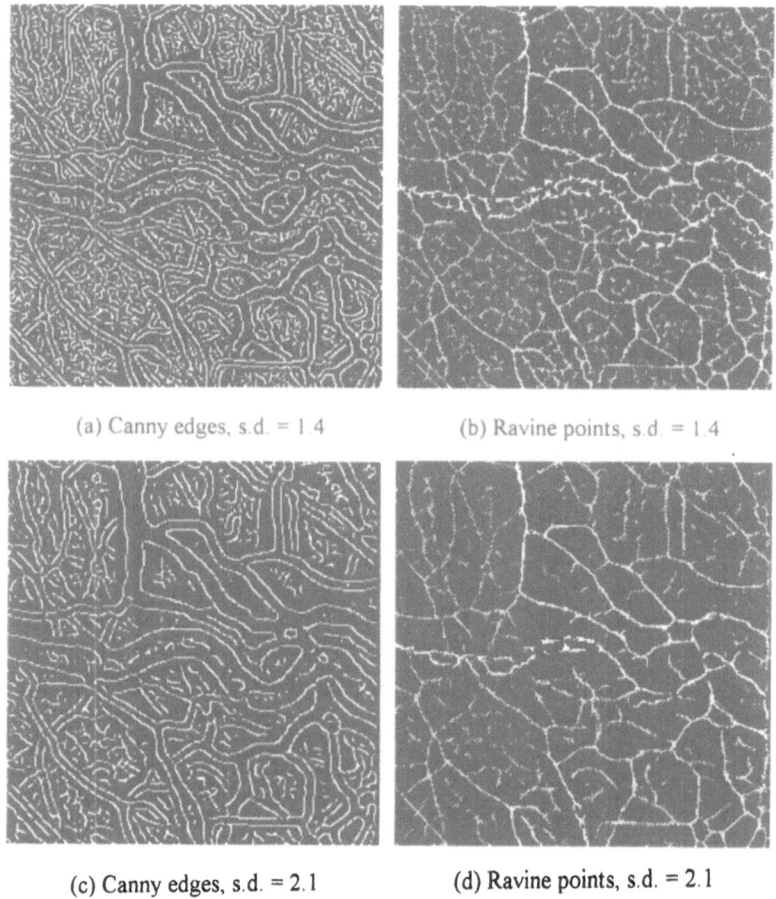

(a) Canny edges, s.d. = 1.4   (b) Ravine points, s.d. = 1.4

(c) Canny edges, s.d. = 2.1   (d) Ravine points, s.d. = 2.1

Figure 6. (a-d). Results of Canny edge detection (a,c) and ridge detection (b,d) on image shown in Figure 3. (a) Canny edges, s.d. = 1.4, (b) Ravine points, s.d. = 1.4, (c) Canny edges, s.d. = 2.1, (d) Ravine points, s.d. = 2.1.

DISCUSSION

The vessel detection algorithm, based on the Canny/Deriche boundary detector and ravine finder, has been shown to produce high quality output for the detection of most of the vessels, other than the smallest and faintest. Where the vasculature becomes dense and of low contrast (middle right of the image) the detection algorithms locate only discontinuous vessel segments. Inevitably, the vessel tracker will be unable to extend these vessels along their length, though the algorithm is still able to make measurements of the vessel widths over the short segments that do exist.

Currently, the tracking algorithm does not reliably extract long lengths of vessel, though it is able to measure a large number of short vessel segments over the image. The problems currently stem from a weakness of the connectivity labeling algorithm, which fails to maintain connectivity at junctions. An adapted version of the algorithm, which will also combine the directional derivative magnitudes, will enable more robust tracking.

Despite these shortcomings this study has shown that there appears to be a higher frequency of larger vessel widths associated with age. Other studies report an increase in

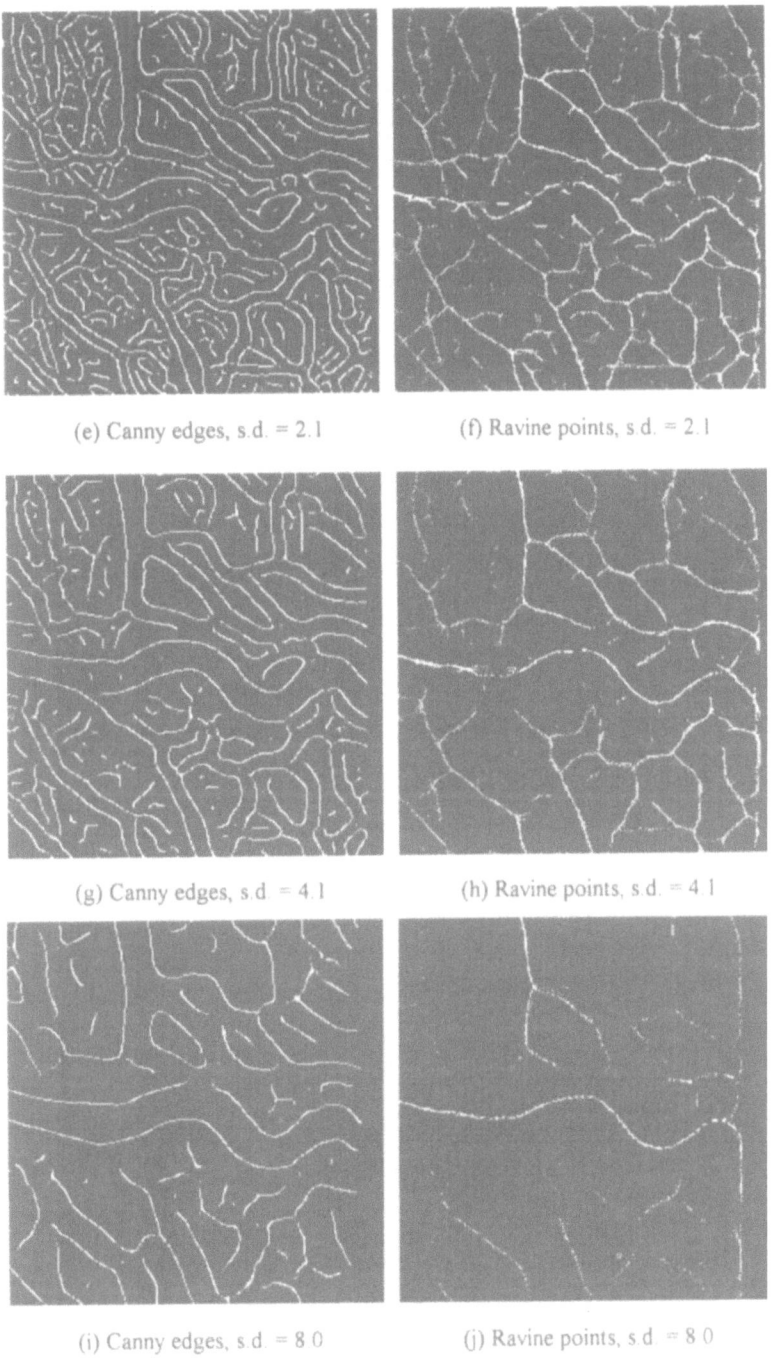

(e) Canny edges, s.d. = 2.1   (f) Ravine points, s.d. = 2.1

(g) Canny edges, s.d. = 4.1   (h) Ravine points, s.d. = 4.1

(i) Canny edges, s.d. = 8.0   (j) Ravine points, s.d. = 8.0

Figure 6. (*Continued*) (e-j). Results of Canny edge detection (e,g,i) and ridge detection (f,h,j) on image shown in Figure 3. (e) Canny edges, s.d. = 2.1, (f) Ravine points, s.d. = 2.1, (g) Canny edges, s.d. = 4.1, (h) Ravine points, s.d. = 4.1, (i) Canny edges, s.d. = 8.0, (j) Ravine points, s.d. = 8.0.

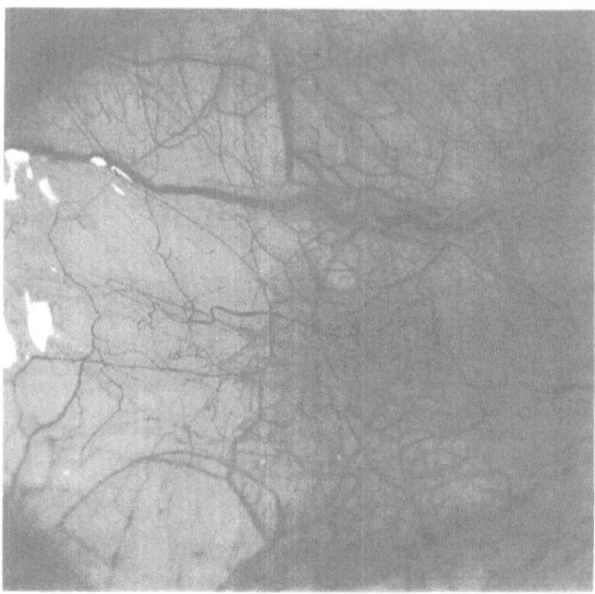

Figure 7. Original full size (512 x 512 pixel) gray scale image.

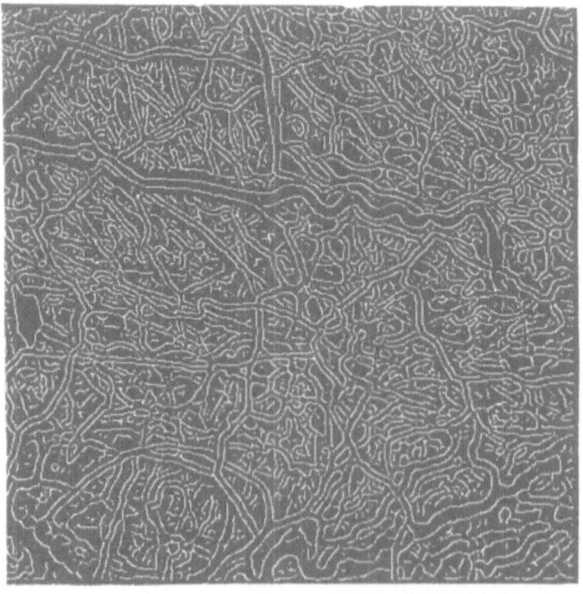

Figure 8. Output of vessel boundary detection using the Canny/Deriche edge detector (s.d.=2.1).

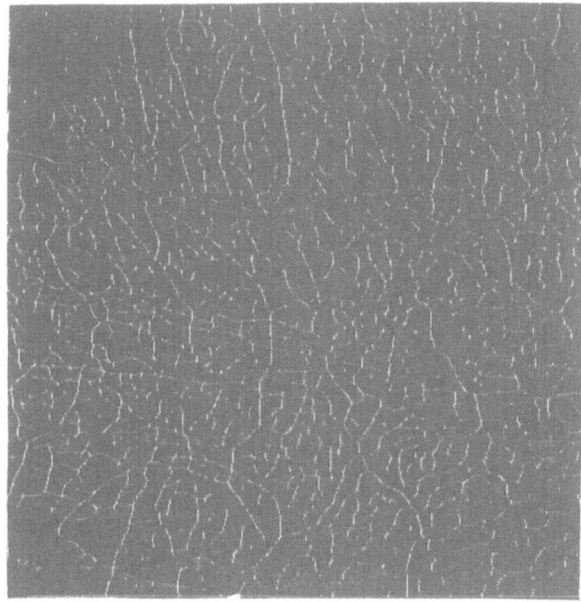

Figure 9. Output of the ravine finder.

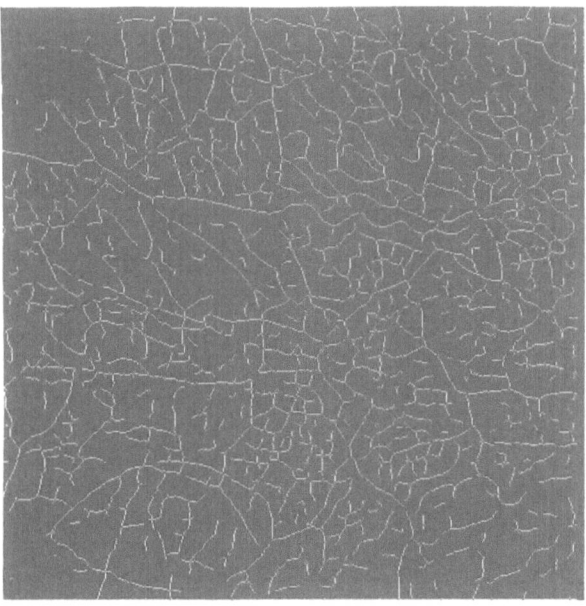

Figure 10. Output of the connectivity labelling algorithm.

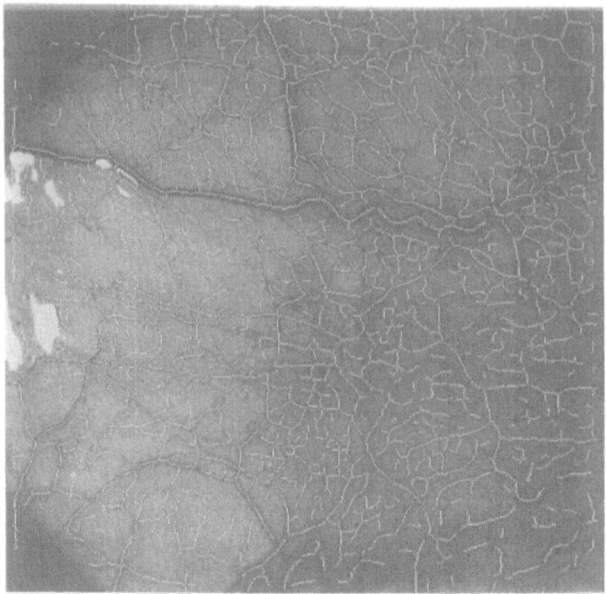

Figure 11. Connected ravine points overlaid on original gray scale image.

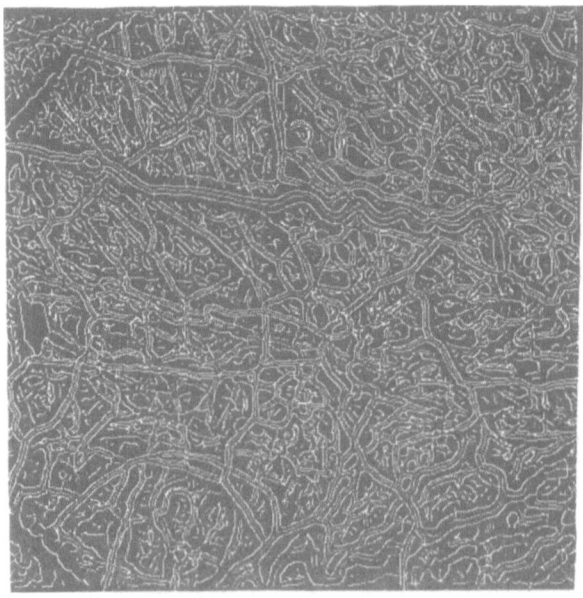

Figure 12. Canny/Deriche edges and connected ravine points.

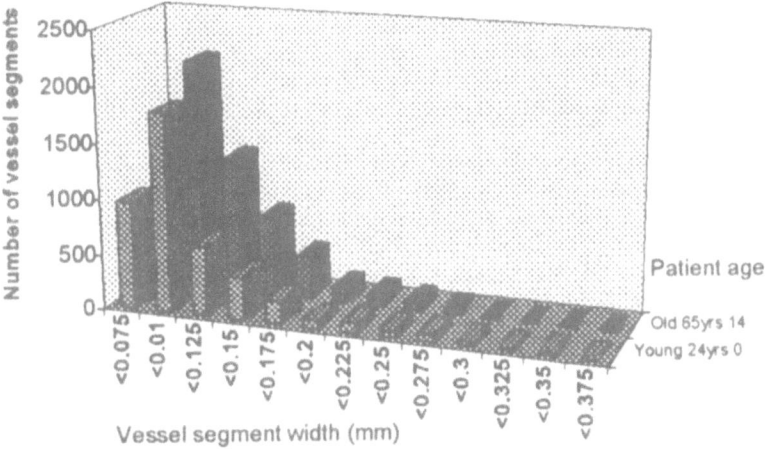

Figure 13. A histogram of the number of vessels segments measured of differing widths for a patient of 65 and 24 years of age.

vessel area with age.[24,25] However, it appears that the increase in vessel area may be due to increased vessel widths. This could represent dilation of the venule population of the conjunctival vasculature network, although further study is needed. The data resulting from this technique is vast and worthy of further investigation. At present, measurements are only taken when vessel segments are identified. With further development of the connectivity algorithm, it is hoped that individual vessels could be tracked allowing further morphometric and morphological characteristics to be quantified. Analysis will include a measure of tortuosity and vessel width variations typified by aneurysms, linear dilations, and arteriolar constrictions etc. Such changes are indicative of disease and/or age.

ACKNOWLEDGMENTS

We wish to thank the Association of Optical Practitioners, The College of Optometrists (UK), and City University for their financial assistance in allowing Chris Owen to attend this conference. The authors are grateful to Dr. Geoffrey West (Dept. Computer Science, Curtin University, Perth, Western Australia) for use of the image filtering and connectivity labeling algorithms used in this work. We also wish to thank Mr. Brian Hull at Pro-Digital Imaging, Leeds, UK, for scanning the images to CD, and Dr. Alicia Rudnicka for her assistance in the preparation of this paper.

REFERENCES

1. A.J. Bron, Mengher, L.S., and Davey, C.C., The normal conjunctivae and its response to inflammation. *Trans. Ophthalmol. Soc. U.K.* 104:424 (1985).
2. P.A.R. Meyer, The circulation of the human limbus. *Eye* 3:121 (1989).
3. P.A.R. Meyer, Patterns of blood flow in episcleral vessels studied by low dose fluorescein videoangiography. *Eye* 2:533 (1988).
4. C.W. McMonnies, and Chapman-Davies, A., Assessment of conjunctival hyperaemia in contact-lens wearers: Part I. *Am. J. Optom. Physiol. Opt.* 64(4):246 (1987).

5. R.S.B. Newsom, Sullivan, P.M., Rassam, S.M.B., et al., Retinal vessel measurement: comparison between observer and computer driven methods. *Graefe's Arch. Clin. Exp. Ophthalmol.* 230, 221 (1992).

6. P.C. Chen, Kovalcheck, S.W., and Zweifach, B.W., Analysis of microvascular network in the bulbar conjunctivae by image processing. *Int. J. Microcirc. Clin. Exp.* 6:245 (1987).

7. J. Villumsen, Rinquist, J., and Alm, A.. Image analysis of conjunctival hyperaemia. *Acta. Ophthalmol.* 69:536 (1991).

8. F.F. Willingham, Cohen, K.L., Coggins, J.M., et al., Automatic quantitative measurement of ocular hyperaemia. *Current Eye Research* 14:1101 (1995).

9. C.W. McMonnies, Chapman-Davies. A., and Holden, B.A., The vascular response to contact-lens wear. *Am. J. Optom. Physiol. Opt.* 59(10):795 (1982).

10. C.W. McMonnies, and Chapman-Davies, A., Assessment of conjunctival hyperaemia in contact-lens wearers: Part II. *Am. J. Optom. Physiol. Opt.* 64(4):251 (1987).

11. B.A. Holden, Sweeney, D.F., Swarbrick, H.A., et al., The vascular response to long-term extended contact lens wear. *Clin. Exp. Optom.* 69(3):112 (1986).

13. J.G. Sivak, Herbert, K.L., and Fonn, D., *In vitro* ocular irritancy measure of four contact lens solutions: damage and recovery. *Contact Lens Assoc. Ophthalmol.* 21(3):169 (1995).

14. P.T. Chew, Watson, P.G., and Chee, C.K., Vascular changes over trabeculectomy blebs. *Eye* 8(4):389 (1994).

15. J. Ditzel, and Sagild, U., Morphological and hemodynalic changes in the smaller blood vessels in diabetes mellitus. *New Eng. J. Med.* 250(14):587 (1954).

16. J.M. Coget, Dupuisuvny, C.H., and Merlen, J.F., Value of the study of the ocular conjunctivae in screening in diabetes. *J. des Malades Vascularies* 14(1):68 (1989).

17. N.G. Davydova, Katsnelson, L.A., Gurtovaya, Y.Y., Changes of the bulbar conjunctivae in essential arterial-hypertension. *Vestnik Ofthamologi.* 5:37 (1990).

18. D. Paton, The conjunctival sign of sickle cell disease. *Arch. Ophthalmol.* 66: 90 (1961).

19. G.R. Sejeant, Sejeant, B.E., and Condon, P.I., The conjunctival sign of sickle cell disease. A relationship with irreversibly sickle cells. *J. Am. Medical Assoc.* 219:1428 (1972).

20. N. Klaasen-Broekema, and van Bijesterveld, O.P., Red eyes in renal failure. *Brit. J. Ophthalmol.* 76:268 (1992).

21. S. Orgül, and Flammer, J., Perilimbal aneurysms of conjunctival vessels in glaucoma patients. *German J. Ophthalmol.* 4(2):94 (1995).

22. S. Chaudhuri, Chatterjee, S., Katz, N., et al., Detection of blood vessels in retinal images using two-dimensional matched filters. *IEEE Trans. Med. Imag.* 8:263 (1989).

23. F.P. Miles, and Nuttall, A.L., Matched filter estimation of serial blood vessel diameters from video images. *IEEE Transactions on Medical Imaging* 12(2):147 (1993).

24. S. Tamura, Okamoto, Y., and Yanashima, K., Zero-crossing interval correction in tracing eye-fundus blood vessels. *Pattern Recognition* 21(3):227 (1988).

25. C.W. McMonnies, and Ho A., Conjunctival hyperaemia in non-contact lens wearers. *Acta. Ophthalmol.* 69:799 (1991).

26. S.W. Kovalchek, Chen, P., and Zweifach, B.W., Microvascular changes associated with age in the bulbar conjunctivae. *International J. of Microcirculation-Clin. Exp.* 3(3–4):530 (1984).

27. N. Efron, Brennan, N.A., Hore, J., and Rieper, K., Temperature of the hyperaemic bulbar conjunctiva. *Curr. Eye Res.* 7(6):615 (1988).

28. J. Aliò, and Padron, M., Influence of age on the temperature of the anterior segment of the eye. *Ophthalmic Res.* 14:153 (1982).

29. J.R. Palmer, Owen, C.G., Ford, A.M., et al., Optimal photographic imaging of the bulbar conjunctival vasculature. *Ophthal. Physiol. Opt.* 16(2):144 (1996).

30. J. Canny, A computational approach to edge detection. *IEEE Trans. Pattern Analysis and Machine Intelligence* 8:679 (1986).

31. R. Deriche, Fast algorithms for low level vision. *IEEE Trans. Pattern Analysis and Machine Intelligence* 12:78 (1990).

9

IMPRESSION CYTOLOGY OF THE CONJUNCTIVA IN AIDS PATIENTS

Goblet and Orange Cells Analysis

A. D. Steck, M. Abreau, M. F. Sartori, and C. Muccioli

Ophthalmology Department
Paulista School of Medicine
Sao Paulo, Brazil

ABSTRACT

Keratoconjunctivitis sicca is one of the most frequent non-infectious ocular manifestations in AIDS patients. This study was performed to prospectively analyze goblet cell density in the conjunctiva of AIDS patients and to correlate orange cells and squamous metaplasia.

In this study conjunctival specimens of 37 patients with AIDS ($CD_4 < 200$ cells/mm^3) and 12 HIV-negative patients were examined by impression cytology in the interpalpebral zone, after clinical evaluation of break-up time, rose bengal staining, and Schirmer test. The AIDS group was subdivided into 19 patients with symptoms of dry eye and 18 patients without symptoms.

Results of this study showed no statistical difference in impression cytology or in evaluation of lacrimal film between the two AIDS groups. There was a statistically significant difference between AIDS patients and the control group in goblet cells counts and in lacrimal function tests ($p < 0.5$). In AIDS patients, goblet cells were absent in 22 (59.45%) eyes. There was a positive correlation between CD_4 and the goblet cell counts in AIDS patients with dry eye symptoms ($p < 0.05$). The orange cells were higher in the two AIDS groups ($p < 0.05$).

In this study decreased goblet cell numbers and the high incidence of orange cells suggested keratinization and metaplasia of conjunctival epithelium. Abnormal lacrimal function tests and damaged conjunctival epithelium, as evidenced by impression cytology, were observed in the two AIDS groups.

INTRODUCTION

Acquired immunodeficiency syndrome (AIDS) has been an important problem in public health care since 1981, when the C.D.C. in Atlanta received the news of homosexual patients and drug abusers who had pneumonia by *Pneumocystis carinii* and Kaposi's sarcoma.[1]

In 1993 some authors in Brazil studied the ophthalmologic alterations that occurred in 445 patients who had the virus.[2] In addition to reduction of T and B cells in patients infected by HIV, the ocular defenses are also compromised and may develop non-infective keratoconjunctivitis, which is observed in 10% of patients. Keratoconjunctivitis sicca appears in 10 to 15% of patients. In many cases it is incidentally discovered and can be controlled easily with artificial tears. However, in the more severe forms, superficial abnormalities and even ocular perforations can occur.[3]

In a 1991 study, the authors treated three AIDS patients with severe dry eye after the Steven-Johnson's syndrome and toxic epidermal necrolysis, which was misdiagnosed as chronic infectious conjunctivitis and did not respond to the use of topical antibiotics but improved with artificial tears. Because these patients have a great propensity for developing infections, it is not surprising that a patient with chronic red eye may be initially diagnosed and treated as infectious conjunctivitis.[4]

Keratoconjunctivitis sicca occurs with some frequency in patients infected by the HIV-virus and aqueous tear deficiency has been observed. For a better study of the conjunctival surface of AIDS patients, impression cytology of the conjunctiva has been used because it is easy to perform, fast, and reproducible. Some authors have diagnosed xerophthalmia by this method.[5]

The objective of this study was to use impression cytology to determine the number of goblet cells in the conjunctiva of AIDS patients with and without dry eye symptoms and compare them to HIV-negative patients. Additional goals are to evaluate, in a quantitative way, the distribution of orange cells of each patient and establish a possible correlation with squamous metaplasia.

METHODS

This study was performed between September 1993 and June 1994 at the Paulista School of Medicine, and Saint Vincent Hospital in Jundiai (Sao Paulo). The study population included 37 group IV AIDS patients with $CD_4 < 200$ cells/mm^3 or who had AIDs definition disease. This population was subdivided into two groups as follows: Group I—19 AIDS patients with dry eye symptoms; Group II—18 AIDS patients without dry eye symptoms; Control Group—12 HIV-negative patients. (See also Table 1).

Criteria for inclusion in this study consisted of the following items: (1) had not used eye drops in the last 6 months; (2) did not use contact lenses; (3) on biomicroscopy presented with no blepharitis, meibomitis, or eyelid alterations of any time; (4) absence of corneal or conjunctival abnormality such as scars, degenerations, infections, or inflammations of any nature; and (5) CD_4 of less than 200 cells/mm^3.

The symptoms established to characterize dry eye (Group I) were at least one of the following: burning, tearing, itching, pain, secretion, red eye, and foreign body sensation.

Blood samples were collected from all patients for HIV testing and CD_4 counting. In all patients the ophthalmologic examination was made by the best corrected visual acuity, biomicroscopy of the lacrimal film done in a TOPCON SL2E (E.U.A.) slit lamp, and indirect ophthalmoscopy (Keeler - England).

Clinical tests performed in this study included tear break-up time (BUT), Schirmer test (Clement Clarke Int. Ltd. 0892/4/5000) done with topical anesthesia (proximetacayne 0.5%) and Rose Bengal test. The BUT was considered normal when values higher than 10 seconds were obtained. The Schirmer test was considered positive when the wet area was 3mm or less in five minutes. Rose Bengal 1% stain, without preservatives and without topical anesthesia, was applied to each eye. The patients were examined after one minute. Each eye was divided into three zones (medial, corneal, and lateral) and the amount of stain in each was recorded and graduated on a scale from 0 to 3. In this way, each eye could receive a maximum score of 9 if it was stained maximally in all three zones. A score of 3 or more for one eye was considered abnormal.

With the prior consent of the patient, a topical anesthetic was instilled into each eye. Cellulose acetate paper (Millipore HAWP 04700 0.45 μm pore) was cut into a 5x5 mm square with a tip in one of the corners of the square. This asymmetric form facilitated grasping it with forceps and transferring the material to the desired area of the conjunctiva without damaging the acetate or the collected material. In the bulbar conjunctiva the paper was aligned tangentially to the nasal and temporal limbar area. This technique facilitated the collection and coloration of the material, thereby identifying the opposite side of the filter and easily locating the material for microscopic reading. After a soft compression of the filter with the back part of the forceps on the desired area for 2 to 3 seconds it was then removed delicately and fixed in absolute alcohol.

The collected material was then stained by the Papanicolaou and PAS methods simultaneously.[6] Then the count of goblet and orange cells was performed by the same experienced pathologist in the Anatomy and Pathology Department of the Federal University of Sao Paulo in this way:

1. Counting of the total number of goblet cells in 40 x and 100 x amplification.
2. For the orange cells, four possibilities were considered:

   a. Total absence of cells (0)
   b. Rare cells (+) - about 10% of the cells/field
   c. Moderate amount of cells (++) - about 50% of the cells/field
   d. Great amount of cells (+++) - more than 50% of the cells/field

RESULTS

The distribution of patients by age, sex, race, and risk factors are shown in Tables 1 and 2. Results of this study verified that the most common complaint was red eye, followed by foreign body sensation that differed significantly from the other symptoms (p<0.05).

With regard to tear break-up time (BUT) and Schirmer test, there was no significant difference between the right and left eyes in the same patient for the three groups. When the three groups were compared there was a significant difference both for the right eye and the left eye. In addition, the values for the control group were significantly higher than in the two AIDS groups (p<0.05), which showed no difference when compared to one another.

There was, however, a significant difference between the two AIDS groups in the Rose Bengal test, with greater epithelial changes occurring in Group I (p<0.05). There was no significant difference between right eye and left eye in all the patients.

There was no significant difference between the nasal and the temporal regions, and neither the right nor the left eyes in the same patient concerning the goblet cell counts. When the three groups were compared there was a significant difference both for the nasal and temporal regions as well as for right and left eyes. In the four cases, the rate of the

Table 1. Age, sex and origin of the patients of the control group, of the patients with AIDS with (group I) and without (group II) dry eye symptoms

Age (years)	Control					Group I					Group II				
	Sex		Origin			Sex		Origin			Sex		Origin		
	M	F	W	B	Y	M	F	W	B	Y	M	F	W	B	Y
20–25	0	1	1	0	0	1	0	0	1	0	2	0	1	1	0
25–30	4	1	5	0	0	5	0	4	1	0	2	0	2	0	0
30–35	3	2	5	0	0	4	2	6	0	0	5	0	4	1	0
35–40	1	0	1	0	0	4	0	4	0	0	7	0	7	0	0
≤ 40	0	0	0	0	0	3	0	3	0	0	1	1	2	0	0
Total	8	4	12	0	0	17	2	17	2	0	17	1	16	2	0

M = male; F = female; W = white; B = black; Y = yellow.

control group was significantly higher than the two AIDS groups (p<0.05) which had no difference between them (Table 3).

When the orange cells in the three groups were compared, there was a significant difference between the two AIDs groups and the control group. The number of orange cells was higher in the two AIDS groups, which showed no difference when compared to one another (p<0.01) (Tables 4 and 5).

Table 6 shows the correlation of the average number of goblet cells, with regard to CD_4 levels. In Group II there was a significant correlation. It was observed that in Group II the lower the CD_4 level, the lower was the goblet cell average (p<0.05). In Group I this correlation was not significant.

DISCUSSION

This work was performed after the observation of AIDS patients who presented with alteration of the lacrimal film verified by diagnostic tests with high frequency. Decreased lacrimal film has been encountered in adults and children infected with HIV.[7] The study sought to correlate this clinical state with the alterations verified by impression cytology. For that, lacrimal function was evaluated by use of tear break-up time, the Rose Bengal

Table 2. Forms of transmission of HIV-virus in group I and II patients

Forms of transmission	Frequency		%	
	I	II	I	II
Homo./Bisexual	10	7	52.6	38.9
Drug abusers	5	4	26.3	22.2
Hetero.	2	4	10.5	22.2
Other cases	2	3	10.5	16.7
Transfusion	0	0	0	0
Total	19	18	100.0	100.0

homo.= homosexual
hetero.= heterosexual

Table 3. The goblet cells in the HIV negative patients (control) and AIDS patients with (group I) and without (group II) dry eye symptoms in the right eye (RE) and left eye (LE) in the nasal and temporal bulbar conjunctiva

Control				Group I				Group II			
RE		LE		RE		LE		RE		LE	
Nasal	Temporal	Nasal	Temporal	Nasal	Temporal	Nasal	Temporal	Nasal	Temporal	Nasal	Temporal
50	12	40	11	0	0	0	0	18	10	2	2
36	135	50	70	2	0	0	0	1	10	40	26
40	31	20	45	0	0	10	0	0	0	60	80
60	36	6	45	0	0	0	0	50	10	35	10
38	50	68	46	0	0	0	0	0	0	0	0
40	20	51	10	0	0	12	0	0	0	0	0
20	60	31	25	13	28	2	10	1	12	20	3
40	76	30	81	0	0	0	0	22	4	1	4
78	62	74	46	0	0	4	2	0	0	0	2
54	61	64	69	7	8	0	0	55	10	25	12
65	76	90	58	7	15	20	1	1	5	2	4
55	24	49	60	5	1	4	12	0	8	2	0
				0	0	0	0	80	10	20	75
				0	2	3	1	5	0	0	6
				3	1	30	33	0	48	1	1
				0	8	0	1	9	40	2	4
				14	11	9	16	67	47	50	75
				0	5	3	2	0	3	0	0
				12	1	8	1				
48.0	53.7	47.8	47.2	3.3	4.2	5.5	4.1	17.1	12.1	14.4	18.2

Wilcoxon Test
1° NASAL X TEMPORAL

CONTROL	GROUP I	GROUP II
RE Tcalc = 38,0	RE Tcalc = 27,0	RE Tcalc=43.5
Tcrit = 14,0	Tcrit = 11,0	Tcrit= 21,0
LE Tcalc = 36,0	LE Tcalc = 28,5	LE Tcalc = 39,0
Tcrit = 14,0	Tcrit = 14,0	Tcrit = 21,0
(p>0,05)	(p>0,05)	(p>0,05)

2° OD X OE

CONTROL	GROUP I	GROUP II
Nasal Tcalc = 32,0	Nasal Tcalc = 33,5	Nasal Tcalc = 40,5
Tcrit = 14,0	Tcrit = 17,0	Tcrit = 21,0
Temporal Tcalc = 30,0	Temporal Tcalc = 27,0	Temporal Tcalc = 41,0
Tcrit = 14,0	Tcrit = 11,0	Tcrit = 21,0
(p>0,05)	(p>0,05)	(p>0,05)

Analysis by Kruskal-Wallis
(Control X Group I X Group II)
H.crítico = 5,99

RE	LE
Nasal H calc = 19,59*	Nasal H calc. = 19,33*
Control > Group I and Group II.	Control > Group I and Group II
(p<0,05)	(p<0,05)
Temporal H calc = 24,47*	Temporal H calc = 20,99*
Control > Group I and Group II(p<0,05)	Control > Group I and Group II. (p<0,05)

Group I x Group II(p> 0,05)

Table 4. Absolute frequencies (FAb), accumulated (FAc) and proportion of accumulated frequencies (PFc) of orange cells in the temporal and nasal conjunctiva, of the right eye in control group and groups I and II

		AUS.	+	++	+++	Total
Orange cells in nasal conjunctiva of the right eye						
Control	FAb	3	8	1	0	12
	FAc	3	11	12	12	
	PFc	0.25000	0.91667	1.00000	1.00000	
Group I	FAb	1	2	12	4	19
	FAc	1	3	15	19	
	PFc	0.05263	0.15789	0.78947	1.00000	
Group II	FAb	0	5	6	7	18
	FAc	0	5	11	18	
	PFc	0.00000	0.27778	0.61111	1.00000	

Group I X Control	$\chi^2 = 16.94$*(p< 0.001)
Group II X Control	$\chi^2 = 11.76$* (p< 0.001) χ^2 critical = 6.64
Group I X Group II	$\chi^2 = 1.18$

		AUS.	+	++	+++	Total
Orange cells in temporal conjunctiva of the right eye						
Control	FAb	4	8	0	0	12
	FAc	4	12	12	12	
	PFc	0.33333	1.00000	1.00000	1.00000	
Group I	FAb	0	3	12	4	19
	FAc	0	3	15	19	
	PFc	0.00000	0.15789	0.78947	1.00000	
Group II	FAb	1	3	7	7	18
	FAc	1	4	11	18	
	PFc	0.05555	0.22222	0.61111	1.00000	

Group I X Control	$\chi^2 = 21.56$* (p<0.001)
Group II X Control	$\chi^2 = 17.42$*(p<0.001) χ^2 critical = 6.64
Group I X Group II	$\chi^2 = 1.18$

Values of calculated χ^2 for the de Kolmogorov-Smirnov test

test, and the Schirmer test in order to estimate the number of goblet cells in the conjunctiva surface by impression cytology.

Although the symptomatology analysis in this study is very subjective, it verified that the most common complaints referred by the patients were red eye and foreign body sensation, followed by burning, itching, and other symptoms.

The symptoms related by the patients in their clinical history are not useful for the diagnosis of dry eye. The patients usually complained of red eye and foreign body sensation. They rarely reported dry eye sensation.[8]

In this work neither the complaint nor the Schirmer test could be evaluated. The tear break-up time and rose bengal test seem to be more sizable for the diagnosis of dry eye considering the comparison of their results with the impression cytology results.

Rose bengal stain and impression cytology are believed to be the best tests for diagnosis in patients presenting with a complaint of dry eye. These findings demonstrate that the rose bengal stain and impression cytology patterns are very convenient examinations for detecting precocious dry eye cases.[9] This conclusion was also observed in this study.

Table 5. Absolute frequency (FAb), accumulated (FAc) and proportion of accumulated frequency (PFc) of the orange cells in the temporal and nasal regions, of the left eye in control group patients groups I and II

		AUS.	+	++	+++	Total
		Orange cells in nasal conjunctiva of the right eye				
Control	FAb	8	3	1	0	12
	FAc	8	11	12	12	
	PFc	0.66666	0.91666	1.00000	1.00000	
Group I	FAb	1	1	7	10	19
	FAc	1	2	9	19	
	PFc	0.05263	0.10526	0.47368	1.00000	
Group II	FAb	0	4	7	7	18
	FAc	0	4	11	18	
	PFc	0.00000	0.22222	0.61111	1.00000	

Group I X Control	$\chi^2=19.37$*(p< 0.001)
Group II X Control	$\chi^2=13.89$* (p< 0.001) χ^2 critical = 6.64
Group I X Group II	$\chi^2 = 0.70$

		AUS.	+	++	+++	Total
		Orange cells in temporal conjunctiva of the right eye				
Control	FAb	6	6	0	0	12
	FAc	6	12	12	12	
	PFc	0.50000	1.00000	1.00000	1.00000	
Group I	FAb	0	1	11	7	19
	FAc	0	1	12	19	
	PFc	0.00000	0.05263	0.63158	1.00000	
Group II	FAb	0	5	5	8	18
	FAc	0	5	10	18	
	PFc	0.00000	0.27777	0.55555	1.00000	

Group I X Control	$\chi^2 = 26.40$* (p<0.001)
Group II X Control	$\chi^2 = 15.02$*(p<0.001) χ^2 critical = 6.64
Group I X Group II	$\chi^2 = 1.87$

Values of calculated χ^2 for the Kolmogorov-Smirnov test.

The fact that Rose Bengal stain revealed a significant difference between the two AIDS groups suggests that the epithelial damage was higher in patients with symptoms.

Much research is appearing on AIDS patients. In this study, even patients without dry eye symptoms (Group II) had altered lacrimal function tests and altered Rose Bengal patterns. This led to investigation of the number of goblet cells and an eventual epithelial damage via impression cytology and simultaneous coloration of PAS and Papanicolau.[6]

The authors chose impression cytology instead of exfoliative cytology primarily because it is painless and permits greater reproducibility. In addition, it is immediately obvious if there has been any error in the collection of the material. This is not possible in exfoliative cytology because there is cell destruction and exfoliation of normal cells when the materials are collected, disturbing the correct cytologic interpretation.

In this study, the density of goblet cells was diminished in 68.4% of the AIDS patients from Group I and in 44.4% in Group II. Probably the incidence of dry eye is very high in patients with AIDS. Total absence of goblet cells was detected in 18.92% of the patients from the two groups, indicating the severity of these cases.

Table 6. Patients of groups I and II, according to goblet
cells average of the patients (XC) and
CD_4 level (cells/mm^3)

Group I		Group II	
XC	CD_4	XC	CD_4
0	47	13.75	65
0.5	80	19	150
2.5	49	35	47
0	70	26.25	100
0	180	0	80
0	60	0	36
13.25	38	8.75	12
0	36	7.5	125
1.5	120	0.5	48
3.75	52	25.5	250
10.5	68	3.0	50
5.5	150	2.5	32
0	228	46.25	210
1.5	7	2.75	47
16.75	200	12.5	168
2.25	44	13.75	75
12.5	12	59.75	280
2.5	120	0.75	166
5.25	160		

Spearman's Coefficient Correlation

XC x CD_4

Group I	Group II
rs calc = 0.03	rs calc = 0.51*
rs crit = 0.39	rs crit = 0.40
(p>0.05)	r^2 = 0.26
	(p<0.05)

Results of this study revealed a significant increase in the number of orange cells in the two AIDS groups when compared with the control group, which can presuppose conjunctival epithelial metaplasia that could be confirmed through a histologic study. The technique utilized does not permit us to give certainty to the diagnosis of metaplasia. Impression cytology is a surface technique that detects goblet cells and keratinized cells, making it more difficult to diagnose morphologic aspects of the deeper layers. For an objective determination of the conditions of dry eye, it is necessary to have an exact observation to qualify the alterations of the ocular surface on the level of the cells. The decrease of the lacrimal function and goblet cells indicates a greater tendency to squamous metaplasia[10] of the conjunctiva, observed in only one patient in the study by impression cytology.[11]

When correlation of the mean number of goblet cells with the CD_4 count was made there was no significant correlation in the symptomatic AIDS group (Group I). It is supposed that in patients the CD4 levels are lower, there would be a greater probability of alterations in the lacrimal film. It is known that there are diminished T and B cells in these patients, compromising local ocular defenses like lacrimal portion deficiency, inadequate eyelid abnormalities, and blink reflexes which was not confirmed.

Based on this clinical study, the ophthalmologist can be aware of the possibility of the existence of lacrimal deficiency in AIDS patients, even when asymptomatic.

REFERENCES

1. H. Masur, Michelis, M.A., Greene, J.B., et al., An outbreak of community-acquired *pneumocystis carinii* pneumonia: initial manifestations of cellular immune dysfunction. *N. Engl. J. Med.* 305:1431 (1981).
2. C. Muccioli, Lottenberg, C., Lima, J., et al., Ophthalmological aspects of 445 HIV infected patients. *Rev. Ass. Med. Brasil.* 40:155 (1994).
3. M.D. DeSmet, Ocular consequences of human immunodeficiency virus infection. *Ophthalmol. Clin. of North America* 6(1):117 (1993).
4. R. Belfort, Jr., DeSmet, M, Withcup, S.M., et al., Ocular complications of Stevens Johnson syndrome and toxic epidermal necrolysis in patients with AIDS. *Cornea* 10(6):117 (1993).
5. J.A. Lucca, Farris, R.L., Bielory, L., and Caputo, A.R., Keratoconjunctivitis sicca in male patients infected with human immunodeficiency virus type 1. *Ophthalmology* 97(8):1008 (1990).
6. S.C.G. Tseng. Staging of conjunctival squamous metaplasia by impression cytology. *Ophthalmology* 92:728 (1995).
7. M. Schiodt, Greenspan, D., Daniels, T.E., et al., Parotid gland enlargement and xerostomia associated with labial sialadenitis in HIV-infected patients. *J. Autoimmun.* 2:415 (1989).
8. D.W. Lamberts, Clinical diseases of the tear film. In, *The Cornea,* G. Smolin and Thoft, R.A., eds., Little Brown, Boston (1994).
9. L. Rivas, Rodriguez, J., Alvarez, M.I., et al., Correlation between impression cytology and tear function parameters in Sjögren's syndrome. *Acta Ophthalmol.* 71:353 (1993).
10. C.A. Paschides, Petroutsos, G., and Psilas, K., et al., Correlation of conjunctival impression cytology results with lacrimal function and age. *Acta Ophthalmol.* 69:442 (1991).
11. E. Takamura, Takano, H., Yoshink, K., et al. Quantitative cellular evaluation of conjunctival squamous metaplasia in the dry eye patient. *Adv. Exper. Med. Biol.* 350:535 (1994).
12. J.P. Dunn, and Holland, G.N., Human immunodeficiency virus and opportunistic ocular infections. *Inv. Dis. Clin. North Amer.* 6:909 (1992).

10

RESPONSE OF THE OCULAR SURFACE TO HISTAMINE

Jack V. Greiner,[1,2] David A. Welter,[3] Charles D. Leahy,[1] Donald R. Korb,[4] Thomas A. Weidman,[3] Stacey L. Hearn,[1] and Thomas Glonek[5]

[1]The Schepens Eye Research Institute
[2]Department of Ophthalmology
 Harvard Medical School
 Boston, Massachusetts
[3]Department of Cell Biology and Anatomy
 Medical College of Georgia
 Atlanta, Georgia
[4]Korb and Associates
 Boston, Massachusetts
[5]MR Laboratory
 Midwestern University
 Chicago, Illinois

ABSTRACT

Eye rubbing results in ocular surface changes, such as irregular epithelial cell morphology, alterations in microprojections, and increased cellular exfoliation. It is unknown whether such changes are related entirely to the mechanical trauma of eye rubbing or manifest secondary to the effects of histamine released from degranulated mast cells associated with eye rubbing. To distinguish between these effects, the present study examines the effects of topical histamine application in the absence of applied mechanical trauma. The bulbar and tarsal conjunctiva of rabbits (n=10) exposed to 25 µl of histamine (25 mg/ml) for 10 minutes were examined using scanning electron microscopy. Contralateral untreated eyes served as controls. Regions studied included the bulbar and tarsal conjunctivae. The bulbar conjunctiva was divided into two regions, the interpalpebral bulbar conjunctiva and that portion unexposed to the environment. In contrast to control eyes, the interpalpebral bulbar conjunctiva of treated eyes had surface cells with irregular morphology and elevated apices. The goblet cell intercellular crypt openings in treated eyes had minimal mucus, while in control conjunctiva most intercellular openings contained mucus. The upper tarsal conjunctiva of treated eyes had an irregular surface and empty intercellular crypt orifices when compared to the smooth tarsal conjunctival surface and mucus-con-

Advances in Corneal Research, edited by Lass
Plenum Press, New York, 1997

taining crypts of control eyes. The lower tarsal conjunctiva had minimal differences in surface cell morphology and did not appear notably altered, in contrast to the upper tarsal conjunctiva. In summary, topical histamine resulted in alteration of the exposed bulbar conjunctiva and upper tarsal conjunctiva, whereas the unexposed bulbar conjunctiva and lower tarsal conjunctiva surfaces exhibited only subtle changes. Perhaps the changes observed in the upper tarsal conjunctiva resulted from the blinking (wiping) action of the upper lid over the chemotic exposed bulbar conjunctiva. The paucity of mucus in the goblet cell orifices after histamine exposure was unexpected.

INTRODUCTION

Eye rubbing has been shown to degranulate more than 50% of the mast cells of the ocular surface.[1] Mast cell degranulation releases vasoactive amines, including histamine, which result in dilation of conjunctival blood vessels, and the migration of great numbers of inflammatory cells (neutrophils and macrophages).[1] A concurrent movement of water into these tissues produces edema and often results in such profound chemosis (swelling) of the bulbar conjunctiva that the normal contour of the conjunctiva is dramatically altered. Such edematous changes might be expected to lead to secondary changes in cell morphology.

Eye rubbing involves mechanical trauma as well as mast cell degranulation. The present study examines the direct effects of histamine on the ocular surface, in the absence of mechanical trauma, in an attempt to determine which ocular surface changes following eye rubbing might be attributed to histamine-mediated (i.e., mast cell-induced) effects.

METHODS

In this study, 25 μl of histamine (25 mg/ml) in balanced salt solution (BSS) was administered to the right eyes of New Zealand white rabbits (n=10, 3–4 kg) with an Eppendorf digital pipette (Brinkman Instruments, Inc.; Westbury, NY) and a sterile tip. The dose was selected following the experimental antigen challenge model.[2] The contralateral eye served as control and was administered 25 μl of BSS. (Normal human tears contain 10.3 ng ± 9.43 ng/ml of histamine.[3]) After 10 minutes, during which animals were restrained in order to avoid eye rubbing, eyes were photographed and animals injected with a lethal dose of pentobarbital sodium, and the eyelids with tarsal conjunctivae and the globes exenterated immediately. In order to minimize artifactual changes during exenteration, the conjunctival sac was anesthetized and irrigated with 3% glutaraldehyde fixative solution in 0.5M cacodylate buffer (pH 7.3), at room temperature.

After a minimum of 1 hour fixation, samples for histology were harvested from the interpalpebral bulbar conjunctiva, unexposed bulbar conjunctiva, upper tarsal conjunctiva, lower tarsal conjunctiva, at the eyelid margin, and the cornea. The unexposed conjunctiva is that portion of the bulbar conjunctiva that is not exposed to the environment while the eyelids are open. The glutaraldehyde-fixed samples were prepared for scanning electron microscopy (SEM) by dehydrating in graded ethyl alcohols, critical-point-dried using CO_2, mounted on aluminum sample stubs using silver paint, coated with gold using a sputtering device, and examined with an AMR-1000 scanning electron microscope. Quantitative morphometric measurements were made from SEM photographs of individual conjunctival areas on Polaroid type NP-55 film.

RESULTS

Biomicroscopy

Following instillation of histamine into the lower tearfilm meniscus, there was an obvious initial conjunctival hyperemia, followed by increasing chemosis of the bulbar conjunctiva. At 10 minutes, the bulbar conjunctiva had minimal to moderate chemosis. With increasing chemosis, the degree of hyperemia appeared to abate (Fig. 1a).

Histology

The cells covering the interpalpebral bulbar portion of the conjunctiva in the histamine-treated samples appeared to retain an approximate polygonal morphology, but the cell apices were elevated (Fig. 1). This is in contrast to the polygonal cells with flat surfaces observed in the control samples (Fig. 2a). The cell borders in both histamine-treated and control samples were marked by microvilli (Figs 1b and 2b). The microprojections

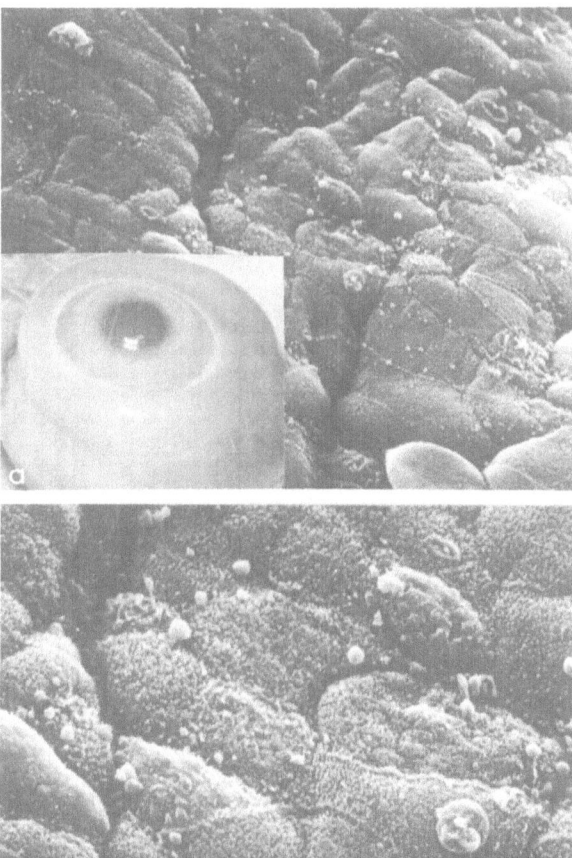

Figure 1. (a) Rabbit eye 10 minutes following instillation of 25 μl of histamine (25 mg/ml). The interpalpebral bulbar conjunctiva is chemotic and mucus is present (inset). Interpalpebral bulbar conjunctival surface demonstrates dome-shaped elevations of epithelial cell apices (x 1600). (b) High magnification showing surface microprojections (x4000).

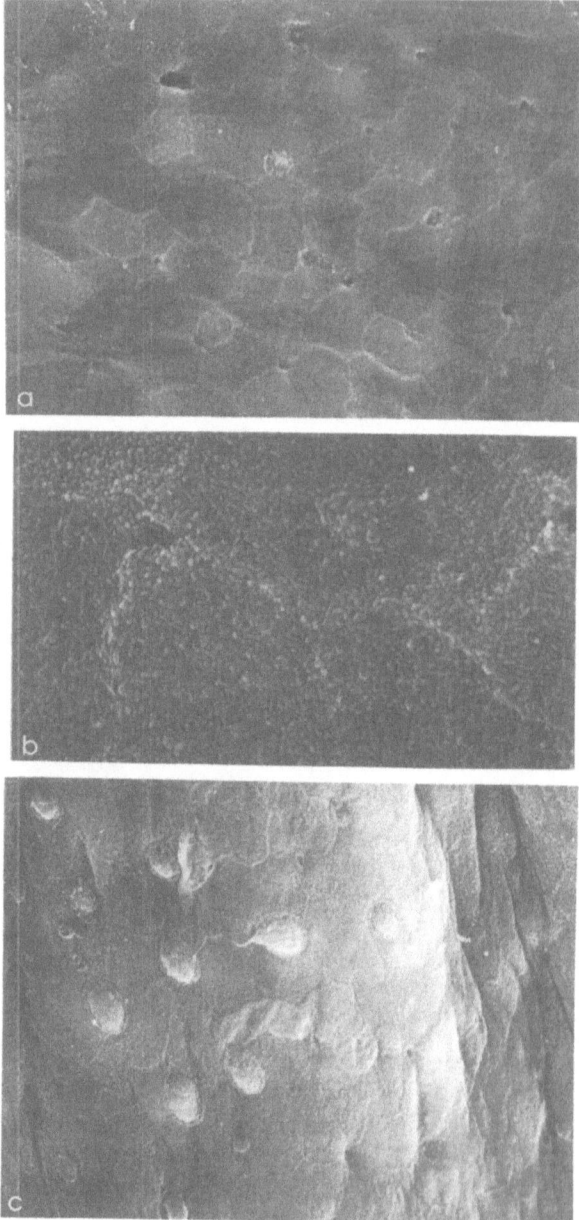

Figure 2. Untreated control eye. (a) Interpalpebral bulbar conjunctival surface demonstrates a smooth, flat surface with typical polygonally shaped cells and small intercellular crypt openings (x1600). (b) High magnification showing surface microprojections (x8000). (c) Interpalpebral bulbar conjunctival surface demonstrating mucus laden intercellular crypts (x1600).

covering the cell surfaces in the histamine-treated samples were not dissimilar to those observed in control samples. The characteristic microvillar morphology was evident (Fig. 1b). The unexposed conjunctiva (Fig. 3a) was not unlike that of the conjunctiva in control samples (Fig. 3b).

The distal (anterior) portion of the upper tarsal conjunctiva in the histamine-treated samples also had surface cells with elevated apices (Fig. 4a), in contrast to control samples where the surface cells were flat. The elevated cells had an irregular morphology. Cells in the more proximal (posterior) portion of the upper tarsal conjunctiva were less developed and had a more regular morphology, similar to those observed in control samples. The microvillus microprojections observed in the histamine-treated samples appeared similar to those of control (untreated) samples (Fig. 4). The lower tarsal conjunctiva in the histamine-treated samples had minimal differences in surface cell morphology, in contrast to the upper tarsal conjunctiva (Fig. 5).

In all histamine-treated samples, but most notably in the interpalpebral bulbar conjunctiva and the upper tarsal conjunctiva, there was evidence of depletion of the contents of the intercellular crypt openings, consistent with the loss of mucus from goblet cell orifices (Figs. 1 and 4). This is in contrast to the mucus-containing crypts of control samples

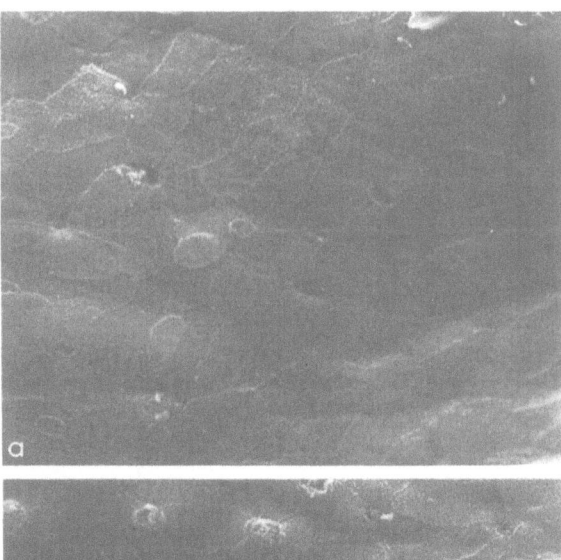
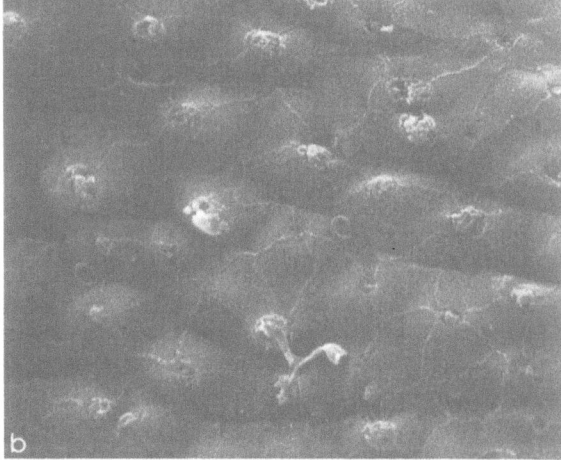

Figure 3. (a) Histamine-treated eye. Unexposed bulbar conjunctival surface demonstrates a smooth, flat surface with typical polygonally shaped cells and small intercellular crypt openings (x1600). (b) Control eye. Unexposed bulbar conjunctival surface demonstrates smooth surface with intercellular crypts containing mucus (x1600).

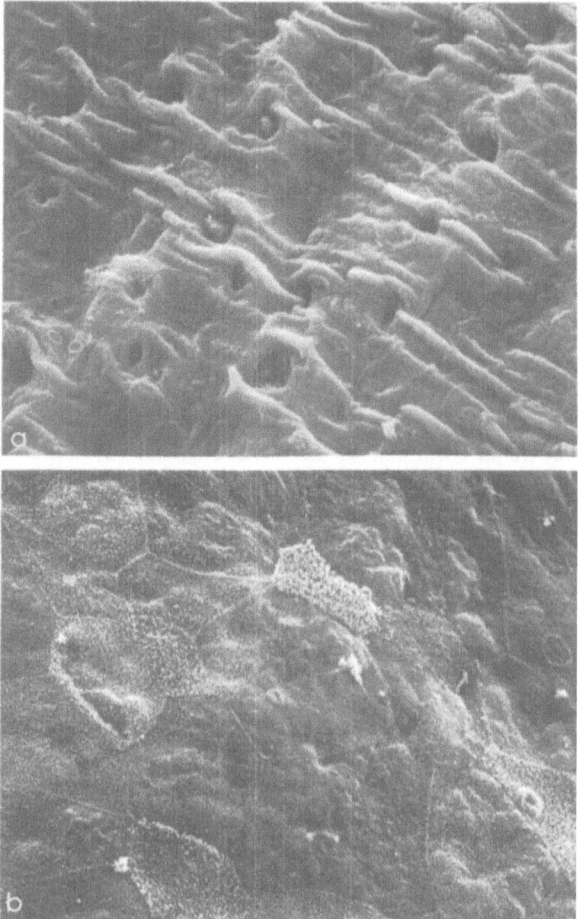

Figure 4. (a) Histamine-treated eye. Upper tarsal conjunctival surface demonstrates irregular surface in the anterior, more distal region, where cell borders are difficult to differentiate (x1600). (b) Upper tarsal conjunctival surface in the posterior, more proximal region demonstrates a regular flatter surface with more distinct cell borders (x1600).

(Fig. 2c). Additionally, mucus strands were often observed over the ocular surface (Fig. 1, inset).

DISCUSSION

Although instillation of histamine immediately caused increased hyperemia, this was followed by increasing conjunctival chemosis that corresponded to a decrease in the degree of hyperemia. This phenomenon has been observed clinically in humans when they are subjected to antigen challenge,[4] and topical instillation of histamine reliably produces the effects of itching and vascular injection in a dose-dependent fashion.[5] Given the degree of chemosis resulting from instillation of histamine, it was expected that the conjunctival surface would be markedly altered along with changes in the morphology of surface

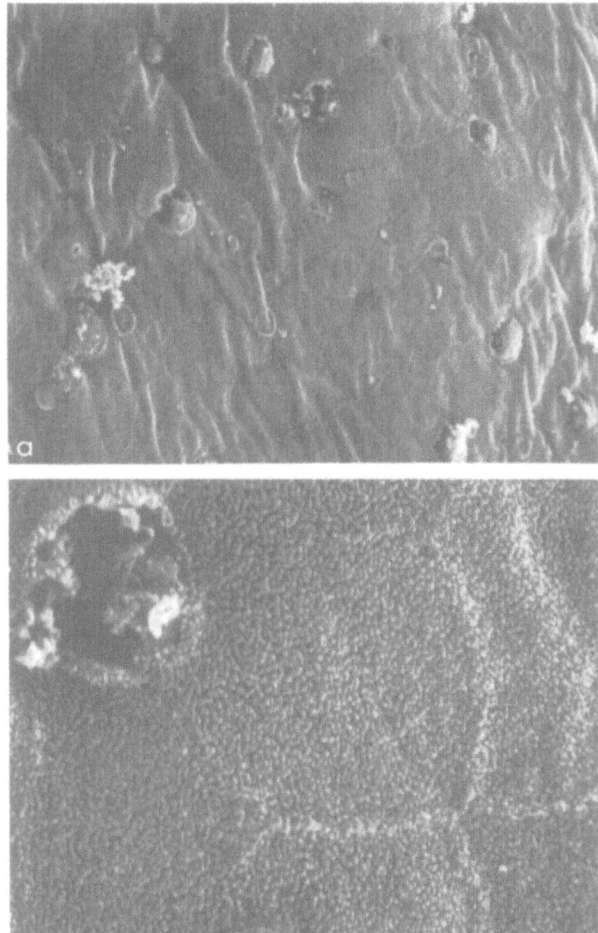

Figure 5. (a) Histamine-treated eye. Lower tarsal conjunctival surface demonstrates a relatively flat surface with recognizable polygonally shaped cells and small intercellular crypt openings (x1600). (b) High magnification showing surface microprojections (x8000).

cells. In fact, the epithelium of the bulbar conjunctiva in the interpalpebral zone, which was directly exposed to the histamine solution, demonstrated the greatest degree of cell surface changes. Although changes in the conjunctival surface were observed, it is remarkable that with chemosis there was no obvious increase in cell surface area of individual cells or changes in the cell borders. Moreover, there was no marked change in the morphology of microprojections of the superficial cells. The microvilli were typical of those described previously in normal conjunctiva.[6–9]

The correspondence of intercellular crypts to goblet cell openings on the ocular surface has been documented previously in human conjunctiva.[7,8,10] The increased number of intercellular crypts that appeared empty or depleted of mucus content following histamine treatment was obvious, but unexpected. This may suggest a possible function of histamine as a mucus secretagogue. However, it cannot be ruled out at present that the concentration of histamine employed in this study was excessively high in a physiological sense and that the observed increase in mucus depleted crypts and mucus present on the ocular surface may be an indirect effect of such a high concentration of histamine. It is interesting to note, however, that preliminary results in our laboratory on rabbit eyes treated with multiple doses of 25 μl of histamine (25 mg/ml) over 30 minutes while under general anesthesia resulted in the accumulation of large amounts of mucus in the interpalpebral space.

Despite the chemosis observed after histamine treatment, the cellular morphology of the conjunctival surface cells was not altered to the degree expected. The changes in the conjunctival surface observed with histamine treatment were dissimilar to those changes observed with eye rubbing.[11] Eye rubbing has been shown to result in degranulation of more than 50% of mast cells,[1] which therefore would result in histamine release. However, the histamine-mediated effects on the ocular surface observed in this study do not mimic those changes observed secondary to eye rubbing.[11] The effects on the tissue reported with eye rubbing would, therefore, appear to be attributed more to mechanical trauma than to histamine release.

ACKNOWLEDGMENTS

The authors wish to acknowledge the contributions of Dr. Mark B. Abelson and Mr. Kevin Richards.

REFERENCES

1. J.V. Greiner, Peace, D.G., Baird, R.S., and Allansmith, M.R. Effects of eye rubbing on the conjunctiva as a model of ocular inflammation. *Am. J. Ophthalmol.* 100:45 (1985).
2. M.B. Abelson, Chambers, W.A., and Smith, L.M., Conjunctival allergan challenge: A clinical approach to studying allergic conjunctivitis. *Arch. Ophthalmol.* 108:84 (1990).
3. M.B. Abelson, Soter, N.A., Simon, M.A., et al., Histamine in human tears. *Am. J. Ophthalmol.* 83:417 (1977).
4. I.J. Udell, and Abelson, M.B., Animal and human ocular surface response to atypical nonimmune mast cell degranulating agent (compound 48/80). *Am. J. Ophthalmol.* 91: 226 (1981).
5. M.B. Abelson, and Allansmith, M.R., Histamine in the eye. In, *Immunology and Immunopathology of the Eye. Proceedings of the Second International Symposium, San Francisco, 1978*, A.M. Silverstein, and O'Connor, G.R., eds., Masson, New York (1979)
6. R.R. Pfister. The normal surface of conjunctiva epithelium. A scanning electron microscopic study. *Invest. Ophthalmol.* 14:267 (1975).
7. J.V. Greiner, Covington, H.I., and Allansmith, M.R., Surface morphology of the human upper tarsal conjunctiva. *Am. J. Ophthalmol.* 83:892 (1977).
8. J.V. Greiner, Covington, H.I., and Allansmith, M.R., The human limbus: a scanning electron microscopic study. *Arch. Ophthalmol.* 97:1159 (1979).
9. J.V. Greiner, Gladstone, L., Covington, H.I., et al, Branching of microvilli in the human conjunctival epithelium. *Arch. Ophthalmol.* 98:1253 (1980).
10. J.V. Greiner, Henriquez, A.S., Covington, H.I., et al. Goblet cells and crypts in the human conjunctiva. *Arch. Ophthalmol.* 99:2190 (1981).
11. J.V. Greiner, Leahy, C.D., Welter, D., et al., Histopathology of the ocular surface after eye rubbing, *Cornea* (in press).

11

BOTULINUM TOXIN TREATMENT FOR FILAMENTARY KERATITIS ASSOCIATED WITH CORNEAL OCCLUSION BY LIDS

Jae Chan Kim,[1] Hanwook Chung,[1] and Scheffer C. G. Tseng[1,2]

[1]Department of Ophthalmology
College of Medicine
Chung Ang University
Seoul, Korea
[2]The Ocular Surface and Tear Center
Department of Ophthalmology
Bascom Palmer Eye Institute
Department of Cell Biology and Anatomy
University of Miami School of Medicine
Miami, Florida 33101

ABSTRACT

Botulinum toxin injections were performed to evaluate its effectiveness in treating filamentary keratitis caused by corneal occlusion by lids in 15 consecutive patients including 13 with essential blepharospasm, one with Meige syndrome and one with paralytic esotropia. After 5.7 ± 1.6 days following the injection, all patients showed subjective improvements with total resolution of corneal occlusion and filaments. Before injections, TBUT was 4.8 ± 3.2 sec and Schirmer I test without anesthetics was 3.9 ± 2.9 mm, both of which were significantly increased to 8.6 ± 3.1 sec and 7.7 ± 3.8 mm, respectively, after injections. A fluorescein clearance test was performed to prove that the increase of tear secretion after injections was caused by further slowing of the preexistent delayed tear clearance after injections. Impression cytology revealed that filaments were composed of a central core surrounded by PAS-positive amorphous materials and small epithelial cells, and the base of the filament was attached to metaplastic superficial epithelial cells. Therefore, it was speculated that excessive lid blinking might have aggravated aqueous tear deficiency, a condition frequently associated with essential blepharospasm, by facilitating tear clearance. Furthermore, filamentary keratitis, a condition associated with diverse diseases, might result from a common vicious cycle established by mechanical trauma from uncontrolled or excessive blinking and corneal occlusion by lids onto the surface epithelial cells with squamous metaplasia. The arrest and breakdown of such a cycle by the botulinum toxin might explain its efficacy in treating filamentary keratitis.

Advances in Corneal Research, edited by Lass
Plenum Press, New York, 1997

INTRODUCTION

Filamentary keratitis is a disorder characterized by the presence of one or more filaments attached to the corneal surface. Formation of filaments on the ocular surface can be associated with many varieties of disorders, among which the most notable are keratoconjunctivitis sicca, superior limbic keratoconjunctivitis, prolonged patching, and following various surgeries (for reviews see [1-3]). Although the exact mechanism remains obscure, two major hypotheses had been put forth to explain the formation of filaments. Based on the histopathologic studies, one theory proposes that the primary abnormality appears to start at the level of superficial stroma which is focally infiltrated with inflammatory cells and associated with focal attenuation of the Bowman's membrane.[4,5] The other theory stresses the important role of excess mucus production[1] and mucus attachment onto abnormal degenerative superficial epithelial cells.[1,6] Without direct evidence, it has further been speculated that the mucus is attached to the intracellular keratins which are exposed after the superficial cell membrane is damaged.[7] Based on these hypotheses, one might speculate that disturbances in the mucus tear film and injuries to the superficial epithelial cells by eyelid blinking might predispose the ocular surface to filament formation.

Another condition leading to filamentary keratitis is essential blepharospasm, a relatively uncommon disease that exhibits variable severity ranging from an increased frequency of eyelid blinking to involuntary spasm of the muscles involved in eyelid closure.[8,9] Such an uncontrolled increase of eyelid blinking may well exert mechanical trauma to superficial ocular surface epithelial cells, acting as a risk factor for the formation of filaments. Furthermore, it has also been noted that the majority of patients with blepharospasm are associated with abnormal tear function tests such as low Schirmer test values,[10] rapid tear break up time, and delayed tear clearance.[11,12] Therefore, it is also likely that these abnormal tear functions might play an important pathogenic role. This article reports on a study of the therapeutic effect of botulinum toxin injection, an accepted standard treatment for essential blepharospasm[10,13] in a group of 15 patients also with filamentary keratitis. Accompanied with relief of subjective symptoms were resolution of filamentary keratitis and significantly increased tear break up time, Schirmer I test value and further delayed tear clearance. The pathogenesis of filament formation is further discussed.

PATIENTS AND METHODS

Botulinum toxin (Botox®, Allergen; Irvine, USA) injections were consecutively performed in 14 female patients and one male patient with ages ranging from 26 to 77 years (52.2 ± 14.9) (mean ± SD) and with filamentary keratitis (Table 1). The state of corneal occlusion caused by lid, i.e., the corneal surface was covered by lid(s), and noted in all patients including 13 with essential blepharospasm (EBS), one with Meige syndrome, and one with paralytic esotropia. Duration of disease was 18.7 ± 20.4 months. A total of 46 to 56 units (50.5 ± 3.7 units) of toxin was injected in 13 blepharospasm patients and 64 units in the patient with Meige syndrome according to a modified Scott's method.[14] In the case of left paralytic esotropia, 10 units of botulinum toxin was injected in the left medial rectus muscle. After botulinum toxin injection, all patients were followed up until filaments disappeared. For each patient, tear break-up time measurement (TBUT), Schirmer I test without anesthetics and fluorescein clearance test were performed before and after the treatment.

Table 1. Summary of clinical data and test results

Case No.	Sex/Age	Diagnosis	Duration of Disease (months)	Disappearance of Filament (days)	TBUT (sec) Pre-	TBUT (sec) Post	Schirmer I (mm) Pre-	Schirmer I (mm) Post-	Type of the Filaments
				3	3	4	4	5	
1	F/39	Paralytic Esotropia	70	3					long large
2	F/65	EBS	25	3	3/3	7/8	1/10	4/5	mixed long & short
3	F/26	EBS	12	6	2/3	6/9	1/2	5/6	diffuse comma-shaped
4	F/64	Meige syndrome	60	6	Not performed		1/0	15/15	long large
5	F/45	EBS	12	6	5/9	13/13	4/4	7/8	diffuse long fine
6	F/57	EBS	8	9	2/0	7/2	2/10	9/13	diffuse comma-shaped
7	M/77	EBS	15	7	12/12	13/13	10/9	11/12	long fine
8	F/54	EBS	1	6	6/9	9/8	3/3	5/4	mixed long & short
9	F/66	EBS	8	6	0/3	3/5	1/1	1/2	mixed long & short
10	F/38	EBS	24	9	5/6	12/10	9/10	13/12	diffuse fine
11	F/47	EBS	7	4	9/7	12/12	5/5	7/9	diffuse comma-shaped
12	F/61	EBS	7	3	7/5	10/7	3/3	7/9	mixed long & short
13	F/70	EBS	4	6	4/4	10/10	1/0	8/10	diffuse comma-shaped
14	F/36	EBS	3	6	5/3	7/6	7/7	13/15	diffuse fine
15	F/38	EBS	24	5	3/0	9/9	2/4	6/6	mixed long & short
Mean ± SD	52.2 ± 18.9		18.7 ± 20.4	5.7 ± 1.6	4.8 ± 3.2 (pre)	8.6 ± 3.1 (post)	3.9 ± 2.9 (pre)	7.7 ± 3.8 (post)	

Tests

The TBUT was performed by adding to the inferior fornix one fluorescein drop obtained by wetting on a fluorescein strip (Chauvin Pharmaceuticals Ltd.; Harold Hill; Ramford, Essex, England) with non-preserved saline, i.e., Unisol® (Alcon Laboratories Inc.; Forth Worth, TX) in a manner similar to those described by Norn[15] and Lemp and Hamill.[16] After a few blinks, the duration in seconds was measured before the precorneal fluorescein tear film broke up, and this was repeated for a total of three times. The mean of these three measurements and the pattern of the film break-up were recorded. The Schirmer I test was performed in a conventional manner without anesthetics. Fluorescein clearance test was performed as briefly described in previous reports[17,18] and resembles that recently reported by Xu et al.[19] In detail, after applying one drop of 0.5% proparacaine (Alcon Laboratories, Inc.; Humacao, PR) to each eye, the inferior fornix was carefully dried with tissue paper. An aliquot of 5 µl of 0.25% fluorescein containing 0.4% benoxinate hydrochloride in a commercial preparation, i.e., Fluoress® (Akorn Inc.; Abita Springs, LA), was then applied to the inferior fornix of each eye through an Eppendorf pipettor (Rainin Instrument Co.; Woburn, MA) without directly touching the conjunctival surface. The patient continued to sit in the examination room under the ambient light and was asked to blink normally. After a lapse of 10 minutes, determined by a timer, a Schirmer paper strip (Alcon Laboratories, Inc.; Fort Worth, TX) was inserted into the inferior fornix of each eye at a position approximately one third lateral to the temporal caruncle. After one minute, during which time normal blinking was allowed, and the strip was removed. The same maneuver was repeated for a total of three times over a prior of 30 min, except that the last measurement was conducted immediately after nasal stimulation similar to that originally described by Jones[20] and recently by Tsubota.[21] The wetting was measured in mm and the intensity of dye staining on the strip was compared to the standard strip colors, and graded from 1 to 4 (grade 0: no staining; grade 4: maximal staining). Impression cytology was performed for all patients using the same methods as previously described.[22]

RESULTS

All 15 patients showed subjective improvements, with disappearance of filaments following resolution of corneal occlusion after botulinum toxin injection. Before injection all patients complained of foreign body sensations, photophobia, increased blinking reflex, episodic tearing, or decreased vision. The appearance of corneal filaments could be classified into the long large type (two patients), the diffuse comma shaped type (three patients), the diffuse fine type (three patients), the mixed small and large type (five patients), and the long fine type (two patients) (Table 1). Generally, the location of filaments were found mainly on the upper or lower nasal corneal surfaces which were occluded by upper or lower lids, respectively, especially at the border between the occluded and non-occluded areas by respective lids (examples see Cases described below). The interval between injection and disappearance of filaments ranged 3 to 9 days (5.7 ± 1.6 days). After injection, the values of TBUT and Schirmer I test without anesthetics were significantly increased when compared with those before injection (p >0.05) (Table 1). Fluorescein clearance test revealed decreased aqueous secretion, i.e., the wetting length less than 3 mm, in 9 cases and delayed clearance, i.e., dye remained to be detected even on the second (20 min) or third (30 min) strips, in 12 cases (Table 2). After injection, there was a

Table 2. Comparison of fluorescein clearance test results before and after injection

	Paper strips	Pre-injection	Post-injection	p-value[a]
Wetting length (mm)	10 min	7.7±3.5	11.0±5.6	<0.01
	30 min	3.8±3.3	6.3±2.3	<0.01
Dye Intensity[b]	10 min	1.8±1.1	2.1±1.8	<0.05
	30 min	1.1±0.6	1.4±0.9	<0.05

[a]Data were analyzed by the univariated paired t-test.
[b]The grading of the dye intensity is described in Methods.

significant increase of wetting length, indicating an increase of aqueous tear secretion (p < 0.001 by univariated paired *t*-test for either 20 min or 30 min strips, Table 2). Furthermore, there was a significantly increase of delayed tear clearance after injection (p < 0.05 by univariated paired *t*-test for 20 min and 30 min strips, respectively, Table 2). Impression cytology revealed that filaments were attached to their bases metaplastic epithelial cells (Fig. 1 A-C) and composed of PAS-positive amorphous mucin-like materials surrounding the central core containing epithelial cells (Fig. 1 D-F).

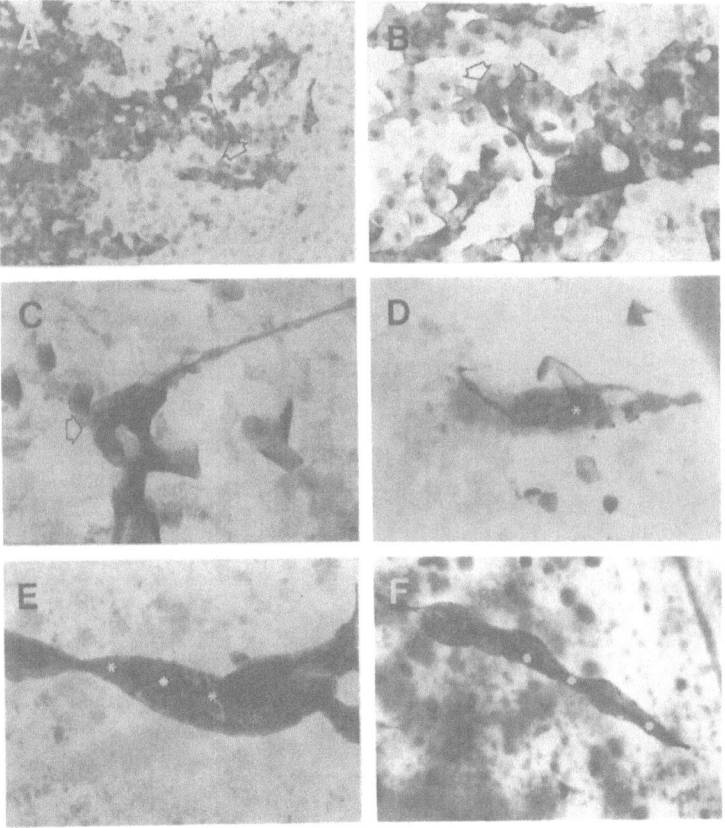

Figure 1. Impression cytology of filaments (diffuse fine type). The base of the filament was attached to metaplastic epithelial cells, which were enlarged and squamous with a large nucleus/cytoplasm ratio (open arrows) (A-C). The long fine type filament was composed of a central core containing epithelial cells, indicated by*, and surrounded by PAS-positive amorphous mucin materials (D-F).

SELECTED CASE REPORTS

Case # 1

A 39-year-old female suffering from a left sixth nerve palsy as a result of a traffic accident sought treatment because of photophobia and foreign body irritation. To treat her left esotropia, she had undergone a Jensen's operation in both eyes 5 years earlier, a bilateral medial rectus muscle recession 4 years earlier, and four times of botulinum toxin injections to the left medial rectus muscle. Slit-lamp examination revealed long, large filaments on her left superonasal cornea, the area occluded by the upper lid because of a 40 prism diopter esodeviation (Fig. 2 A, B). The value of Schirmer I test without anesthetics was 9 mm in the right eye and 3 mm in the left eye. Ten units of botulinum toxin was injected into her medial rectus muscle. Filaments and esodeviation resolved completely

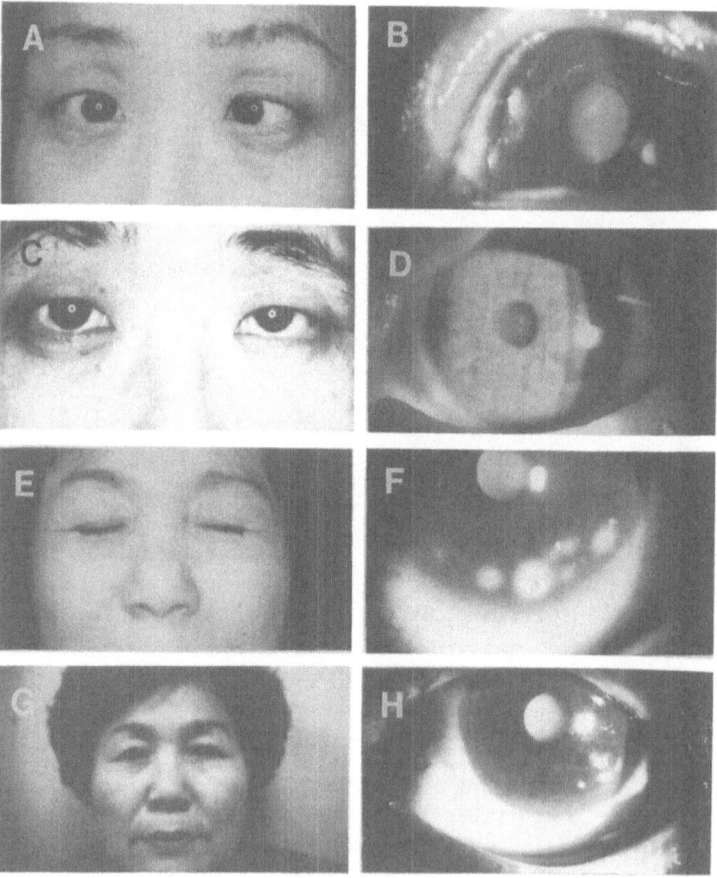

Figure 2. A–D: External appearance of Case #1 showing esodeviation before injection (A), which disappeared and became orthophoric after injection (C). Slit-lamp examination showed long large filaments on her lower cornea (B), which disappeared after injection (D). E–G: External appearance of Case #2 showing involuntary spasm of both eyelids before injection (E) which resolved after injection (G). Slit-lamp examination showed mixed long and short filaments on her lower cornea (F), which disappeared after injection.

three days later (Fig. 2 C, D) with resolution of ocular discomfort. Values of TBUT, Schirmer I test without anesthetics and fluorescein clearance test were not notably changed before and after the injection.

Case # 2

A 65-year-old female complained of foreign body irritation and photophobia for 2 years and had not responded to artificial tears and debridements directed to persistent corneal filaments. The external examination revealed involuntary lid spasm compatible with the diagnosis of essential blepharospasm (Fig. 2E). The slit-lamp examination showed mixed long and short filaments on both lower corneas, especially at the border where preferentially covered by lids (Fig. 2F). The value of Schirmer I test without anesthetics was 1 mm in the right eye and 0 mm in the left eye, and TBUT was 3 seconds bilaterally. Three days after the botulinum toxin injection, corneal filaments on both eyes completely disappeared together with the resolution of lid occlusion (Fig. 2G,H). The Schirmer I test value increased to 4 mm in the right eye and 5 mm in the left eye, and TBUT increased to 7 seconds in the right eye and 8 seconds in the left eye. Fluorescein clearance test showed decreased secretion with delayed tear clearance before injection, but after injection, aqueous secretion was increased as reflected by increased wetting length, albeit the tear clearance was further delayed (not shown).

Case # 3

A 26-year-old female with hyperthyroidism complained of ocular irritation and involuntary spasms of both eyelids compatible with the diagnosis of essential blepharospasm. The slit-lamp examination revealed Rose Bengal-stained diffuse, comma-shaped filaments on both corneas (Fig. 3A). The value of Schirmer I test without anesthetics was 1 mm in the right eye and 2 mm in the left eye. TBUT was 2 seconds in the right eye and 3 seconds in the left eye. Two days after the botulinum toxin injection into orbicular muscles, there was complete relief of symptoms and resolution of filaments (Fig. 3B). Schirmer I test value became 5 mm in the left eye and 6 mm in the left eye. TBUT was 6 seconds in the right eye 9 seconds in the left eye. Fluorescein clearance test showed decreased secretion with delayed tear clearance before injection, but after injection, aqueous secretion was increased as reflected by increased wetting length, albeit the tear clearance was further delayed (Fig. 3C).

Case # 4

A 64-year-old female had not responded to treatments with a tranquilizer and a herb medicine for five years because of Meige syndrome. She continued to complain of ocular irritation and involuntary spasm of the her eyelid, face, and neck muscles (Fig. 3D). The slit-lamp examination showed long, large filaments on both corneas (not shown). The value of Schirmer I test without anesthetics was 1 mm bilaterally. TBUT could not to be performed in this patient because of severe lid spasm. Two days after the botulinum toxin injection, filaments resolved and ocular irritation disappeared (Fig. 3E). Schirmer I test value increased to over 10 mm. Fluorescein clearance test showed decreased secretion with delayed tear clearance before injection, but after injection, aqueous secretion was increased as reflected by increased wetting length, albeit the tear clearance was further delayed (Fig. 3F).

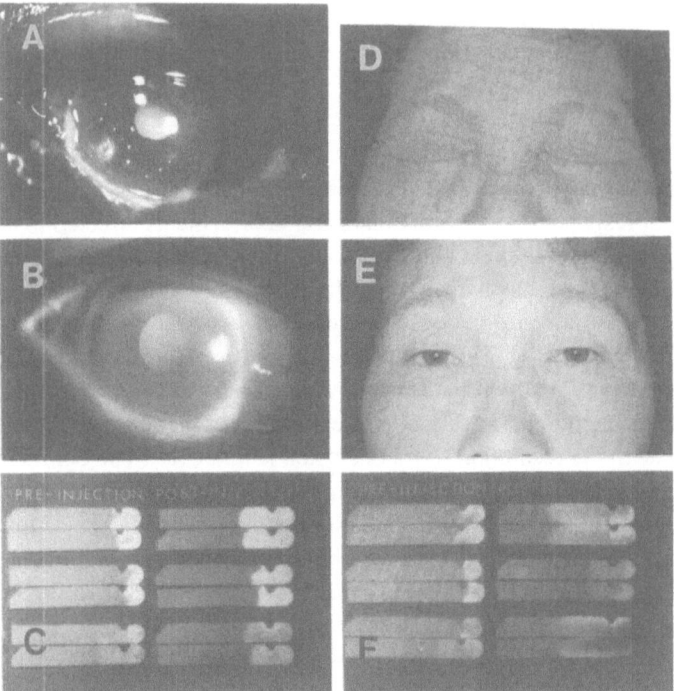

Figure 3. A–C: Slit-lamp examination of Case #3 showed diffuse comma shaped filaments before injection (A), which disappeared after injection (B). Fluorescein clearance test showed decreased secretion with delayed tear clearance before injection and increased aqueous secretion with further delayed tear clearance after injection (C; Top: 10 min.; Middle: 20 min.; Bottom: 30 min.). D–F: External appearance of Case #4 showing involuntary spasm of facial muscles on both eye lids before injection (D), which disappeared after injection (E). Fluorescein clearance showed decreased secretion with delayed tear clearance before injection, and increased aqueous secretion with further delayed tear clearance after injection (F; Top: 10 min; Middle: 20 min.; Bottom: 30 min).

DISCUSSION

Filamentary keratitis, frequently leading to annoying ocular irritation, is a disease associated with diverse causes (reviews[1–3]). Although many treatments (including artificial tears, 0.5% silver nitrate, mechanical debridement, punctal occlusion[23] and bandage contact lens[24]) have been tried, none has been consistently successful. Such a variety of associated diseases and treatment modalities might have also prompted two different theories to explain the pathogenesis of filament formation. One theory proposes that the primary abnormality appears to start at the level of superficial stroma which is focally infiltrated with inflammatory cells and associated with focal attenuation of the Bowman's membrane.[4,5] The other theory stresses the important role of excess mucus production[1] and mucus attachment onto abnormal degenerative superficial epithelial cells.[1,6] Impression cytology results showed that filaments were attached to superficial metaplastic epithelial cells (Fig. 1). This is based on the fact that the filter paper used for impression cytology can only remove superficial desquamating corneal epithelial cells and not basal cells attached to the basement membrane. Therefore, it can be concluded that corneal filaments, at least those caused by corneal occlusion, are not attached to the basement membrane.

For the same reason, the likelihood that there might be stromal inflammation focally associated with the filaments examined cannot be ruled out. Because impression cytology also revealed that all filaments were composed of a central "core" surrounded by PAS-positive amorphous materials and desquamated epithelial cells (Fig. 1), an observation consistent with that by Wright[1], this result suggests that cytoskeletons might be involved in the formation of this core, as speculated by Maudgal and Missotten.[7] Future studies are needed to characterize the component of this core material.

Concerning the pathogenesis, one important aspect of corneal filament formation noted in this group of patients is the uniform presence of corneal occlusion by lids. Occlusion of the corneal surface by lids has been recognized by others as a risk factor for filament formation,[25] and is consistent with the previous reports that filamentary keratitis can be associated with pressure patching[26] and contact lens.[27] Because corneal occlusion by lids or other means is not always associated with filament formation, there is some speculation about whether excessive blinking is important to its pathogenesis. As shown in this study, such excessive lid blinking was noted in all cases with uncontrolled blepharospasm. But even for the one case with large paralytic esotropia, which was similarly reported by Good,[25] there is some question as to whether excessive blinking might have secondarily been induced by annoying ocular irritation into a vicious cycle.

The other important contributing factor to the filament formation is the presence of aqueous tear deficiency, i.e., dry eyes, as shown by the Schirmer I test without anesthetics in the majority of cases (Table 1) and by the fluorescein clearance test (Table 2). As first reported by Nelson et al.[28] and subsequently by others[22] using impression cytology, various dry states are associated with squamous metaplasia, a finding also confirmed in this report by impression cytology (Fig. 1). The frequent association of dry eyes with filament formation has been recognized causes (reviews[1-3]). Interestingly, aqueous tear deficiency is also frequently associated with essential blepharospasm,[10] a finding also supported by this study. Previously, one speculative cause of aqueous tear deficiency in blepharospasm has been related to general dysfunction of the facial nerve including its parasympathetic function causes (reviews[1-3]). This study, however, showed that arrest of excessive lid blinking by botulinum toxin injections led to a significant improvement of aqueous tear secretion as evidenced by both Schirmer I test without anesthetics (Table 1) and fluorescein clearance test (Table 2). Because this treatment also resulted in further delayed clearance (Table 2), this result further suggests that it is excessive blinking aggravating aqueous tear deficiency by increasing tear clearance. This notion is supported by works of Doane[29] and others,[30-32] who all have shown that lid blinking is the primary driving force for clearing tears from the ocular surface into the nasolacrimal drainage system. Nevertheless, it remains unclear why patients with essential blepharospasm are prone to have delayed tear clearance (turnover). Without knowing the causes of this delayed tear clearance, recent work has provided evidence that this abnormality is intrinsically pathogenic in causing ocular irritation.[33] Taken together, these results strongly suggest that aqueous tear deficiency and delayed tear clearance can aggravate unstable tear film, evidenced by short TBUT, leading to various symptoms of ocular irritation.

The existence of surface epithelial cell squamous metaplasia and excessive blinking can lead to the cell membrane damage to reveal intracellular cytoskeletons, which then facilitate the filament formation. In examining the accuracy of this line of thinking, it is important to consider the use of botulinum toxin injections to break up the vicious cycle built in the setting of corneal occlusion and excessive blinking with or without the inciting cause of ocular irritation in the management of some forms of filamentary keratitis.

ACKNOWLEDGMENT

This research was supported by Chung-Ang University special research grant in 1996.

REFERENCES

1. P. Wright, Filamentary keratitis. *Trans. Ophthalmol. Soc. (U K)* 95:260 (1975).
2. F.H. Theodore, Filamentary keratitis. *Contact and Intraocular Lens Med. J.* 8:138 (1982).
3. B.M. Kowalik, and Rakes, J.A., Filamentary keratitis - the clinical challenges. *J. Am. Optom. Assoc.* 62:200 (1991).
4. C. Weskamp, Parenchymatous origin of filamentary keratitis. New histopathologic concepts. *Am. J. Ophthalmol.* 42:115 (1956).
5. G.W. Zaidman, Geeraets, R., Paylor, R.R., and Ferry A.P., The histopathology of filamentary keratitis. *Arch. Ophthalmol.* 103:1178 (1985).
6. P.C. Maudgal, Missotten, L., and Van Deuren, H., Study of filamentary keratitis by replica technique. *Graefes Arch. Klin. Exp. Ophthalmol.* 211:11 (1979).
7. P.C. Maudgal, and Missotten, L. Cytology of the superficial keratinised cells in experimental keratitis sicca. *Ophthalmologica* 176:113 (1978).
8. T.H. Wonjo, Essential blepharospsm: diagnosis and treatment. *Ophthalmic Practice* 5:1085 (1989).
9. D.R.Jodan, Patrinely, J.R., Anderson, R.L., and Thiese, S.M., Essential blepharospasm and related dystonias. *Surv. Ophthalmol.* 34:123 (1989).
10. J. Price, and O'Day, J., A comparative study of tear secretion in blepharospasm and hemifacial spasm patients treated with botulinum toxin. *J. Clin. Neuro-Ophthalmol.* 13:67 (1993).
11. H.N. Koo, Kim, J.C., and Koo, B.S., The clinical study of the effective treatment of blepharospasm and hemifacial spasm with botulinum toxin A (I). *J. Korean. Ophthalmol. Soc.* 31:59 (1990).
12. J.C. Kim, Chun, J.S., Hong, R.S., and Koo, B.S., Delayed tear clearance induced by botulinum toxin injection in essential blepharospasm and hemifacial spasm. *J. Korean Ophthalmol. Soc.* 36:1084 (1995).
13. J.D. Wirtshafter, and Rubenfeld, M., Botulinum toxin injections for treatment of blepharospasm and hemifacial spasm. *Int. Ophthalmol. Clin.* 31:117 (1991).
14. R.H. Kennedy, Treatment of blepharospasm with botulinum toxin. *Mayo Clin. Proc.* 64:1085 (1989).
15. M.S. Norn, Desiccation of the precorneal film. I. Corneal wetting-time. *Acta Ophthalmol.* 47:865 (1969).
16. M.A. Lemp, and Hamill, J.R., Factors affecting tear film breakup in normal eyes. *Arch. Ophthalmol.* 89:103 (1973).
17. S.C. Pflugfelder, Tseng, S.C.G., Pepose, J.S., et al., Epstein-Barr virus infection and immunological dysfunction in patients with aqueous tear deficiency. *Ophthalmology* 97:313 (1990).
18. S.C. Pflugfelder, Huang, A.J.W., Schuchovski, P.T., et al., Conjunctival cytological features of primary Sjögren syndrome. *Ophthalmology* 97:985 (1990).
19. K. Xu, Yagi, Y., Toda, I., and Tsubota, K., Tear function index. A new measure of dry eye. *Arch. Ophthalmol.* 113:84 (1995).
20. L.T. Jones, The lacrimal secretory system and its treatment. *Am. J. Ophthalmol.* 62:47 (1966).
21. K. Tsubota, The importance of the Schirmer test with nasal stimulation. *Am. J. Ophthalmol.* 111:106 (1991).
22. S.C.G. Tseng, Staging of conjunctival squamous metaplasia by impression cytology. *Ophthalmology* 92:728 (1985).
23. A.W. Tuberville, Punctal occlusion in tear deficiency syndrome. *Ophthalmology* 89:1170 (1982).
24. S.E. Bloomfield, Gasset, A.R., Forstot, S.L., and Brown, S.I., Treatment of filamentary keratitis with the soft contact lens. *Am. J. Ophthalmol.* 76:978 (1973).
25. W.V. Good, Filamentary keratitis caused by corneal occlusion in large angle strabismus. *Ophthal. Surg.* 23:66 (1992).
26. H.T. Dodds, and Laibson, P.R., Filamentary keratitis following cataract extraction. *Arch. Ophthalmol.* 88:609 (1972).
27. V. Dada, and Zsman, Z., Contact lens induced filamentary keratitis. *Am. J. Optom. & Physiol. Optics.* 52:545 (1976).
28. J.D. Nelson, Havener, V.R., and Cameron, J.D., Cellulose acetate impressions of the ocular surface; dry eye states. *Arch. Ophthalmol.* 101:1869 (1983).

29. M.G. Doane, Blinking and the mechanics of the lacrimal drainage system. *Ophthalmology* 88:844 (1981).

30. F.T. Fraunfelder, Extraocular fluid dynamics: how best to apply topical ocular medication. *Tr. Am. Ophth. Soc.* 74:457 (1976).

31. W.L. White, Glover, A.T., and Buckner, A.B., Effect of blinking on tear elimination as evaluated by dacryoscintigraphy. *Ophthalmology* 98:367 (1991).

32. M.A. Lemp, and Weiler, H.H., How do tears exit? *Invest. Ophthalmol. Vis. Sci.* 24:619 (1983).

33. P. Prabhasawat, and Tseng, S.C.G., The pathogenic role of delayed tear clearance. *Invest. Ophthalmol. Vis. Sci.* 37:S851 (1996).

12

CLINICAL USES OF HUMAN AMNIOTIC MEMBRANE FOR OCULAR SURFACE DISEASES

Jae Chan Kim, Dohyting Lee, and Kywig Hwan Shyn

Department of Ophthalmology
Yongsan Hospital, Chung-Ang University
College of Medicine
65–207, Hangangro 3-Ga, Yongsan-Gu
Seoul 140-757, Korea

ABSTRACT

This study evaluated the clinical efficacy of amniotic membrane transplantation with or without limbal graft in the management of ocular surface disease (11 primary pterygia, nine recurrent pterygia, one limbal choristoma, three chemical injuries, and one cryotherapy to the limbal region). In addition, eight patients underwent the temporary amniotic membrane anchoring flap surgery for two chronic stromal herpetic keratitis, two non-healing corneal ulcer, two corneal perforation, and two chemical burns. The average duration of follow-up ranged from 3 to 40 months (mean 24.3 ± 10.4 months). In pterygium, the recurrence rate was 18% (2/11) after amniotic membrane transplantation. In recurrent pterygium and pseudopterygium, amniotic membrane transplantation with a small piece of limbal autograft resulted in an improved ocular surface without recurrence in all of the cases, and symblepharon and ocular motility were significantly improved postoperatively. Complications included submembrane hemorrhage (12%, 3/25) and early detachment or dissolution of the membrane (4%, 1/25). No major complications such as infection and rejection were encountered. In selected cases, a temporary amniotic membrane flap anchored onto the corneal surface led to rapid epithelial wound healing in unresponsive ulcerative keratitis. These results indicate that extracellular matrix components provide a good cell basement membrane interaction that is critical for cytoskeletal changes or differentiation. Furthermore, the amniotic membrane can also protect the ocular surface from being exposed to the unwanted inflammatory cytokines, derived from tears, and subconjunctival inflammatory cells. These procedures are thought to be clinically useful for ocular surface reconstruction.

INTRODUCTION

The normal ocular surface is covered by conical, limbal, and conjunctival epithelia, each of which has a distinct cellular phenotype. This differentiated phenotype influences the stability of the preocular tear film, which in turn dictates the normal health of the ocular surface.[1,2] Limbal stem cells can be considered as the ultimate source of conical epithelial regeneration and serve as the conjunctival barrier between conical and conjunctival epithelium.[1,2] Depending on the pathogenic nature of limbal involvement, destruction can come from chemical and thermal injuries, Stevens-Johnson syndrome, multiple surgeries or cryotherapies to the limbal region. The rare situation of contact lens-induced keratopathy and long standing recalcitrant conical ulceration can also cause limbal stem cell damage. All of these ocular surface disorders are characterized by the loss of limbal stem cells, a condition termed limbal deficiency.[2] Even for a focal and milder form of conical diseases with limbal deficiency such as pterygium, and other diseases such as aniridia, there is a gradual loss of stem cell population presumably because of poor stromal microenvironmental support.[2,3]

Experimentally, limbal autograft for conical surface reconstruction has been reported to be superior to conjunctival transplantation,[4] and useful for treating human patients with severe ocular surface damage[5-7] and pterygium.[8,9] For those with dysfunctional stromal microenvironment due to intense limbal inflammation that may lead to hypofunction of limbal deficiency, ideal treatments should be directed to maintaining and activating the remaining stem cell population and corneal basal cells. Therefore, it is conceivable that improvement of limbal microenvironments by protecting against inflammatory insults from tears and inflammatory cells by replacing the diseased substrate or by combining with conjunctiva-limbal transplantation will be ideal to reconstruct the ocular surface. Kim and Tseng[10] had previously shown that morphological transformation of the conjunctiva epithelium to a cornea-like epithelium with inhibition of neovascularization can be achieved by providing the basement membrane containing glycerin-preserved human amniotic membrane in severely damaged rabbit corneas.

This paper reports the first human clinical attempt of transplanting preserved human amniotic membrane with or without a small piece of conjunctiva-limbal graft, and temporary amniotic membrane anchoring flap on diseased cornea or conjunctival surface as an alternative to improve the stromal microenvironment and hence the ocular surface.

MATERIALS AND METHODS

Surgical Indications

Simple amniotic membrane transplantation was consecutively performed on 11 eyes of nine patients (10 primary and one recurrent pterygium), aged from 40 to 70 years old. Amniotic membrane transplantation combined with small conjunctiva-limbal autograft was performed in 14 eyes of 14 patients (eight male and six female patients), aged from 4 to 60 years old. These 14 eyes could be subdivided into: (a) recurrent pterygium (>3 months after operation) (n=8); (b,) pseudopterygium due to thermal or chemical burns or cryotherapies to the limbal region (>6 months after injury) (n=4); (c) limbal choristoma (n=1); and (d) conical perforation in corneal ulcer due to intractable increased intraocular pressure (n=1).

In addition, eight patients (six males and two females) underwent temporary amniotic membrane anchoring flap surgery for two chemical burns, four recalcitrant conical ulcer (two herpetic ulcers and two sterile unresponsive ulcerations) and two conical perforations. Other pertinent clinical information such as history of prior surgery and other abnormal findings are also detailed in Tables 1 and 2. All the procedures followed the tenets

Table 1. Demographic, clinical, and surgical data on 22 patients with Amniotic Membrane Transplantation with or without Conjunctival Autograft

Patient No.	Age / Sex	Disease (injury)	Other abnormal findings	preoperative		procedure			postoperative			follow-up: month revascular graft(day)	comment
				Visual Acuity	EOM Degree of limitation	AMT or / with CG (size of CG)	Medial rectus dissection	Fornix reconstruction	Visual Acuity	EOM	Recurrence		
1	60 / F	Primary pterygium (OD)	None	20 / 30	Full	AMT	No	No	20 / 30	Full	No	28 (4)	
2	60 / F	Advanced primary (OD)	Lipid deposition, DE Symblepharon	20 / 50	Full	AMT	No	No	20 / 50	Full	Yes	38 (7)	Subamniotic hemorrhage for 14 days
3	57 / F	Recurrent(OS) Excision X 2	Diplopia Intrastromal invasion	20 / 50	Abduction (-3)	AMT with CG (3 X 6 mm)	Yes	Yes	20 / 50	Full	No	15 (11)	
4	62 / F	Recurrent(OD) Excision X 4	Diplopia Fornix shortening DE	20 / 50	Abduction (-3) Supraduction (-1)	AMT with CG (3 X 6 mm)	Yes	Yes	20 / 70	Full	No	19 (3)	
5	65 / F	Primary (OS)	DE	20 / 20	Full	AMT	No	No	20 / 20	Full	No	12 (5)	
6	65 / M	Recurrent(OD) Excision X 1	DE	20 / 30	Full	AMT (OD) with CG (3 X 6 mm)	Yes	Yes	20 / 30	Full	No	25 (7)	
7	55 / M	Primary (OD) Advanced (OS)	None None	20 / 30 20 / 30	Full	AMT AMT	No No	No No	20 / 30 20 / 30	Full	No	24 (5) 38 (4)	
8	65 / F	Recurrent(OD) Excision X 2	Diplopia Partial symblepharon	20 / 400	Abduction (-2)	AMT with CG (3 X 6 mm)	Yes	Yes	20 / 100		No	5 (3)	

Table 1. (*Continued*)

No.	Age/Sex	Diagnosis	Associated findings	VA	Motility	Operation			VA			Follow-up mo (visits)	Complication
9	40 / M	Primary (OD)	None	20 / 20	Full	AMT	No	No	20 / 20	Full	No	5 (3)	Early dissolution with dehiscence
10	23 / M	Pseudopterygium (OS)	Diplopia Deep stromal neovascularization	20 / 400	Abduction (- 3)	AMT with CG (3 X 12 mm)	Yes	Yes	20 / 50	Full	No	36 (5) Regressed neovascularization	Chronic alkali burn Subconjunctiotic hemorrhage for 9 days
11	11 / M	Limbal choriostoma (OD)	Diplopia Deep stromal neovascularization	20 / 200	Adduction (- 2)	AMT with CG (3 X 9 mm)	Yes	Yes	20 / 100	Full	No	6 (5) Regressed neovascularization	Large choriostoma across the corneal surface
12	70 / F	Recurrent(OD) Excision X 1	Lipid deposition Pupillary involvement Cataract	HM	No	AMT ECCE	Yes	Yes	20 / 40	Full	Yes	36 (9)	Subconjunctiotic membrane hemorrhage for 14 days
13	63 / F	Primary (OD)	-	20 / 20	No	AMT	No	No	20 / 20	Full	No	30 (5)	
		Primary (OS)	-	20 / 20	No	AMT	No	No	20 / 20	Full	No	29 (5)	
14	61 / M	Primary (OD)	-	20 / 20	No	AMT	No	No	20 / 20	Full	No	28 (5)	
		Primary (OS)		20 / 20	No	AMT	No	No	20 / 20	Full	No	27 (6)	
15	4 / F	Pseudopterygium (OS)	ROP Symblepharon	20 / 50	Adduction (- 2)	AMT LKP CG (3 X 7 mm)	Yes	Yes	20 / 30	Full	No	24 (6)	Multiple cryo-therapies on temporal limbus

Table 1. (Continued)

No	Age/Sex	Diagnosis		Preop VA	Preop EOM	Operation			Postop VA	Postop EOM	Result	Follow-up	Complication
16	44 / M	Corneal ulcer perforation (OD)	Increased IOP pannus formation	HM	No	AMT Gundersen's flap Cryodestruction of ciliary body	No	No	HM	Full	Reduced painful condition	28 (3)	Pain eye corneal ulcer
17	32 / M	Pseudopterygium (OS)	Partial symblepharon (inferior)	HM	No	AMT LKP(inferior-nasal) CG (3 X 7 mm)	No	No	20 / 200	Full	Cosmetically improved / No	25 (14)	Chronic alkali injury
18	45 / M	Recurred Excision X 1 advanced (OD)	Diplopia Lipid deposition	20 / 30	Abduction (- 2)	- AMT with CG (3 X 7 mm)	Yes	Yes	20 / 20	Full	No	28 (5)	
19	35 / F	Recurrent(OD) Excision X 3	-	20 / 30	No	AMT with CG (3 X 6 mm)	No	No	20 / 30	Full	No	27 (3)	
20	59 / F	Recurrent(OD) Excision X 3	Diplopia Symblepharon	20 / 50	Abduction (- 2)	AMT with CG (3 X 6 mm)	Yes	Yes	20 / 50	Full	No	28 (3)	
21	62 / M	Recurrent(OD) Excision X 1	-	20 / 70	No	AMT with CG (3 X 8 mm)	No	No	20 / 70	Full	No	8 (4)	
22	32 / M	Pseudopterygium (OD)	Diplopia Symblepharon	20 / 50	Adduction (- 2)	AMT with CG (3 X 11 mm)	Yes	Yes	20 / 30	Full	No	38 (6)	Acid burn

AMT : Amniotic membrane transplantation, CG : Conjunctival autograft, DE : Dry eye, OD : Right eye, OS : Left eye, EOM : Extraocular movement

HM : Hand motion, LP :Light perception, LKP : Lamellar keratoplasty, ROP : Retinopathy of prematurity

Table 2. Temporary Amniotic Membrane flap cases summaries

pa-tient No	Age / Sex	Disease (Etiology?)	Combined abnormal findings (limbal injury : degree)	Persistent epithelial defect	Prior treatment with complication	TAMF	VA change	Stromal epithelial healing completely (days)	Complications	Follow up (months)	Comment
23	46/M	Corneal perforation(trauma)	Cataract (absence)	2	Primary suture leakage	Flap covered by 10-0 nylon purse string suture	LP → 20/70	10	None	3	No leakage
24	28/M	Persistent sterile corneal ulcer (Pseudomonas)	Corneal melting with epithelial defect (absence)	25	Antibiotics topical & systemic Gundersen flap : failed(dissolved flap)	Covered by 10-0 nylon purse string suture	HM → 20/70	14	None	7	
25	44/M	Epithelial defect (chemical burn)	Limbal damage(200°)	7	Hyaluronic acid eyedrop Topical steroid & antibiotics (topical)	Covered whole cornea limbal by 10-0 nylon interrupted suture	20/200 → 20/30	8	Mild hazziness	13	Acute thermal burn
26	18/M	Persistent limbal corneal epithelial defect (absence)	Limbal damage (200°)	3	Topical antibiotic & steroid	Covered, burned corneal limbal lesion by interrupted suture	20/400 → 20/30	10	Corneal infiltration of cement substance	10	Reduced myopia -2.5 D → 0.25 D
27	55/M	Persistent herpetic corneal ulcer	Stromal melting (absence)	30	Antiviral agent Chemical cautery	Covered 10-nylon interrupted suture	20/800 → 20/50	3	Mixed corneal opacity	15	Induced hyperopia (+2.5 D)
28	77/F	Buttonhole of filtering bleb, flat chamber	None (absence)	3	Glaucoma Filtering surgery of Glaucoma	Covered with histoacryl	20/400 →20/200	5	None	3	
29	66/F	Strerile interstitial keratitis(?)	Stromal immune ring melting (absence) DE	35	ECCE & IOL Excimer laser to Treat herpetic keratitis	Covered by 10-0 nylon purse-string suture	20/400 → 20/40	7	Mild hazziness	40	Induced hyperopia (+3.0D)
30	24/M	Peripheral corneal ulcer with perforation (Excimer laser)	Imbedded iron particle Wound leakage 1x1.5mm round stromal defect° (absence)	15	Topical antibiotics eyedrop	Removal of foreign body Covered by histoacryl	FC → 20/30	10	Marked astigmatism	30	Transpositional auto KP: succeed

TAMF : Temporary amniotic membrane anchoring flap D : Diopter LP : Light perception CF : Counting finger HM : Hand movement

ECCE : Extracapsular Extraction IOL : Intraocular lens DE : Dry eye of Declaration of Helsinki, and consents were obtained after the explanation of the nature of the possible consequence of the treatment method.

Preparation of Human Amniotic Membrane

The procedure of preparation was similar to that previously described.[10] In brief, human placentas were obtained shortly after elective Cesarean sections. Screening test against human immunodeficiency virus (HIV), hepatitis C virus (HCV), hepatitis B virus (HBV), and Venereal Disease Research Laboratory (VDRL) test were performed before use. Under laminar-flow hood, the placenta was first washed of blood clots with balanced salt solution. The semitransparent amniotic membrane was separated from the chorion by blunt dissection and then flattened onto a nitrocellulose membrane filter with the epithelial surface up. The membrane with filter was washed three times with phosphate buffered saline containing vancomycin 9.5 mg/ml and gentamycin 10 mg/ml, cut into 3 cm diameter discs and stored at -70°C in 50% Dulbecco's modified Eagle's medium (DMEM) and 50% glycerin before transplantation. Amniotic membrane was used within two months of storage.

Surgical Techniques

Amniotic Membrane Transplantation with or without Conjunctival Autograft. The operative procedure usually involved the transfer of amniotic membrane with or without small free grafts of limbal conjunctiva from the uninjured or less injured eye to the diseased eye. Surgery was performed with an operating microscope under topical or subconjunctival anesthesia (amniotic membrane transplantation with conjunctival autograft cases with only retrobulbar anesthesia). The amniotic membrane was washed and immersed with antibiotic-containing saline for 30 min. and then transferred to the injured eye. Amniotic membrane transplantation in pterygium is schematically illustrated in Fig. 1 (A, B). In brief, the procedures include the following three key points: (1) prevention of the loss of corneal substance by using blunt dissection; (2) removal of subconjunctival tissue in an area greater than that covered by the pterygium; and (3) covering of the exposed sclera (Fig. 1A) or cornea (Fig. 1B) with amniotic membrane graft.

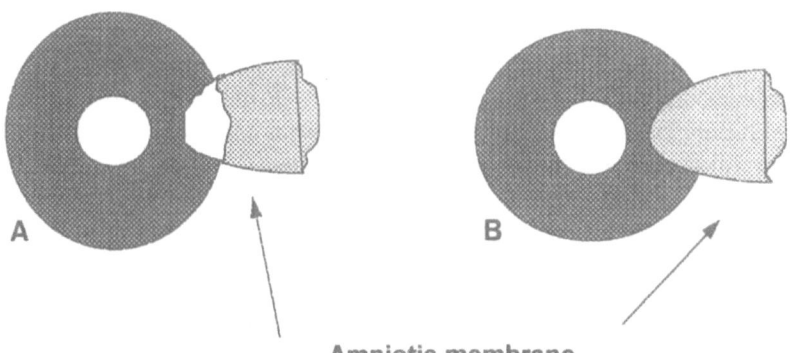

Amniotic membrane

Figure 1. Diagram of simple amniotic membrane transplantation. Following bare sclera excision of pterygium, amniotic membrane of required dimension was cut, transferred to cover exposed sclera and medial rectus muscle (A) or denuded cornea (B) and secured (C, arrows indicate transplanted amniotic membrane).

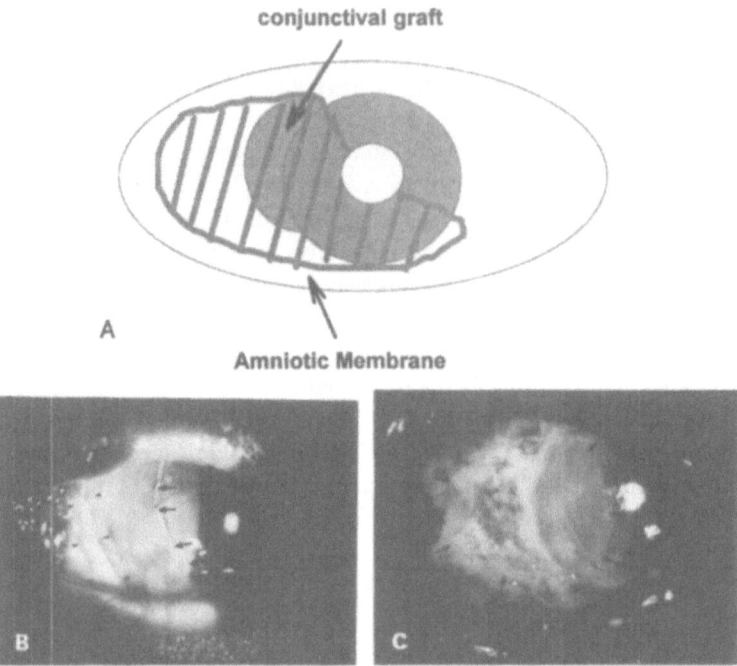

Figure 2. Diagram of amniotic membrane transplantation with conjunctiva-limbal graft. Following superficial keratectomy with excision of diseased bulbar conjunctiva, uninvolved superotemporal bulbar conjunctiva or opposite eye (A) are thinly dissected, transferred to cover amniotic membrane in limbal lesion, and secured (B; arrow heads indicate conjunctival flap, and arrows indicate amniotic membrane).

The surgical procedure of amniotic membrane transplantation with conjunctival autograft (Fig. 2 A, B) was similarly performed. In brief, the injured eye was first cleared of superficial vascularized scar tissue including diseased bulbar conjunctiva with Tenon's capsule and cicatrix. The bare sclera and rectus muscle were exposed. The adjacent limbus and cornea arc were scraped and polished in recurrent pterygium and pseudopterygium due to chemical bums. Conjunctival margins were recessed to restore the fornix. Conjunctiva was sutured to sclera with absorbable suture on spatula model (e.g., 84 Vicryl®). For amniotic membrane transplantation, the size of the membrane was cut to replace exposed sclera and horizontal rectus muscle or to reconstruct the symblepharon by recreating the fornix area with the membrane that was removed from the nitrocellulose filter paper. Transferred membrane was secured to the entire keratectomized corneal surface and exposed sclera with rectus muscle. The membrane was secured both by interrupted 10–0 nylon sutures at the corneal margin and by interrupted 84 Vicryl® at the scleral and conjunctival margin. Several approaches had been reported previously to obtain donor conjunctival epithelium.[11,12] The technique chosen to obtain the conjunctival graft resembled that described by Kenyon et al,[13] which contained some stem cells and provided an additional advantage in surface reconstruction. In brief, small rectangular grafts of limbal conjunctiva that do not contain clean cornea and extend approximately 3 mm into bulbar conjunctiva were obtained. We took small graft (3 x 6 – 3 x 12 mm) which is schematically illustrated in Fig 2 (A,B). This small graft just covered amniotic membrane of limbal region (Fig 2.B). This conjunctiva-limbal graft is thought to maintain a barrier function between conjunctiva and cornea. The small graft was secured by interrupted 10–0 nylon suture at the corneal and limbal conjunctival margins and the free edge of the conjunctival margin was anchored to the amniotic membrane and episcleral tissue using 8–0 vicryl. After surgery, topical Maxitrol® eyedrops were applied four times a day. There were no restrictions on patient activity. Conjunctival grafts were recanalized within three to seven days, and became adherent to the amniotic membrane and sclera. Topical steroid eye drops were continuously applied for about two weeks postoperatively, or shorter if inflammation did not persist.

Temporary Amniotic Membrane Anchoring flap. Gundersen,[14] in 1958, described a tech-nique and a number of surgical indications for conjunctival flaps. This procedure remains effective for recalcitrant corneal ulceration and poor epithelialization caused by many different underlying diseases, including herpetic infection, neurotrophic keratopathy, sterile ulceration from a recent infectious keratitis, and a refractory bullous keratopathy. Huang and Tseng[1,3] reported that the use of pedicle (hinged) conjunctival flaps yielded better success than conjunctival transplantation in absence of limbal deficiency. Therefore, temporary amniotic membrane anchoring flap may be substituted for a conjunctival flap in aforementioned indications, especially in the absence of limbal deficiency or impending limbal deficiency.

For the procedure of temporary amniotic membrane flap surgery (Fig.5., C,F), the membrane was first removed from the nitrocellulose filter paper, and transferred to the recipient eye, covering the debrided stromal wound. A purse-string or interrupted 10–0 nylon fixation suture was performed at the peripheral cornea (e.g., recalcitrant corneal ulcer) or 4 mm behind the surgical limbus (e.g., acute chemical burn). Other surgical indications included impending corneal perforation, corneal perforation, and button hole of filtering bleb after glaucoma surgery. In these cases, amniotic membrane was temporarily (2 weeks-3 months) transplanted with histoacryl glue or with a purse-string amniotic-corneal anchoring suture. In case of perforated wound, we used lyophilized amniotic membrane with histoacryl glue (cases 27, 30). Topical Maxitrol® eye drop was applied four times a day and the ointment of the same kind applied at night. Amniotic membrane to corneal anchoring fixation sutures was removed between postoperative 5th day and in the 2nd week. All cases were performed only by one of us (JCK).

RESULTS

We have performed amniotic membrane transplantation with or without conjunctiva-limbal autograft on 25 eyes of 22 patients. The clinical and surgical details of this series are summarized in Table 1. Recipient age ranged from 4 to 70 years old (mean, 48.6 + 18.7 years). Postoperatively, all patients receiving amniotic membrane transplantation had less pain compared to those who underwent bare-sclera technique operation alone. We did not encounter any microbial infections.

Among 25 eyes, 10 eyes with primary pterygium and one eye with recurrent pterygium received amniotic membrane transplantations alone. Epithelial outgrowths resurfaced the denuded corneal area and the surface of amniotic membrane, usually within 7 days of surgery. Among 11 simple amniotic membrane transplantation, two early cases (cases 2, 12) recurred (2/11, 18%), and were associated with subamniotic membrane hemorrhage that lasted for 10 days more than those in other cases.

Of the other 14 eyes receiving combined amniotic membrane transplantation and conjunctival autograft, six eyes with the recurrent pterygia and three pseudopterygia had marked cicatrization with loss of the medial fornix (cases 3, 4, 8, 10, 15, 18, 20, 22), or temporal fornix (case 15), and mechanical restriction of the horizontal rectus muscle, resulting in symptomatic diplopia. The rapidity of epithelial resurfacing was striking in the conjunctival autograft group in which revascularization of the conjunctival graft also occurred within seven days, but in case 17, the corneal epithelial defect persisted for 14 days but eventually healed. Among various depths of keratectomy, we encountered one case of microperforation (case 17), created by a 10–0 nylon needle through a thin stromal area during amniotic membrane transplantation. This microperforated hole was sealed with an amniotic membrane anchoring suture around the hole. We did not encounter graft rejection or severe inflammation. Except for case 9 showing early dissolution with dehiscence of amniotic membrane on postoperative day five (1/25, 4%), the remaining 24 eyes showed integration of amniotic membrane with the surrounding conjunctiva. In the group receiving conjunctival autografts, improvement of vision and diplopia were also substantial in most cases. Among nine recurrent pterygium, three pseudopterygium and other cases, five patients had visual acuity improvement (7/14, 50%), but no change showed in the remaining eye (7/14, 50%). The patients who had diplopia were totally improved.

We also performed a temporary amniotic membrane anchoring flap onto the diseased corneal wound in eight eyes of eight patients. The clinical and surgical details of this series are summarized in Table 2. Recipient ages ranged from 18 to 77 years old. The length of follow-up ranged from three months to 40 months (mean 15.1 ± 13.3). The maintenance of anchoring flap of amniotic membrane was determined by complete epithelial covering and no wound leakage. Postoperatively, visual acuity improvement and a stable ocular surface were noted in all cases. In cases 5 and 7, with follow-up of more than 1 year, the patients developed hyperopia (+2.5 D) and reduced myopia (-2.OD) respectively. Leakages due to corneal perforation (case 23, 30), and the button hole in the filtering bleb (case 28) was easily sealed by histoacryl and a purse-string suture with amniotic membrane flap. In cases with acute chemical burns (cases 26, 30), rapid corneal epithelialization occurred with visual acuity markedly improved.

SELECTED CASE REPORTS

Case 4: Recurrent Pterygium

A 62-year-old female housewife had a recurrent pterygium in right eye. She had undergone four surgical excisions of a medial pterygium and at least two times received topical mitomycin. She had experienced increasing diplopia for more than three years. She was examined on December 12, 1994 and noted to have a visual acuity 20/50(OD). Externally, the right eye showed marked limitation of abduction (Fig.3A) with diplopia upon attempted right abduction gaze. Objectively, the right eye could abduct 10° lateral and supraduct 15° to primary position. Slit-lamp biomicroscopy revealed a thick and dense band of scar tissue uniting the caruncle to the limbus with partial symblepharon in the inferonasal fornix (Fig.3B). On December 13, 1994, amniotic membrane transplantation with conjunctiva-limbal autograft was performed. At that time, forced duction testing demonstrated almost total mechanical restriction of the right medial rectus and mild restriction of inferior rectus muscle. A bare sclera excision of the pterygium was done with difficulty, and the medial rectus and inferior rectus were enmeshed with dense fibrovascu-

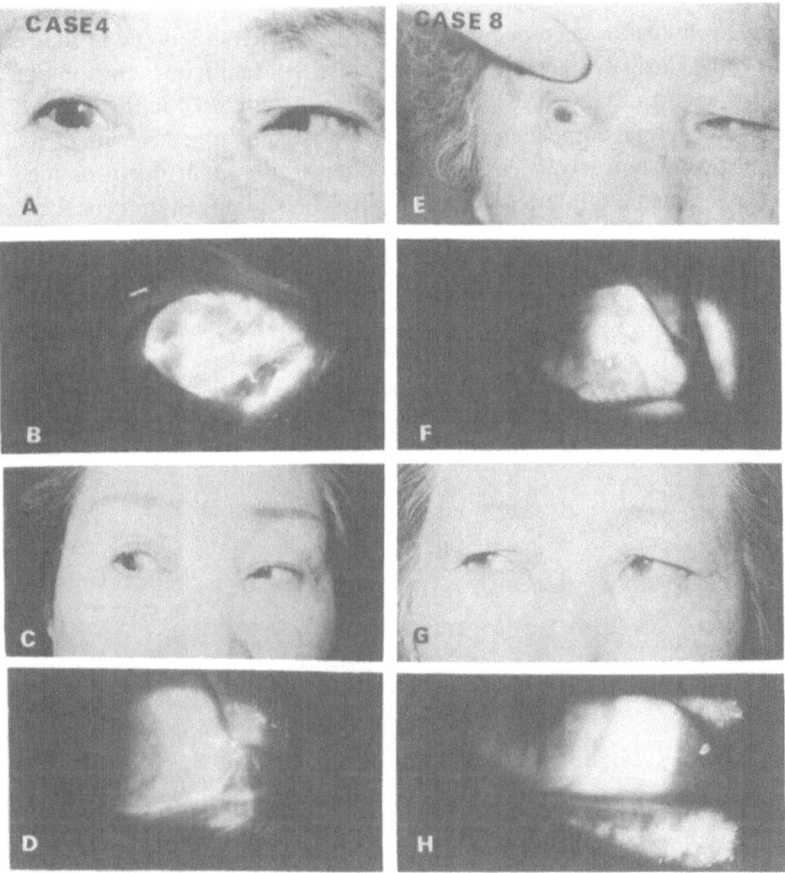

Figure 3. Case 4: A 62-year old female housewife had undergone four previous pterygium excision in right eye. There is marked restriction of right abduction with clinical significant diplopia (A). A dense band of scar tissue obliterates the medial fornix and displaces the caruncle nearby to the limbus (B). Two weeks after amniotic membrane transplantation with conjunctival autograft, transplanted tissue was vascularized and ocular motility was improved (C). One and one-half years after surgery, the operated eye was uninflamed, and pterygium had not recurred and conjunctival graft remains nearly indistinguishable from adjacent conjunctiva (D). Case 8: this 65-year-old woman had two previous pterygium excision failures. There was diplopia upon attempted right gaze with restriction (E). A recurrent pterygium was of dense thick band with large elevated nodule formation (F). Two weeks postoperatively, there was no limitation of movement (G). Three months after surgery, operated wound was relatively stable ocular surface (H) with neither pterygium recurrence nor diplopia.

lar scar tissue. After the medial rectus muscle and inferior rectus muscle were freed, the globe could be fully abducted, supraducted and the diseased bulbar conjunctiva was treated with lysis of symblepharon, and remaining bulbar conjunctiva recessed to reconstruct the inferonasal fornix and reposition the caruncle. Amniotic membrane was transplanted on the exposed bare sclera, medial, and inferior rectus muscle. A 3 x 11 mm free conjunctival graft was taken from the uninvolved superotemporal quadrant and covered only the limbal region. During the ensuing 16 months, she experienced neither diplopia nor recurrence. The recent follow-up examination disclosed improved visual acuity (20/50–20/70) and ocular motility (Fig.3A) with a stable ocular surface (Fig.3D).

Case 10: Chronic Unilateral Alkali Burn

A 23-year old man was burned with potash and bleach to left eye in June 1992. Although the eye was irrigated copiously immediately, upon initial examination on the day of the injury, visual acuity was 20/200 in the right eye and 20/20 in the left eye. By slit-lamp examination, a total corneal epithelial defect was noted together with devitalized inferonasal limbal and bulbar conjunctiva Two weeks after injury, a near total corneal epithelial defect containing inferonasal conjunctiva-limbal epithelium persisted, and by 4

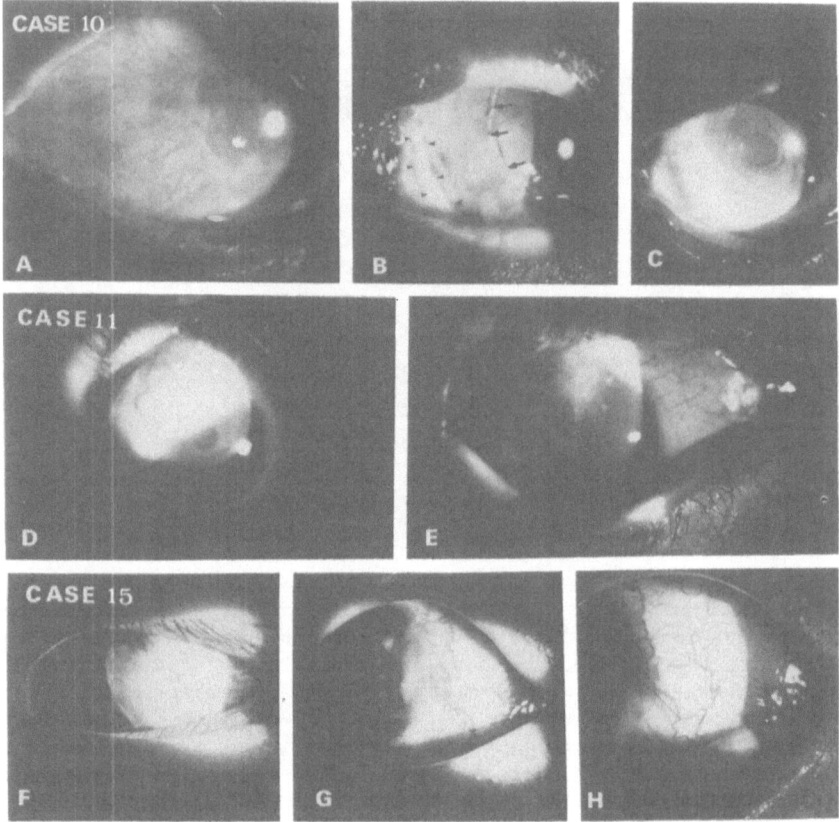

Figure 4. Case 10: A 23-year-old had an alkali injury to his left eye 9 months age, the cornea scarred with recurrent neovascularization, especially in inferonasal par (A). Three days after superficial lamellar keratectomy, amniotic membrane transplantation (arrows) and 3 × 12 mm conjunctiva limbal graft (arrow heads), subamniotic membrane hemorrhage still remained (B). Three years after surgery, visual acuity improved from 20/200 to 20/70. Stromal neovascularization much regressed but peripheral corneal opacity still remained (C). Case 11: An 11-year-old boy had choristoma with chronic recurrent keratoconjunctivitis which led to protruded soft mass on the cornea, limbal and bulbar conjunctiva (D) and visual acuity of 20/200. Two months after superficial keratectomy, amniotic membrane transplantation, 3 × 9 mm small conjunctival autograft, and visual acuity improved to 20/100 and relatively stable ocular surface (E). Case 15: A 4-year-old girl had a temporal pseudopterygium in left eye due to cryotherapy for retinopathy of prematurely. The fibrovascular dense band of scar tissue nearly united the temporal canthal skin to the limbus (F). Two years after superficial lamellar keratectomy with graft, amniotic membrane transplantation and 3 × 7 mm small conjunctival graft, visual acuity improved 20/30 to 20/70 and the operated eye is uninflamed and has not recurred and conjunctival graft remains nearly indistinguishable from adjacent conjunctiva (G, H).

weeks, vision was 20/400. During the next 8 months, chronic irritation, photophobia, and diplopia were accompanied by fibrovascular ingrowth and deep stromal neovascularization with scarring which were especially noted from the 5 to 11 o'clock position (Fig.4A). Nine months later, a superficial lamellar keratectomy, lysis of symblepharon and amniotic membrane transplantation with conjunctival autograft (Fig.4B) were performed. Postoperatively, subamniotic hemorrhage developed; it persisted for 9 days but eventually was absorbed. The epithelialization was rapid in the amniotic membrane, occurring within 5 days, and at that time deep stromal neovascularization began to regress. Extraocular movement had totally improved although the peripheral stromal opacity still remained 3 years after transplantation. Visual acuity had improved to 20/70 in the involved eye that was not inflamed, and had a smooth and stable ocular surface with complete involution of stromal neovascularization (Fig.4C).

Case 26: Acute Unilateral Alkali Injury

An 18-year-old boy was splashed in the left eye with liquefied cement (calcium hydroxide) in January, 1995. The eye was irrigated copiously immediately. Upon initial examination on the day of the injury his visual acuity was 20/20 with glasses in the right eye and 20/400 with glasses in the left eye, and he wore -2.5 Diopter myopic glasses for both eyes. By slit-lamp examination, the total corneal defect was seen and inferior bulbar conjunctival epithelium was devitalized (Fig 5A), the corneal stroma was diffusely hazy (Fig. 5B) and tenaciously adherent cement seen on the low fornix and corneal and conjunctival surface. Initial management included removal of cement deposition with topical antibiotic and steroid, and with oral ascorbate. Five days after injury, the corneal epithelial defect still persisted, and marked adherent cement substance on the entire corneal and limbal conjunctival was also noted. The next day, debridement of deposited cement substance on the cornea and a large amniotic membrane anchoring flap on the denuded corneal and limbus were performed. The epithelial defect gradually decreased and many cement substance deposits were noted on the stromal side of amniotic membrane (Fig.5C). Nine days after the amniotic membrane anchoring flap surgery, the membrane was removed, and the epithelial defect was nearly covered. Three days after removal of membrane, epithelial healing was completed and his vision improved to 20/50 with myopic glasses. The most recent examination disclosed that his visual acuity was 20/20 without myopic glasses in the left eye and he did not require myopic glasses in the left eye because of reduced myopia, but tiny small cement deposits in the peripheral cornea remained (Fig. 5D).

Case 27: Persistent Herpetic Ulceration

A 55-year-old man had persistent herpetic ulceration in the left eye. He had undergone mechanical debridement with antiviral therapy twice and experienced chemical cauterization due to persistent recurrent herpetic epithelial keratitis. When initially evaluated, his visual acuity was hand movement. Slit-lamp biomicroscopy revealed dendrogeographic ulceration that had gray, thickened borders formed by heaped-up epithelium unable to cross or adhere to melted the stromal bed with brownish pigmentation in upper part of covered epithelium (Fig. 5E). Diffuse corneal edema and fine KP on the endothelium were also noted. Subsequently, we performed debridement of melted stromal tissue with diseased epithelium and then also performed a temporary amniotic membrane anchoring flap using 10–0 nylon interrupted suture on the denuded corneal surface (Fig. 5E).

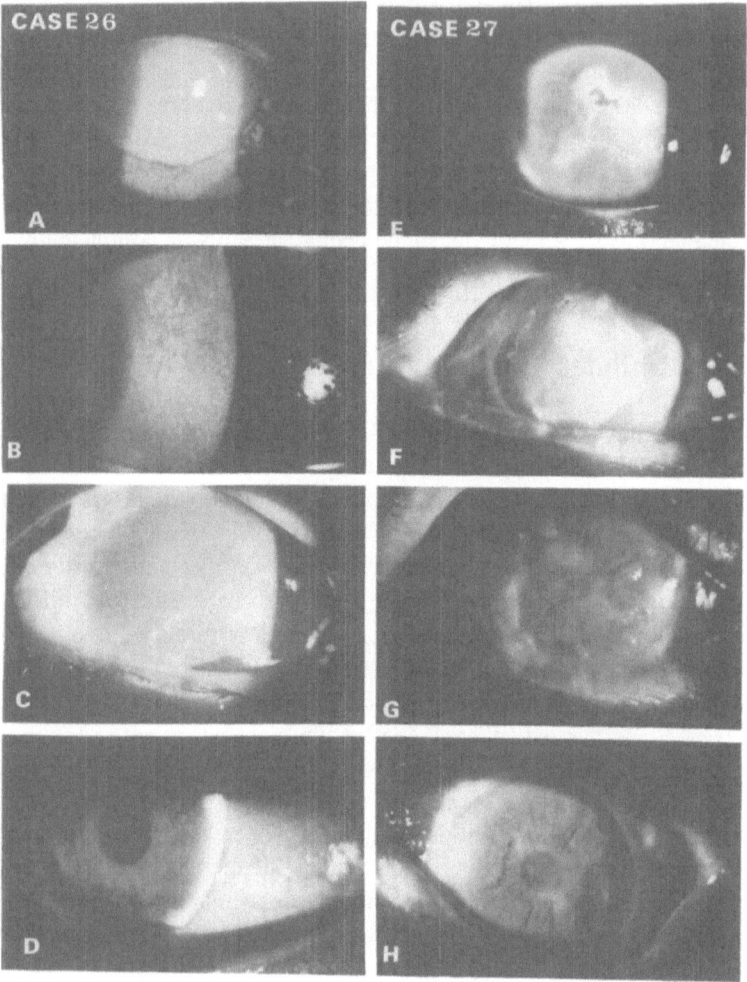

Figure 5. Case 26: An 18-year-old myopic boy was splashed in the left eye with liquefied cement (calcium hydroxide). Slit-lamp biomicroscopy revealed subtotal corneal epithelial defect and inferior limbal bulbar conjunctival epithelium devitalized (A), and the corneal stromal edema. Five days after injury, corneal epithelial defect persisted and marked adherent cement cast on the entire corneal surface (B). One day after temporary amniotic membrane flap with epithelial side down, many cement particles cast deposited on the amniotic membrane surface (C). Nine months after injury, visual acuity improved 20/400 to 20/20 without myopic glasses, but tiny small cement deposition in the peripheral corneal subepithelium remained (D). Case 27: A 55-year-old man had persistent herpetic ulceration in the left eye. Slit-lamp biomicroscopy revealed dendrogeographic ulceration which had gray, thickened borders formed by heaped-up epithelium unable to be across or adhere to melted stromal bed with brownish pigmentation in corneal epithelium (E), and diffuse corneal edema and fine KP on the endothelium were also noted. After 2 days, debridement of melted stromal tissue with diseased epithelium and temporary amniotic membrane anchoring flap were revealed (F). Three days after surgery, corneal healing was completed but superficial punctuate erosion stil remained (G). One year later, his visual acuity improved hand movement to 20/30 with hyperopic glasses but still remained mild superficial abnormal opacity (H).

Topical trifluorothymidine and Maxitrol® eye drop were applied four times a day. Three days later, corneal epithelial healing was completed (Fig. 5G) but superficial punctate keratitis still remained. At that time, his visual acuity improved to 20/200. One year later, he had a visual acuity 20/30 with +2.5 Diopter glasses, mild superficial stromal opacity and a stable ocular surface (Fig. 5H).

DISCUSSION

A literature review indicates that amniotic membrane has previously been used as a graft for skin burn, ulcer and artificial vagina, as a dressing for full thickness skin wound and repair of omphalocele, and as a means of preventing tissue adhesion surgery of head, abdomen, pelvis, and otolarynx.[15] In 1940, De Roth[16] first reported the use of amniotic membrane in the eye for the repair of conjunctival symblepharon and defects. Kim and Tseng[10] have previously reported the efficacy of amniotic membrane transplantation in restoring the corneal surface severely damaged by chemical and surgical means in a rabbit model. We present here the first detailed report of amniotic membrane transplantation with or without conjunctival-limbal autograft for advanced recurrent pterygium and pseudopterygium. We also report that temporary amniotic membrane flap can be used to acute chemical burn injury, for recalcitrant ulceration, and for corneal perforation.

Successful corneal surface reconstruction was noted by amniotic membrane transplantation, especially when combined with conjunctiva-limbal autograft, which yielded better results than did simple amniotic membrane transplantation. Although the recurrence rate (18%) was relatively high with simple amniotic membrane transplantation, compared with conjunctival autograft reports,[9,18] the rate was lower than that seen with bare excision technique.[17] In amniotic membrane transplantation with conjunctival grafts, all cases had no recurrence and had achieved rapid surface healing, stable ocular surface without persistent epithelial defect, progressive regression of corneal neovascularization, restoration of a smooth and optically improved ocular surface which resulted in improved visual acuity, and probably increased success for subsequent keratoplasty. These clinical findings are further supported by other human data showing that conjunctiva-limbal autograft transplantation carries a lower recurrence rate[8] in pterygium and pseudopterygium. In the present study, amniotic membrane replaced by removal of abnormal basement membrane and inflamed stromal tissue provide suitable basement membrane substrate and might maintain a better microenvironment. Furthermore, transplanted conjunctiva-limbal graft provides stem cells and restores the barrier function to protect abnormal conjunctival epithelial growth. Taken together, amniotic membrane transplantation with conjunctiva-limbal graft on the limbal region provides a strong and potent healing source, a feature compatible with stem cell properties.

The phenomenon that the migrating conjunctival epithelium on the corneal surface can morphologically transform into a corneal epithelium has been termed conjunctival transdifferentiation.[18,19] Previously, conjunctival transdifferentiation was modulated by corneal vascularization and by change in the local supply of vitamin A or retinoid.[20–23] In addition to reported results[24–29] of conjunctival transdifferentiation that could be influenced by the extracelluar environment, the in vivo study by Kim and Tseng[10] further indicated that transplanting amniotic membrane-containing basement membrane could facilitate such a phenotypic change. That basement membrane could be another important environment factor that was first speculated by Rodriguez et al.[30] and confirmed by Kurpakus et al.,[31] who showed that corneal basement membrane stimulates cultured conjunctival epithelial cells to express corneal epithelium phenotype (K12 keratin). In this clinical study, all successful transplanted cases had no or minimal vascularization. It is also speculated that avascularity might have a synergistic effect with that of the basement membrane in modulating such a phenotypic change. Transplanted amniotic membrane might contain a component similar to that of corneal basement membrane, and act as a good extracellular substrate. Previously, disappearance of the basement membrane after an alkali injury has been noted.[32] Therefore, the restoration of a basement membrane by amniotic membrane transplantation in part contributes to the recovery of the healthy normal corneal and conjunctival epithelium. Clinically, severe corneal surface destruction can occur in number of diseases, including those mentioned in the Introduction, characterized by a clear history of limbal cell loss. We also consider another potential impending conditions of limbal cell damage by inflammatory insults which can occur in a various condition such as recalcitrant corneal ulceration and initial stage of chemical bums. For the former conditions with unilateral or focal involvement, autograft limbal transplantation is effective for corneal surface reconstruction.[3,5-18] For the latter cases, we need to improve the microenvironment by preventing inflammatory insults such as inflammatory cytokines,[33] and inflammatory cells[32] from gaining access to the ocular surface. Results indicate that temporary amniotic membrane flap treatment for recalcitrant corneal ulceration and acute phase of chemical burns can induce rapid epithelial and stromal wound healing with a stable ocular surface.

Amniotic membrane that contains a high concentration of b-FGF reported by Shinozaki at al.,[34] basement membrane components,[10-13] and unknown trophic factors, can provide good cell basement membrane interaction that is critical for epithelial proliferation and differentiation.[26,27,29-31]

We prefer that the present results for various ocular surface diseases might also be viewed in a broader context, as amniotic membrane transplantation with or without conjunctiva-limbal autograft now offers anatomically and functionally satisfaction, and, in some cases, visually spectacular results. Furthermore, transplantation of preserved human amniotic membrane should circumvent the need of immunosuppressive agents because no viable cells are transplanted, and these procedures are technical straightforwardly require no additional surgical skills or instrumentation, and have multiple applications. We envision that amniotic membrane transplantation will be useful for effective ocular surface reconstruction.

ACKNOWLEDGMENTS

The authors thank Dr. Scheffer CG Tseng for scientific advice and critical review of the manuscript.

REFERENCES

1. S.C.G. Tseng, Chen, J.J.Y., Huang, A.J.W., et al., Classification of conjunctival surgeries for corneal disease based on stem cell concept. *Ophthalmol. Clin. North Am.* 3:595 (1990).
2. S.C.G. Tseng, Concept and application of limbal stem cells. *Eye* 3:141 (1989).
3. S.C.G. Tseng, Conjunctival grafting for corneal disease. In, *Duane's Clinical Ophthalmology*, W. Tasman, and Jaeger, E.A., eds., (1994).
4. R.J.F. Tsai, Sun, T-T., and Tseng, S.C.G., Comparison of limbal and conjunctival autograft transplantation in corneal surface reconstruction in rabbits. *Ophthalmol.* 97:446 (1990).

5. K.R. Keynon, and Tseng, S.C.G., Limbal autograft transplantation for ocular surface disorder. *Ophthalmol.* 96:709 (1989).

6. R.A. Copeland, and Char, D.H., Limbal autograft reconstruction after conjunctival squamous cell carcinoma. *Am. J. Ophthalmol.* 110:412 (1990).

7. C. Jonkins, Tuft, S., Lin, C., and Buckley, R., Limbal transplantation in the management of chronic contact-lens-associated epitheliopathy. *Eye* 7:629 (1993).

8. K.H. Kenyon, Wagoner, M.D., and Hettinger, M.E., Conjunctival autograft transplantation for advanced and recurrent pterygium. *Ophthalmology* 92:1461 (1985).

9. J.M. Koch, Mellin KB, and Waubke, T.N., The pterygium, autologous conjunctiva-limbus transplantation as treatment. *Ophthalmology* 89(2):143 (1992).

10. J.C. Kim, and Tseng, S.C.G., Transplantation of preserved human amniotic membrane for surface reconstruction in severely damaged rabbit corneas. *Cornea* 14:473 (1995).

11. R.A. Thoft, Conjunctival transplantation. *Arch. Ophthalmol.* 95:1425 (1977).

12. W.K. Herman, Doughman, D.J., and Lindstrom, R.L., Conjunctival autograft transplantation for unilateral ocular surface disease. *Ophthalmology* 90:1121 (1983).

13. K.H. Kenyon, Wagoner, M.D., and Hettinger, M.E., Conjunctival autograft transplantation for advanced and recurrent pterygium. *Ophthalmology* 92:1461 (1985).

14. T. Gundersen, Conjunctival flap in the treatment of corneal disease with reference to a new technique of application. *Arch. Ophthalmol.* 60:880 (1958).

15. J.D. Telford, and Trelford-Sauder, M., The amnion in surgery, past and present. *Am. J. Obstet. Gynecol.* 134:833 (1979).

16. A. DeRoth, Plastic repair of conjunctival defects with fetal membrane. *Arch. Ophthalmol.* 23:522 (1940).

17. M. Fine, Recurrent pterygium: mucous membrane grafts. In, *Symposium on Medical and Surgical Diseases of the Cornea; Transsection of the New Orleans Academy of Ophthalmology* C.V. Mosby, St. Louis (1980).

18. J. Friend, and Thoft, R.A., Functional competence of regenerating ocular surface epithelium. *Invest. Opthalmol. Vis. Sci.* 17:135 (1979).

19. R.A. Thoft, and Friend, J., The X, Y, Z, hypothesis of corneal epithelial maintenance. *Invest. Ophthalmol. Vis. Sci.* 24:1442 91983).

20. A.J.W. Huang, Watson, B.D., Hernan deg, E., and Tseng, S.C.G., Induction of conjunctival transdifferentiation by photothrombotic occlusion of corneal neovascularization. *Ophthalmology* 95:228 (1988).

21. S.C.G. Tseng, Hirst, L.W., Faradaghi, M., and Green, W.R., Goblet cell density and vascularization during conjunctival transdifferentiation. *Invest. Ophthalmol. Vis. Sci.* 25:1168 (1984).

22. S.C.G. Tseng, Hirst, L.W., Faradaghi, M., and Green, W.R., Inhibition of conjunctival transdifferentiation by topical retinoids. *Invest. Ophthalmol. Vis. Sci.* 28:537 (1987).

23. S.C.G. Tseng, Faradaghi, M., and Rider, A.A., Conjunctival transdifferentiation induced by systemic vitamin A deficiency. *Invest. Ophthalmol. Vis. Sci.* 28:1497 (1987).

24. S.C.G. Tseng, and Faradaghi, M., Reversal of conjunctival transdifferentiation by retinoids. *Cornea* 7:273 (1988).

25. A. Schermer, Galvin S., and Sun, T-T., Differentiation-related expression of a major 64K corneal keratin *in vivo* and in culture suggests limbal location of corneal epithelial stem cells. *J. Cell. Biol.* 103:49 (1986).

26. W.Y.W. Chen, Mui, M-M, Kay, WW-Y, et al., Conjunctival epithelial cells do not transdifferentiate in organotipic cultures: expression of K_{12} keratin is restricted to corneal epithelium. *Curr. Eye. Res.* 13:765 (1994).

27. S. Kinoshita, Nishida, K., Kiritoshi, A., et al., Keratin expression in the conjunctival epithelium can be greatly influenced by the external environment. *Invest. Ophthalmol. Vis. Sci.* 33(S):1176 (1992).

28. A. Kiritoshi, Nishida, K., Ohashi, Y., et al., 64 kd keratin expression in normal conjunctival epithelium. *Invst. Ophthalmol. Vis. Sci.* 34(S):1490 (1993).

29. Z-G. Wei, Wu, R-L., Lavuka, R.M., and Sun, T-T., *In vitro* growth and differentiation of rabbit bulbar, fornix, and palpebral conjunctival epithelia. Implications on conjunctival epithelial transdifferentiation and stemcell. *Invest. Ophthalmol. Vis. Sci.* 34:1814 (1993).

30. M. Rodriguez, Ben-Zvi, A., Krachmer, J., et al., Suprabasal expression of a 64 kilodalton keratin in developing human corneal epithelium. *Differentiation* 34:60 (1987).

31. M.A. Kurpakus, Stock, E.L., and Jones, J.C.R., The role of the basement membrane in differential expression of keratin proteins in epithelial cells. *Dev. Biol.* 150:243 (1992).

32. R.R. Pfister, and Berstein, N., The alkali-burned cornea. I. Epithelial and stromal repair. *Exp. Eye Rcs.* 23:519 (1976).

33. D.T. Jones, Munroy, D., Ji, Z., et al., Sjögren's syndrome: cytokine and Epstein-Barr viral gene expression within the conjunctival epithelium. *Invest. Ophthalmol. Vis. Sci.* 35:3493 (1994).

34. N. Shinozaki, Shoda, A., Shimazaki, J., et al., Detection of basic fibroblast growth factor (b-FGF) from amniotic membrane. *Invest. Ophthalmol. Vis. Sci.* 36(S):131 (1995).

13

DIFFERENTIAL DIAGNOSIS BETWEEN CORNEAL INTRAEPITHELIAL NEOPLASIA AND CONJUNCTIVAL EPITHELIAL INVASION BY IMPRESSION CYTOLOGY

Keiko Matsumoto, Kohji Nishida, and Shigeru Kinoshita

Department of Ophthalmology
Kyoto Prefectural University of Medicine
Kyoto, Japan

ABSTRACT

The differential diagnosis of noninflammatory peripheral corneal epithelial haze of unknown etiology includes corneal intraepithelial neoplasia and conjunctival epithelial invasion. However, on the basis of the clinical manifestations alone, it is difficult to distinguish between these two entities. The purpose of this study was to evaluate the efficacy of impression cytology in the differential diagnosis of these two conditions. Six eyes from six consecutive patients with noninflammatory peripheral corneal epithelial haze of unknown etiology, who presented to our clinic between September 1993 and December 1995, were enrolled in this study. In all of the eyes, the haze mainly affected the epithelial layers and arose at the limbus. To determine whether goblet cells were present in the involved epithelium, impression cytology was performed. In three eyes, a large number of goblet cells were found in the affected regions, thus indicating that the etiology was conjunctival epithelial invasion. In contrast, in the other three eyes, larger squamous cells, but not goblet cells, were found; this was suggestive of corneal epithelial neoplasia. In two of the latter cases, a pathological examination of the tissues excised at surgery confirmed the above diagnosis. These results indicate that impression cytology of the affected region is important to the accurate diagnosis of noninflammatory peripheral corneal epithelial haze.

INTRODUCTION

Corneal intraepithelial neoplasia is a rare pathological condition that affects corneal epithelium unilaterally or bilaterally.[1] This disease almost always arises at the limbus of the eye, with or without a limbal mass, and extends into the cornea. The abnormal epithelium appears frosted or opalescent. Recently, based on the concept that dysplasia and carcinoma *in situ* are actually part of a single disease entity, the term "intraepithelial neoplasia" has replaced the terms dysplasia, carcinoma *in situ*, Bowen's disease, intraepithelioma, etc. This terminology can be applied to both the conjunctival epithelium[2] and the corneal epithelium.[1,3] Recently, this pathological condition has been reported to be caused by human papilloma virus (HPV) types 16 and 18.[4,5]

In cases of noninflammatory peripheral corneal epithelial haze of unknown etiology, the difficulty is in differentiating between corneal intraepithelial neoplasia and conjunctival epithelial invasion on the basis of their clinical manifestations alone, especially when the corneal intraepithelial neoplasia has no limbal mass. Previously, the removal or debridement of the abnormal region was performed for a pathological examination.[3] However, this procedure is invasive, and cannot be repeated easily. Impression cytology is a noninvasive method for the pathological examination of the ocular surface epithelium.[6-8] The present study evaluated the efficacy of impression cytology for the differential diagnosis of these two conditions.

PATIENTS AND METHODS

In this study six eyes from six consecutive patients with noninflammatory peripheral corneal epithelial haze of unknown etiology were studied. These patients were examined at the outpatient clinic of the Department of Ophthalmology at the Kyoto Prefectural University of Medicine between September 1993 and December 1995. The six patients consisted of four males and two females who ranged in age from 39 to 83 years. Of these six patients, two had bilateral abnormalities and only the more involved eye was enrolled in this study. The other four patients had unilateral involvement. Two patients had surgical histories. Table 1 summarizes the patient profiles, including surgical treatment for the corneal abnormality. This study was approved by the Institutional Review Board (IRB) on Human Experiments of the Research Committee of the Kyoto Prefectural University of Medicine.

Slit-lamp biomicroscopic examinations were performed to observe the area of corneal opacification and the fluorescein staining pattern, as well as to confirm the presence or absence of a limbal mass. Following fully informed consent, involved peripheral corneal epithelial specimens were collected from all six subject eyes using the impression cytology technique previously reported. (Fig. 1).[8] Briefly, filter paper with a pore size of 0.22 μm was obtained commercially (MF Millipore filter VS). Circular sheets of this material were cut into strips measuring approximately 5 x 8 mm. After impression cytology, the eye was stained with fluorescein and photographed with a blue filter. The photograph

Table 1. Patient profile

Patient no.	Age (gender)	Bilateral (B) or unilateral (U)	Subject eye	Surgical history	Surgical treatment
1	73(M)	U	Right	None	—
2	69(F)	U	Right	None	Keratoepithelioplasty
3	39(M)	B	Left	None	Keratoepithelioplasty
4	74(F)	U	Left	ICCE	Keratoepithelioplasty
5	45(M)	B	Left	None (Light eye)	—
6	83(M)	U	Left	ECCE (Both eyes)	Keratoepithelioplasty

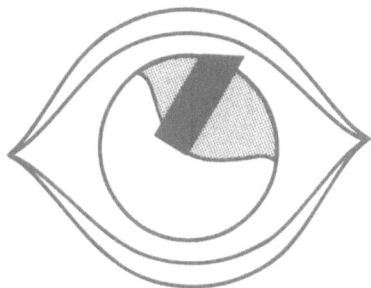

Figure 1. Schematic representation of the impression cytology technique. Superficial layer of involved epithelium was collected by this method.

was then used to double-check the position of the strip on the abnormal epithelium. The specimens thus obtained were fixed in 10% neutral buffered formaldehyde for at least 24 hours, stained with periodic acid-Schiff stain for 15 minutes and hematoxylin for two minutes, cleared with xylene, and then permanently mounted. Finally, the strip was observed to determine whether goblet cells were present in the involved epithelium.

For treatment, surgical removal and keratoepithelioplasty were performed in four eyes (patients 2, 3, 4, and 6)(Table 1). A definite pathological diagnosis was obtained in two of these cases (patients 2 and 4), but not in the others (patients 3 and 6) because of a loss of the sample morphology following surgery.

RESULTS

In all six subject eyes, the corneal epithelial haze extended from the limbus to the visual axis without neovascularization, and resulted in a decrease in visual acuity. One eye (patient 4) had a limbal mass, but the other five did not. The involved epithelium exhibited strong staining to fluorescein (Table 2, Fig. 2).

The impression cytology study (Table 2) revealed that many goblet cells were present in the involved epithelium in three eyes (patients 1, 5, and 6) (Fig. 3a), indicating that the etiology in these cases was conjunctival epithelial invasion. In these cases, the size and morphology of the involved epithelium collected was similar to the normal conjunctival epithelium. In contrast, in the other three eyes (patients 2, 3, and 4), larger squamous cells but no goblet cells were found (Fig. 3b). This was suggestive of corneal intraepithelial neoplasia. In two of the latter cases (patients 2 and 4), a pathological examination of the tissues excised at surgery confirmed the above diagnosis by demonstrating moderate squamous cell dysplasia in patient 2 and carcinoma *in situ* in patient 4 (Fig. 4).

In patients 1 and 5, after impression cytology, a normal-appearing epithelium without any haze recovered on the area where the impression cytology had been performed, resulting in an improvement in visual acuity. In patients 2, 3, 4, and 6 the surgical removal and keratoepithelioplasty resulted in no recurrence and improved visual acuity.

DISCUSSION

It is generally believed that noninflammatory peripheral corneal haze of unknown etiology is due either to corneal intraepithelial neoplasia[1,3] or to conjunctival epithelial invasion. In the six eyes studied here, the involved epithelium had a very similar appear-

Table 2. Clinical and histological findings

Patient No.	Corneal Haze Area	Presence or Absence of Limbal Mass	Fluorescein Staining	Best-Corrected Visual Acuity Pre-ope	Post-ope	Impression Cytology Presence or Absence of Goblet cell	Histopathologic Examination	Differential Diagnosis
1	1/3	Absence	+	20/300	20/50*	Presence	–	conjunctival epithelial invasion
2	1/2	Absence	+	20/50	20/25	Absence	moderate dysplasia	corneal intraepithelial neoplasia
3	1/3	Absence	+	20/100	20/20	Absence	–	corneal intraepithelial neoplasia
4	1/2	Presence	+	20/200	20/20	Absence	carcinoma in situ	corneal intraepithelial neoplasia
5	1/2	Absence	+	20/300	20/20*	Presence	–	conjunctival epithelial invasion
6	1/2	Absence	+	20/200	20/20	Presence	–	conjunctival epithelial invasion

* post-impression cytology visual acuity

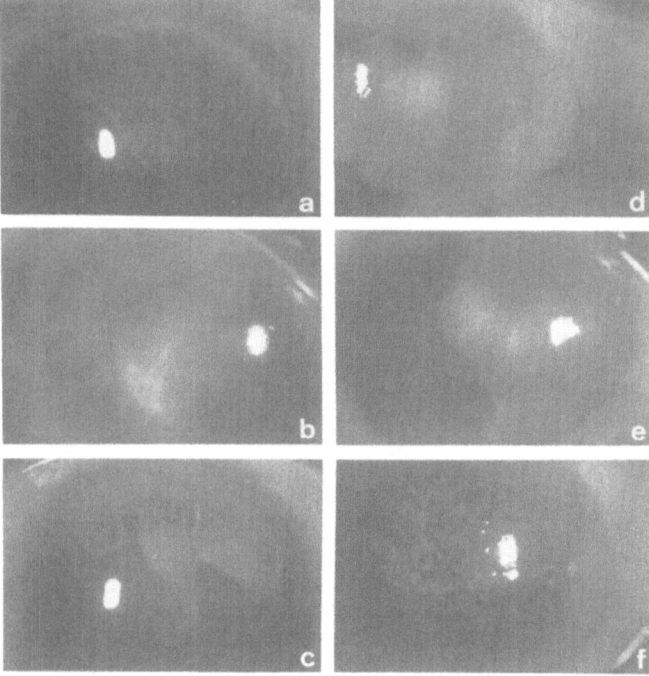

Figure 2. Representative slit lamp photomicrographs with fluorescein staining. (a-f) Indicate patients 1–6, respectively. In all six eyes, the involved epithelium exhibited strong staining to fluorescein.

ance; the epithelium was opalescent without neovascularization, extending from the limbus to the corneal center, and exhibited strong staining to fluorescein. Judging from the clinical appearance alone, it is difficult to differentiate between the above diseases. However, the existence of a limbal mass in case 4 suggested that this abnormality was corneal and conjunctival intraepithelial neoplasia.[1,3] Of these six patients, the abnormality was bilateral in two patients and unilateral in the other four. Two patients had eye surgery history. Since both of the above conditions can be either bilateral or unilateral, and both can be induced by eye surgery, this information is not very useful for making a differential diagnosis.

Based on the results from the impression cytology examination, these eyes could be divided into two groups. In one group (patients 1, 5, and 6), goblet cells were found, while no goblet cells were found in the other group (patients 2, 3, and 4). Since the presence of goblet cells is specific for the conjunctival epithelium on the ocular surface, these results indicate that the etiology of the former group was conjunctival epithelial invasion, whereas the latter group was suffering from corneal intraepithelial neoplasia. In addition, in two eyes (patients 2 and 4) from the latter group, a pathological examination confirmed the above diagnosis. Impression cytological study of the affected region is therefore important in accurately diagnosing noninflammatory peripheral corneal epithelial haze.

In patients 1 and 5, the impression cytology resulted in a therapeutic effect as well as diagnostic information. Since this technique removes the superficial layers of the epithelium, it was likely that in these eyes, the abnormality was present only in the superficial layers of the affected region. In addition, since the dysplastic changes are more

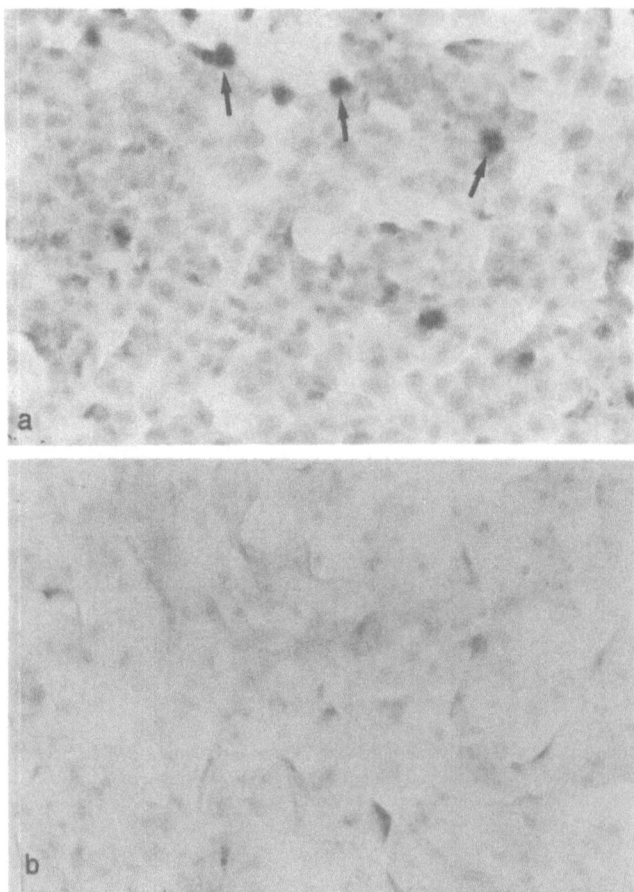

Figure 3. Histologic examination using impression cytology. (a) In patient 1, goblet cells (arrows) were present; (b) in patient 4, larger squamous cells but not goblet cells were found (PAS staining, magnification x50).

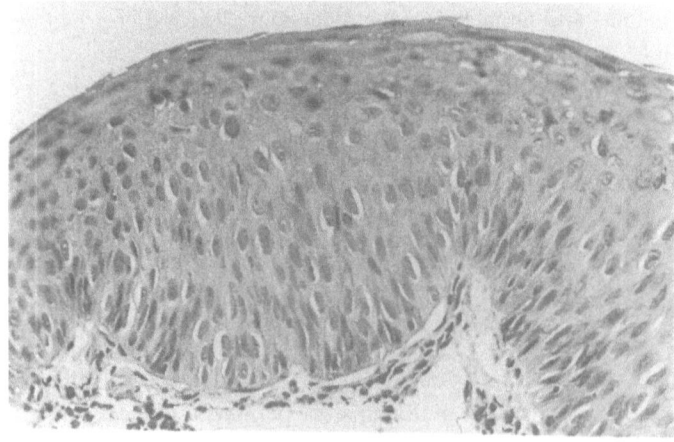

Figure 4. Histopathology in patient 4. In the epithelial layers, there was a considerable number of undifferentiated dysplastic cells which showed significant nuclear pleomorphism and dyskeratosis. Some inflammatory cells were also seen in the subepithelial region (hematoxylin and eosin staining, magnification x66).

pronounced in the deeper epithelial layer,[1] the improvements seen after impression cytology also suggested that these eyes suffered from conjunctival invasion rather than corneal intraepithelial neoplasia. From both diagnostic and therapeutic viewpoints, impression cytology is an important tool in diagnosing noninflammatory peripheral corneal epithelial haze.

ACKNOWLEDGMENTS

Supported in part by a grant in-aid for scientific research (07771557) from the Ministry of Education, Culture, and Science of Japan, a research grant from the Kyoto Foundation for the Promotion of Medical Science, and by a grant from the intramural research fund of the Kyoto Prefectural University of Medicine.

REFERENCES

1. G.O. Waring, III, Roth, A.M., and Ekins, M.B., Clinical and pathologic description of 17 cases of corneal intraepithelial neoplasia. *Am. J. Ophthalmol.* 97:547 (1984).
2. L.D. Pizzarello, and Jacobiec, F.A., Bowen's disease of the conjunctiva: a nismoner. In, *Ocular and Adnexal Tumors*, Aesculapius, Birmingham (1978).
3. J.C. Erie, Campbell, R.J., and Liesegang, T.J., Conjunctival and corneal intraepithelial and invasive neoplasia. *Ophthalmology* 93:176 (1986).
4. S.A. Lauer, Malter, J.S., and Meier, J.R., Human papillomavirus type 18 in conjunctival intraepithelial neoplasia. *Am. J. Ophthalmol.* 110:23 (1990).
5. M.G. Ordich, Jakobiec, F.A., Lancaster, W.D., et al., A spectrum of bilateral squamous conjunctival tumors associated with human papillomavirus type 16. *Ophthalmology* 98:628 (1991).
6. J.D. Nelson, Havener, V.R., and Cameron, J.D., Cellulose acetate impressions of the ocular surface. Dry eye states. *Arch. Ophthalmol.* 101:1869 (1983).
7. S.C.G. Tseng, Staging of conjunctival squamous metaplasia by impression cytology. *Ophthalmology* 92:728 (1985).
8. M. Ohji, Ohmi, G., Kiritoshi, A., and Kinishita, S., Goblet cell density in thermal and chemical injuries. *Arch. Ophthalmol.* 105:1696 (1987).

14

FROZEN SECTION GUIDED LAMELLO-LAMELLAR SCLEROKERATOPLASTY IN SQUAMOUS CELL CARCINOMA OF CONJUNCTIVA AND CORNEA

Anita Panda, Namrata Sharma, Supriyo Ghose, J. S. Titiyal, S. K. Angra, and Seema Sen

All India Institute of Medical Sciences
New Delhi, India

ABSTRACT

Twenty-one eyes with conjunctival and corneal squamous cell carcinoma underwent microscopically controlled, frozen section guided excisions. Fresh/M.K./glycerine-preserved donor corneas were used to cover the defect with a lamellar graft. No recurrence was seen over a mean follow up of 5.5 ± 2 years (range 1–15 years). Useful visual acuity of $\geq 6/24$ was achieved in 67% of the eyes and no eye had astigmatism >4D at the end of 1 year. Poor visual acuity (<6/24) in 33% of the eyes studied was due to associated cataract. All grafts remained clear to partially clear at the end of minimum follow up and good cosmesis was achieved in all the cases. No complication was seen, except in one case in which postoperative symblepharon occurred and was managed successfully.

INTRODUCTION

The primary modality and most accepted method of treatment of squamous cell carcinoma of the conjunctiva and cornea is excision with wide surgical margins.[1-3] Recurrence following excision is the most ominous complication encountered and has been reported at a rate of 15–69% in the literature.[2-5] Other therapies that have been evaluated are adjuvant cryotherapy and radiotherapy; these modalities have achieved variable results.[6,7] In addition, other treatment modalities, like chemotherapy and immunotherapy are still in infancy stages.[2] Frozen section controlled excision and modified Moh's microsurgical excision have been undertaken in isolated cases in limited studies.[1,8,9]

Advances in Corneal Research, edited by Lass
Plenum Press, New York, 1997

This paper presents experience in microscopically-controlled, frozen section guided excision of 21 patients with squamous cell carcinoma of the conjunctiva and cornea, followed by lamello-lamellar sclerokeratoplasty over a period of the last 15 years.

PATIENTS AND METHODS

Twenty-one patients with clinical diagnosis of squamous cell carcinoma of the conjunctiva and cornea reported to the Cornea Service at Dr. Rajendra Prasad Centre for Ophthalmic Sciences from 1980 to 1995. All patients had large, exophytic, unilateral limbal masses which extended well onto the cornea and were adhered to the underlying tissues (Fig. 1). No patient had evidence of any intraocular or intraorbital extension. All but one eye had a history of more than one previous excision; one eye had been subjected to more than four excisions. Minimal to moderate lenticular opacities were present in 16 eyes. Routine ophthalmologic examination included visual acuity, slit lamp biomicroscopy, photography, and posterior segment evaluation in each patient. Gonioscopy to rule out angle involvement, keratometry, and specular microscopy were undertaken in these eyes, wherever possible. Systemic examination was apparently normal with no preauricular and cervical lymphadenopathy in any patient. Maximum conjunctival and corneal involvement of the growth was measured from the limbus in each eye (Table 1). The conjunctival extent varied from 3 mm to a maximum of 6 mm and no muscle was involved in any eye. Corneal extent was noted and near total corneal involvement was seen in two eyes. Limbal involvement of various degrees was also noted in each eye, which revealed that the temporal limbus was most commonly involved (nine eyes), followed by superior (eight eyes), and nasal (four eyes); no lesion was seen inferiorly.

Surgical Technique

The surgery was performed under local anesthesia. Peritumor conjunctival incision was made 5 mm away from the tumor mass. The underlying bleeders were cauterized and

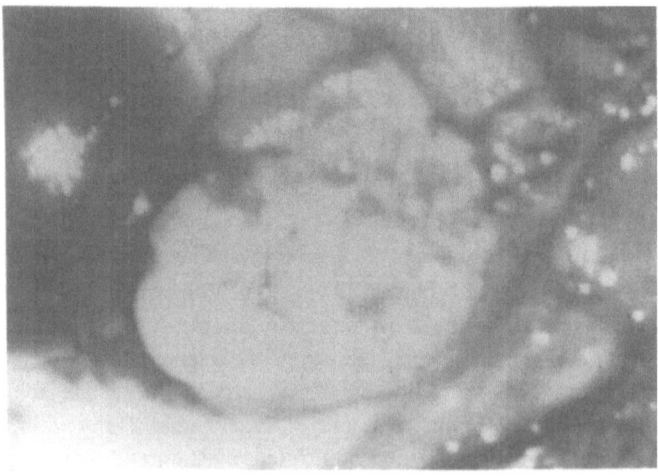

Figure 1. Preoperative squamous cell carcinoma.

Table 1. Conjunctival, corneal, and limbal extent of squamous cell carcinoma

	No. of eyes
Conjunctival extent (mm)	
3	2
4	4
5	9
6	6
Corneal extent (mm)	
3–4	7
5–6	7
7–8	5
9–10	2
Limbal extent (degrees)	
>90°	6
90–180°	9
180–270°	4
>270°	2

the tumor mass was undermined gently. The separation of the mass was carried out from the unaffected to the affected zone. The whole mass was sent for histopathological evaluation. A 0.2 mm deep corneoscleral mark was made 2 mm from the microscopically identified tumor margin, either with the help of trephine or free hand dissection. This first layer of corneoscleral/corneal tissue was dissected lamellarly and was also sent for histopathological studies. Thereafter, a second layer of corneoscleral tissue 0.1 mm thick was dissected lamellarly; this layer had the same horizontal dimensions as the first layer. This layer was placed on absorbent paper (filter paper) to prevent any curling of the edges, and hence its proper assessment. The tissue was properly oriented and sent for frozen section evaluation. The tissue margins, as well as the undersurface, were scanned by an ocular pathologist for the presence of residual malignant cells. The next step was frozen section dependent. If the under-surface revealed the presence of tumor cells, a 0.1 mm thick layer was again dissected and the specimen underwent a repeat frozen section evaluation. If, however, both edges and the undersurface showed the presence of malignant cells, the horizontal extent was increased by 2 mm further and depth of removal was increased by 0.1 mm. When the tissue margins and under-surface were declared free of tumor cells, a size and depth matched corneal tissue was dissected lamellarly from fresh/MK/glycerine-preserved donor corneas. Non-viable corneas not fit for penetrating keratoplasty were used. Interrupted sutures with 10–0 monofilament were used to fix the donor cornea to the host bed and the knots were buried (Fig. 2). The patients were followed up regularly.

RESULTS

Twenty-one patients with squamous cell carcinoma consisted of twelve females and nine males. The mean age was 56 ± 9 years (range 47–73 years). Sixteen eyes had associated cataract. All patients were followed up for a minimum of 1 year. The maximum follow up was 15 years (mean 5.5 ± 2 years). Sixty-seven percent of the eyes had a useful visual acuity of 6/24 or more at the end of 1 year of follow up (Table 2) and no eye had an

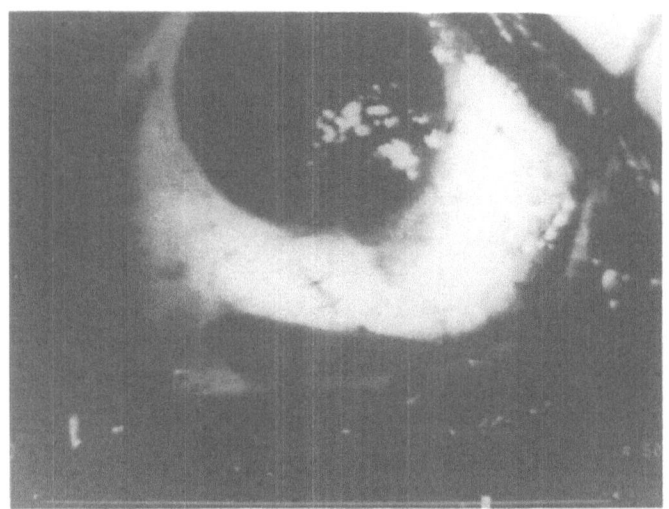

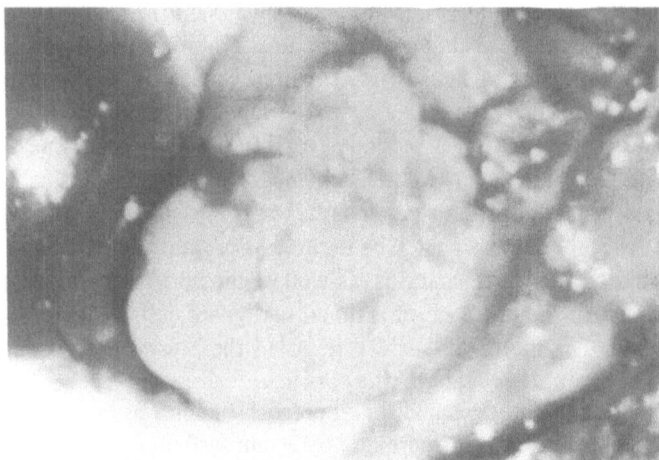

Figure 2. Excised tumor with a lamello-lamellar sclerokeratoplasty.

Table 2. Visual acuity

	Pre-op (No. of eyes)	Post-op (No. of eyes)
<6/60	17	1
6/60	1	2
6/36	1	4
6/24	2	10
6/18	–	3
6/12	–	1

Table 3. Graft clarity grading[10]

Grades	A/c details	Corneal thickness
4[+]	Clearly visible	Normal
3[+]	Clearly visible	Increase up to 20%
2[+]	Faintly visible	Increase 21–40%
1[+]	Faintly visible	Increase >40%
0	Not visible	Not possible

astigmatism of more than 4 D. Graft clarity was graded based on anterior chamber details and corneal thickness (Table 3).[10] and all grafts remained clear to partially clear at the end of 1 year (Table 4). One eye developed symblepharon postoperatively, which was managed successfully by release of the same followed by symblepharon ring.

PATHOLOGICAL EVALUATION

Preoperatively, the dissected margins of the corneoscleral layer and the undersurface were declared free of the tumor cells in all but two eyes. In one eye, the tissue margins were positive for tumor cells, hence an additional 2 mm of the corneoscleral extent was dissected. In another eye, the margins and the undersurface showed evidence of malignancy and further 2 mm of corneoscleral extent with 0.1 mm thickness was dissected. Repeat frozen section evaluation, however, did not reveal any tumor cells. All the specimens of tumor masses subjected to histopathological evaluation confirmed the diagnosis of well-differentiated invasive squamous cell carcinoma (Fig. 3).

DISCUSSION

Surgical excision, cryotherapy, and radiation therapy have been utilized to treat squamous cell carcinoma of the cornea and conjunctiva with variable rates of recurrence and complications.[2,3,6,7] Simple excision of squamous cell carcinoma is associated with high rates of recurrence.[2] However, histologically verified tumor-free tissue margins is not assured by excision alone.[1,2] Recurrence rate varying from 5% in verified free surgical margins to 53% in incompletely excised margins have been known.[1,5] Microscopically controlled excision reported no recurrence after excision.[1] However, a second stage repeat surgery was required in 21% of cases when the histopathological presence of tumor cells in the excised tissue was confirmed.[1] In this series, larger tumors with deeper invasion of the underlying tissues were encountered, thus necessitating a lamellar corneoscleral graft.

Table 4. Post-op graft clarity

Grades	No. of eyes
4[+]	3 (14.29%)
3[+]	9 (42.86%)
2[+]	7 (33.31%)
1[+]	2 (9.54%)

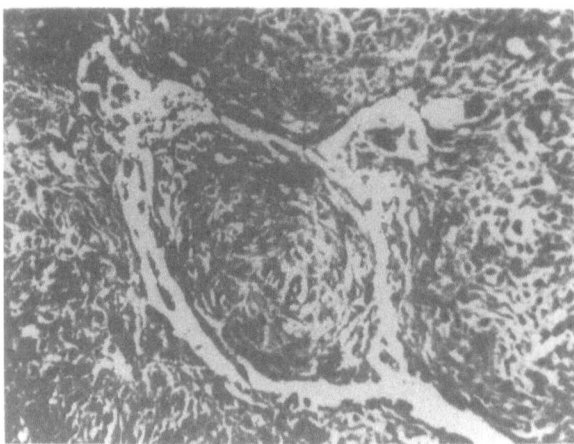

Figure 3. Histopathology: well-differentiated squamous cell carcinoma.

This is attributed to the repeated incomplete excisions that were seen in 20 out of 21 eyes. Incompletely excised tumors presented more aggressively after each recurrence.[3] Thus, a lamellar graft following surgical excision was required in all eyes in the present series.

Frozen section guided excision has been undertaken previously, but only in isolated cases in limited studies.[8,9] The purpose of microscopically controlled, frozen section guided excision was to locate the a slender "silent" cancerous outgrowths and to follow them selectively to their terminations, which may be beyond the clinically or microscopically visible borders of the tumor mass. The precision of microscopic control provides not only the maximal eradication of tumor but also ensures maximum sparing of the adjacent normal ocular tissue. Modified frozen section analysis done for the tumor cells from the margins as well as the undersurface eliminated the malignant cells not only from its horizontal extent but also along its depth. Thus, there was no recurrence seen in any eyes in this series after an average follow up of 5.5 ± 2 years (range 1–15 years).

Useful visual acuity of 6/24 or more was attained in 67% of eyes at the end of one year. Poor visual acuity following surgery was attributed to cataract and presence of incision line and suture marks in front of the pupillary axis. Of 16 eyes with associated cataract, nine underwent a subsequent cataract extraction with good vision. However, no eye had an astigmatism of more than 4D postoperatively, even when the tissue dissection was performed by free-hand technique. Besides, good cosmesis was achieved in all eyes following a lamellar graft. Minimal complications were seen, with successfully managed symblepharon in one patient.

Thus, frozen section guided excision followed by lamello-lamellar sclerokeratoplasty in cases of squamous cell carcinoma of conjunctiva and cornea is a feasible and reliable procedure, especially where intraocular invasion has been ruled out. Although no recurrence was seen in this study, a regular and careful follow-up is mandatory in all of these patients.

REFERENCES

1. D.R. Buuns, Tse, D.T., and Folberg, R., Microscopically controlled excision of conjunctival squamous cell carcinoma. *Am. J. Ophthalmol.* 117:97 (1994).
2. G.A. Lee, and Hirst, L.W., Ocular surface squamous neoplasia. *Surv. Ophthalmol.* 38(6):429 (1995).
3. W.J. Iliff, Marback, R., and Green, W.R., Invasive squamous cell carconima of conjunctival. *Arch. Ophthalmol.* 93:119 (1975).
4. J.C. Eric, Campbell, R.J., and Liesgang, J., Conjunctival and corneal intraepithelial and invasive neoplasia. *Ophthalmology* 93:176 (1986).
5. D.D. Pizzarello, and Jakobiec, F.A., Bowen's disease of the conjunctiva. A misnomer. In *Ocular and Adnexal Tumors*, F.A. Jakobiec, ed., Aescul Splue, Birmingham, (1978).
6. J.R. Goldberg, Becker, S.C., and Rosenbaum, H.D., Gamma radiation in the treatment of squamous cell carcinoma of limbus. *Am. J. Ophthalmol.* 55:811 (1976).
7. G. Peksayer, Soyturk, M.K., and Demiryout, M., Long term results of crytotherapy on malignant epithelial tumours of the conjunctiva. *Am. J. Ophthalmol.* 15:337 (1989).
8. D.H. Char, Crawford, J.B., Howes, E.L., and Weinstein, A.J., Resection of intraocular squamous cell carcinoma. *Br. J. Ophthalmol.* 76:123 (1992).
9. W.J. Glasson, and Hirst, W.L., Invasive squamous cells carcinoma of the conjunctiva. *Arch. Ophthalmol.* 112:1342 (1994).
10. A. Panda, and Kumar, S.T., Penetrating keratoplasty in viral keratitis. *Ann Ophthalmol.* 23:272 (1991).

SESSION I: OCULAR SURFACE, LIDS, TEARS

Abstracts of Other Conference Presentations and Posters

CONJUNCTIVAL EPITHELIAL HEALTH AND ITS MORPHOLOGIC ASSESSMENT

J. D. Nelson

Departments of Ophthalmology, Ramsey Clinic and St. Paul-Ramsey Medical Center, St. Paul, MN and the University of Minnesota, Minneapolis, MN

The conjunctiva, in particular the epithelium and goblet cells, is critical for maintaining the health of the eye. Conjunctival epithelium is histologically and biochemically quite different from the corneal epithelium. It is an important source of tear mucins which arise from the goblet cells and from the conjunctival epithelium. Goblet cells account for 5-10% of ocular surface cells. The ideal conjunctival surface is one in which there are small compact epithelial cells which are well adherent to adjacent cells, with a nuclear/cytoplasmic ratio of 1:2. In addition, goblet cells are plentiful (1000-56,00 cells/mm^2). Squamous metaplasia is a term used to describe the surface changes where there is a loss of goblet cells and a trend toward keratinization. In an individual without symptoms or clinical findings of dry eye (a "normal" individual), there is little change in the conjunctival surface morphology over time. However, there are variations in surface morphology between normal individuals. Some "normal" individuals may have a decrease in goblet cell density and epithelial cell changes consistent with mild squamous metaplasia. Patients with aqueous tear deficiency, often show more severe stages of squamous metaplasia, but like normal individuals, show little individual variation over time. It is likely that there is a regulatory mechanism which is responsible for maintaining the health and integrity of the conjunctival surface. When this regulatory mechanism goes awry, squamous metaplasia follows.

CONFOCAL IMAGES OF THE HUMAN TEAR FILM AND THEIR CORRELATION WITH TEAR FUNCTION

William D. Mathers, James K Lane, and Bridget Zimmerman

Department of Ophthalmology, The University of Iowa, Iowa City, Iowa

Purpose: To examine the human tear film with confocal microscopy and correlated the appearance with multiple physiologic functions. **Methods:** We used confocal microscopy to examine 55 patients with several forms of blepharitis (MGD) and dry eye: obstructive MGD (8), sehorrheic MGD (10), dry eye (10), seborrheic MGD/dry eye (5), seborrheic MGD/obstructive (5) and normals (17). Each patient was also examined for: tear osmolarity, fluorometric tear flow, Schirmers test, meibomian gland expression, ocular surface evaporation, and meibomian gland morphology. A clinical diagnosis was based on our previously published age-adjusted normal data,. The confocal microscope was fitted with a 10X objective and focused on the tear film surface. The tear film was evaluated in masked fashion using non-parametric scales: lipid thickness (1 thin-10 thick), linear pattern (1 linear-10 nonlinear), tear film debris (1 rare-10 heavy), pattern stability (1 stable-10 unstable), dry spots (1 few-10 many). **Results:** We found that the evaporative rate of both eyes in ten subjects was significantly reduced following digital expression. The evaporative rate pre-expression was $29.57 \pm 9.9 \times 10^{-7}$ gms/cm^2/sec and post expression decreased to 14.75 ± 4.0. The average decrease was $48 \pm 12\%$. Post expression the tear film lipid layer also showed significant changes in appearance. Lipid thickness increased from 3.2 ± 1.5 to 8.0 ± 1.0. The pattern became more linear from 7.8 ± 1.7 to 4.4 ± 3.0. Debris increased from $1.8 \pm .87$ to 3.6 ± 2.2. The stability improved from 5.0 ± 1.9 to 1.7 ± 0.9. The dry spots did not change (1.0). We also found the appearance of the tear film correlated with physiologic variables. Linearity correlated with osmolarity (+.44), Schirmers test (-.30), lipid volume (-.45) and viscosity (+.32). Pattern stability correlated with decay constant (-.37), lipid volume (+.35). Dry spots correlated with evaporation (-.32), decay constant (+.33) and lipid viscosity (+.27). Lipid thickness correlated with tear flow (+.28), lipid viscosity (+.27), and lipid volume (+.27). The bight correlations for debris were with evaporation (-0 .21), tear flow (+.21), gland dropout (-0.28). We also found that the appearance of the tear film correlated with the clinical/physiologic diagnosis. The highest non-linear pattern score was in dry eye patients (9.0 ± 1.2) and in obstructive MGD patients (8.3 ± 2.7). The pattern was most linear in seborrheic patients (6.0 ± 2.8). Debris was lowest in obstructive MGD (2.0 ± 1.6) and dry eye patients (2.5 ± 2.3) and highest in seborrheic patients (3.4 ± 2.9). The lipid pattern was most stable in dry eye patents (1.6 ± 0.8), obstructive MGD (1.7 ± 0.7) and normals (1.9 ± 1.3). It was the most unstable in seborrheic patients (3.6 ± 2.4). **Conclusions:** This study demonstrates that the tear film can be successfully examined with confocal microscopy and that the appearance correlates with the physiologic functions of the tear film and clinical diagnoses based on these physiologic functions.

MEIBOMIAN SECRETIONS IN CHRONIC BLEPHARITIS

James P. McCulley and Ward Shine

Department of Ophthalmology, The University of Texas Southwestern Medical Center at Dallas

Chronic blepharitis represents a complex group of diseases with differing pathophysiological mechanisms. Over the years we have demonstrated that staphylococcal species appear to have a direct role in both staphylococcal and mixed seborrheic/staphylococcal blepharitis. We have also demonstrated that several different types of bacteria may share common pathways in contributing to disease, i.e., the production of lipolytic exoenzymes in the majority of the forms of chronic blepharitis including the above mentioned, seborrheic blepharitis with meibomian seborrhea or secondary meibomianitis and primary meibomianitis. We not only characterized the normal composition of meibomian secretions in individuals but in individuals with each of the forms of chronic blepharitis. We have demonstrated an association of abnormality in patients who have meibomian gland involvement as a part of the chronic blepharitis. Similarly we have demonstrated that fatty waxes and cholesterol esters differ in several of the disease categories. We have also demonstrated that there are two groups of normals, i.e., those that have cholesterol and cholesterol esters in their secretions and those that do not; whereas, all patients with chronic blepharitis have these compounds. We also have demonstrated differences in the triglycerides and polar lipids in several of the disease sub-groups. We currently are completing our analysis of the lipids and evaluating the effect of tetracycline on both normal and abnormal secretions. (Supported by unrestricted grant from Research to Prevent Bindness and NEI EYO3650.)

CORNEAL EPITHELIAL DAMAGE INDUCED BY PROSTAGLANDIN F2a DERIVATIVE (ISOPROPYL UNOPROSTONE) IN COMBINATION WITH B-BLOCKER

N. Kokawa, A. Niiya, A. Komuro, Y. Matsumoto, N.Yokoi and S. Kinoshita

Department of Ophthalmology, Kyoto Prefectural University of Medicine, Kyoto, Japan

Prostaglandin F2a (isopropyl unoprostone), a novel anti-glaucoma agent, has been used in Japan since 1994. We encountered 5 cases of corneal epithelial damage induced by topical application of isopropyl unoprostone in combination with B-blocker. Case histories of these five glaucoma patients with severe corneal epithelial damage were reviewed. They were all males with a mean age of 56.2 years (range, 45-65 years), treated with B-blocker and/or other topical anti-glaucoma agents, based on the diagnosis of primary open-angle glaucoma. These patients developed corneal epithelial damage shortly after additional application of isopropyl unoprostone. 4 cases showed corneal epithelial damage characterized by highly enhanced fluorescein permeability and one was persistent corneal epithelial defect. This clinical study implies that combined usage of prostaglandin F2a and B-blocker affects corneal epithelial metabolism.

IN VIVO CONFOCAL MICROSCOPIC CHARACTERIZATION OF SLIGHT, MILD AND MODERATE SURFACTANT-INDUCED OCULAR IRRITATION

J. K. Maurer,[1] H. F. Li,[2] J. V. Jester,[2] W. M. Petroll,[2] R. Parker,[1] and H. D. Cavanagh[2]

[1]The Procter & Gamble Co., Cincinnati, OH and [2]UT-Southwestern Medical Center, Dallas, TX

Purpose: We have previously demonstrated the application of non-invasive, *in vivo* confocal microscopy (CM) to characterize qualitatively and quantitatively the pathobiology of ocular irritation *in situ*. The purpose of this study was to further establish unique histopathologic correlates distinguishing ocular injury occurring with anionic surfactants (AS) of different irritancy, using a standard ocular irritation test. **Methods:** Representative AS causing slight, mild, or moderate ocular irritation were applied to the corneas of rabbits (6/group) at a dose of 10 μl. Eyes and eyelids of each animal were examined macroscopically and scored for irritation beginning at 3 hr after dosing and periodically through day 35. Concurrently, the same corneas were evaluated by *in vivo* CM; 3-D data sets from 4 areas extending from the surface epithelium to the endothelium in 50 μm steps were collected; and epithelial thickness, corneal thickness, and depth of stromal injury determined. **Results:** The maximum average scores for the slight, mild, and moderate irritants were 6.0, 41.3 and 48.5, respectively, out of a possible 110. All eyes were macroscopically normal by day 35, except for 2 animals dosed with the moderate irritant. *In vivo* CM revealed corneal injury with the slight irritant to be limited to the epithelium; epithelial thickness was 82.4% of controls (33.6 μm vs 40.8 μm, $p<0.005$) at 3 hr and returned to normal by day 7. For the mild irritant the epithelium was absent at 3 hr and keratocyte necrosis occurred to an average depth of 5.4 μm; these parameters were essentially normal by day 35. For the moderate irritant, the epithelium was absent at 3 hr and remained significantly thinner than controls ($p<0.05$) at day 35. Additionally, keratocyte necrosis extended to an average depth of 19.7 μm, which was statistically greater than that observed for the mild irritant ("<0.05). **Conclusion:** These findings demonstrate that significant differences in the area and depth of injury occur with surfactants of differing irritancy at 3 hr, and suggest differences at 3 hr can be used to predict ocular irritation. Data such as this will be important in the development and evaluation of future mechanistically-based *in vitro* alternatives for ocular irritancy testing. (Supported by The Procter & Gamble Co and a Senior Scientist Award from Research to Prevent Blindness, Inc.)

ADHESION-CYTOLOGY OF CONJUNCTIVAL EPITHELIUM AFTER SURGICAL RECONSTRUCTION OF SEVERE BURNS WITH TENON PLASTY

Martin Reim, Jakob Becker, Christiane Genser, and Sabine Salla

Eye Clinic, Faculty of Medicine, Technical University (RWTH) Aachen, Germany

Purpose: Tenon plasty has been used to reconstruct the conjunctival surface in severe burns, where ischemic sclera was exposed or undergoing ulceration. Adhesion cytology allowed to investigate the epithelium in larger series of patients. The quality of the regenerated epithelium on the advanced Tenon sheets was assessed.

Methods: Twenty five severely burnt eyes in 21 patients between 6 weeks and 5 years after surgery, and 53 normal eyes of 31 healthy volunteers were examined. A 25 mm^2 Biopore membrane (Millipor Catalogue PICM 01250) was placed on the conjunctival surface in the lower temporal quadrant, 3–5 mm distant from the limbus till it was soaked with fluid. The ablated cell sheets were stained with PAS.

Results: In all cases an intact conjunctival epithelium was observed. In healthy eyes 2337,5 epithelial cells/mm^2 and 154,8 goblet cells/mm^2 were found. Eyes after surgical reconstruction with Tenon plasty resulted only in 1575 epithelial cells/mm^2 and 71 ,5 goblet cells/mm^2. The differences were highly significant. The ratio of epithelial/goblet cell counts revealed an increase of goblet cells with time.

Conclusion: Tenon plasty provides regeneration of fully intact conjunctival epithelium. Goblet cells are present from 6 weeks after surgery, their number increased with time. The difference from heterotopic epithelial transplants was evident in the cytological examination as well as in the clinical aspect. Dry eye symptoms persist. Stimulation of goblet cell mucous secretion has to be discussed.

LIMBAR GRAFTS FOR EARLY TREATMENT OF SUPERFICIAL CORNEO-LIMBAR BURNS

Francisco Barcaquer

Early detection of the extension and intensity of corneo-limbar burns requires biomicroscopy and anterior segment fluorescein angiography. The presence and permeability of the limbar vascular mesh can be used as an index of the viability of the corneal stem cells, given its close relationship with the limbar vessels. This allows us to identify patients who are able to benefit with free limbar grafts from the contralateral eye. The early reconstruction of the epithelial surface of the cornea, favors the return to a normal homeostatic state of the corneal stroma, speeding the healing process and minimizing the scarring sequelae.

DYE SPREAD VIA GAP JUNCTIONS IN THE CORNEAL EPITHELIUM OF THE RABBIT

K. Keven Williams and Mitchell A. Watsky

Department of Physiology and Biophysics, University of Tennessee, College of Medicine, Memphis, TN

Purpose: We used microelectrode dye injection to investigate intercellular communication via gap junctions in the epithelium of the isolated rabbit cornea. **Methods:** Microelectrodes coupled to a piezoelectric micromanipulator were used to inject 5,6-carboxyfluorescein (CF) into epithelial cells of isolated rabbit corneas bathed in NaCl Ringer's. Injections started in the first (superficial) layer and proceeded stepwise into the underlying epithelial layers until spread was observed. Intracellular $[Ca^{2+}]$ was manipulated by either exposing the cornea to the Ca^{2+} ionophore A23 187 or increasing the $[Ca^{2+}]$ in the injection electrode. Intracellular pH was manipulated by either exposing the cornea to nigericin in a low pH KCl Ringer's or lowering the pH in the injection electrode. Heptanol was tested in the bath for its ability to uncouple the gap junctions. **Results:** The degree of gap junctional communication was based on the layer at which spread was first observed, and the distance traveled by the dye from the point of injection.

	Control (n=8)	1 mM Ca^{2+} in electrode (n=6)	100μM Ca^{2+} in electrode (n=6)	A23187 in bath (n=5)	pH 5 in electrode (n=S)	pH 6 in electrode (n=5)	Nigericin bath pH 5 (n-5)	Heptanol (2.5mM) (n=4)
Average spread layer	3	2	2	4	3	3	3	no spread
Dye travel (μm/20min)	74±5	61±5	64±2	59±8	69±7	68±2	61±7	

(mean± SEM)

Conclusions: We have provided direct evidence for gap junctional communication in the corneal epithelium. Under control conditions, initial dye spread occurs in or below the third layer. when the $[Ca^{2+}]$ of the electrode solution is increased, the average initial dye spread occurred in the second layer. By contrast, when the $[Ca^{2+}]$ is increased globally as is the case with A23187, dye spread did not occur until the fourth layer. Dye travel is less but not significantly different from control with increased intracellular Ca^{2+}. Lowering the pH does not affect the spread layer or distance traveled by the dye. Dye coupling via gap junctions in the corneal epithelium is blocked by 2.5 mM heptanol. (Supported by NIH Grant EY10178)

TEAR FUNCTION IN OCULAR SURFACE DISEASE

K. Barton, A Nava, R. Naqui, D.C. Monroy, and S.C. Pflugfelder

Ocular Surface and Tear Center, Bascom Palmer Eye Institute, University of Miami School of Medicine

Purpose: Patients with keratoconjunctivitis sicca secondary to Sjögren's syndrome, non-Sjögren's aqueous tear deficiency and meibomian gland dysfunction secondary to rosacea suffer from severe ocular irritation. In more than 50% of cases, conjunctival epithelial cells demonstrate aberrant expression of MHC class II antigens, although these conditions are characterised by marked differences in the clinical appearance of the ocular surface. Recent studies have demonstrated that the bulbar conjunctival epithelium can produce mRNA specific for tumor necrosis factor-alpha (TNF-α), interleukins -1α, -6 and -8 (IL-1α, IL-6 and IL-8) in response to acute microtrauma in normal individual. Additionally mRNA-specific for TNF-α, IL-1α, IL-6, IL-8 and IL-10 has been detected in the bulbar conjunctiva of patients with Sjögren's syndrome but not in controls. However, it is likely that the local effects of these cytokines will be dependent on tear function. **Methods:** In order to investigate the role of tear function in these types of disease, 14 patients with severe meibomian gland disease associated with facial rosacea and moderate to severe symptoms of ocular irritation were examined for ocular surface disease, reduced tear break-up the and delayed tear clearance (tear function index [TFI]). 15 ideal normal controls, with no ocular symptoms and normal tear function were assessed using the same parameters. Non-stimulated tears samples (20μl) were drawn from each subject and analysed using a sandwich ELISA to detect the presence of IL-1α, TNF-α and epidermal growth factor (EGF). **Results:** A significant delay in tear clearance was observed in rosacea when compared with controls in association with a significantly higher level of EGF ($p<0.05$) and IL-1α ($p<0.05$) TNF-α was not detected in patients or controls, indicating levels of less than <10pg/ml. **Conclusion:** Significantly higher levels of the inflammatory cytokine IL-1α were observed in the tears of patients with ocular rosacea. Elevated TFI and tear EGF concentrations indicate reduced tear turnover and it is likely that the resultant pooling of IL-la and other cytokines in a relatively stagnant tear film may contribute to the associated ocular surface disease.

RECURRENT EROSION SYNDROME: THE RELATIONSHIP BETWEEN AETIOLOGY AND PROGNOSIS – A 4 YEAR FOLLOW-UP OF 117 PATIENTS

P. Heyworth

We aimed to investigate the relationship between the aetiology and natural history of recurrent erosion syndrome. One hundred and seventeen patients with recurrent erosion syndrome were enrolled consecutively and treated with topical lubricants*. Inclusion criteria included epithelial basement membrane dystrophy (EBMD), focal epithelial abnormalities or normal corneal appearance, all either with or without a history of trauma. Patients were surveyed 4 years later with regard to symptoms, frequency, pain and ongoing treatments. 86/117 (74%) were contacted. Mean age at follow-up was 44.1(±12.1 SD) years with a mean follow-up of 46.9(± 4.0) months. 50/86(58%) were still symptomatic and 27/50 (54%) of those still required topical treatment Recurrent attacks occurred at a mean frequency of 64.16 (± 64.4) days. The mean pair score was 3.7 (± 2.7) on a 10 point analogue scale. Those with EBMD were more likely to be symptomatic than those with a traumatic aetiology [(77% Vs 45%) p=0.009] and those with EBMD were more likely to have a continuing requirement for topical medication [(75% Vs 40%) p=0.034]. Frequency of attacks and associated pain scores were similar between aetiological groups. Establishing the cause of recurrent erosion; particularly distinguishing between EBMD and traumatic cases offers a valuable guide to longterm prognosis. (*Hykin et al. The natural history and management of recurrent erosion. *Eye* (1994) 8:35-40.)

MICROSURGICAL APPROACH TO CONJUNCTIVAL FLAP

Ali Khodadart

Conjunctival flap provides support to the cornea when medical therapy fails to control disorders of this vital tissue. The most accepted technique described by Gundersen involved 360 degree peritomy, mobilizing tissue from upper bulbar conjunctiva, removing corneal epithelium and securing the flap to lower limbal conjunctiva. This technique covers the entire cornea. Visualization of the anterior segment is difficult at immediate post-op, can cause ptosis and is difficult in patients with short fornices.

During the past 20 years, we have applied micro-surgical techniques for a selective, pedunculated partial conjunctival flap tailored to cover the desired part of the diseased cornea. This technique enables good visibility of anterior segment, does not cause ptosis, and is applicable in all patients. This technique of conjunctival flap and the result of its application in 40 consecutive patients with various corneal disorders will be presented.

ALLOGRAFT LIMBAL-CONJUNCTIVAL TRANSPLANTATION FOR BILATERAL OCULAR SURFACE DISORDERS

Sergio Kwitko

A prospective study of allogenic limbal-conjunctival transplantation with HLA typing and crossmatching was undertaken in 17 eyes of 13 patients with bilateral surface disorders, to evaluate its efficacy for such diseases. Nine eyes suffered from Stevens-Johnson Syndrome, three Lyell Syndrome, three bilateral alkali bum, one bilateral thermal burn, and one ectodermal dysplasia. Fifteen of 17 eyes (88.2%) had improved visual acuity, corneal transparency and surface lubrication, stabilization of corneal epithelia, and decreased corneal neovascularization and photophobia, after an average follow-up of 29.2 months. Five cases (29.4%) presented conjunctival rejection episodes with no disturbance of corneal surface in 3 of them. Two of these 5 cases had 100% incompatible HLA donor-recipient pairs, two had haploidentical pairs (50% identity), and HLA of the fifth case 'was not available. Disturbance of corneal surface in the other two cases of graft rejection led to descemetocele in one of them, requiring a therapeutic contact lens, and corneal perforation in the other one that required a corneal patch to restore eye integrity. Patients with favorable evolution were either HLA identical or haploidentical with their donors. Donor eyes did not present any epithelial problems during the follow-up period. HLA-matched allogenic limbal-conjunctival transplantation proved to be an adequate method of treatment for severe bilateral surface disorders, with minimal complications.

DIAMOND BURR KERATECTOMY FOR THE TREATMENT OF RECURRENT CORNEAL EROSION SYNDROME

S. Lance Forstot, R.E. Damiano, Rhea Witters, Jan Sevier, and Robert B. Keyser

Thirty-six eyes of 32 patients underwent a superficial keratectomy with a 5mm diamond burr for recurrent corneal erosions. All patients had previously failed on medical therapy. With a minimum follow-up of 2 years (26 months) and maximum of 6 years (74 months), all patients were completely free of symptoms and no patients had any recurrent erosions during the follow-up period. 100% of patients had less than 1D of change in their previous refraction.

Diamond burr keratectomy is a safe, effective treatment for recurrent corneal erosion syndrome. This treatment uses less expensive technology than either excimer or Yag laser treatment for this condition and may be more cost effective. It is a simple, in-office procedure. Pathology of donor corneas undergoing diamond burr keratectomy will be presented.

COLLAGEN PRODUCTION INHIBITORS INHIBIT THE MIGRATION OF CORNEAL EPITHELIUM

Natsuko Hashizume, Shizuya Saika, Yoshitaka Ohnishi, andAkira Ooshima

Department of Ophthalmology and Pathology; Wakayama Medical College; Wakayama, 640, Japan

Purpose: To examine the effects of collagen production inhibitors on the migration of rabbit corneal epithelium. These chemicals inhibit collagen secretion by suppressing triple-helix formation. **Methods:** Corneal epithelial migration was evaluated in vitro using a rabbit corneal block (Nishida, et al. J Cell Biol. 97:1653–1657, 1983) in the presence or absence of a prolyl hydroxylase inhibitor,ethyl-3,4-dihydroxybenzoate, or a lysyl hydroxylase inhibitor, minoxidil. The effects of an inhibitor of lysyl oxidase, beta-amino-propionitrile, were also examined. Previous reports have revealed that the concentrations of the chemicals used are not cytotoxic. **Results:** Minoxidil and ethyl-3,4-dihydroxyben-zoate inhibited the migration of corneal epithelium in a dose-dependent manner. Beta-aminopropionitrile had no effect on epithelial migration. **Conclusions:** The exact mechanism of action of these chemicals is still unknown. It is possible that collagen production is closely related to the migration of sqamous epithelium. Cross-linking of collagen in extracellular spaces may not he required for such epithelial migration. Further detailed studies are needed to identify the specific proteins, including collagen types, involved in corneal epithelial migration.

THE TWYMAN-GREEN INTERFEROMETER AND LATERAL SHEARING INTERFERENCE TECHNIQUES FOR IN VIVO MEASUREMENTS OF THE TEAR FILM STABILITY ON A CORNEA AND A CONTACT LENS

T. J. Licznerski, H. T. Kasprzak, and J. J. Jaronski

Institute of Physics, Technical University, Wroclaw, Poland

Purpose: To present and compare two different interferometry techniques for evaluation of the break-up characteristic of the tear film, the non-invasive tear break-up time (NITBUT) value, and examining the dynamic changes in its distribution.

Methods: The Twyman-Green interferometer (TGI) and shearing technique were applied in two separate set-ups. The sequence of interferograms were recorded with a TV frame speed and synchronized with a shutter released HeNe laser beam. The selected frames were acquired by the Frame Grabber, die "Stop Motion" and "Median" filters were applied to improve images. Such an arrangement enables the observation dynamic effects on unstable biomedical objects like the eye. In addition die TGI provides precise and detailed information of the topography of the tear film overlaying the cornea or contact lens.

Results: A series of interferograms of *in vivo* precorneal tear film break-up formation are presented. The 3D plots of selected frames obtained from interferograms representing break-up are given. The steps of creation of the tear film rupture due to its evaporation are shown in a sequence of frames. The interferograms from TGI technique contain precise information about a wave-front reflected from the tear film. TGI, however, has also severe drawbacks such as blurred fringes which correspond to fast moving objects. Interferometer of the shearing type is more stable but gives less sensitivity and has some difficulties of the fringe pattern interpretation.

Conclusions: The proposed method has the advantage of being non contact and applies the low energy laser beam in interferometric set-up. This provides non invasive testing of the human cornea *in vivo* and enables observation the kinetic of its tear layer deterioration. NITBUT could be easily evaluated using these methods by simply observing the first appearance of the break-up. Even very small ruptures in the tear film could be detected. The analysis of deformation of the interference fringes allows to find fine topography of the tear's layer surface. Furthermore the proposed method gives possibilities of precise quantitative diagnostics of the tear film condition.

Session II

Corneal Transplantation and Eye Banking

15

STROMAL HYDRODELAMINATION TECHNIQUE IN DEEP LAMELLAR KERATOPLASTY WITH COMPLETE REMOVAL OF PATHOLOGIC STROMA

Juntaru Sugita

Sugita Eye Hospital
Nagoya, Japan

ABSTRACT

Lamellar keratoplasty may result in poor postoperative visual acuity. To eliminate this drawback, deep lamellar keratoplasty was performed to completely remove the diseased corneal stroma, leaving only Descemet's membrane in the optical zone. The deeper corneal stroma was excised with spatula-delamination and corneal scissors while it was swelling with a balanced salt solution (BSS) injected deeply. Hydrodelamination allows safe excision of the deep stroma as well as determination of the normality of the stroma.

STROMAL HYDRODELAMINATION TECHNIQUE IN DEEP LAMELLAR KERATOPLASTY

Deep lamellar keratoplasty is a surgical intervention used to restore visual acuity for stromal opacification with no epithelial or stromal edema, and in cases where it is thought that endothelial function is preserved. Postoperative interface opacity is minimized by complete removal of the diseased stroma, limitation of the pupillary region at least to Descemet's membrane (Fig. 1), and use of a graft without endothelial cells.

This technique offers favorable recovery of visual acuity comparable with that obtained after penetrating keratoplasty.[1,2] Advantages of this procedure include the fact that because the recipient's endothelial cells are retained there is no need for the donor's and there is no postoperative endothelial rejection. Excision of the stroma down to Descemet's membrane usually requires highly sophisticated surgical skill,[1-3] but hydrodelamination technique provides a safe approach by injection of a balanced salt solution (BSS) in between collagen fibers in the deep stroma for swelling.

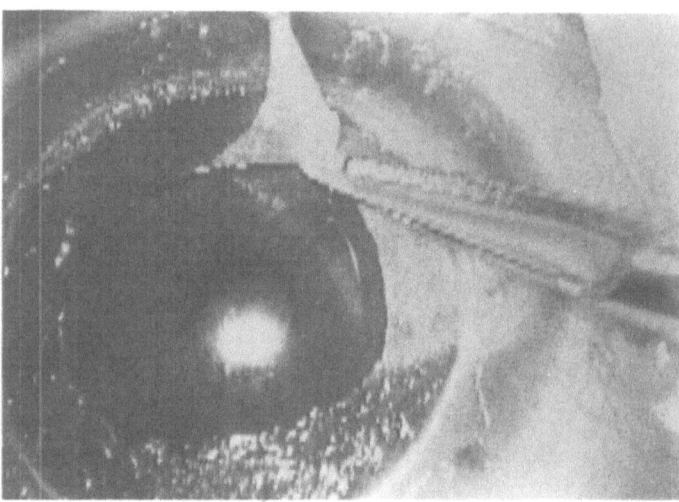

Figure 1. Descemet's membrane with the diseased stroma completely removed from optical zone.

After the cornea is excised to approximately two-third thickness as in regular lamellar keratoplasty, further incision is made with a golf knife confirming the thickness of the remaining stroma. BSS is injected through a blunt needle, like an anterior chamber injector, applied to the base of this incision. With BSS penetrating the collagen fibers, the stroma swells and whitens. The deeper the stroma, the coarser the stromal fibers, and only a single injection provides an extensive range of swelling. The stroma, which has been very thin and unlikely to be removed, now increases its thickness dramatically by this hydrodelamination technique (Fig. 2) to facilitate safe excision.

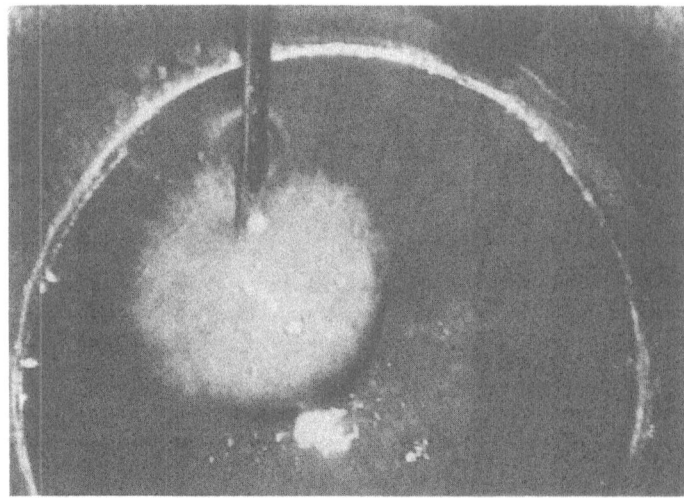

Figure 2. Water injected into a healthy stroma evenly disperses. The stroma swells and whitens.

With this hydrodelamination, disposition of the stromal collagen fibers can be known to some extent. As seen in Fig. 2, if the water injected disperses evenly in all directions, the collagen fibers are disposed uniformly. A diseased, opacified stroma does not have such disposition.

For excision, a thin spatula is advanced in a straight fashion for ablation, or a Paufique knife or thin corneal scissors are used carefully. Excision should be done patiently, little by little, and a single deep cut should be avoided.

Descemet's membrane is extremely smooth and uniform, being clearly distinguished from the stroma, consisting of collagen fibers. When Descemet's membrane is exposed partially, this part is extended to approximately 5 mm in diameter, including the pupillary region. Descemet's membrane adheres loosely to the adjacent stromal boundary membrane. This adhesion is separated with corneal scissors with the stroma lifted with forceps. If the corneal stroma is severely degenerated or there is scarring from corneal herpes, collagen fiber construction is lost and hydrodelamination is difficult. However, the boundary between the stroma and Descemet's membrane is clear, which makes excision easy.

Descemet's membrane thickens with aging and is fairly strong in middle-aged or elderly patients, or in those who have sever stromal degeneration. However, care should be taken in younger patients whose Descemet's membrane is rather thin and easy to perforate. The strength of Descemet's membrane is similar to that which one feels at the time of anterior capsulotomy in the extracapsular cataract extraction: in younger patients thin and elastic while thicker and less elastic in the elderly.

REFERENCES

1. G.K. Chau, Dilly, S.A., Sheard, C.E., and Rostron, C.K., Deep lamellar keratoplasty on air with lyophilised tissue. *Br. J. Ophthalmol.* 76:646 (1992).
2. J. Sugita, and Kondo, J., Lamellar keratoplasty and deep lamellar keratoplasty. *Folia. Ophthalmol. Jpn.* 45:1 (1994).
3. E.A. Archila, Deep lamellar keratoplasty dissection of hist tissue with intrastromal air injection. *Cornea* 3:217 (1985).

16

INDICATIONS AND RESULTS OF KERATOPLASTY "A CHAUD"

C. Macêdo, R. W. Macêdo, D. Freitas, and M. Cunha

Department of Ophthalmology
Paulista School of Medicine
Federal University
São Paulo, Brazil

ABSTRACT

When a keratoplasty is indicated in the presence of important inflammation, cases with no responses to clinical treatment, it is called keratoplasty "a chaud." One year of keratoplasty "a chaud" was analyzed regarding its indications, visual acuity (VA) in the postoperative period, complications, and clinical outcome.

This study analyzed 20 eyes of 19 patients from the Cornea Sector who had submitted to keratplasty "a chaud," with regard to indications, visual acuity, complications, and clinical cure. Infectious keratitis was the major indicating cause (n = 11 eyes, 55%). Clinical cure was observed in 19 eyes (95%). In only one case was there recurrence of the pathology that originally indicated the surgery (fungal keratitis). The main complication was the absence of clear graft. Also observed were glaucoma, cataract, synechiae formation, and inflammatory pupillary membrane formation, among other complications. In 95% of these cases the final visual acuity was below 0.1. It was concluded that keratplasty "a chaud" achieved good results regarding the disease eradication, but that another surgery was necessary to re-establish visual acuity.

INTRODUCTION

Keratoplasty "a chaud" is the term used for surgeries performed in inflamed eyes that are either non responsive to clinical treatment or at risk for perforation.

In 3% of bacterial keratitis cases clinical treatment is not effective,[1] whereas in the mycotic ones this rate can be as high as 20 to 29%.[2,3,4] Less common pathogens, such as Acanthamoeba and Nocardia, traumas, chemical agents, and persistent epithelial defects can also represent major threat to ocular integrity and may lead to perforation and endophthalmitis.

Advances in Corneal Research, edited by Lass
Plenum Press, New York, 1997

PURPOSE

In the present study one year of keratoplasty "a chaud" was analyzed regarding its indications, visual acuity (VA) in the postoperative period, complications, and clinical outcome.

PATIENTS AND METHODS

Twenty eyes of 19 patients (7 female and 12 male) were retrospectively studied. Patients' ages ranged from 1 to 73 years (mean 41.7). The postoperative follow up period varied from 1 to 18 months (mean 4.9 months).

Cases 5 and 13 reported vegetable matter trauma (Table 1). Eight patients had perforation at the moment of surgery (cases 2, 5, 7, 8, 11, 12, 14 and 15) (Table 1). Only five eyes (25%) received preoperative treatment in the Corneal Service, two receiving antibiotic therapy; one, tissue adhesive; one conjunctival flap; and, finally, one corneal suture. Cases suspected of infection had corneal smears performed before surgery and microscopically examined on Gram and Giemsa stain, and cultivated in blood agar, chocolate agar, Sabouroud, and soya medium (cases suspected of Acanthamoeba). The removed corneas were analyzed by culture and cytological examination.

In perforation cases systemic antibiotic therapy was administered prior to surgery. Surgeries were performed under general anesthesia. A Flieringa ring was used whenever the eye was perforated. Conventional trephine was used, and with the perforations trephination was performed free hand; trephine used only to delimit the area to be removed. The button size ranged so as to remove all affected area, with a donor recipient difference never smaller than 0.5 mm. Peripheral iridectomies and interrupted 10–0 nylon sutures were performed. At the end of surgery, subconjunctival injection of dexamethasone in the cases of known etiology and non-fungal infections and either garamycin or other antibiotic based on the smear exams was administered. Postoperative supportive therapy was based on clinical findings, varying from antibiotics to topical and/or systemic corticosteroids, acethazolamide, and timolol maleate, in the cases that developed increase of intraocular pressure (IOP), and 1% atropine.

RESULTS

Of the 20 necrotic keratitis cases studied (11 eyes) only two eyes had preoperative positive cultures. The agents identified were *Staphylococcus* sp. and a filamentous fungus. In five additional corneas the diagnosis of mycotic keratitis (four eyes) and *Acanthamoeba* keratitis (one eye) was obtained either by culture or cythologic analysis. In four eyes, however, the etiological diagnosis was not possible. Additional causes were use of anesthetic eye drops in four eyes (20%), descemetocele in two eyes (10%), trophic ulcer in one eye (5%), trauma with loss of tissue in one eye (5%) and progressive thinning following graft failure in one eye (5%).

The most frequent complications were rejection and endothelial decompensation, which occurred in 11 cases (55%) (Figure 3) and mostly accounting for the low final visual acuity. Four cases presented IOP (intraocular pressure) increase (see Figure 3). In cases 14 and 20 a filtering surgery was required. Case 16 developed malignant glaucoma, controlled after vitreous puncture. Persistent epithelial defect or sterile ulcer occurred in five cases. Such cases were well controlled with therapeutic contact lenses or tarsorrhaphy.

Table 1. Age, sex, diagnosis, complications and postoperative visual acuity

Case	Age (years)	Sex	Diagnosis	VA 1st month	Last VA (time)	Major complications
1	58	f	necrotic keratitis, no ethiology	HM 50cm	HM 50cm (3.5 months)	Endothelial decomp.
2	66	f	necrotic keratitis, no ethiology	LP	LP (3 months)	Phthisis, sterile ulcer
3	28	m	anesthetic eyedrop keratitis	20/60	FC 1m (6 months)	Endothelial decomp.
4	28	m	anesthetic eyedrop keratitis	20/40	FC 1m (6 months)	Endothelial decomp.
5	54	m	perforating trauma	HM 50cm	FC 1 m (6 months)	Endothelial decomp., IOP increase
6	44	m	mycotic keratitis	HM 50cm	HM 50cm (18 months)	Endothelial decomp., hyphema
7	10	f	post-transplant thinning	HM 50cm	HM 50cm (3 months)	Endothelial decomp.
8	41	m	anesthetic eyedrop keratitis	FC 4 m	FC 4 m (1 month)	IOP increase
9	49	m	mycotic keratitis	HM 50cm	LP (1.5 months)	Endothelial decomp., epithelial defect, hyphema, sterile hypopyon
10	42	m	anesthetic eyedrop keratitis	HM 50cm	LP (3 months)	Endothelial decomp., epithelial defect
11	1	m	descemetocele	unmeasurable	unmeasurable	Endothelial decomp., ocular hypotension
12	64	m	descemetocele	LP	LP (5 months)	Epithelial defect
13	70	m	necrotic keratitis, no etiology	LP	LP (5 months)	Cataract, 360° synechiae, endothelial decomp.
14	31	f	trophic ulcer post-transplantation	HM 50cm	FC 10 cm (5 months)	Glaucoma, 360° synechiae, endothelial decomp.
15	73	m	necrotic keratitis, no etiology	FC 50 cm	HM 50cm (3 months)	Epithelial defect, cataract
16	66	m	mycotic keratitis	LP	· LP (1.5 months)	Recurrence, hyphema, malignant glaucoma, endothelial decomp.
17	33	m	necrotic keratitis, no etiology	HM 50cm	LP (7.5 months)	Retina detachment, sterile hypopyon
18	15	f	Staphylococcus keratitis	0,1	0,2 (4 months)	Synechiae
19	33	f	mycotic keratitis	0,2	FC 10 cm (5 months)	360° synechiae, cataract, rejection
20	37	f	Acanthamoeba keratitis	FC 1 m	FC 3 m (11 months)	IOP increase, synechiae, rejection

Legend: VA - visual acuity, LP - light perception, HM - hand movement, FC - finger count, m - meters, cm - centimeters, m - male, f - female, PO - postoperative, IOP - intraocular pressure, decomp - decompensation.

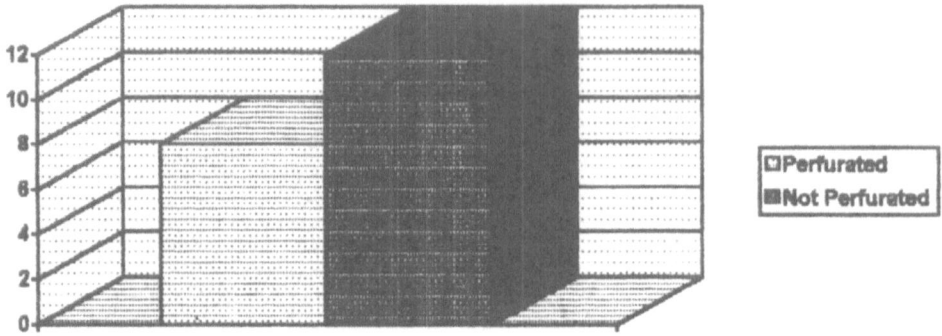

Figure 1. Conditions of the cornea before surgery.

Other complications such as fibrinous anterior chamber reaction (cases 5, 10, 13, 14, 16 e 17), cataract and sterile hypopyon among others were also observed (Figure 3).

Only one of the infectious cases (case 16) recurred on the button, and was controlled with a new keratoplasty. Visual acuity, however, was lower than 20/400 following a 3-month follow up.

Only case 2 developed phthisis bulbi. Patients' potential visual acuity is represented in Figure 2.

DISCUSSION

In the present study infectious keratitis was the major factor in the surgical treatment decision, in agreement with the literature.[5,6,7] In cases in which an etiologic agent was isolated, fungal ulcers were the most prevalent (20% of all cases), in disagreement with other works[2] that show bacteria as the major causative agent. Infection recurred in only one case (mycotic ulcer) which was controlled with a second keratoplasty, showing the procedure as therapeutically successful, as in other series.[5,8,9] Despite the pessimistic prognosis regarding transplantation in cases of *Acanthamoeba*,[10] the only such case in this study was successful.

Of the 20 eyes studied 20% required surgery due to an excessive use of anesthetic eyedrops, showing this still to be an important cause of surgical treatment decision in our country.

Only one eye had better than 0.1 vision. The low visual acuity resulted from complications, among which endothelial decompensation was the major one. Other series, how-

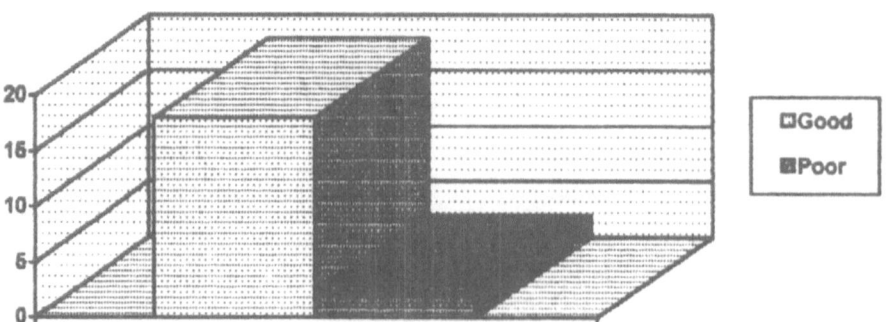

Figure 2. Potential visual acuity.

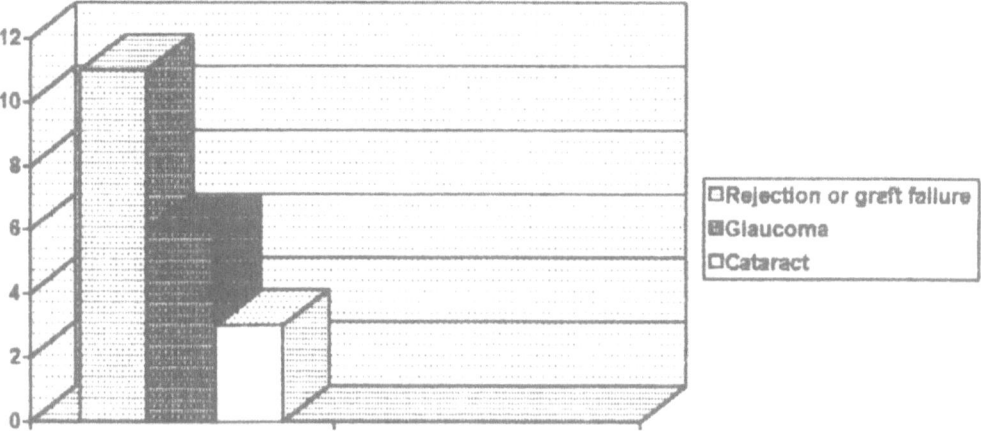

Figure 3. Major complications.

ever, show better results such as a 60 to 77% clear cornea rate following therapeutic infectious keratoplasty[4,5,8] and 75% of patients with a better than 0.1 VA.[2]

It should be emphasized that surgical decision in such cases does not first aim to replace vision but rather saving an eye about to perforate or develop endophthalmitis.

Further complications as cataract, increase in IOP, retinal detachment and formation of pupillary membrane were also observed. Most of these complications are of inflammatory origin rather than related to the surgical procedure. All our patients had obvious ocular inflammation at the time of surgery, which might account for the larger number of complicated cases and consequent worsening of visual acuity.

Case 5 had a perforating trauma in which a perfect coaptation of the edges failed to be obtained after suture and transplantation was the only choice for laceration closure. The literature shows that success in post trauma keratoplasty is directly proportional to the time spent for its performance[7] due to the deleterious effect of inflammatory reaction. The intense inflammatory reaction that followed the surgical act accounted for the increase in IOP and consequent button failure.

Finally, in cases of corneal thinning clinical treatment with contact lenses and tissue adhesives must be tried; keratoplasty is a choice only when such treatment alternatives are not successful.

CONCLUSION

In this study keratoplasty "a chaud" proved to be effective in the control of severe inflammatory corneal diseases non responsive to clinical treatment, however the postoperative complications of a surgery performed in a inflammed eye highly affect the clearness of the cornea, impairing the final visual acuity.

REFERENCES

1. R.K. Foster, The role of excisional keratoplasty in microbial keratitis. In, *The Cornea: Transactions of the World Congress on the Cornea III.* Cavanagh HD, ed., New York: Raven Press (1988).

 2. F.M. Polack, Kaufman, H.E., and Newmark, E., Keratomycoses: medical and surgical treatment. *Arch Ophtalmol.* 85:410 (1971).
 3. R.K. Foster, and Rebell, G., The diagnosis and management of keratomycoses. II. Medical and surgical management. *Arch. Ophthalmol* 93:1134 (1975).
 4. R.K. Foster, and Rebell, G., Therapeutic surgery in failures of medical treatment for fungal keratitis. *Br. J. Ophthalmol.* 59:366 (1975)
 5. D.W. Killingsworth, Stern, G.A., Driebe, W.T., et al., Results of therapeutic keratoplasty. *Ophtalmol.*100:534–541 (1993).
 6. M.P. Tragakis, Rosen, J., and Brown, S.I., Transplantation of the perforated cornea. *Am. J. Ophthalmol.* 78:518–522 (1974).
 7. J.R. Nobe, Moura, B.T., Robin, J.B., and Smith, R.E., Results of penetrating keratoplasty for the treatment of corneal perforations. *Arch Ophthalmol.* 108:939 (1990).
 8. N.Z. Du, Chen, J.Q., Gong, X.M., et al., Therapeutic keratoplasty in the menagement of purulent corneal ulceration: report of 100 cases. *Jpn. J. Ophthalmol.* 23:412 (1979).
 9. E.H. Sato, Rigueiro, M.P., Burnier, Jr., M., and Belfort Mattos, R., Transplante de córnea "a quente" em úlcera micótica: estudo clínico, microbiológico e histopatológico. *Arq. Bras. Oftalmol* 52:52–56 (1989)
10. J.D. Auran, Starr, M.B., and Jakobiec, F.A., *Acanthamoeba* keratitis: a review of the literature. *Cornea* 6:2 (1987).

17

LANGERHANS CELLS IN THE RECIPIENT CORNEA AS PROGNOSTIC INDICATOR IN CORNEAL TRANSPLANTATION

Wolfgang Philipp and Lilly Speicher

Department of Ophthalmology
University of Innsbruck
Anischstraße 35
A-6020 Innsbruck, Austria

ABSTRACT

The aim of the present study was to investigate whether there is a correlation be-tween the density of Langerhans cells (LC) in the recipient cornea (graft bed) and the inci-dence of immunologically caused graft failures.

In this study 60 human corneas were obtained at the time of penetrating keratoplasty in various degenerative and inflammatory corneal diseases. Monoclonal antibodies, anti-HLA-DR, and anti-CD1 were used for the detection of LC by immunohistochemical tech-niques. The densities of LC in the recipient corneas were correlated with the frequency of irreversible allograft rejections.

Results revealed that high densities of LC in the recipient corneas were associated with a high frequency of graft failures (65.2%) while low densities were associated with a favorable outcome (13.3% graft failures) (p<0.01). These results suggest that high densi-ties of LC in the recipient cornea may be responsible—at least in part—for the increased frequency of graft failures in inflammatory corneal diseases.

INTRODUCTION

Corneal transplantation is the most successful form of tissue transplantation with a success rate of more than 90% in avascular corneas, although HLA typing and systemic immunosuppressive therapy usually are not performed.[1,2] The reasons for this so-called immunological privilege of the cornea are not fully understood. It is estimated, however, that besides avascularity and the lack of lymphatics in the graft bed,[3,4] the absence of Langerhans cells (LC) in the central portion of the cornea may contribute to this phenome-non.[4] Nevertheless, allograft rejection is the leading cause of graft failure, particularly in patients with vascularized and inflamed corneas, where the immunological privilege

Table 1. Density of Langerhans cells (LC) in the recipient cornea in various degenerative and inflammatory corneal diseases

Number of corneas (n=60)	Diagnosis	Duration of disease	Number of LC
10	Keratoconus		–/+
4	Fuchs' dystrophy		–/+
4	Bullous keratopathy		–/+
4	Corneal scars		–/+
2	Bacterial keratitis	5–24d	+/+++
7	Herpetic stromal keratitis	0.5–5y	+/+++
5	Phlyctenular keratoconj.	1–7y	+/+++
2	Zoster keratitis	2–9m	+/+++
2	Rheumatoid corneal ulcers	6–12m	+/+++
6	Chronic allograft rejection	6–14m	+/+++
14	Chemical burns	1–6y	+/+++

Results indicate the number of LC per linear 5 mm of central corneal epithelium: –, negative; +, 1–5; ++, 6–10; +++, >10. d: day; m: month; y: year.

breaks down.[5,6] In former studies it has been shown that LC may be present in high densities in the center of vascularized and inflamed corneas.[7,8.]

The aim of the present study was to investigate whether there is a correlation between the density of LC in the recipient cornea (graft bed) and the incidence of immunologically-caused graft failures.

MATERIALS AND METHODS

Patients with various degenerative or inflammatory corneal diseases who underwent penetrating keratoplasty were included in the study (Table 1). According to clinical findings, patients with avascular corneas were assessed to be at low risk for allograft rejection (low-risk group) whereas patients with two or more quadrants of corneal stromal vascularization or a history of previous graft rejection were considered to be at high risk for graft failure (high-risk group).

Indications for grafting in the low-risk group were keratoconus (10 patients), Fuchs' dystrophy (four patients), bullous keratopathy (four patients), posttraumatic corneal scars (four patients) (Table 1). The high-risk group included patients with bacterial keratitis (two patients), herpetic stromal keratitis (seven patients), phlyctenular keratoconjunctivitis (five patients), zoster keratitis (two patients), corneal ulcers due to rheumatoid arthritis (two patients), graft failure from chronic allograft rejection (six patients), and chemical burns (14 patients) (Table 1). All patients were treated with topical betamethasone dinatriumphosphate 0.1%, five times daily for the first postoperative period. Topical steroid therapy was reduced to three times daily at 1 month, to twice daily at 4 months, and to once daily from 6 months up to one year after keratoplasty.

Allograft rejections were treated with topical betamethasone dinatriumphosphate hourly for two weeks and intravenous methylprednisolone (1.5 mg/kg) for 4 days, which was followed by prednisone (1 mg) orally for 5 days.

The diagnosis of allograft rejection was made by typical clinical findings such as diffuse endothelial precipitates or a rejection line, edema of the stroma and epithelium, and anterior chamber flare and cells.[5] Graft rejection was defined as irreversible if corneal edema or opacities did not clear despite intensive topical and systemic steroid therapy.

Tissue Preparation

Immediately after trephination the corneal buttons were bisected with a razor blade. One half was embedded in OCT compound (Tissue-Tek) and stored in liquid nitrogen for immunohistochemical staining. The other half was fixed in buffered formalin for routine histopathology to confirm morphologic observations made on the immunohistochemically stained slides.

Antibodies

Two monoclonal antibodies, anti-HLA-DR (Dako-HLA-DR/alpha) and anti-T6 (Dako-T6; Dakopatts, Copenhagen Denmark), were used for the detection of LC. The specificity and characteristics of these antibodies were reported previously.[9,10] In brief, Dako-HLA-DR/alpha reacts with the alpha chain of monomorphic histocompatibility antigen class II (HLA-DR), which can be detected on various cells, including monocytes, B-cells, activated T-cells, and LC. Dako-T6 reacts with 60% of the cortical thymocytes and has been recognized as a highly specific marker for intraepidermal LC. In addition, a panel of mAbs (Dakopatts) was used to characterize the composition of the inflammatory infiltrates in the inflamed corneas. Dako-T11 was used to detect mature peripheral T cells; Dako-T4, to mark helper/inducer T cells; Dako-T8, to detect cytotoxic/suppressor T cells; Dako-EBM 11, to detect monocytes/macrophages; and Dako-CD22, to mark B cells. In order to confirm the presence of neovascularization in the inflamed we used a mAb to the von Willebrand factor (Factor VIII-related antigen, Dako) which selectively stains vascular endothelial cells.

Immunohistochemical Staining Technique

Six-micrometer-thick frozen sections were cut from the specimens in a Reichert Jung cryostat (Leica-Reichert Co., Vienna, Austria) at -20°C and mounted on poly-L-lysine-coated slides. The sections were air-dried over night, fixed in acetone at 4°C for 10 min and stained with the streptavidin-biotin-peroxidase method, which has been described previously in detail.[11] In brief, sections were rehydrated in Tris-buffered saline (TBS) for 5 minutes and then immersed in a solution of 0.3% H_2O_2 in distilled H_2O for 20 minutes to block endogenous peroxidase activity. After a buffer wash (three 5-minute washes in TBS) the sections were incubated in 20% normal rabbit serum diluted in TBS for 20 minutes to reduce background staining. Excess serum was shaken off and the sections were then incubated with the selected primary mouse mAb for 60 minutes at room temperature. The optimal dilution of antibody in TBS containing 0.1% bovine serum albumin was determined by titration. The sections were then incubated for 30 minutes with biotinylated rabbit anti-mouse immunoglobulins (diluted 1:300 in TBS; Dakopatts, Copenhagen, Denmark), and finally a freshly prepared streptavidin-biotin-peroxidase complex (Dakopatts) was added for a 30-minute incubation at room temperature. All steps were separated by three 5 minute washes in TBS at room temperature. Finally, the sections were immersed in a solution of 3-amino-9-ethylcarbazole, dimethylformamide, and H_2O_2 in acetate buffer (pH 5.2; Dakopatts) for 5 minutes at room temperature, rinsed in TBS, counterstained with Mayer's hematoxylin for 2 minutes and coverslipped with glycerine gelatin. The slides were examined under an Olympus microscope (Olympus Co., Vienna, Austria). Sections of normal skin, processed identically, served as positive controls. Negative controls were prepared by substituting non-immune mouse serum or equivalent amounts of irrelevant mouse mAbs (of the same IgG classes as the primary mAbs) for the primary antibodies. Any T6- or HLA-DR-positive intraepithelial cells with definite dendritic morphology were classified as LC. The LC were counted in a total of 5 mm of the corneal epithelium from the sections of each cornea using an ocular micrometer on an Olympus microscope. At least five sections of each specimen were examined. According to former investigations, LC densities from 1 to 5 cells per linear 5 mm of corneal epithelium were classified as low while densities of more than five cells were arbitrarily classified as high.[8] The incidence of graft failures between recipient corneas with low and high densities of LC were statistically compared using the Chi-square test.

RESULTS

Patients with various degenerative and inflammatory corneal diseases were followed up after penetrating keratoplasty for 12 months to three years, and the densities of LC in the recipient corneas were correlated with the frequencies of irreversible allograft rejections. As was to be expected, LC were found only sporadically in avascular corneas (Table 1). The success rate of corneal transplantation was 92% in this low-risk group one to three years after corneal transplantation. In contrast, LC were found in various high densities in vascularized and inflamed corneas (Table 1; Figure 1). The most numerous of such cells were found in rejected corneal allografts, in corneas with herpetic stromal keratitis, and particularly in corneas with severe alkali burns with a density similar to that in normal epidermis.

As regards the success rate of corneal transplantation in the high-risk group, irreversible allograft rejections occurred in 44.7% of patients two months to three years after grafting (Table 2). The success rates of corneal transplantation in these vascularized and inflamed corneas depended on the density of LC in the recipient corneas. The success rate was 86.7% in corneas with low LC densities, but only 34.8% in corneas with high LC den-

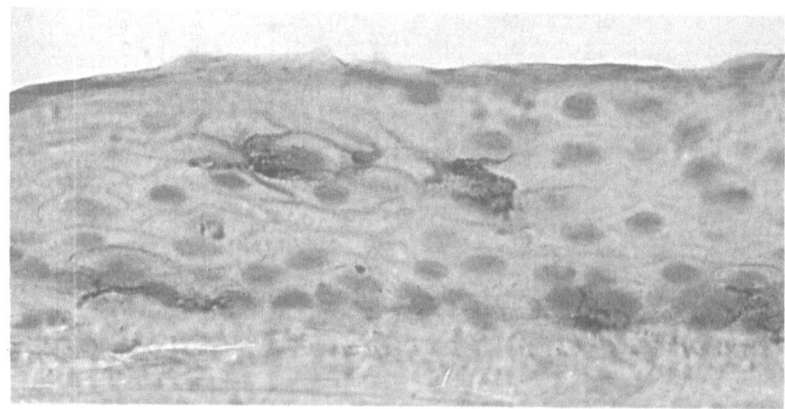

Figure 1. Central cornea from a patient 12 months after alkali burn. Langerhans cells at high density are seen in the epithelium.

Table 2. Results of corneal transplantation in patients with vascularized corneas depending on the density of Langerhans cells (LC) in the recipient cornea

Density of LC[1]	Favorable outcome	Graft failure	Number of patients (n)
1–5 LC/5mm	13 (86.7%)*	2 (13.3%)	15
>5 LC/5mm	8 (34.8%)*	15 (65.2%)	23
Number of patients (n)	21 (55.3%)	17 (44.7%)	38

[1]Results indicate the number of LC per linear 5mm of central corneal epithelium.
*$p<0.01$.

sities (Table 2). This difference was statistically significant ($p < 0.01$). In this context, it must be mentioned that corneas from the high density group with irreversible allograft rejections contained more than 10 LC per linear 5 mm of central corneal epithelium in most cases (89%) and very high densities of more than 15 LC/5 mm of corneal epithelium in 30%.

With regard to corneal neovascularization, there was no clear correlation between the degree of vascularization and the density of LC in the recipient cornea. However, most LC were found independently of corneal vascularization in corneas with dense mononuclear cell infiltrates while corneas with moderate cell infiltrates disclosed only low densities of LC in the epithelium. In alkali-burned corneas, mononuclear cell infiltrates consisted mainly of varying densities of macrophages, and, to a lesser extent, of helper/inducer T cells and cytotoxic/suppressor T-cells. The cellular infiltrates in corneas with herpetic stromal keratitis and in rejected corneal allografts also were composed predominantly of macrophages and helper-inducer and cytotoxic/suppressor T cells, most of which were T-helper/inducer cells. However, there was considerable individual variation in the density and composition of the cellular infiltrates, probably according to the time course and severity of the disease.

DISCUSSION

The present study showed that the incidence of immunologically-caused graft failures was significantly higher in recipient corneas with high densities of LC than in those with low densities. A clear correlation between the degree of corneal neovascularization and the density of LC could not be found. A possible explanation for this interesting finding may be the observation that corneas often showed various degrees of neovascularization but only sparse LC infiltrates after the inflammatory process had declined. Although various stimuli may induce both corneal neovascularization and LC migration from the limbus to the center of the cornea,[7,12] these two processes may not always occur together. In this context, an interesting finding was made by Niederkorn and coworkers,[13] who found that corneas of nude and hairless mutant mice contained blood vessels that extended into the centermost portion of the cornea but were not populated with LC. Thus, factors responsible for corneal neovascularization did not induce LC migration into the cornea in these animals.

How, then, can the increased incidence of graft failures in recipient corneas with dense LC infiltrates be explained?

LC belong to the dendritic cells (DC), which are important antigen presenting cells essential for the induction of primary immune responses of resting T cells in several tissues.[14,15] Furthermore, DC are recognized as so-called passenger leukocytes, which are defined as bone marrow-derived cells in a graft being responsible for sensitizing the host against graft antigens.[15]

As regards corneal transplantation, the absence of LC in the central cornea may explain, at least in part, the immunological privilege of corneal allografts.[4] In this context, it was also shown in experimental animals that the abnormal presence of allogenic LC that were induced to infiltrate the graft before transplantation greatly increased the risk of allograft rejection.[16]

However, according to Lechler and Butchelor,[17] there may be two routes of sensitization to a graft. The first may be direct activation of host T cells by allogenic dendritic cells from the graft. The second pathway may be activation of host T cells by alloantigens presented by host DC. Evidence for this second pathway has been obtained by Golding and Singer[18] in vitro and by Sherwood and co-workers[19] in experimental animals. As regards corneal allograft rejection, it possibly is the second route of sensitization that may play an important role, since the central portion of the cornea, and thus the corneal graft, is presumably devoid of allogenic LC.[4] It has been shown that host LC may also be found in high densities in the center of the cornea and thus in the graft bed in various inflammatory corneal disease.[7,8] After corneal transplantation these dendritic cells may lie in the immediate vicinity of the graft and may be stimulated to invade the graft. Various stimuli were shown to induce LC migration, including mechanical irritations and corneal sutures.[7,12] Thus, it is possible that host LC may pick up shed HLA-antigens of the transplant and may present them to host T cells, thus initiating the rejection process.

Investigating the incidence of graft failures in various corneal diseases, Williams and co-workers[20] have shown that the frequency of irreversible graft failures was statistically higher in corneas with dense leukocyte infiltrates in the graft bed than in corneas with only low or moderate infiltrates. Although these authors investigated the densities of different leukocytes in the graft bed, they did not analyze which leukocyte population might have been responsible for the increased frequency of allograft rejection in these corneas.[20]

Several risk factors for the survival of corneal allografts have been well established, including the degree of corneal neovascularization, the diameter of the graft, the underlying disease, HLA matching, and previous allograft rejection.[1,21–23] Although in the present study it was not possible to take into consideration several risk factors of corneal allograft rejection due to the relatively small number of patients with inflamed corneas, it was evident that a high density of Langerhans cells in the recipient cornea—independent of the degree of neovascularization—was definitely a high risk factor for irreversible allograft rejection. Thus, determining the density of LC in the recipient cornea before grafting may be a good means of evaluating the possible risk of graft failure in vascularized corneas.

REFERENCES

1. S.E. Wilson and Kaufman H.E., Graft failure after penetrating keratoplasty. *Surv. Ophthalmol.* 34: 325–356 (1990).
2. Council on Scientific Affairs. Report on the organ transplant panel: Corneal Transplantation. *JAMA* 259: 719–722 (1988).
3. M.H. Friedlaender, Corneal transplantation. In, *Allergy and Immunology of the Eye.* Harper and Row, New York. (1979).

4. J.Y. Niederkorn, Immune privilege and immune regulation in the eye. *Adv. Immunol.* 48: 191 (1990).

5. A. A. Khodadoust, The allograft reaction: the leading cause of late failure of clinical corneal grafts. In: *Corneal Graft Failure* (Ciba Foundation symposium) B.R. Jones, ed., Elsevier, Amsterdam. (1973).

6. D.J. Coster, Factors affecting the outcome of corneal transplantation. *Ann. R. Coll. Surg. Eng.* 63: 91 (1981).

7. T.E. Gillett, Chandler J.W., and Greiner J.V., Langerhans cells of the ocular surface. *Ophthalmology* 89: 700 (1982).

8. W. Philipp and Gottinger W., T6-positive Langerhans cells in diseased corneas. *Invest. Ophthalmol. Vis. Sci.* 32: 2492 (1991).

9. T.E. Adams, Bodmer, J.G., and Bodmer, W.F., Production and characterization of monoclonal antibodies recognizing the alpha-chain subunits of human Ia alloantigens. *Immunology* 50: 613 (1983).

10. J.A. Thomas, Janossy, G., Chilosi, M., et al., Combined immunological and histochemical analysis of skin and lymph node lesions in histiocytosis X. *J. Clin. Pathol.* 35: 327 (1982).

11. C. Bonnard, Papermaster, D.S., and Kraehenbuhl J.P., The streptavidin-biotin bridge technique: application in light and electron microscope immunocytochemistry. In *Immunolabelling for Electron Microscopy,* J.M. Polak and Varndell, I.M., eds., Elsevier Science Publishers, Amsterdam (1984).

12. M.J. Jager., Corneal Langerhans cells and ocular immunology. *Reg. Immunol.* 4: 186 (1992).

13. J.Y. Niederkorn, Ubelaker, J.E., and Martin, J.M., Vascularization of corneas of hairless mutant mice. *Invest. Ophthalmol. Vis. Sc.i* 31: 948 (1990).

14. J.M. Austyn, Lymphoid dendritic cells. *Immunology* 62: 161 (1987).

15. J.M. Austyn and Steinman, R.M., The passenger leukocyte-a fresh look. *Transplant. Rev.* 2: 139 (1988).

16. D. Callanan, Peeler, J.S., and Niederkorn, J.Y., Characteristics of rejection of orthotopic corneal allografts in the rat. *Transplantation* 45: 437 (1988).

17. R.I. Lechler, and Batchelor J.R., Restoration of immunogenicity to passenger cell-depleted kidney allografts by the addition of donor strain dendritic cells. *J. Exp. Med.* 155: 31 1982).

18. H. Golding, and Singer, A., Role of accessory cell processing and presentation of shed H-2 alloantigens in allospecific cytotoxic T lymphocyte responses. *J. Immunol.* 133: 597 (1984).

19. R.A. Sherwood, Brent, L., and Rayfield, L.S., Presentation of alloantigens by host cells. *Eur. J. Immunol.* 16: 569 (1986).

20. K.A. Williams, White, M.A., Ash, J.K., and Coster, D.J., Leukocytes in the graft bed associated with corneal graft failure: analysis by immunohistology and actuarial graft survival. *Ophthalmology* 96: 38–44 (1989).

21. T.H. Mader, and Stulting, R.D., The high-risk penetrating keratoplasty. *Ophthalmol. Clin. North Amer.* 4: 411 (1991).

22. J.R. Batchelor, Casey, T.A., Gibbs, D.C., et al., HLA matching and corneal grafting. *Lancet* 1: 551 (1976).

23. H.J. Volker-Dieben, *The Effect of Immunological and Non-immunological Factors on Corneal Graft Survival.* Dr. W. Junk Publishers, Dordrecht, (1984).

18

TAMPA TREPHINE PENETRATING KERATOPLASTY

Results of the First 35 Cases

J. James Rowsey,[1] Juan Camilo Sanchez-Thorin,[2] Antonio Maglione,[2]
Guillermo Rocha,[2] Bradley Fouraker,[2] and Scott X. Stevens[2]

[1]James P. and Heather Gills Professor and Chairman
Cornea Section
University of South Florida
Tampa, Florida
[2]Cornea Section
University of South Florida
Tampa, Florida

ABSTRACT

The Tampa Trephine penetrating keratoplasty technique (TTPK) provides a 7.0 mm corneal donor button with six rectangular tabs of Bowman's layer and anterior stroma, 50 microns in thickness, which are inserted into the recipient corneal stroma beneath Bowman's layer. TTPK offers the hypothetical advantages over standard penetrating keratoplasty of a more stable donor-host interface, the presence of fewer sutures (12 interrupted), lower astigmatism, a shorter visual acuity recovery period, and additional tectonic support in thin recipient beds. This article reports the results from the first 35 patients operated on within a four month follow-up period. The patients in this study were submitted to TTPK and evaluated postoperatively at 1, 7, and 15 days, as well as 1, 2, 3, and 4 months. Retrospective evaluations included visual acuity, computerized corneal topography, ultrasonic pachymetry, slit lamp examination, and intraocular pressure. The tab presence induced a clinically stable donor-host interface by four months postoperatively. Early suture removal accomplished in nine cases in the postoperative time frame between 110 and 145 days reflected in minimal astigmatism only in three sutureless corneas. A myopic postoperative sphere was usually observed, especially when early complete suture removal was accomplished. Early postoperative complications included transient donor epithelial defects and corneal edema, inadequate wound closure, wound dehiscence, superficial neovascularization directed towards the tabs, epithelial inclusion in the stromal pocket, and contamination of the donor button. Late complications included one primary graft failure, one endothelial graft rejection, and one crystalline keratopathy.

Advances in Corneal Research, edited by Lass
Plenum Press, New York, 1997

Results indicate that Tampa Trephine penetrating keratoplasty is a viable surgical technique offering potential theoretical benefits and risks over the standard penetrating keratoplasty technique. However, a comparative assessment of risks and benefits of this procedure needs to be addressed through randomized clinical trials. This case series includes examples in which a sutureless cornea with minimal astigmatism was achieved within the first four postoperative months. This study also shows examples of several complications that could be inherent to this surgical technique.

INTRODUCTION

Penetrating keratoplasty is routinely performed by transplanting a round donor corneal button incised with standard stainless steel corneal trephines. The recently described Tampa trephine penetrating keratoplasty technique (TTPK) (paper at the American Academy of Ophthalmology; Atlanta, GA; October 31, 1995) utilizes a 7.0 mm corneal donor button with six rectangular 1 x 2 mm tabs of Bowman's layer and anterior stroma, 50 microns in thickness generated with the *Tampa Trephine*. The tabs are inserted into the recipient stroma beneath Bowman's layer and the corneal button is secured with 12 interrupted sutures, six sutures through, and six sutures between the tabs. Previous studies have demonstrated the reproducibility of corneal buttons obtained with the Tampa Trephine (poster and paper presentation at the Association for Research in Vision and Ophthalmology; May, 1995; Ft. Lauderdale, FL.), a localized peripheral endothelial cell loss during the trephination process[1] and the procedure's surgical viability and safety in the cat animal model (paper and poster presentation at the Association for Research in Vision and Ophthalmology; May, 1995; Ft. Lauderdale, FL). Theoretical advantages of TTPK include a more stable donor-host interface with more precise wound coaptation due to the tab presence, the potential for earlier suture removal as compared to the standard penetrating keratoplasty, the presence of fewer corneal interrupted sutures decreasing the time to minimal postoperative astigmatism, and additional tectonic support in thin stromal beds. Additionally, the donor-host interface stability provided by the tabs may provide a sutureless penetrating keratoplasty in the future, with the aid of collagen- or fibrogen-based biological glues that could substitute for sutures.

This report presents the results of a retrospective case series of 35 patients who underwent TTPK with a follow up time of 4 months. Preliminary results have been previously presented (paper at the American Academy of Ophthalmology; Atlanta, GA, October 31, 1995, submitted for publication).

PATIENTS AND METHODS

Indications for TTPK are the same as for penetrating keratoplasty. Patients ineligible for TTPK included those with a history of previous incisional keratotomy, presence of active corneal or ocular infection, or evidence of corneal perforation and consequent ocular hypotony. Data was reviewed retrospectively and included uncorrected and best corrected visual acuity, refraction, ultrasonic pachymetry (utilizing a DGH ultrasonic pachymeter; DGH Technology, Inc.; Frazer, PA), intraocular pressure (Tono-PenXL tonometer, Mentor; Norwell, MA) slit lamp examination, and computerized corneal topography (CCT) using the EyeSys Corneal Analysis System (EyeSys Laboratories, Inc.; Houston, TX). Examinations were performed preoperatively, as well as postoperatively at day 1, weeks 1 and 2, month 1, and then monthly in the postoperative period. Patients included in this report completed a minimum four month postoperative period. Informed consent was obtained from every patient.

Donor Button Trephination

Fulfilling the established criteria for the Eye Bank Association of America, donor corneas were obtained from the Lions Eye Bank (Tampa, FL) using the routine acquisition process.

The *Tampa Trephine* (Martin Marietta Specialty Components; Largo, FL), as shown in Figure 1, consists of two metallic bases on which the donor corneoscleral rim is submitted to prescribed trephination steps as previously reported[1] (poster and paper presentation at the Association for Research in Vision and Ophthalmology; May, 1995; Ft. Lauderdale, FL). In brief, a six-tab donor punch is initially performed, providing a 7.0 mm graft with six 2.0 x 1.0 mm full thickness tabs. These tabs are grooved at the 7.0 mm optical zone to a 400 micron depth leaving Bowman's layer intact. A second trephination shaves the residual tab tissue, leaving only Bowman's layer and anterior stroma for subsequent imbrication into the recipient bed. The result is a 7.0 mm corneal donor button with six tabs, 50 to 100 microns in thickness, 2 mm wide x 1 mm long attached to it (Fig. 2).

Surgical Technique

A detailed description of the surgical technique has been presented previously (paper presentation at the Association for Research in Vision and Ophthalmology; May, 1995; Ft. Lauderdale, FL). Briefly, the following steps are included. The visual axis is marked with a Sinskey hook. A six-incision radial keratotomy marker is placed around the visual axis to prescribe the tab pocket positions. A 7.5 mm Hessburg-Barron vacuum trephine (Jedmed Instruments Company; St. Louis, MO) is placed on the cornea and suctioned into place. The trephine is rotated one full revolution following epithelial

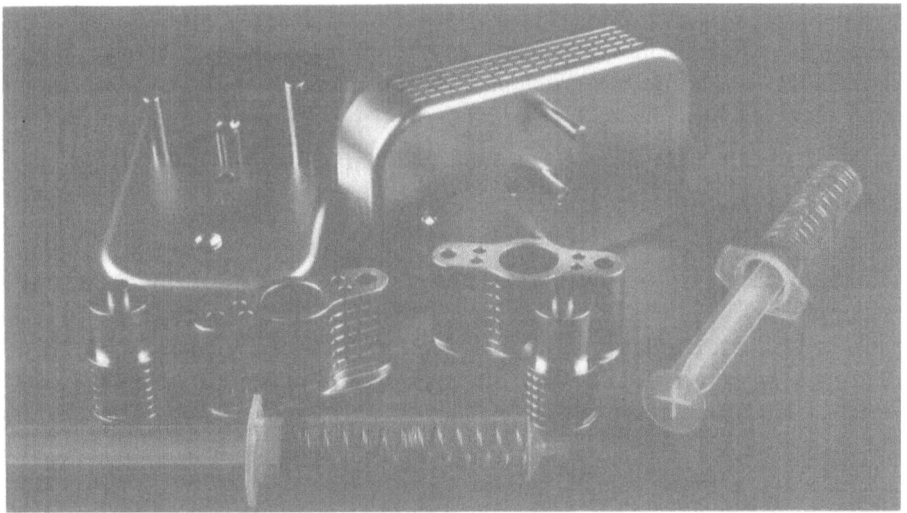

Figure 1. The Tampa Trephine (Martin Marietta Speciality Components, Largo, FL).

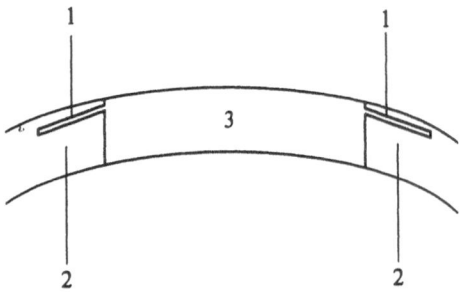

1. Tabs in stromal pockets
2. Recipient stroma
3. Donor cornea

Figure 2. Schematic demonstration of the Tampa Trephine penetrating keratoplasty. Six stromal tabs from the donor cornea, 50 to 75 microns in thickness, are inserted into the recipient stromal pockets.

engagement (250 micron depth), after which the Hessburg-Barron Trephine is removed by releasing suction. The groove is verified to be equivalent in all quadrants. A 2.5 mm, 30° angled diamond blade (KMI Surgical Products; West Chester, PA) creates six pockets, 60 degrees apart, just beneath Bowman's layer, 2.5 mm x 2.0 mm in size. Globe fixation and pressure elevation for sectility are accomplished with a Thornton ring during this maneuver. The anterior chamber is entered with a 15 degree sharp blade (Storz Instruments Co.; St. Louis, MO). Standard left-going and right-going Troutman Katzen corneal scissors are used to remove the host cornea. The host Descemet's rim is minimized using Vannas scissors. Sodium hyaluronate [Healon] (Pharmacia; Piscataway, NJ) is placed over the host rim. Six interrupted radial 50% depth 10–0 nylon sutures (Alcon CU-5 N66016; Alcon Pharmaceutical; Fort Worth, TX) secure the donor and the host corneas between the tabs. Residual epithelium over the corneal tabs is manually debrided with a feather blade and an iris sweep for support. Each tab is marked with a sterile marking pen for future verification of final intra-pocket positioning. The tabs are inserted within the host pocket simply by rolling the tissue tab into the pocket with a Sinskey hook. This process is repeated for the remaining five tabs. The cornea is secured into position with six additional sutures passed around the tabs. Residual Healon is irrigated out of the anterior chamber and the sutures are tied. The anterior chamber is filled with balanced salt solution (Alcon Pharmaceutical; Fort Worth, TX) and corneal sphericity is verified. Topical fluorescein confirms a secure incision. Postoperative subconjunctival gentamicin (20 mg) and dexamethasone (20 mg) are injected to complete the procedure.

RESULTS

A profile of the TTPK recipient population is shown in Table 1. Thirty eight patients were submitted to TTPK, and 35 patients ages 20 to 85 (mean 60.44) are discussed in this paper, due to inadequate follow-up data from three. Twenty-one right and 14 left eyes received grafts. Clinical examples of the normal postoperative course of several patients at different time points can be seen on Fig. 3.

Intraoperative Events

The following significant intraoperative difficulties were documented:

Table 1. Demographic data of patients receiving Tampa Trephine penetrating keratoplasty

Donor factors	
Mean endothelial cell count	2783 cells/mm^2
Mean age	48.2 years
Median death to enucleation time	5 hours
Mode preservation to surgery time	5 days
Causes of donor death	
Acute myocardial infarction	29
Pulmonary embolism	3
Lung Cancer	1
Gun shot wound	1
MVA	1
Recipient Information	
Mean age in years (+/-SD)	60.44 (±18.08)
Preoperative Systemic conditions	
Arthritis	9
Acne roseacea	2
Diabetes mellitus	3
Thyroid disease	1
Hepatitis B+	1
Muscular dystrophy	1
Heart disease	1
Preoperative Corneal Diagnosis	
Pseudophakic bullous keratopathy	12
Fuchs endothelial dystrophy	9
Herpetic corneal disease	4
Keratoconus	4
Traumatic corneal scarring	4
Corneal blood staining following hyphema	1
Corneal Scarring (trichiasis)	1
Graft failure	2
Keratoglobus	1
Other Preoperative Ocular Conditions	
Amblyopia	2
Glaucoma	4
Proliferative Diabetic Retinopathy	1
Cystoid macular edema	1
Cataract	8
Cogan's map-dot-fingerprint dystrophy	1
Age-related maccular degeneration	2
Ptosis	1
Previous lens status	
Pseudophakic	15
Anterior chamber	4
Posterior chamber	11
Phakic	19
Aphakic	1
Surgocal factors	
Combined surgeries	
Anterior vitectomy	10
Lens Surgery	
Extraction with IOL implant	12
IOL removal or exchange	4

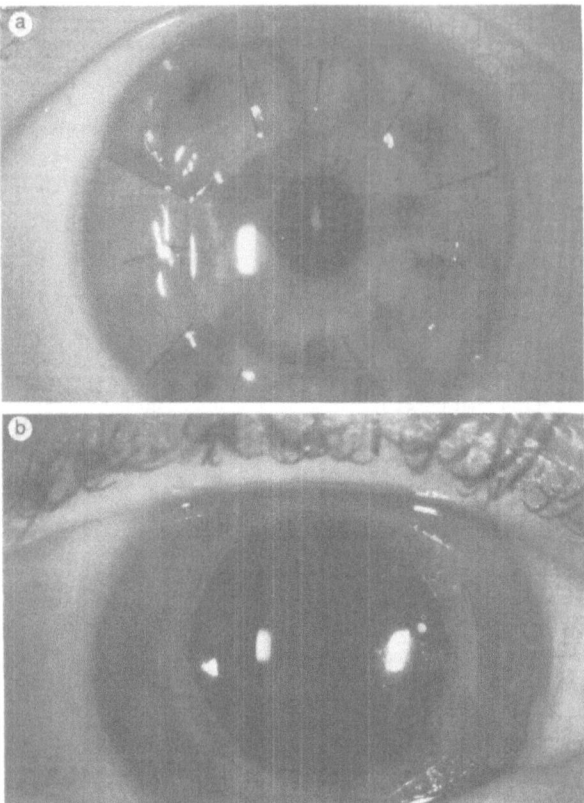

Figure 3. a) Normal postoperative status one month following TTPK. (T): Area of tabs. b) Normal postoperative status four months after TTPK. Notice some peripheral Descemet's folds.

1. Tab pocket preparation: Pocket preparation into the host tissue resulted in recipient bed extension of the pocket through the surface on two occasions. These pockets were uneventfully repaired with simple interrupted sutures.
2. Inadequate tab placement: Two tabs were not completely secured into the pockets, a finding that was only noted postoperatively. Inadequate marking of the tabs and placement into the host stromal pockets was the source of this complication, which was corrected by adequate repositioning and suturing of the tab under local anesthesia.

Postoperative Uncorrected and Best Corrected Visual Acuity

Uncorrected and best corrected visual acuity data can be seen on Table 2. The proportion of patients with uncorrected and best corrected visual acuity grater or equal to 20/200 increased during the first two months and then stabilized. The most frequently observed uncorrected and best corrected visual acuities after two post-surgical months were 20/200 and 20/150, respectively. The proportion of patients with best corrected visual acuity equal or greater than 20/40 also increased during the first two months and then stabilized. At all time points less than 20% of patients had uncorrected visual acuity equal to or

Table 2. Visual acuity following Tampa Trephine penetrating keratoplasty

Postoperative day	Day 15	Mon. 1	Mon. 2	Mon. 3	Mon. 4	PCSR
n	35	35	33	28	26	9
UVA						
Range	HM- 20/50	CF- 20/30	CF-20/30	CF-20/30	CF-20/50	CF-20/100
Mode	CF	20/200	20/200	20/200	20/150	20/200
≥ 20/200 (%)	29.41	61.76	78.79	67.86	61.54	60
BVA						
Range	HM-20/25	CF-20/25	CF-20/30	CF-20/30	CF-20/30	CF-20/30
Mode	CF	20/150	20/150	20/150	20/80	20/100
			20/100			
≥ 20/200 (%)	47.06	67.64	81.81	78.57	77.78	70
≥ 20/40 (%)	2.9	5.8	15.15	14.29	18.52	10

n: Number of patients
UVA: Uncorrected visual acuity
BVA: Best corrected visual acuity
≥ 20/200: Equal or better than 20/200
≥ 20/100: Equal or better than 20/100
PCSR: Post complete suture removal

better than 20/40. Non-corneal causes for low visual acuity were present in several patients (Table 1).

Corneal Refractive Power and Astigmatism

Four patients were not included, two because of early Tampa Trephine transplant replacement and two because of media opacities. From the 31 patients on whom manifest refraction could be performed, nine were submitted to early complete suture removal and will be discussed later. Among the 22 remaining patients with at least one suture present, 15 were myopic with a mean sphere of -1.15 diopters. Table 3 shows the latest postoperative refraction of these 22 patients.

Corneal astigmatism, as measured by manifest cylinder and computerized corneal topography at several time points, is described in Table 4. Astigmatism could be evaluated consistently by computerized corneal topography one month after surgery. As observed, the mean postoperative astigmatism four months postoperatively was 5.39 (95% confidence intervals 4 to 6.78 diopters) as measured by corneal topography. At this time point, mean refractive cylinder was 4.37 diopters (95% confidence intervals 3.5 to 5.2).

Corneal Healing and Early Complications

A list of intraoperative and postoperative complications is provided in Table 5.

Epithelial Corneal Healing. On the first postoperative day, 31 patients presented an epithelial defect comprising 10 to 100% of the donor epithelium. One week after surgery (mode 6 days), 8 patients demonstrated an epithelial defect, and one week later (mode 13 days postoperatively) eight patients still disclosed incomplete epithelial healing. One month after surgery (mean 30 days), six patients persisted with small and variable epithelial defects, all of which were healed at all further evaluations. At two months (mean 58 days) postoperatively, two patients presented small epithelial defects after complete epithelialization, which subsequently healed with medical management.

Table 3. Postoperative refraction of 22 patients after TTPK

No.	SPH	CYL	Axis	Time
1	-4.00	1.75	135	4M
2	-1.00	4.50	60	2M
4	-2.50	2.00	150	4M
5	1.50	4.75	65	4M
14	-3.25	6.00	20	4M
15	-3.25	3.00	180	4M
16	-5.75	6.50	142	4M
17	Plano	3.00	10	4M
18	-3.75	7.00	55	4M
19	-5.75	5.50	45	3M
21	-4.25	4.75	120	4M
22	-2.75	3.25	10	4M
26	1.75	2.00	135	4M
27	-4.25	8.00	110	3M
28	-5.75	5.75	140	4M
29	3.00	6.00	15	4M
30	-4.00	6.00	170	4M
31	2.00	8.50	153	4M
32	2.25	0.50	155	3M
33	-1.50	1.75	15	3M
34	7.00	2.75	55	3M
35	4.75	0.75	175	4M
X	1.34	4.27		4M*
SD	3.61	2.32		

NT: Not tested
LFU: Loss to follow-up
PGF: Primary graft failure
X: Mean
SD: Standard deviation
*: Mode

Table 4. Mean and standard deviation of postoperative refractive cylinder and computerized corneal topography astigmatism

	Month 1	Month 2	Month 3	Month 4	PCSR
n	17	26	22	22	9
Cylinder	3.28	5.44	4.16	4.37	4.17
Mean (SD)	(2.36)	(2.86)	(2.29)	(2.06)	(3.40)
Cylinder Range	0.5–4.75	3.0–12.50	0.5–7.50	0.75–8.50	1.00–12.00
n	24	23	15	12	5
TCC AST	6.63	6.09	4.63	5.39	4.69
Mean (SD)	(3.17)	(2.93)	(2.15)	(2.46)	(4.06)
TCC AST Range	1.87–14.42	1.21–11.28	1.7–8.48	3.11–9.63	1.8–9.23

n: Number of patients available
TCC AST: Computerized cornealtopography astigmatism
SD: Standard Deviation
PCSR: Post complete suture removal

Table 5. Complications associated with Tampa Trephine
Penetrating Keratoplasty

Intraoperative
  Button trephination
    1. Endothelial detachment secondary to blade torquing
    2. Peripheral endothelial detachment, tears, and folds
  Corneal button placement in host tissue
    1. Pocket exteriorization
    2. Anterior chamber penetration during pocket formation
    3. Inadequate tab positioning
Early postoperative [Days 1 to 30]
    1. Donor epithelial defects
    2. Inadequate non-tab wound closure
    3. Wound dehiscence in non-tab area
    4. Corneal edema
    5. Positive culture of donor rim
    6. Intraocular pressure elevation
    7. Donor button fungal contamination
Late postoperative [After day 30]
    1. Wound dehiscence following early suture removal
    2. Neovascularization to tab tissue
    3. Epithelium inclusion in stromal pockets
    4. Primary graft failure
    5. Endothelial graft rejection
    6. Crystallin keratopathy
Post early suture removal [After Day 110]
    1. Wound dehiscence topographic pattern
    2. Dellen
    3. Increase in astigmatism

Corneal Thickness and Edema. The corneal deturgescence rate starting at postoperative Day 1 is shown in Fig. 4. The day following surgery, corneal edema was noted in 30 patients, and folds in Descemet's membrane were observed in 28. Six days after surgery, 24 corneas still displayed residual stromal edema and Descemet's folds. Two weeks postoperatively edema persisted in 17 patients. Forty percent of the corneas were less than 600 microns thick at this time. One month postoperatively, 46.7% of patients showed a central pachymetry below 600 microns (six patients were lost to follow-up at this time point). Descemet's folds persisted in 13 of 30 patients (43.33%). Two and three months after surgery, 19 of 25 (76%) and 19 of 24 (79.6%) corneas, respectively, had a thickness below 600 microns. Four months postoperatively, 69.6% (16 of 23) of the corneal grafts were under 600 microns thick. One month postoperatively, 46.7% of patients showed a central pachymetry below 600 microns (six patients were lost to follow-up at this time point). Descemet's folds persisted in 13 of 30 patients (43.33%). Two and three months after surgery, 19 of 25 (76%) and 19 of 24 (79.6% of corneas, respectively had a thickness of less than 600 microns. Four months postoperatively, 69.6% (16 of 23) of the corneal grafts were under 600 microns thick.

Host-Donor Interface Healing

Adequate wound healing and progressive amalgamation of tab and host corneal tissues were consistently observed in all patients at different time points as observed in Figure 5, save for the following events.

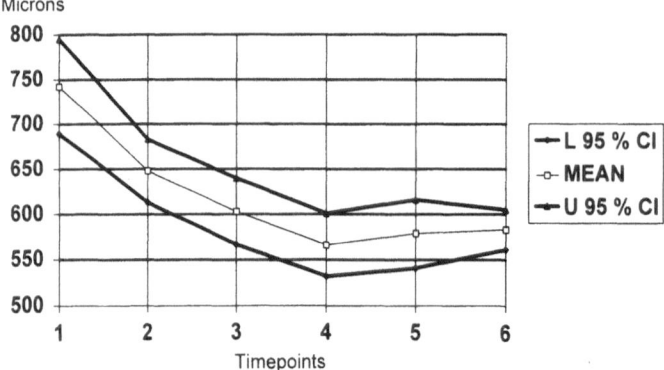

Figure 4. Graph showing the deturgescence rate of corneas following TTPK at different timepoints. Timepoint (T) 1 is day 1 (95% confidence intervals [CI] 689.19 to 795.29), T2 is day 7 (95% CI 682.95 to 764.29), T3 is day 15 (95% CI 613.49 to 683.91), T4 is month 1 (95% CI 567.93 to 639.72), T5 is month 2 (95% CI 532.57 to 600.93), T6 is month 3 (95% CI 541.71 to 616.71) and T7 is month 4 (95% CI 561.31 to 605.91).

On the first postoperative day, four patients presented inadequate wound closure requiring suture placement. These defects were consistently located between two of the tabs. One week after surgery, two other patients presented spontaneous wound dehiscences with Seidel positive phenomena, and two weeks postoperatively two patients presented a second episode of spontaneous wound dehiscence, and one *de novo*. These were also consistently located in an area between the tabs. At this time, one patient developed a dellen adjacent to a tab at the 4:00 position. Two months postoperatively, one patient presented a spontaneous wound dehiscence, and two presented wound dehiscences following early suture removal. Poor epithelial healing had been present preoperatively in one of these latter patients, a controlled non-insulin-dependent diabetic with rosacea-induced surface failure phenomenon. At day 72, one patient presented another spontaneous wound dehiscence. All wound dehiscences were treated satisfactorily with 10–0 nylon interrupted sutures across the leaking area. Corneal superficial neovascularization directed toward the corneal pockets was observed in only one patient, two weeks after surgery.

Postoperative Infections

Six days after surgery, one patient presented a stromal infiltrate inside the 9:00 position pocket, with a satellite lesion located peripherally in the donor-host interface at the 10:30 position. At this time her donor corneal rim culture was positive for *Candida albicans* and the corneal button was uneventfully replaced through a standard penetrating keratoplasty. Another patient developed a crystalline keratopathy located at the host-donor interface in an area between the tabs at postoperative day 110. Bacterial and fungal cultures were negative, and the patient was successfully treated with subconjunctival vancomycin plus topical vancomycin and ceftazidine.

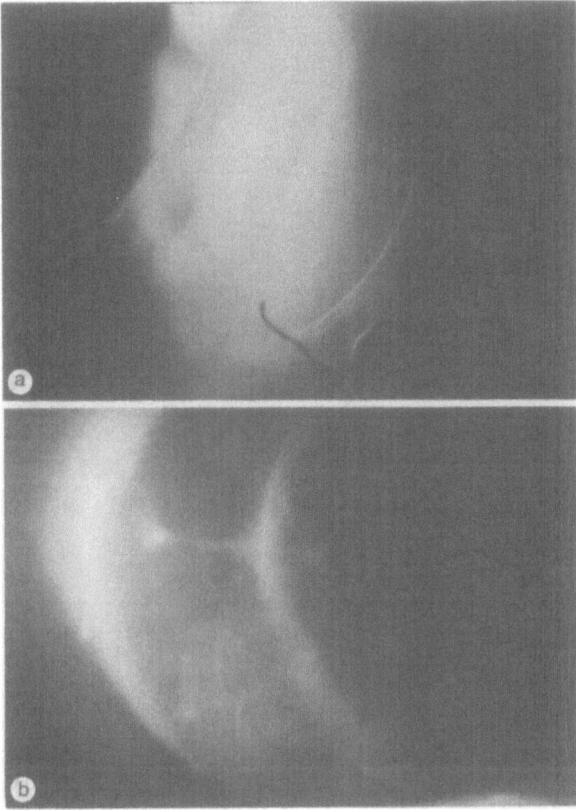

Figure 5. a) Adequate amalgamation of tab tissue into the recipient stroma two months after TTPK. b) Adequate host-donor interface healing in an area between tabs, at 3 months postoperatively.

Elevated Intraocular Pressure

Seven patients presented elevated intraocular pressure on the first two week postoperative course, all were successfully managed with topical beta-blockers. Occasional intraocular pressure elevations were documented later on, although none were present at three months postoperatively.

Other Late Postoperative Complications

One patient experienced an endothelial graft rejection three months after surgery, successfully treated with topical steroids. Another patient demonstrated a primary donor failure with a pachymetry over 800 microns at postoperative week 8. Her donor button was replaced with a routine penetrating keratoplasty. Peripheral localized endothelial detachments and Descemet's folds were consistently observed in patients undergoing this technique, as shown in Figure 6.

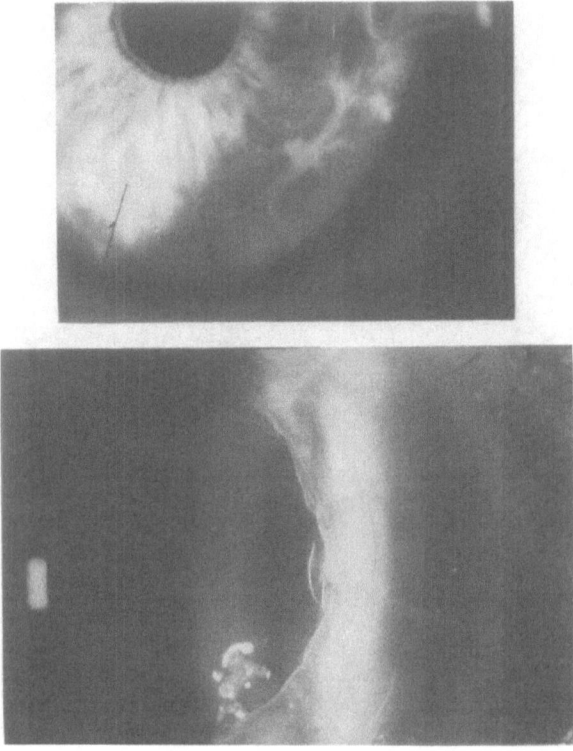

Figure 6. Peripheral localized endothelial detachments following TTPK.

Suture Removal

Healing of the tab tissue into the host cornea was observed in patients at a four-month postoperative period. In the patients with previous pseudophakic bullous keratopathy, this healing pattern was evident even in the presence of significant host corneal edema associated with previous pseudophakic bullous keratopathy. The observation of advanced wound healing prompted removal of all sutures from nine patients at a time range between 110 and 145 days after surgery. The latest available manifest refraction after complete suture removal (range of seven 50 42 days after suture removal) is presented in Table 6. As noted, the mean sphere in this group of eyes was -5.27 diopters, and seven of nine cases showed a myopia of at least -2.75 diopters. In one patient, early complete suture removal induced a wound dehiscence pattern in an area between the tabs, requiring new suture placement. Three of the nine cases showed a post-suture removal astigmatism of less than 2 diopters.

DISCUSSION

This report presents a case series of 35 patients undergoing a new surgical technique, the Tampa Trephine penetrating keratoplasty. A valid comparison between the

Table 6. Postoperative refractive status of patients
submitted to TTPK and early complete
suture removal

No.	Sphere	Cylinder	Axis	PSRD
1	-2.75	1.00	90	17 D
2	-15.00	12	45	7 D
3	-8.00	3.25	53	7 D
4	-8.25	5.5	165	7 D
5	-8.00	3.25	53	7 D
6	-6.25	6.00	45	30 D
7	-4.75	3.25	175	42 D
8	1.75	1.25	37	28 D
9	4.00	2.00	135	14 D
Mean	-5.27	4.17		17.7 D
SD	5.71	3.39		

SD: Standard Deviation

standard and the new technique of TTPK will only be available in the future through randomized clinical trials designed to compare specific safety and efficacy issues.

Experience with these first cases shows that uneventful TTPK is a successful technique. However, TTPK has inherent potential wound healing risks which require early recognition and appropriate management.

Severe epithelial defects on the donor tissue were observed on the first operated cases, probably induced by the use of methylene blue for tab staining. This step of the procedure was abandoned with subsequent improvement in results. In the presence of donor corneal tabs, a clinically stable donor-host interface along the tabs can be observed three to four months after surgery. This stability may not be present in the early postoperative period, when researchers observed a number of wound dehiscences, both spontaneous and following early suture removal, all of them located in the non-tab areas. Four months may not be adequate host-donor interface coaptation time in the non-tab areas. The presence of the tabs has induced a stable interface in the presence of recipient edematous corneal beds, permitting early complete suture removal with minimal astigmatism, a setting difficult to replicate following standard penetrating keratoplasty.

Future controlled studies may address the hypothesis that following TTPK, visual acuity recovers faster in the presence of minimal corneal sphere and astigmatism in a transparent sutureless cornea. Interestingly, more than 60% of patients submitted to TTPK are myopic postoperatively, despite the presence of a 7.0 mm diameter donor button placed on a 7.5 mm host bed. This could be secondary to an anterior bowing of the corneal button or to a tissue addition phenomenon. Of interest also is the observation that seven of nine patients were myopic following early complete suture removal, in ranges between -2.75 and -15 diopters. Following TTPK and early complete suture removal operated corneas did not necessarily have low astigmatism. Astigmatism less than 2 diopters was observed in only three of nine patients following early complete suture removal. The occurrence of two post-TTPK corneal infections of known etiology but unknown source requires further evaluation. One infection was due to corneal donor button contamination, which might have occurred anytime before the donor rim was placed into culture. Another infection occurred two months after surgery, in the presence of a persistent epithelial defect. It is believed that the Tampa Trephine technique does not have an increased risk for postoperative corneal infections in and of itself.

The presence of the tabs close to the limbal antigen presenting dendritic cells can, in theory, increase the risk of graft rejection. One case of neovascularization directed towards the tab area was observed, as was one case of endothelial graft rejection. Four patients with preoperative keratoconus and one with keratoglobus gained tectonic support by tab stromal tissue addition, a variable that has not been objectively evaluated. For any new surgical technique, prospective, randomized clinical trials addressing specific issues are required to determine comparative benefits and risks as compared with the best standard of care. Because of the lack of controls, this study cannot suggest that TTPK is a better option than standard penetrating keratoplasty. A future clinical trial will compare the standard penetrating keratoplasty technique utilizing 16 interrupted sutures and a 24-bite running suture with the Tampa Trephine technique, with postoperative residual astigmatism as the primary endpoint. Patients with keratoconus, advanced corneal scarring (including secondary infectious, dystrophic, and degenerative diseases), aphakic and pseudophakic bullous keratopathy, and previous graft failures will be included in the study.

ACKNOWLEDGMENTS

Supported in part by Technology Deployment Center, Department of Energy (Grant No. 6124061LO) and an unrestricted grant from Research to Prevent Blindness. Dr. Sanchez-Thorin is supported by Colciencias (Colombia).

NOTE

The University of South Florida (Tampa, FL) and Martin Marietta Specialty Components (Largo FL) have patent pending rights to the Tampa Trephine instrumentation. The authors do not have any proprietary interest in any of the products used in this study.

REFERENCE

1. J.C. Sanchez-Thorin, Rocha, G., Bowyers, B., et al., Effects on the cat corneal endothelium following trephination using the Tampa Trephine technique. *Cornea* In press.

19

PENETRATING KERATOPLASTY FOR PSEUDOPHAKIC BULLOUS KERATOPATHY

An Indian Experience

Anita Panda, Namrata Sharma, and S. K. Angra

Dr. Rajendra Prasad Centre for Ophthalmic Sciences
All India Institute of Medical Sciences
New Delhi, India

ABSTRACT

A retrospective analysis of 198 eyes with pseudophakic bullous keratopathy undergoing penetrating keratoplasty with or without intraocular (IOL) exchange was performed over an 11-year period. The 198 eyes evaluated consisted of 86 anterior chamber (AC), 27 iris fixated (IF), and 85 posterior chamber (PC) lenses. Patients were followed up for an average of 3.2 ± 1.3 years. The mean intervals between initial cataract surgery and penetrating keratoplasty were 38 ± 4, 44 ± 3, and 3 ± 1.2 months with AC, IF and PC lenses, respectively. Pre-existing endothelial changes in fellow eyes were present in 56% of cases. Anterior vitrectomy was performed in 93% of AC, 54% of IF, and 35% of PC lenses. More than half of the PC lenses (58.8%) were retained as opposed to 1.7% of AC lenses and 0% of IF lenses. Maximum grafts remained clear with posterior chamber implants (83%) at the time of mean follow up. Visual acuity of 6/18 or more was achieved in 15% of eyes with AC, 17% with IF, and 45% PC with implants respectively. The most common cause of graft failure was raised intraocular pressure with all types of pseudophakos. The leading causes of non-improvement of vision in the presence of clear graft were cystoid macular edema (40%) and glaucomatous optic atrophy (37.1%).

INTRODUCTION

Pseudophakic bullous keratopathy is one of the leading indications for penetrating keratoplasty worldwide.[1-5] The incidence of corneal edema after extracapsular cataract extraction and posterior chamber lens implantation is less than 1%, which reflects improvement in surgical technique, intraocular lens design, and use of viscoelastic substances.[3] A number of authors have described the results of keratoplasty and discussed various approaches for the intraoperative management of intraocular lenses.[6-13]

Advances in Corneal Research, edited by Lass
Plenum Press, New York, 1997

This study was undertaken to assess the magnitude of disease in a referral eye care center in a developing country. Patients who had undergone penetrating keratoplasty for pseudophakic bullous keratopathy were evaluated. The spectrum of associated intraocular lenses and results following penetrating keratoplasty were analyzed with regard to visual acuity and graft clarity.

PATIENTS AND METHODS

This study evaluated the case records of 198 consecutive eyes with pseudophakic bullous keratopathy undergoing penetrating keratoplasty from January 1, 1984 to December 31, 1994. Of 198 eyes evaluated, 86 had intracapsular cataract extraction (ICCE) with AC IOL, 27 had ICCE with IF IOL, and 85 had ICCE with PC IOL. Relevant history and examination findings, including slit lamp biomicroscopy, were recorded in all patients from the case records. The type of intraocular lens and the interval between cataract extraction and corneal transplantation was noted in each case. Specular microscopy of the unoperated fellow eyes were also evaluated wherever possible.

A standard penetrating keratoplasty was undertaken for all eyes. Cases requiring anterior vitretomy, pupilloplasty, and angle reconstruction were recorded. The operative management of intraocular lens was correlated with the visual outcome and graft clarity. The size of the recipient bed varied from 7.0–8.5 mm and the donor buttons used were 0.5–1 mm larger than the recipient bed, depending upon whether the eye was left pseudophakic or aphakic. Decision of IOL retention, removal, or exchange was made depending on the fellow eye status and patient's motivation. Lenses associated with iritis, recurrent hyphaema, or chronic macular edema were removed. Lens exchange was performed if there was no history of glaucoma and chronic ocular inflammation.

All patients received topical corticosteroid-antibiotics post-operatively. Antiglaucoma medication and systemic corticosteroids were given wherever indicated. Best corrected visual acuity, slit lamp biomicroscopy, and tonometry were noted from each follow-up visit. Graft clarity grading was based on anterior chamber details and corneal thickness (Table 1). The follow-up period varied from 1 to 8.5 years (mean 3.2 ± 1.3 years). Sutures were removed six months after surgery or earlier if there were suture-related problems. Spectacles or contact lenses had been fitted to achieve best corrected visual acuity and latest visual acuity, rather than the best visual acuity obtained at any time, were noted. Associated complications like cystoid macular edema, retinal detachment, and glaucomatous optic atrophy were also noted. Cystoid macular edema was diagnosed on ophthalmoscopy or contact lens examination in 40% of cases and only 8% had fluorescein angiographic confirmation of diagnosis.

Table 1. Graft clarity grading

Grades	A/C details	Corneal thickness
4+	Clearly visible	Normal
3+	Clearly visible	Increase up to 20%
2%	Faintly visible	Increase 21%–40%
1+	Faintly visible	Increase > 40%
0	Not visible	Not possible

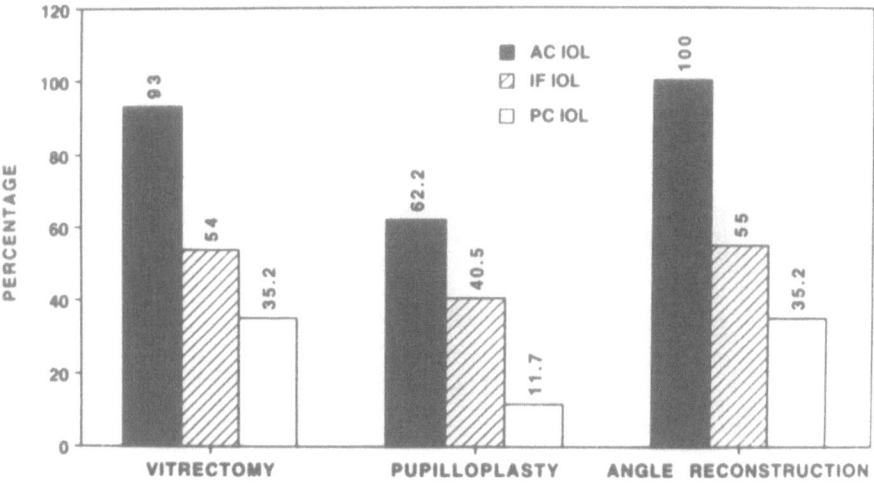

Figure 1. Adjuvant procedures with penetrating keratoplasty for pseudophakic bullous keratoplasty.

RESULTS

The average age of the patients included in this study was 49 ± 4.8 years (range, 28 to 62 years). The 198 eyes in 188 patients included ten bilateral cases; 90 patients were male and 98 were female. Of 86 AC intraocular lenses, 76 were Kelman multiflex open loop and 10 were closed loop semiflexible lenses. Twenty seven IF lenses included 25 iris claw lenses and two iris sutured lenses with prolene. The follow-up ranged from 1 to 8.5 years (mean 3.2 ± 1.3 years). The average time taken for development of bullous keratopathy following cataract surgery was 38 ± 4, 44 ± 3, and 3 ± 1.2 months in eyes with AC, IF, and PC lenses, respectively. Anterior vitrectomy was required in 93% of AC, 54% of IF, and 35% of PC lenses (Fig. 1). Intraoperative complications such as hyphaema and vitreous loss were more frequent with AC and IF lenses as compared to PC lenses. More than half of the PC lenses (58.8%) were retained as opposed to 1.7% of the AC and none of the IF lenses (Fig. 2). Graft clarity of 3+ or more reached a maximum of 83% in the PC group, followed by 52% in the IF and 50% in the AC IOL groups (Fig. 3). Final best corrected visual acuity of 6/18 or better was seen in 17%, 15%, and 45% in AC, IF, and PC intraocular lenses, respectively (Table 2).

The most common cause of graft failure was increased intraocular pressure, followed by severe iridocyclitis and graft rejection (Table 3). The major cause of visual acuity ≤6/60 was graft opacification (54%). Causes of non-improvement of vision in a clear graft included cystoid macular edema, glaucomatous optic atrophy, ARMD, and retinal detachment (Table 4).

Of 146 unoperated fellow eyes, 82 showed presence of guttata with low cell count and pleomorphism (Table 5). Both cell density and pleomorphism were statistically significant in comparison with normal controls. Thirty-four eyes had low cell count and specular microscopic evidence of guttata. Slit lamp examination in these eyes appeared normal. Thus, 58.5% of contralateral eyes had definite evidence of clinical or subclinical endothelial decompensation. Thirty eyes were, however, almost identical to 30 age- and sex-matched normal controls. Because 52 fellow eyes were either pseudophakic or aphakic, no comparison was made with age/sex-matched corneas.

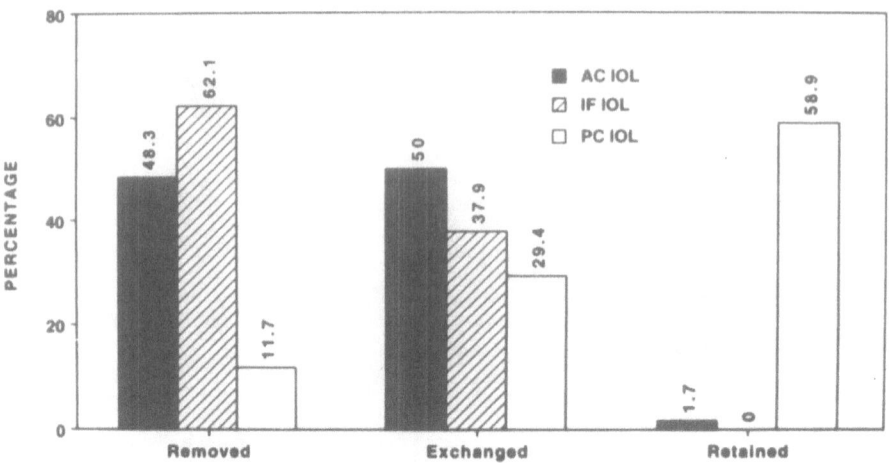

Figure 2. Intraocular lenses removed, exchanged, and retained.

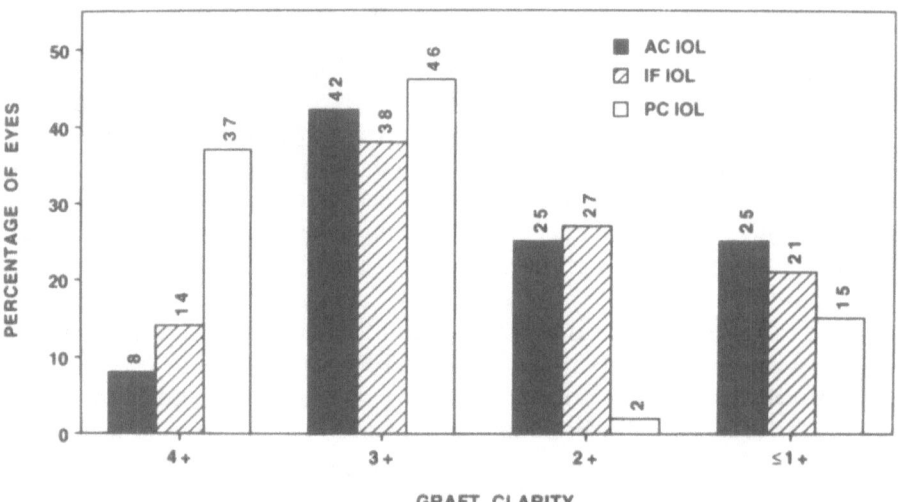

Figure 3. Graft clarity at the end of 1 year.

Table 2. Post PK visual acuity

	AC	IF	PC
≥ 6/12	11%	10%	35%
6/18	6%	5%	10%
6/24	36%	18%	16%
6/36	17%	17%	13%
≤ 6/60	30%	50%	26%

Table 3. Causes of graft failure

	AC IOL	IF IOL	PC IOL
Raised IOP	40%	54%	38%
Severe Iridocyclitis	15%	18%	8%
Graft Rejection	3%	5%	3%

Table 4. Causes of visual acuity ≤ 6/60 (N = 76)

1. Opaque graft	41	(54%)
2. Clear graft	35	(46%)
a) Clinical CME	14	(40%)
b) Glaucomatous optic atrophy	13	(37.1%)
c) ARMD	6	(17.1%)
d) RD	2	(5.7%)

DISCUSSION

Bullous keratopathy continues to be the most common blinding complication of cataract surgery with or without intraocular lens insertion.[6,7] Surgical trauma was considered to be one of the major causes of bullous keratopathy, others being intraocular lens type and quality.[8] Among the various types of pseudophakes, a relatively high incidence of bullous keratopathy is reported with anterior chamber lens and iris fixated lenses.[3,9]

In this series, the early onset of corneal decompensation with posterior chamber lenses (mean 3 ± 1.2 months), late onset with iris fixated lenses (mean 44 ± 3 months), and intermediate onset with anterior chamber lenses (mean 38 ± 4 months) correlates with the pathogenesis of corneal decompensation. A similar pattern has also been noted by other authors.[2,10] Iris supported lenses can intermittently traumatize the endothelium on a chronic basis with rapid eye movements, which has been substantiated by Rao et al., using specular microscopy to document progressive loss of endothelium up to 2 years following the date of implant surgery.[11] This mechanism accounts for a longer latent period for corneal decompensation with these lenses.

Previous studies have demonstrated the importance of primary endothelial disease in the development of pseudophakic bullous keratopathy after intracapsular cataract extraction.[10–14] In this series, clinical or subclinical endothelial decompensation in contralateral eyes was present in 58.5% of cases. A similar figure of 50% has also been reported by Arentson.[8] The relatively rapid onset of corneal edema with posterior chamber pseudophakes

Table 5. Specular microscopy of fellow eyes (n = 146)

Group (No. of Eyes)	Slit lamp	Specular microscopy	Mean cell density (cells/mm^2)	Pleomorphism	Significance**
A (82)	Guttata	Guttata	1587±40	+	D vs. A–HS
B (34)	Normal	Guttata	1884±23	+	D vs. B–S
C (30)	Normal	Normal	1980±82	–	D vs. C–NS
D (30)*	Normal	Normal	2080±66	–	

*Group D is normal controls.
**HS = Highly Significant, S = Significant, NS = Not Significant.

suggests that primary endothelial dystrophy is an important predisposing factor in the development of pseudophakic bullous keratopathy following cataract surgery.

In 1987, problems with closed loop semiflexible anterior chamber lenses were stressed in the literature and their removal recommended.[13,15-18] Despite high rates of graft clarity, visual outcome was often disappointing.[15-18] Retained posterior chamber lenses were associated with the best visual outcome[8,12,19-20] and 58.6% of such lenses in this series were retained as opposed to 1.17% of anterior chamber and none of the iris fixated lenses. Pupilloplasty was required in 66.2% of patients with IF lenses and 40.5% of patients with anterior chamber lenses.

Although clear corneal grafts were obtained in 86% of eyes, visual acuity of 6/12 or better was achieved in only 21% of eyes. Previous series of transplantation for pseudophakic bullous keratoplasty report a visual acuity of 6/12 or better in 17 to 76% of cases (Table 6). As reported in the literature, the three most common causes of decreased visual acuity after penetrating keratoplasty for pseudophakic bullous keratopathy are cystoid macular edema, glaucoma, and graft failure.[14] Cystoid macular edema was diagnosed by ophthalmoscopy or contact lens examination in 40% of cases and only 8% of eyes underwent fluorescien angiography. Maculopathy is attributed to intraoperative inflammation and vitritis during cataract surgery and subsequent penetrating keratoplasty and vitrectomy.[21] Patients with iris supported and anterior chamber lenses often require vitrectomy at the time of keratoplasty. However, the records of original cataract surgery were not available in all patients. Nevertheless, many patients had anterior vitrectomies at the time of cataract surgery. Kramer has demonstrated a direct association between vitrectomy and cystoid macular edema following keratoplasty.[22] Thus, the high incidence of single or multiple vitrectomies in this series explains an increased cystoid macular edema and decreased visual acuity.

Glaucomatous optic atrophy was responsible for visual acuity of <6/60 in 37.1% of cases with clear grafts. This occurs more frequently with anterior chamber and iris fixated lenses and has been attributed to a number of factors: anterior chamber lenses may occlude the angle; they may be associated with increased formation of peripheral anterior synechia; and obviously, they are more often required in cases predisposed to glaucoma, such as those who have undergone vitrectomy.

This study outlines the visual results and functional outcomes of penetrating keratoplasty for pseudophakic bullous keratopathy in a referral center of a developing country and suggests that the results are similar to those of advanced countries (Table 6). This re-

Table 6. Pseudophakic bullous keratopathy visual acuity
(comparative study) at 1 year

	6/6-6/12	6/18-6/36	≤ 6/60
Meyer & Sugar (1980)	50%	14%	36%
Charlton (1981)	–	75%	25%
Arentson (1982)	33%	52%	14%
Waring (1983)	17%	60%	23%
Kozarsky (1983)	38%	28%	33%
Koenig (1988)	76%	12%	12%
Insler (1988)	40%	35%	25%
Cohen (1988)	31%	33%	36%
Hassan (1991)	39%	–	–
Present study (1996)	21%	41%	38%

view suggests that eyes undergoing intraocular implant should have a pre-operative specular microscopy done routinely. Moreover, intraoperative manipulation like anterior vitrectomy, pupilloplasty, and angle reconstruction, more often required with anterior chamber and iris fixated pseudophakes, predisposes to post-operative cystoid macular edema and glaucoma and is thus responsible for compromised visual outcome, despite a clear graft.

REFERENCES

1. R.E. Smith, McDonald, H.R., Nesburn, A.B., and Minckler, D.S., P.K., Changing indications 1947 to 1978. *Arch. Ophthalmol.* 98:1226 (1980).
2. J.B. Robin, Gindi, J.J., Koh, K., et al., An update of the indications for keratoplasty 1979 through 1983 *Arch. Ophthalmol* 104(1):87 (1986).
3. D.M. Taylor, Atlas, B.F., Romanchuk, K.G., and Stern, A.L., Pseudophakic bullous keratopathy. *Ophthalmology* 90(1):19 (1983).
4. P. Haaman, Jensen, O.M., and Schmidt, P., Changing indications of penetrating keratoplasty. *Acta Ophthalmol.* 72(4):443 (1994).
5. F.W. Price, Whitson, W.E., Collins, K.S., and Marks, R.G., Five year corneal graft survival. A large, single-center patient cohort. *Arch. Ophthalmol.* 111(6):799 (1993).
6. R.F. Meyer, and Sugar, A., P.K. in pseudophakic bullous keratopathy 90:677 (1980).
7. K.H. Charlton, Binder, P.S., and Perl T., Visual prognosis in pseudophakic corneal transplants. *Ophthalmic Surg.* 12(6):411 (1981).
8. J.J. Arentsen, and Laibson, P.R., Surgical management of pseudophakic corneal edema: complications and visual results following penetrating keratoplasty. *Ophthalmic Surg.* 13(5):371 (1982).
9. W.R. Fagadau, Maumenee, A.E., Stark, W.J., and Datiles, M., Posterior chamber intraocular lenses at the Wilmer Institute: a comparative analysis of complications and visual results. *Br. J. Ophthalmol.* 68(1):13 (1984).
10. E.J. cohen, Brady, S.E., Leavitt, K.L., et al., Pseudophakic bullous keratopathy. *Am. J. Ophthalmol.* 106:264(1988).
11. G.N. Rao, Aquavella, J.V., Goldberg S.H., and Berk, S.L., Pseudophakic bullous keratopathy. Relationship to pre-operative endothelial status. *Ophthalmology* 91(10):1135 (1984).
12. S.B. Koenig, and Schultz, R.O., Penetrating keratoplasty for pseudophakic bullous keratopathy after extracapsular cataract extraction. *Am. J. Ophthalmol* 105:348 (1988).
13. M. Lugo, Cohen, E.J., Eagle, R.C., et al., The incidence of preoperative endothelial dystrophy in pseudophakic bullous keratopathy. *Ophthalmic Surg.* 19:16 91988).
14. S.R. Waltman, Penetrating keratoplasty for pseudophakic bullous keratopathy. Visual results. *Arch. Ophthalmol.* 99(3):415 (1981).
15. M. Busin, Arffa, R.C., McDonald B., and Kaufman, H.E., Intraocular lens removal during penetrating keratoplasty for pseudophakic bullous keratopathy. *Ophthalmology* 94:505 (1987).
16. P.W. Smith, Wong, S.K., Stark, W.J., et al., Complications of semiflexible, closed loop anterior chamber intraocular lenses. *Arch. Ophthalmol.* 105:52 (1987).
17. G.O. Waring, Stulting, R.D., and Street, D., Penetrating keratoplasty for pseudophakic corneal edema with exchange of intraocular lenses. *Arch. Ophthalmol.* 105:58 (1987).
18. D.J. Apple, and Olson, R.J., Closed loop anterior chamber lenses. *Arch. Ophthalmol.* 105:19 (1987).
19. A.M. Kozarsky, Stopak, S., Waring, G.O., et al., Results of penetrating keratoplasty for pseudophakic corneal oedema with retention of intraocular lens. *Ophthalmology* 91(10:1141 (1984).
20. M.S. Insler, Craig, J., Helm, B.S., and Kaufman, B.E., Visual results after keratoplasty in patients with P/C IOL. *Am. J. Ophthalmol.* 106:72 (1988).
21. G.O. Waring, Welch, S.N., Cavanagh, H.D., and Wilson, L.A., Results of penetrating keratoplasty in 123 eyes with pseudophakic or aphakic corneal edema. *Ophthalmology* 90(1):25 (1983).
22. S.G. Kramer, Cystoid macular edema after aphakic penetrating keratoplasty. *Ophthalmology* 88(8):782 (1981).

20

PENETRATING KERATOPLASTY FOR BULLOUS KERATOPATHY AFTER ARGON LASER IRIDOTOMY

Aoi Komuro, Norihiko Yokoi, Kohji Nishida, Chie Sotozono, and
Shigeru Kinoshita

Department of Ophthalmology
Kyoto Prefectural University of Medicine
Kyoto, Japan

ABSTRACT

Recently, bullous keratopathy has been reported as a devastating late-onset complication after argon laser-iridotomy (ALI). This study investigated the results of penetrating
keratoplasty for bullous keratopathy after ALI.

In this study, 17 patients (17 eyes) who had undergone penetrating keratoplasty between April, 1992 and August, 1995 were retrospectively evaluated. The mean age was
73.2 years, with a range of 63 to 85 years. Five eyes received ALI for primary angle-closure glaucoma attack and 12 eyes for prophylaxis. Five eyes with Fuchs' endothelial dystrophy were included in this study. The triple procedure, consisting of penetrating
keratoplasty with cataract extraction and intraocular lens implantation was performed in
11 eyes. The average postoperative follow-up was 1.5 ± 0.1 years. All grafts were clear at
the latest examination. Corrected visual acuity improved in 16 (94.1%) of the 17 eyes. Notable complications were transient shallow anterior chambers (three eyes) in the early
postoperative period and anterior chamber fibrin response (eight eyes) at the postoperative
period. Although penetrating keratoplasty was successful in bullous keratopathy after
ALI, anterior chamber fibrin response was observed at high incidence. The presurgical
systemic administration of corticosteroid may be effective.

INTRODUCTION

Argon laser iridotomy (ALI) has been widely accepted as a relatively safe procedure
for treating chronic and acute closed-angle glaucoma.[1] Reported complications include
transient intraocular pressure elevation, anterior chamber inflammation, iris hemorrhage,
pupillary distortion, and focal burns to lens, retina, and cornea.[2,3] In recent years, however,

there have been several reports regarding bullous keratopathy induced by ALI[4-8] and even in Japan, such cases are increasing in number.

As predisposing background, previous studies have indicated those episodes of angle-closure glaucoma with pressure elevation,[9] inflammation, high laser energy, diabetes,[10] and corneal guttata. In such cases, penetrating keratoplasty (PKP) is sometimes performed. However, little is known about the long-term results and intraoperative and postoperative complications in ALI-induced bullous keratopathy.

This study reports on the problems in PKP regarding ALI-induced bullous keratopathy, and refers to the aspects of the patients' backgrounds that predispose them to occurrence of bullous keratopathy.

PATIENTS AND METHOD

The subjects of this study were 17 eyes of 17 patients with bullous keratopathy after ALI who underwent PKP between April, 1992 and August, 1995 at the Department of Ophthalmology, Kyoto Prefectural University of Medicine, and who were studied retrospectively. The study included 15 females and two males whose ages ranged from 63 to 85 years (mean 73.2) at the time of PKP. The follow-up period from corneal transplantation to latest examination was 1.5 ± 0.1 (range, 0.1 to 3.0 years). All patients were subjected to careful slit-lamp examination; best corrected visual acuity was measured at follow-up.

RESULTS

The clinical features of the 17 cases are summarized in Table 1. ALI was performed prophylactically on 12 of these eyes, because gonioscopy had demonstrated occluded angle (10 eyes), and on seven eyes because the fellow eye had experienced an acute glaucoma attack. In the fellow eye, five eyes of five patients had corneal guttata; corneal endothelial cell densities in nine eyes of nine patients were decreased to less than 1,000 cells/mm^2; and nine eyes of nine patients had received laser energy exceeding 10J.

Notable complications associated with PKP were transient shallow anterior chamber (three eyes) within the early postoperative period and anterior chamber fibrin response at the time of operation, continuing into the postoperative period (three eyes) and only in the postoperative period (eight eyes) (Figs. 1 and 2).

No graft rejection occurred; all grafts in this series remained clear at the latest follow-up period. The final corrected visual acuity improved two lines in 16 (94.1%) of the 17 subject eyes.

DISCUSSION

These results demonstrate that episodes of angle-closure glaucoma with pressure elevation and inflammation, high laser energy, ALI, and corneal guttata were predisposing risk factors in the backgrounds of patients in this study. It is noted that ALI was performed prophylactically rather than for acute attack. Moreover, in about 50% of the cases, the fellow eye's corneal endothelial cell density decreased to less than 1,000 cells/mm^2 and five eyes of five patients had corneal guttata. Therefore, it is expected that in the cases show-

Table 1. Summary of cases

Case NO.	Age	Sex	DM	Operative Eye Episode of acute attack	Operative Eye Laser energy (J)	Fellow Eye Episode of acute attack	Fellow Eye Laser Energy (J)	Corneal endothelial Cell Density (cells/mm²)	Guttata
1	67	F	–		6.1	O	no data	500	
2	81	F	–		2.0		2.0	664	
3	71	M	–	O	12.0		10.6	457	
4	81	F	–		21.9		16.6 (2 times)	946	
5	71	F	–	O	no data	O	no data	932	
6	63	F	–	O	74.9*	O	31.7*	593	
7	75	F	–	OO	50.7	O	6.6	1183	
8	68	F	–		41.0 (3 times)		22.4	no data	
9	77	F	–		72.2		no deta	2965	
10	72	F	–		7.4	O	7.4	no data	OO
11	85	F	–		no data		no data	no deta	
12	73	F	–		55.0*		41.8*	481	OO
13	72	F	–		19.4 (2 times)	O	0	no data	
14	70	F	–		5.4		4.8	2244	
15	71	M	–		6.9		8.6	300	
16	70	F	–		23.4	OO	0	845	O
17	77	F	–	O	no data		no data	no data	

* Cases performed ALI without Abraham lens

Table 2. Summary of complications

Case No.	Surgical procedure	Transient flat anterior chamber	Fibrin response Intra operative	Fibrin response Post operative	Episode of acute attack
1	Triple				
2	Triple			○	
3	PKP+vitrectomy			○	○
4	Triple				
5	Triple		○	○	
6	Triple			○	○
7	PKP	○	○	○	○
8	PKP+lensectomy				○
9	PKP				○
10	Triple				
11	Triple	○		○	
12	PKP				
13	Triple				
14	PKP				
15	Triple				
16	Triple				
17	Triple	○	○	○	○

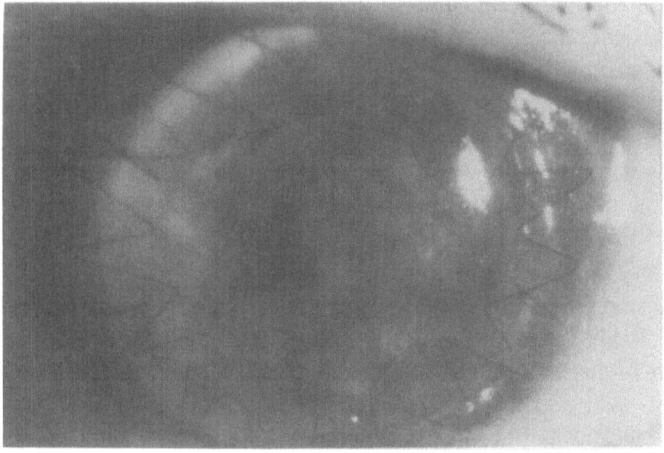

Figure 1. Representative case of fibrin response in anterior chamber early postoperatively. In this case (case 5), anterior chamber massive fibrin response at the time of operation continued into the postoperative period. Fibrin mass disappeared by systemic administration of betamethasone and installation of dexamethasone eyedrops 4 times a day for 2 weeks.

ing diminished corneal endothelial density in the fellow eye, the pre-existing corneal endothelial abnormalities are responsible for the pathogenesis of bullous keratopathy. In one bullous keratopathy case (case 13) corneal endothelial cell density in the fellow eye exceeded 2,000 cells/mm^2 and ALI was performed with minimal energy (5.4J). In such a case, the possibility of ALI inducing long-standing inflammation becomes a contributing factor to late onset endothelial decompensation.

Among the problems complicating the operation, a high incidence of anterior chamber fibrin foi nation was found (eight of 17 eyes, 54.9%). Common causative factors in-

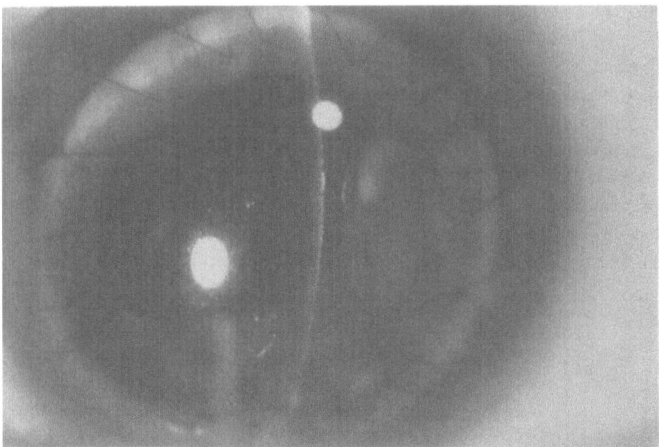

Figure 2. Slit-lamp photomicrograph in case 5 six months after the penetrating keratoplasty showing that graft clarity was maintained.

cluded both ALI and long-term administration of pilocarpine; these induced long-standing blood-aqueous barrier damage,[11] resulting in intra- and/or post-operative fibrin response.

Transient shallow anterior chamber occurred in three eyes (15.4%) from the intraoperative period, continuing into the postoperative period. Possible reasons for this finding included: presence of a shallow anterior chamber before the operation, and an abrupt decrease in intraocular pressure at trephination of the host cornea and subsequent forward movement of the iris-lens diaphragm. In addition, a massive fibrin response might cause angle closure. To overcome this complication, the selection of disparate size trephines and anti-inflammatory therapies are required.

In conclusion, this study reveals that relatively long-term graft survival and visual outcome are favorable following PKP for bullous keratopathy after ALI, although anterior chamber fibrin formation and shallow anterior chamber are observed at high incidence. This study also indicated the importance of corneal endothelial cell density evaluation. Abnormalities, such as guttata, are also important findings to evaluate before ALI.

ACKNOWLEDGMENTS

Supported in part by a research grant from the Kyoto Foundation for the Promotion of Medical Science, and the intramural research fund of the Kyoto Prefectural University of Medicine.

REFERENCES

1. H.A. Quigley, Long-term follow-up of laser iridotomy. *Ophthalmology* 88:218 (1981).
2. R.M. Mandelkorn, Mendelsohn, A.D., Olander, K.W., and Zimmerman, T.J. Short exposure times in argon laser iridotomy. *Ophthalmic Surgery* 12:805 (1981).
3. A.L. Robin, and Pollack, I.P., A comparison of neodymium: YAG and argon laser iridotomies. *Ophthalmology* 91:1011 (1984).
4. I.P. Pollack, Current concepts in laser iridotomy. (Review). *International Ophthalmology Clinics* 24:153 (1984).
5. A.L. Schwartz, Martin, N.F., and Weber, P.A., Corneal decompensation after argon laser iridotomy. *Arch. Ophthalmol.* 106:1572 (1988).
6. S. Jeng, Lee, J.S., and Huang, S.C., Corneal decompensation after argon laser iridectomy — a delayed complication. *Ophthalmic Surgery* 22:565 (1991).
7. K.R. Wilhelmus, Corneal edema following argon laser iridotomy. *Ophthalmic Surgery* 23:533: 1992).
8. R.W. Zabel, Macdonald, I.M., and Mintsioulis G., Corneal endothelial decompensation after argon laser iridotomy. *Can. J. Ophthal.* 26:367 (1991).
9. F. Bigar, and Witmer R., Corneal endothelial changes in primary acute angle-closure glaucoma. *Ophthalmology* 89:596 (1982).
10. R. Schultz, Matsuda, M., and Yee, R., Corneal endothelial changes in type I and II diabetes mellitus. *Ophthalmology* 98:401 (1984).
11. T.J. Zimmerman, and Wheeler, T.M., Miotics: side effects and ways to avoid. *Ophthalmology* 89:76 (1984).

21

INTRAOPERATIVE USE OF TISSUE PLASMINOGEN ACTIVATOR FOR CORNEA TRANSPLANT SURGERY

Mark D. Sherman

Cornea/External Disease/Uveitis Service
Department of Ophthalmology
Anaheim Hills, California

ABSTRACT

Cornea transplant surgery is occasionally necessary for diagnostic and therapeutic purposes in patients with progressive ulcerative keratitis. These cases can be technically difficult as fibrin begins to deposit during suture placement, and postoperative glaucoma is a serious complication which frequently mandates subsequent medical treatment and further surgical procedures. Tissue plasminogen activator (tPA) has been used for the treatment of post-operative fibrin deposition following cornea transplant surgery. Its use *during* cornea transplant surgery has not previously been described.

Six consecutive cases of progressive ulcerative keratitis are reported. Cases were assigned to tPA or no-tPA groups in a random fashion. Informed consent was obtained from each patient receiving intraoperative tPA. All cases were referred with a progressive corneal infiltrate with hypopyon and stromal thinning unresponsive to maximal medical therapy. The decision to perform surgery was made when scleral involvement was threatened, perforation was imminent, or perforation had occured. Culture-negative cases underwent corneal biopsy prior to surgery. Outcome measurements included post-operative visual acuity and intraocular pressure as well as any post-operative complications necessitating further medical or surgical treatment.

For the tPA group, the underlying corneal disease included *Candida* keratitis, *Lactobacillus* keratitis, and *S. aureus* perforation. One of these patients required a conjunctival flap six months after surgery due to self-inflicted corneal erosions. None of the patients required treatment for postoperative glaucoma. For the no-tPA group, the underlying disease included two patients with topical anaesthetic abuse, and one unknown etiology. Two of these patients had postoperative complications from glaucoma. One required laser iridotomy and subsequent tube-shunt surgery. The other is maintained on topical glaucoma medications. The third patient required a conjunctival flap for a persistent epithelial defect.

Intracameral instillation of tPA during penetrating keratoplasty is an effective method for reducing the risk of postoperative glaucoma in cases of progressive ulcerative keratitis with hypopyon. Its routine use is limited by its significant cost. However, the cost of managing postoperative complications may justify its use in high-risk cornea transplant surgery.

INTRODUCTION

Intraocular fibrin deposition can cause serious and sight-threatening complications. The mechanism for an excessive intraocular fibrin reaction involves increased permeability of the blood-ocular barrier as well as dysfunction of the coagulation system and fibrinolytic pathways. These changes are related to the production of endogenous chemical mediators that are part of the normal intraocular inflammatory response. Tissue plasminogen activator (tPA) is a 70,000-dalton protein that converts plasminogen to plasmin in the presence of fibrin. Plasmin then acts on fibrin to degrade it into soluble split products. Intraocular administration of human recombinant tPA has been used successfully for the treatment of postoperative complications resulting from fibrin exudation following vitrectomy, glaucoma filtering surgery, and penetrating keratoplasty (PKP). This report investigates the use of intracameral tPA *during* cornea transplant surgery for the management of intraoperative fibrin exudation and prevention of postoperative complications related to fibrin deposition.

METHODS

The Cornea/External Disease Service at the Anaheim Medical Offices (Orange County, CA) serves a member population of over 800,000 individuals. This study describes six consecutive patients referred for management of progressive ulcerative keratitis with hypopyon. Each patient had a documented history of poor medical compliance from the referring ophthalmologist and each patient was traveling from outside of the Orange County area for specialty care. Cases were assigned to the tPA group or no-tPA group in a randomized fashion. All cases were referred with a progressive corneal infiltrate, hypopyon and stromal thinning unresponsive to maximal medical therapy. Cases referred without an etiological diagnosis underwent repeat corneal cultures. Culture-negative cases underwent corneal biopsy prior to PKP. Surgery was indicated when scleral involvement was threatened, perforation was imminent, or perforation had already occurred. Informed consent for use of intraoperative tPA was obtained from each patient in the tPA group. All surgery was performed in an identical fashion by one surgeon (MDS) except for the use of tPA in randomized cases. Each patient received a pulse dose of intravenous hydrocortisone during surgery and a tapering dose of Prednisone (1 mg/kg tapered over two weeks) following surgery. Each patient received an identical regimen of topical steroids and antibiotic following surgery. When necesssary, postoperative medications were individualized to treat the particular etiologic diagnosis. All grafts were oversized by 0.5 mm, had four peripheral iridotomies created during surgery, and were sutured with 16 interrupted 10-nylon sutures with the knots buried. Subconjunctival antibiotics and steroids were administered at the completion of each case. Following the placement of eight cardinal sutures to establish a closed anterior chamber, tPA (15 µg) was injected between the graft-host margin into the anterior chamber. The eye was allowed to settle for

five minutes before proceeding with surgery. The anterior chamber was irrigated periodically with BSS to remove inflammatory breakdown products and maintain a clear
aqueous fluid. Outcome measurements included visual acuity, intraocular pressure at 6
weeks and 6 months, postoperative complications such as graft failure, glaucoma and cataract, and need for chronic medical treatment or surgical procedures resulting from the intraocular inflammatory response.

CASE REPORTS

Case 1

A 32-year-old female home-health nurse was treating herself for a "stye" with
Maxitrol. After noticing a white corneal opacity and increasing pain, she sought attention
from an ophthalmologist. Cultures and smears were reported as "negative." She was referred when a hypopyon appeared. A corneal biopsy revealed *Candida albicans*. Despite
vigorous use of antifungal agents, the corneal thinning progressed and the stroma began to
necrose. A therapeutic corneal transplant was performed with intraoperative tPA. Postoperatively, the graft healed without clouding, the anterior chamber remained deep, and the
intraocular pressure remained under control. At six weeks, the visual acuity was count fingers, intraocular pressure was 16 mm Hg and the patient returned to work. Long term, the
patient began to miss follow-up appointments and admitted to self-medicating the eye.
She ultimately developed a central bacterial ulcer and the graft failed.

Case 2

A 43-year-old female with a history of herpes simplex keratitis in her left eye was
referred for progressive ulceration in the right eye following contact lens wear. Corneal
cultures were negative and a corneal biopsy was nondiagnostic. Penetrating keratoplasty
was performed for progressive thinning and impending perforation. Intraoperative tPA
was *not* used. Her immediate postoperative course was complicated by elevated intraocular pressure and pupillary block glaucoma. She required laser iridotomy and chronic oral
and topical hypotensive medications. Six weeks following surgery, her visual acuity was
hand motion and intraocular pressure was 39 mm Hg. She ultimately developed graft failure and a cataract requiring repeat PKP combined with cataract extraction and intraocular
lens placement. She subsequently required a glaucoma tube-shunt procedure.

Case 3

A 33-year-old female "crack" cocaine addict was referred with a flat anterior chamber and necrotic central cornea. *S. aureus* had been cultured from the progressive ulcer by
the referring ophthalmologist. Penetrating keratoplasty was performed with intraoperative
tPA. On postoperative day #1 and #7, the graft was clear, the intraocular pressure was 12
mm Hg and the anterior chamber was deep with minimal inflammatory activity. The patient did not return for follow-up for 6 weeks. She had discontinued all medications. Visual acuity was count fingers and the intraocular pressure was 18 mm Hg. The corneal graft
remained clear. The anterior chamber was deep and quiet. She returned six months later
with an opacified graft. The peripheral rim of cornea was still clear, allowing visualization
of the anterior chamber, which was deep and quiet. Visual acuity was hand motion and the

intraocular pressure was 18 mm Hg. (Comment: The patient returned requesting a repeat cornea transplant. She explained that she had quit her cocaine addiction and now used only "speed." At the time, she was eight months pregnant.)

Case 4

A 32-year-old unemployed railroad worker presented to the emergency room with a foreign body sensation in his right eye. He developed a persistent epithelial defect and infiltrate which was culture negative. He was treated with topical fortified antibiotics and referred when a ring infiltrate and hypopyon formed. The patient's mother is a nurse suggested that she "may have given him" Ophthetic eyedrops. Corneal biopsy was nondiagnostic. A therapeutic/diagnostic PKP was performed *without* the use of tPA. Histopathologic examination of the corneal button showed no organisms. At six weeks, the patient's vision improved to 20/100 and the intraocular pressure was 32 mm Hg. At six months, the patient remains on topical hypotensive medications.

Case 5

A 34-year-old female with a diagnosis of "delusions of parasitosis" was referred complaining of "worms" crawling out of her eyes and nose. She had undergone a PKP four months earlier for a corneal perforation. Culture of the corneal infiltrate demonstrated *Lactobacillus sp.*, which was also identified on histopathologic examination of the corneal button. She received intraoperative tPA. The patient did well postoperatively with a best visual acuity of 20/100 and intraocular pressure of 16 mm Hg at six weeks. At that time, the limbus to limbus graft was clear, the anterior chamber was deep and quiet and the lens was clear. Three months later the patient returned complaining of a foreign body sensation and feared the eye was "infested again." An epithelial defect was noted. Soon afterward, she underwent conjunctival flap surgery and has been stable since then.

Case 6

A 38-year-old man with a history of porphyria cutanea tarda was referred for management of a central corneal ulcer with hypopyon. Cultures and biopsy were unrevealing. A descemetocele formed and PKP was performed without tPA. Postoperatively the patient did well and intraocular pressure remained under control. At six weeks, his visual acuity was count fingers and intraocular pressure was 15 mm Hg. He had formed a persistent central epithelial defect and was noted to have "pocketed" Ophthetic eyedrops from the exam room. Upon confrontation, he returned the Ophthetic drops, as well as other medications taken from the exam rooms. A conjunctival flap was performed for treatment of the surface disorder and the patient has done well since then.

RESULTS

The individual case histories and data tabulation appear above. In summary, the tPA group consisted of three females. Their average age was 33 years (range = 32–34). The no-tPA group consisted of two men and one woman. Their average age was 38 (range = 32–43). Placement into the tPA or no-tPA group was random. However, the two groups differ preoperatively in an important manner. All of the tPA cases were found to have an underlying infectious process (*Candida, S. aureus, Lactobacillus*) whereas the no-tPA group had no underlying infectious etiology identified.

Postoperative visual acuity results are similar for both groups. Long-term intraocular pressure control and need for subsequent pressure management was significantly better for the group receiving intraoperative tPA. None of the tPA cases demonstrated signs of intraocular toxicity from the medication. There were no intraoperative complications related to the use of tPA.

DISCUSSION

Intraocular fibrin deposition is a serious complicaton of eye surgery that may increase the risk of surgical failure. It is a common event when performing surgery on actively inflamed eyes. Cases such as those described in this investigation with progressive ulcerative keratitis that require penetrating keratoplasty for emergent therapeutic or diagnostic purposes are particularly prone to an excessive fibrin response. Traditionally, postoperative fibrin deposition was treated by administration of steroids. This standard treatment was aimed at re-establishing the integrity of the blood-ocular barrier. However, chemical mediators formed in response to the inflammatory stimulus cause alterations in the coagulation system and fibrinolytic cascade as well. Therefore, stabilization of the blood-ocular barrier alone is generally ineffective at preventing a fibrin reaction.[1,2]

The value of intraocular tPA for postoperative fibrinolysis has now been described for several clinical situations including severe postvitrectomy fibrin formation in diabetics,[3] postvitrectomy pupillary membrane formation,[4,5] hyphema,[6] postoperative trabeculectomy,[7,8,9] and postoperative penetrating keratoplasty.[10,11] Potential toxicity to intraocular tissues has been examined by several investigators. Intraocular doses below 25 ug appear to be relatively safe for the cornea and retina.[12,13] Possible complications related to intraocular bleeding have also been reported following use of tPA.[14] The current study investigates the use of tPA as an intraoperative treatment to reduce fibrin exudation during the surgical procedure and prevent postoperative complications related to fibrin deposition.

The results of this investigation are remarkable for the effectiveness of intraoperative tPA at reducing the incidence of postoperative glaucoma, the absence of intraoperative complications related to the use of tPA, and the absence of postoperative signs of toxicity related to tPA. Unfortunately, the number of cases is still small and a selection bias is present. While the cases selected for the study were randomized to a tPA or no-tPA group, each patient had a known history of noncompliance and a severe ocular condition that prevents reliable judgement concerning long-term visual prognosis. However, the data indicate a significant trend towards long-term intraocular pressure control when intraoperative tPA is used compared to similar cases without tPA. The clinical impression is that intraoperative fibrinolysis using tPA simplified the surgery as a fibrin membrane did not have to be repeatedly pealed or irrigated out of the anterior chamber as the graft was being secured. Further studies, for example using corneal topography, may reveal an improved symmetry of the graft-host margin as an indicator of improved healing and ease of surgery. Such a study would require selecting patients with a better compliance record.

REFERENCES

1. F.H. Lambrou, Snyder, R.W., Williams, G.A., and Lewandowski, M., Treatment of experimental intravitreal fibrin with tissue plasminogen activator. *Am. J. Ophthalmol.* 104:619 (1987).

2. R.W. Snyder, Lambrou, F.H., and Williams, G.A., Intraocular fibrinolysis with recombinant human tissue plasminogen activator. *Arch. Ophthalmol.* 105:1277 (1987).
3. G.A. Williams, Lambrou, F.H., Jaffe, G.A., et al., Treatment of postvitrectomy fibrin formation with intraocular tissue plasminogen activator. *Arch. Ophthalmol.* 106:1055 (1988).
4. G.J. Jaffe, Lewis, H., Han, D.P., et al., Treatment of postvitrectomy fibrin pupillary block with tissue plasminogen activator. *Am. J. Ophthalmol.* 108:170 (1989).
5. D.F. Williams, Bennett, S.R., Abrams, G.W., et al., Low-dose intraocular tissue plasminogen activator for treatment of postvitrectomy fibrin formation. *Am. J. Ophthalmol.* 109:606 (1990).
6. F.H. Lambrou, Snyder, R.W., and Williams, G.A., Use of tissue plasminogen activator in experimental hyphema. *Arch. Ophthalmol.* 105:995 (1987).
7. J.R. Piltz, and Starita, R.J., The use of subconjunctivally administered tissue plasminogen activator after trabeculectomy. *Ophthalmic. Surg.* 25:51 (1994).
8. R.C. Tripathi, Tripathi, B.J., Park, J.K., et al., Intracameral tissue plasminogen activator for resolution of fibrin clots after glaucoma filtering procedures. *Am. J. Ophthalmol.* 111:247 (1991).
9. J.R. Ortiz, Walker, S.D., McManus, P.E., et al., Filtering bleb thrombolysis with tissue plasminogen activator. *Am. J. Ophthalmol.* 106:624 (1988).
10. D.G. Heidemann, Williams, G.A., and Blumenkranz, M.S., Tissue plasminogen activator and penetrating keratoplasty. *Ophthalmic Surg.* 21:364 (1990).
11. R.W. Snyder, and Sherman, M.D., Intracameral tissue plasminogen activator for treatment of excessive fibrin response after penetrating keratoplasty. *Am. J. Ophthalmol.* 109:483 (1990).
12. M.L. McDermott, Edelhauser, H.F., Hyndiuk, R.A., and Koenig, S.B., Tissue plasminogen activator and the corneal endothelium. *Am. J. Ophthalmol.* 108:91 (1989).
13. W.D. Irvine, Johnson, M.W., Hernandez, E., and Olsen, K.R., Retinal toxicity of human tissue plasminogen activator in vitrectomized rabbit eyes. *Arch. Ophthalmol.* 109:718 (1991).
14. C.K. Dabbs, Aaboerg, T.M., Aguilar, H.E., et al., Complications of tissue plasminogen activator therapy after vitrectomy for diabetes. *Am. J. Ophthalmol.* 110:354 (1990).

22

SURGICAL TREATMENT OF CASTROVIEJO URRETS-ZAVALIA SYNDROME

Walton Nosé,[1,2] Regina M. Nosé,[2] Luciene B. Sousa,[1,2] and Adriana S. Forseto[1,2]

[1]Sao Paulo Federal University
Paulista School of Medicine
Sao Paulo, Brazil
[2]Eye Clinic Day Hospital
Sao Paulo, Brazil

ABSTRACT

The purpose of this study was to evaluate the efficacy of pupiloplasty in postkeratoplasty patients with dilated and fixed pupil (Castroviejo Urrets-Zavalia Syndrome). This study analyzed four patients submitted to keratoplasty due to keratoconus complaining of photophobia, glare, and decreased vision since their first surgery. Graft failure and cataract were responsible for the blurred vision. The pupillary diameter ranged from 8 to 9 mm. A circular iris suture technique with 10.0 mersylene was performed in all cases (by the same surgeon: W.N.). Regrafts were necessary in two cases, and the sutures were made open-sky. The other two that had cataract underwent phacoemulsification with intraocular lens implantation and the sutures were performed by peripheral paracentesis. The results were followed by an average of 6 months. Results indicated that patients were asymptomatic regarding photophobia and there was a reduction in glare symptoms. Slit lamp examination revealed a pupillary diameter ranging from 4 to 5 mm. There were no complications such as glaucoma, hyphema, iridocyclitis, synechiae, or clinical signs of graft rejection. All the patients presented an improvement in corrected and uncorrected visual acuity at the last follow-up. These results led to the conclusion that circular iris suture with 10.0 mersylene seems to be an efficient technique for the treatment of Castroviejo Urrets-Zavalia Syndrome, as a single procedure or in association with another one.

INTRODUCTION

The incidence of paralytic mydriasis following penetrating keratoplasty due to keratoconus was first reported by authors such as Castroviejo and Paufique.[1] Later, Urrets-

Zavalia published his first results, in which he indicated his belief that the association of paralytic mydriasis, iris atrophy, and secondary glaucoma following keratoplasty represented a specific syndrome, which became known and named after him.[2]

The objective here is to present a pupiloplasty technique for surgical correction of mydriasis in those patients and to assess its value regarding the presence of symptoms such as photophobia and glare.

MATERIALS AND METHODS

Four patients who had penetrating keratoplasty due to keratoconus and complained of photophobia, glare, and reduction of visual acuity were assessed over a 3 to 12 year period (average 7.25 ± 4.03 years).

At the ophthalmologic examination, these patients presented uncorrected visual acuity of $\leq 20/400$. Slitlamp examination presented corneal edema with button failure in two cases, cataract in the other two, and paralytic mydriasis in all of them, with pupil diameter ranging from 8 to 9 mm (average = 8.375 ± 0.47). Intraocular pressure was normal in all cases (Exam 1).

A technique of circular iris suture with 10–0 mersylene was used under peribulbar blockade with 6 ml of an anesthetic mixture of 0.5 bupivacaine without vasoconstrictor and 2.5 µg/ml fentanyl citrate. Two injections for the blockade were performed, one on the lower temporal orbit margin and the other on the upper nasal border.

Surgical Technique

The circular iris suture was performed in two different ways:

• As a procedure associated with penetrating keratoplasty: Regrafting was necessary on patients presenting button failure. On those patients, the iris suture was done following trephination and removal of the button. The procedure was performed in an open sky pattern, introducing the straight needle with the mersylene thread about 2 mm from the mydriatic pupil border—through its anterior region, transfixing and returning to the surface. Such movement was repeated until the whole iris perimeter had been run through, always with due care so as not to injure the lens. The knot was then tied so as to carefully pull the iris, thus closing the pupil (Figure 1). Afterwards the new button was placed and sutured with a conventional technique.

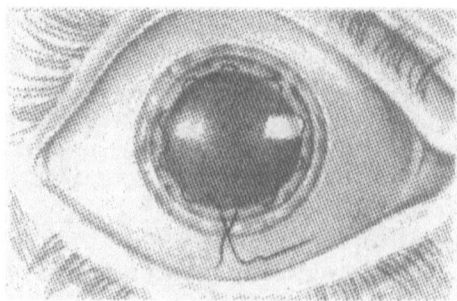

Figure 1. Open-sky iris suture technique associated with regrafting.

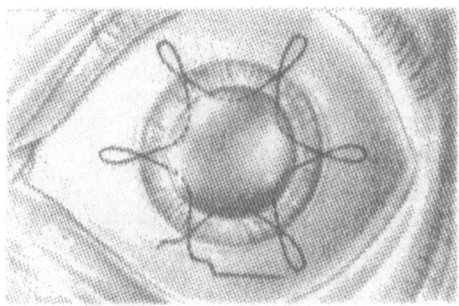

Figure 2. Iris suture technique associated with phacoemulsification, using peripheral paracentesis.

• As a procedure associated with cataract surgery: Two patients with cataract were submitted to phacoemulsification and iris suture was made using 6 peripheral paracentesis following intraocular lens implantation. The needle was introduced from the first to the second paracentesis, thus performing double iris transfixation, from the anterior to the posterior surface, again coming out anteriorly. The procedure was repeated until all six paracentesis had been run through, when the needle was brought out through the initial site so that the knot could be tied, always taking care not to injure the iris through pulling (Figure 2).

All surgeries were performed by the same surgeon (W.N.). In the postoperative period, no mydriatics were prescribed and the patients were instructed to use a topical corticosteroid and antibiotic solution (Maxitrol[R]: 0.1% dexamethasone acetate, neomycin, and polymixin B), one drop every 4 hours for 30 days in cases of phacoemulsification. As the regrafted ones needed the medication for a longer period, it was gradually reduced. A non-hormonal anti-inflammatory also was used, only for patients who had cataract surgery (Still[R]: sodium diclophenac, 1 drop every 4 hours for 30 days).

Patients were followed for 3 to 12 months (average = 6 ± 4.08 months) and in their last examination they were assessed for visual acuity, alteration of photophobia and glare complaint, and presence of complications (Exam II).

RESULTS

All patients were male with ages ranging from 28 to 34 years (average = 31 ± 2.58 years). Corrected and uncorrected visual acuity assessment over the last examination shows significant vision improvement. Before surgery, uncorrected visual acuity was $\leq$ 20/400 in all cases and in the last examination, the visual acuity was 20/30, 20/40, 20/80, and 20/200 (Graphic 1).

Corrected visual acuity was 20/200 at Exam I in two cases and 20/50 in the remaining two cases. In the postoperative period, all patients showed corrected acuity of 20/30 or higher (Graphic 2).

An average pupil diameter reduction from 8.375 ± 0.47 mm to 4.5 ± 0.40 mm was observed in Exam II (ranging from 4 to 5 mm). Patients reported subjective improvement in the photophobia and glare symptoms (Figure 3).

No complications such as glaucoma, hyphema, iridocyclitis, synechiae, or rejection were noted during the story.

Pre and Post-operative UCVA

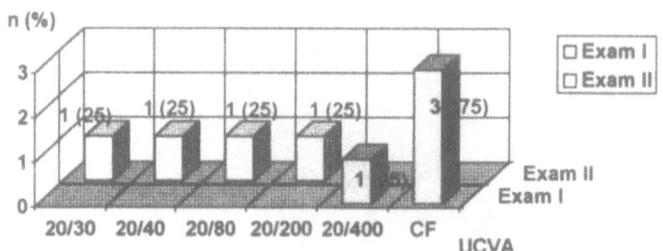

Graphic 1. Pre- and postoperative uncorrected visual acuity.

DISCUSSION

A number of theories have been proposed in an effort to explain the origin of Castroviejo Urrets-Zavalia syndrome. Urrets believed that medicamentous mydriasis accounted for the syndrome pathogenesis, with a parallel role of pupil blockade. Ocular hypertension would be an event secondary to the formation of goniosynechiae.[2] Thus, he was against the use of mydriatics in such patients' postoperative period and recommended the performance of peripheral iridectomy.[2] Likewise, Flament et al., did not notice mydriasis in their patients when peripheral iridectomy was performed; others presented it without the use of mydriatics and one when miotic was used.[3]

A further theory considers the syndrome as the outcome of the neurovegetative system balance rupture, leading to the sympathetic system hyperfunction, suggesting the use of sympatholytic substances (5% guanethidine) in the pre- and postoperative periods to prevent it.[4] Lagoutte obtained reduction of mydriasis in one case, through Ismelin[R] instillation (5% guanethidine sulphate) every 4 hours for 24 hours, immediately after noticing pupillary dilatation, which occurred on the sixth postoperative day.[5] In this study the patients already had the condition previously installed.

Ischemic atrophy of the muscle sphincter of the pupil secondary to iris strangulation during surgery, following removal of the receptor button and even formation of the anterior chamber has been proposed to explain the origin of alterations in such patients.[1]

A further explanation would be the presence of a mesodermic defect in the keratoconus not always confined to the cornea, often associated with hypoplasia of the iris stroma which may account for paralytic mydriasis.[6]

Pre and Post-operative BCVA

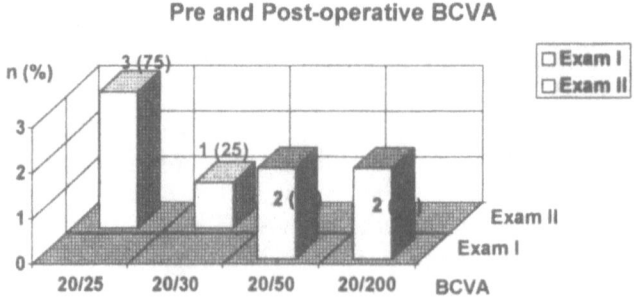

Graphic 2. Pre- and postoperative best corrected visual acuity.

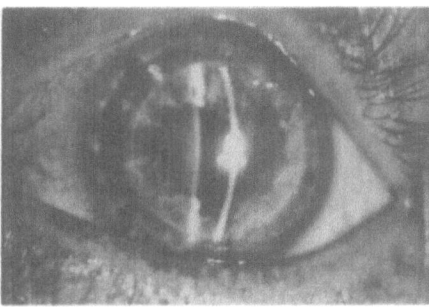

Figure 3. Postoperative of the surgical treatment of Castroviejo Urrets-Zavalia Syndrome. Note the pupil diameter.

Irrespective of the involved mechanism, once the syndrome is installed, treatment leading to symptomatology relief for such patients should be attempted. Subjective improvement of photophobia and glare symptoms was noticed in all of the included patients.

Lack of glaucoma in these patients is in keeping with its incidence in the literature, in which authors believe it to be normally secondary to the presence of goniosynechiae, due to extended periods of shallow anterior chamber. Albert and Schnitzler reported eight cases, none with glaucoma, out of a series of 80 penetrating keratoplasties.[7] Urrets reported five in 225 surgeries, of which complete syndrome was found in two cases.[2]

No surgical correction techniques for the syndrome were found in the literature. The lack of complications suggests the procedure to be safe, despite technical difficulties, provided it is performed by experienced surgeons.

CONCLUSION

Circular iris suture for paralytic mydriasis secondary to penetrating keratoplasty by means of keratoconus proved to be an effective technique, which may be performed as an isolated procedure or in association with an additional ocular procedure as shown in this study.

REFERENCES

1. P.D. Davies, and Ruben, M., The paretic pupil: its incidence and aetiology after keratoplasty for keratoconus. *Brit. J. Ophthal.* 59:223 (1975).
2. A. Urretz-Zavalia, Jr., Fixed dilated pupil, iris atrophy and secondary glaucoma. Distinct clinical entity following penetrating keratoplasty in keratoconus. *Am. J. Ophthalmol.* 56:257 (1963).
3. J. Flament, Schraub, M., Guimeraes, R., and Bronner, A., Syndrome d'Urrets-Zavalia et cataract glaucomatosa. Discussion étiopathogènique et nosologique. *Ophthalmologica, Basel.* 189:186 (1984).
4. M. Bonnet, Lemarchands, H., and Martin, J., Prophylaxie et traitement du syndrome "mydriase irrèductible-atrophie irienne progressive" succèdant a une keratoplastie perforante pour keratocone. *Annals Oculist.* 202:1139 (1969).
5. F. Lagoutte, Thien pont, Ph., and Comte, P., Proposition de traitement du syndrome d'Urrets-Zavalia. A propos d'un cas reversible. *J. Fr. Ophthalmol.* 6(3):291 (1983).
6. T.I. Bertelsen, and Seim, V., The cause of irreversible mydriasis following keratoplasty in keratoconus: a preliminary report. *Ophthalmic Surg.* 5:56 (1974).
7. B. Alberth, and Schnitzler, A., Irreversible mydriase nach keratoplastik bei keratokonus. *Klin. Mbl. Augenheik.* 159:330 (1971).

23

POSTOPERATIVE ENDOPHTHALMITIS AND INTRAOCULAR VANCOMYCIN

Thomas O. Wood,[1] Vickie A. Nix,[1] Judith Mohay,[2] and B. J. McLaughlin[2]

[1]Associated Ophthalmic Specialists, Inc.
Memphis, Tennessee
[2]Department of Ophthalmology and Visual Sciences
University of Louisville School of Medicine
Louisville, Kentucky

ABSTRACT

This study reviewed 570 consecutive corneal transplants done in one hospital by one ophthalmologist. In 480 of these transplants, vancomycin, 1 mgm/BSS 1 ml, was used to store the donor cornea for 5–10 minutes after removal from Optisol or Optisol GS and as an irrigating solution throughout the procedure. Ninety donors stored in Optisol only were used as a control. The vancomycin solution also was used to fill the anterior chamber, posterior chamber, and vitreous cavity, when indicated, at the end of surgery. Donor rims stored in the vancomycin/BSS before transplantation had 5% positive cultures. Prior to vancomycin immersion 16.6% of donor rims grew bacteria. The decrease to 5% is statistically significant (p = 0.00036). Vancomycin/BSS storage reduced the incidence of streptococcus cultured from the donor from 3.3% to 0.2%. The study found that 0.6% (3/480) patients with vancomycin treated corneas developed postoperative endophthalmitis. All of their donor cultures were negative. Three additional eyes developed endophthalmitis following suture adjustment (0.6%). Previous lens surgery, glaucoma, regrafting, and postoperative suture manipulation were found to be associated with postoperative endophthalmitis. In the nonvancomycin eyes, two eyes (2.2%) developed endophthalmitis.

INTRODUCTION

Endophthalmitis following corneal transplantation occurs in approximately 1% of cases.[1] It has been characterized as usually occurring within the first 72 hours and bacteria cultured from the donor are frequently the causative agent.[1–3]

Vancomycin added to storage media inhibits the growth of *Streptococcus pneumoniae* and is stable in preservative for several months.[4–6] Optisol GS (GS = gentamicin and streptomycin) is the most frequently used short-term corneal preservation media in the United States. Prior to this, Optisol with gentamicin was used for corneal preservation.

The purposes of this study were: (1) to determine the incidence of positive cultures from corneas stored in Optisol or Optisol GS and soaked in vancomycin/balanced salt solution (BSS); (2) to examine a consecutive series of patients who underwent corneal transplantation with Optisol and Optisol GS corneal preservation, to determine the effect of vancomycin, 1 mgm/BSS 1 ml, used during corneal transplantation; and (3) to identify factors that make eyes more susceptible to endophthalmitis following corneal transplantation.[7]

METHODS AND RESULTS

In this study, 570 consecutive corneal transplants done by one surgeon in one hospital were examined. All of the corneas had been preserved in Optisol or Optisol GS. One hundred ninety six corneas had been stored in Optisol then vancomycin and 284 corneas in Optisol GS then vancomycin. Four hundred seventy five of the 480 donor rims were cultured (Tables 1, 2). A solution of BSS with 1 mgm/ml of vancomycin was routinely used to store the donor for 5–10 minutes before transplantation. The donor corneas were examined prior to suturing and foreign particles were removed by dripping the vancomycin/BSS solution on the cornea. Ninety donor rims preserved in Optisol and not stored in the vancomycin/BSS solution were used as a control (Table 3).

The donor rims were placed on chocolate agar in the operating room and transferred to the bacteriology laboratory. The corneas were ground in thioglycollate broth then inoculated with thioglycollate and on blood, chocolate, and MacConkey agar. Cultures are held for 7 days. We considered any growth a positive culture. Six percent of the corneas stored in Optisol followed by vancomycin and 5% in Optisol GS followed by vancomycin

Table 1. Twelve donor corneas out of 196 (6%) stored in Optisol then vancomycin were culture positive. All staphylococcus tested were sensitive to vancomycin

Patient	Organism	Vancomycin	Gentamicin	Streptomycin
1	Rare *Staphylococcus aureus*	1S	NA	ND
	Rare *Pseudomonas aeruginosa*	NA	2S	ND
2	Rare coagulase-negative staphylococci	1S	ND	ND
3	Rare *Streptococcus intermedius*-Type 1	S	ND	ND
	Rare *Streptococcus intermedius*-Type 2	S	ND	ND
4	Rare *Staphylococcus epidermidis*	1S	ND	ND
5	Rare *Pseudomonas aeruginosa*	NA	4S	ND
	Rare coagulase-negative staphylococci	1S	NA	ND
6	Rare *Corynebacterium* species	S	ND	ND
7	Rare coagulase-negative staphylococci	1S	ND	ND
8	Rare coagulase-negative staphylococci	1S	ND	ND
	Rare *Micrococcus* species	ND	ND	ND
9	Rare coagulase-negative staphylococci	1S	ND	ND
10	Rare *Staphylococcus epidermidis*	S	S	S
	Corynebacterium species	S	S	R
11	Rare *Pseudomonas aeruginosa*	ND	2S	ND
12	Rare *Serratia liquefaciens*	ND	<=0.5 S	ND

*196 donor rims stored in Optisol and immersed in vancomycin, 1 mgm/ml, BSS.

Table 2. Fourteen of 284 (5%) donor corneas stored in Optisol GS then vancomycin were culture positive. Vancomycin was effective against all staphylococcus tested; note resistant strain to streptomycin (patient 17)

Patient	Organism	Vancomycin	Gentamicin	Streptomycin
13	Rare coagulase-negative staphylococci	S	S	S
14	1 CFU coagulase-neg staphylococci	ND	ND	ND
15	Rare coagulase-negative staphylococci	S	S	S
16	Rare *Citrobacter freundii*	ND	<=0.5 S	ND
	Rare *Serratia marcescens*	ND	<=0.5 S	ND
17	Rare coagulase-negative staphylococci	S	S	R
	Rare *Micrococcus* species	S	S	S
18	*Chryseomonas luteola*	R	S	S
19	Rare coagulase-negative staphylococci	S	R	S
	Beta lactamase-positive	ND	ND	ND
20	*Propionibacterium* species	ND	ND	ND
	Beta lactamase-negative	ND	ND	ND
21	Rare coagulase-negative staphylococci	1S	ND	ND
22	Rare *Staphylococcus epidermidis*	ND	ND	ND
23	Rare coagulase-negative staphylococci	S	R	S
	Beta lactamase-positive	ND	ND	ND
24	Rare *Bacillus megaterium*	S	S	S
25	Rare *Candida albicans*	ND	ND	ND
26	Rare *Propionibacterium acnes*	ND	ND	ND
	Beta lactamase-negative	ND	ND	ND

*284 donor rims stored in Optisol GS and immersed in vancomycin, 1 mgm/ml, BSS.

were culture positive (Tables 1, 2). In the 90 donor eyes stored in Optisol, but not immersed in vancomycin, 16.6% were culture positive; three grew a streptococcus species.

Scanning electron microscopy was used to determine the endothelial storage effect of the vancomycin. Corneas were immersed in 1 mg/BSS 1 ml, as well as BSS alone, for up to 2 hours. The endothelium exhibited normal morphology and appeared healthy (Fig. 1).

In corneas that were placed in vancomycin, 1 mg/BSS 1 ml, the same solution was used for irrigation during the procedure. The posterior chamber, anterior chamber, and vitreous cavity, when indicated, were filled with the vancomycin/BSS solution at the conclusion of surgery.

A profile of the patients that had undergone corneal transplantation, with vancomycin stored corneas, revealed 44% (213) were patients with pseudophakic bullous keratopathy, 7% (33) aphakic bullous keratopathy, 15% (74) keratoconus, 16% (79) endothelial dystrophy, and 16% (81) other categories. During the postoperative period, three (0.6%) eyes developed endophthalmitis (Table 4). Three eyes (0.6%) developed endophthalmitis following suture adjustment. All of the eyes that developed endophthalmitis had undergone previous lens surgery. Five were pseudophakic and one was aphakic. Five of the eyes had preoperative glaucoma and four were regrafts. The time for development of endophthalmitis varied from six days to five months.

Two eyes with Optisol-vancomycin storage developed endophthalmitis, and four eyes with Optisol GS-vancomycin developed endophthalmitis. Staphylococcus was the only bacteria cultured and accounted for 50% of the endophthalmitis. All of the vancomycin eyes that developed endophthalmitis had a negative donor culture. Four of the six eyes with endophthalmitis were treated without loss of functional vision. The one eye eviscerated with endo-

Table 3. Fifteen of 90 donor corneas stored in Optisol were culture positive. Three of the donors cultured a streptococcus species

Patient	Organism	Vancomycin	Gentamicin	Streptomycin
27	Rare bacillus species	S	ND	ND
28	Rare *Staphylococcus epidermidis*	1S	ND	ND
29	Rare *Staphylococcus epidermidis*	1S	ND	ND
30	Rare coagulase-negative staphylococci	S	ND	ND
31	Rare *Staphylococcus aureus*	S	ND	ND
32	Rare coagulase-negative staphylococci	1S	ND	ND
33	Rare *Moraxella* species	ND	S	ND
34	Rare *Streptococcus intermedius* (2 types)	S	ND	ND
35	Rare *Staphylococcus epidermidis*	S	ND	ND
36	Rare *Streptococcus pneumoniae*	S	ND	ND
37	Rare *Streptococcus mitis*	S	ND	ND
38	Rare coagulase-negative staphylococci	1S	ND	ND
39	Rare coagulase-negative staphylococci	1S	ND	ND
40	Rare *Corynebacterium* species	S	ND	ND
41	Rare coagulase-negative staphylococci	1S	ND	ND

*90 donor rims stored in Optisol and not immersed in vancomycin.

phthalmitis had an expulsive choroidal hemorrhage during surgery. Two eyes (2.2%) in the control group developed endophthlamitis, both were pseudophakic (Table 5).

DISCUSSION

In this study, endophthalmitis developed in six (1.25%) out of a total of 480 patients undergoing corneal transplantation in which donor corneas were immersed in vancomycin. Each eye with endophthalmitis had an extenuating factor: previous lens surgery (100%), glaucoma (83%), previous graft (66%), and suture adjustment (50%).

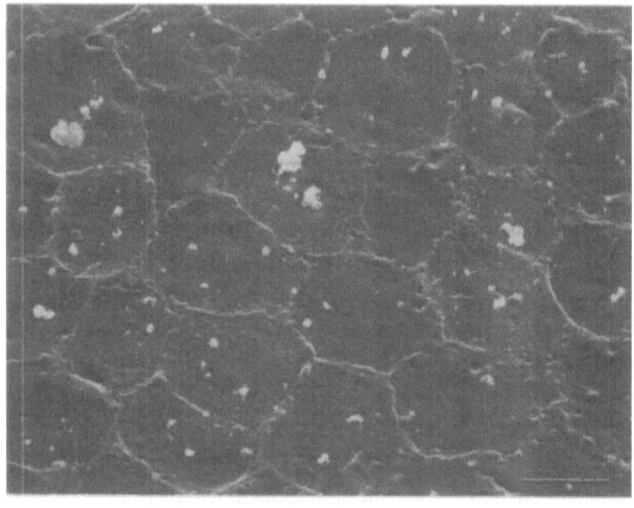

Figure 1. Scanning electron micrograph of human endothelial cells after immersion in vancomycin, 1 mg/BSS 1 ml, for 2 hours. Cells look normal. Scale bar = 10μm.

Table 4. Staphylococcus was the only bacteria cultured

Case #	Preop DX	S/P factors	Time[*]	Lab results	Outcome
1	pseudophakic bullous keratopathy open angle glaucoma	none	6 days PO	C&S negative for vitreous and aqueous	CF
2	aphakic corneal scar open angle glaucoma	none	33 days PO	stain: gram + cocci culture: staph coag -	20/50
3	regraft pseudophakic	suture adjustment for astigmatism	19 days PO 7 days PSA	stain:gram + cocci culture: staph coag +	20/80
4	regraft pseudophakic open angle glaucoma	suture adjustment for astigmatism	5.5 mos PO 55 day PSA	stain:gram + cocci culture:staph EPI	20/40
5	regraft pseudophakic open angle glaucoma	suture adjustment for wound leak	29 days PO 19 day PSA	C&S negative	LPO
6	regraft open angle glaucoma	expulsive choroidal hemorrhage	18 days PO	no C&S	enucleation

[*]PO = postoperative
PSA = post suture adjustment

The endophthalmitis associated with suture manipulation was probably unrelated to intraocular inoculation of bacteria during the surgery. The eyes undergoing suture adjustment are believed to have developed the endophthalmitis (Cases 3, 4, and 5) secondary to postoperative introduction of bacteria into the wound or anterior chamber.

Positive cultures were obtained from 16.6% of donor corneas stored in Optisol but not vancomycin.[8] Immersing the corneas in vancomycin for 10 minutes prior to corneal transplantation reduced the positive cultures from 16.6% to 5% (p = 0.00036).[*] Vancomycin/BSS storage reduced the incidence of streptococcus cultured from the donor from 3.3% (3/90) to 0.2% (1/475) (p = 0.014)** (Tables 1, 2, 3). Optisol GS did not lower the incidence of endophthalmitis or positive donor cultures when compared to Optisol, when the corneas were immersed in vancomycin prior to transplantation.

The host should be considered as a possible source of bacteria in endophthalmitis, especially with staphylococcus. In our initial study, 7% (6/86) of the host corneas grew staphylococcus after betadine preparation.[8]

With this information, positive donor cultures linked to postoperative endophthalmitis can be reduced significantly. It is possible to identify patients who are prone to developing endophthalmitis after corneal transplantation and further reduce the incidence of endophthalmitis with use of postoperative antibiotics, particularly after suture adjustment.

Table 5. Two pseudophakic eyes in the control group developed endophthalmitis

Case #	Preop DX	S/P factors	Time[*]	Lab results	Outcome
7	regraft pseudophakic bullous keratopathy	none	2 days PO	stain:negative culture:staph species	20/400
8	pseudophakic bullous keratopathy	none	6 days PO	not available	CF

[*]PO = postoperative

ENDNOTES

* Statistical significance determined by using the Chi square, two-tailed test.
** Statistical significance calculated with Fisher's Exact test because the numerator was less than 5.

ACKNOWLEDGMENTS

Supported by Baptist Memorial Hospital; Memphis, Tennessee.

REFERENCES

1. L.P. Aiello, Javitt, J.L., and Canner, J.K., National outcomes of penetrating keratoplasty. *Arch. Ophthalmol.* 111:509 (1993).
2. A.S. Leveillie, McMullan, F.D., and Cavanagh, H.D., Endophthalmitis following penetrating keratoplasty. *Ophthalmology* 90:38 (1983).
3. J.C. Baer, Nirankari, V.S., and Glaros, D.S.: Streptococcal endophthalmitis from contaminated donor corneas after keratoplasty. *Arch. Ophthalmol.* 97:560 (1984).
4. F.J. Garcia-Ferrer, Pepose, J.S., Murray, P.R., et al., Antimicrobial efficacy and corneal endothelial toxicity in DexSol corneal storage medium supplemented with vancomycin. *Ophthalmology* 98:863 (1991).
5. T.L. Steinemann, Kaufman, H.E., Beuerman, R.W., et al., Vancomycin-enriched corneal storage medium. *Am. J. Ophthalmol.* 113:555 (1992).
6. T.D. Lindquist, Brian, P.R., and Fritsche, T.R., Stability and activity of vancomycin in corneal storage media *Cornea* 12:222 (1993).
7. R.B. Guss, Koenig, S., LaPena, W., et al., Endophthalmitis after penetrating keratoplasty. *Am. J. Ophthalmol.* 95:651 (1983).
8. T.O. Wood, Mohay, J., and McAlughlin, B.J., Vancomycin in corneal transplantation. *Trans. Amer. Ophthal. Soc.* 91:391 (1993).

SESSION II: CORNEAL TRANSPLANTATION AND EYE BANKING

Abstracts of Other Conference Presentations and Posters

EYE BANKING IN THE WORLD COMMUNITY

Paul J. Dubord

Vancouver, Canada

Eye Banking on a global basis varies dramatically. With world wide increasing demand superimposed on decreasing resources, different solutions are being employed to resolve problems. The structure and function of eye banking systems and their response to different health care systems will be reviewed. Medical standards are of primary importance in the development of an efficient responsive eye banking system. They must reflect local needs, cultural differences and access to resources.

Access to a safe adequate supply of transplant tissues is crucial. Increasing awareness of quality assurance superimposed on demands of governments, the public, and the medical community, and how these issues are being addressed will be reviewed.

RISK FACTORS FOR CORNEAL GRAFT FAILURE

Penetrating keratoplasty is one of the most common and successful ophthalmic procedures. However, controversy and uncertainty still call to question the significance of certain risk factors for graft failure.

A consecutive series of 1819 penetrating keratoplasties at a single center was studied to determine donor and recipient risk factors for graft failure. Mean follow up was 2.3 years (range, 1 to 96 months) with 139 (7.7%) eyes lost to follow up.

Previous graft failure was the most significant risk factor for secondary failure (P = .003). The risk of failure significantly decreased with increased postoperative time. Significant patient risk factors for secondary failures in initial grafts included race (P = .01), age (P = .004), iris color (P = .02), use of preoperative glaucoma medications (P = .0008), deep stromal vascularization (P = .002), and host horizontal diameter (P = 0.007).

Significant risk factors for failures associated with immunologic allograft reactions in initial grafts included horizontal corneal diameter (P = .002), donor size (P = .05), differences between horizontal corneal diameter, and both donor size (P = .02) and recipient trephination size (P = .01). However, deep stromal vascularization was only marginally significant (P = .09). A history of preoperative glaucoma medication usage was not a significant risk factor.

The relationship of the recipient's horizontal corneal diameter to immunologic graft rejection is a new risk factor that surgeons can directly control and thereby help avoid graft failure.

QUALITY OF LIFE ASSESSMENT AFTER CORNEAL TRANSPLANTATION

David C. Musch[1,2] and Roger F. Meyer[1]

Departments of Ophthalmology[1] and Epidemiology[2]
The University of Michigan, Ann Arbor, MI

Health-related quality of life (QOL) is increasingly being recognized as an outcome that can and should be measured in studies of the effects of diseases and their treatments on patients. In ophthalmology, this recognition has arisen primarily in assessing cataract surgery outcome, and has led to the development of a number of questionnaires to assess visual function, which is one aspect of health-related QOL. We selected one of these questionnaires, the VF-14, and a more general QOL measure, the SF-36, to determine the extent to which commonly-used clinical measures of corneal transplantation outcome are related to aspects of visual function and health-related QOL.

Clinical outcomes were obtained from routine, follow-up examinations that took place at least one year after surgery. Within one to four weeks of this examination, patients were contacted by telephone at their homes, and the QOL questions were asked by a trained interviewer. Complete information was obtained on 77 patients whose average age was 72 years at the time of contact, and who were on average five years postcorneal transplantation. Patients' assessment of their visual function and QOL were evaluated relative to pre-defined outcome categories for three clinical measures of corneal transplantation success: best-corrected visual acuity, emmetropia, and astigmatism.

There was a highly significant association (P<0.0001) of the VF-14 outcome with VA — those with 20/50 or worse VA in both eyes had the poorest visual function. Best-corrected VA was also directly related to the patients' assessment of their emotional role limitations (P=0.04), emotional well-being (P=0.08), and social functioning (P=0.02). Those with a high degree of keratometric astigmatism showed an impact on social functioning (P=0.005). The extent of anisometropia, age, and time since surgery were not associated with the patients' reported visual function or QOL assessments. Upon stepwise, linear regression, the single most important factor in the patients' reported visual function was their VA in the better eye, followed by the extent of keratometric astigmatism. We conclude that there is a high degree of criterion validity in using the VF-14 questionnaire to assess the outcome of corneal transplantation, whereas the more generic SF-B 6 questionnaire's application shows effects of visual disability on aspects of corneal transplant patients' emotional and social functioning.

APPLICATION OF CONFOCAL MICROSCOPY IN CORNEAL TRANSPLANTATION

M. Böhnke, B. R. Masters, B. Frueh, and A. Thaer

Background: Confocal microscopy allows for a visualization of all layers of the cornea including basal epithelial and wing cells, thus introducing a new diagnostic tool to the established techniques of slit lamp and specular microscopy. **Aim**: To apply confocal microscopy for the investigation of donor corneas. **Materials and methods**: *Instrument*: A flying slit confocal microscope, which produces real time video pictures on SVHS videotape. Single frames were either photographed directly off the monitor screen or digitized and exposed on slide film without further image processing. *Tissues:* 10 donor globes were studied between 6 and 35 hours post mortem. 10 corneo scleral discs were studied under various conditions of corneal organ culture or refrigerated storage. 20 patients were studied 1–120 months after penetrating keratoplasty. **Results**: In the *enucleated donor eyes,* the anterior layers of the donor cornea are clearly visible in confocal microscopy. With increasing post mortem time, posterior stromal details and the corneal endothelium decreased in visibility. Beyond 12 hours post mortem, a useful picture of the corneal endothelium could not be obtained. In *donor discs,* cellular layers can be investigated either from the epithelial or endothelial side. In vitro epithelial and endothelial wound healing and regeneration, as well as keratocyte morphology can be visualized under the conditions of organ culture. In grafted tissue, all corneal layers could be documented (epithelial cell layers including basal cells, the process of corneal reinnervation, stromal wound healing, endothelial cell morphology). In selected cases, specific findings like poor epithelial differentiation, pannus formation, stromal infiltrates/deposits, and endothelial cell pathologies could be found. **Conclusion**: Confocal microscopy adds a wide spectrum of morphological findings to the current knowledge. While some aspects of the donor corneas' morphology can be visualized with less elaborate methods, confocal microscopy may improve our understanding of the events taking place in corneal donor tissue before and after grafting.

WHEN GLAUCOMA PRESSURES THE GRAFT

Helene Boisjoly,[1,2] Isabelle Brunette,[1] Manon Charest,[1] Marjolaine-Marie Gagnon,[1] Marcel Amyot,[1] Raynald Roy,[2] and Richard Bazin[2]

Ophthalmology Research Units, Maisonneuve-Rosemont Hospital[1], Montreal and Laval University Medical Center[2], Quebec, Canada

Based on a single-center observational study, 539 adult recipients of a corneal graft were followed for a median time of 30 months. Survival analysis was carried out. Relative risks of graft failure for 12 risk factors were calculated. Recipients with glaucoma as a co-morbidity factor to corneal disease had a threefold increased risk of graft failure (RR = 3.0 [1.9–4.8]). The risk of failure was greater for glaucoma than for other important risk factors such as repeat graft in the study eye and presence of recipient corneal vessels. This failure rate could be related to postoperative IOP fluctuation with IOP peaks that repeatedly damage the corneal graft endothelium. This is supported by the fact that the risk of failure tended to increase significantly beyond 24 months after transplantation up to five-fold at 36 months.

We went on to study the association between glaucoma and corneal endothelial cell vitality indicators. 102 glaucomatous patients were compared to 52 nonglaucomatous patients of the same age group with clear corneas. Specular microscopies were performed on central corneas. Corneal endothelial cell counts were significantly lower in patients with glaucoma (2154 ± 419 cells/mm^2) compared to nonglaucomatous controls (2560 ± 306 cells/mm^2) (t-test, $p<0.0001$). In the glaucoma group, cell counts were inversely proportional to the means of IOPs. Patients receiving three or four glaucoma medications had lower cell counts than those receiving one or two medications. This study presents evidence that glaucoma is associated with corneal endothelial cell anomalies.

Lastly, 21 patients with ocular hypertension were compared to 21 age-matched controls. These patients never received any glaucoma medication nor laser treatment. The mean IOP was significantly higher in the hypertensive group (mean, 24.5; range 23–28) compared to the normotensive group (mean, 15.5; range 12–21). Corneal endothelial cell counts were significantly lower in patients with ocular hypertension (2254 ± 277 cells/mm^2) compared to controls (2496 ± 418 cells/mm^2; $p = 0.03$). This study demonstrates that corneal endothelial cell counts are lower in glaucoma suspects that present with ocular hypertension in the 23 to 28 mm range.

The proposed mechanisms are direct endothelial damage from intraocular pressure or congenital alteration of the corneal endothelium in patients with glaucoma or ocular hypertension. Enhanced surveillance in recipients with glaucoma is therefore recommended for prevention of late corneal graft failure.

Supported in part by the Quebec Eye Bank Foundation and the FRSQ Network for Research in Vision and Ophthalmology.

TOPICAL CYCLOSPORINE A IN THE MANAGEMENT OF POST-KERATOPLASTY GLAUCOMA

Henry D. Perry,[1,2] Eric D. Donnenfeld,[1,3] Anastasios J. Kanellopoulos,[4] and Gayle Grossman[1]

[1]North Shore University Hospital, Manhasset, New York, [2]New York Eye and Ear Infirmary, New York, [3]Manhattan Eye, Ear and Throat Hospital, New York, [4]Massachusetts Eye and Ear Infirmary Boston, Massachusetts

PURPOSE: Cyclosporine A (Sandimmune,® Sandoz Pharmaceuticals, East Hanover, NJ) a highly specific immunomodulator that affects primarily T-lymphocytes, does not inhibit the phagocytic system as much as steroids, allowing the antimicrobial arm of the immune system to fight infection. Furthermore, Cyclosporine A 0.5% does not inhibit wound healing, increase the intraocular pressure, or produce lens changes. The experience with Cyclosporine A appears to be equal to topical corticosteroid in preventing graft rejections in high risk patients. These factors led us to substitute topical Cyclosporine A for corticosteroids in treating post-keratoplasty patients with glaucoma.

METHODS: Topical Cyclosporine A was prospectively substituted for topical corticosteroids in 60 patients with post-keratoplasty glaucoma.

RESULTS: Forty-seven of 60 patients showed a reduction in intraocular pressure (2 to 28 mm Hg) with a mean of 8.4 mm Hg. Follow-up ranged from 4 to 21 months, with a mean of 9.8 months. Graft clarity was maintained in 59 patients, with 2 patients having allograft rejection episodes. Twenty-one patients were able to discontinue one or more glaucoma medications.

CONCLUSION: Topical Cyclosporine A may be safely substituted for topical corticosteroids in post-keratoplasty glaucoma patients with a resultant decrease in intraocular pressure. (No proprietary interest.)

PENETRATING KERATOPLASTY FOR HERPETIC KERATITITS

R. Doyle Stulting

Emory Eye Center, Atlanta, Georgia

Herpes simplex keratitis (HSK) is the primary diagnosis for about 5% of patients undergoing keratoplasty in the United States. It was second only to pseudophakic and aphakic corneal edema as a primary diagnosis among high-risk patients who were subjects of the Collaborative Corneal Transplantation Studies. Recurrent herpetic ocular disease and allograft rejection are often the causes of graft failure. This presentation will review the results of penetrating keratoplasty for HSK, emphasizing postoperative complications and their management.

SURGICAL MANAGEMENT OF SEVERE OCULAR SURFACE DISEASE

Edward J. Holland

Cornea Service, Department of Ophthalmology
University of Minnesota, Minneapolis, Minnesota

Conditions that result in limbal stem deficiency can result in profound morbidity for patients. These etiologies include aniridia, chemical and thermal burns, Stevens-Johnson Syndrome (SJS), ocular cicatricial pemphigoid, severe contact lens induced keratopathy, as well as multiple surgical procedures. Routine penetrating keratoplasty for these patients typically result in ocular surface failure and subsequent graft failure.

Recently epithelial transplantation procedures have been developed to stabilize the ocular surface prior to penetrating keratoplasty in limbal stem cell deficiency patients. Epithelial transplantation procedures can be classified as one of the following procedures: conjunctival autograft, conjunctival allograft, conjunctival limbal autograft, cadaveric conjunctival limbal allograft, living related conjunctival limbal allograft, or keratolimbal allograft.

Twenty-five eyes of 21 patients who underwent a keratolimbal allograft for severe ocular surface disease were evaluated. Ocular surface stability, improvement of visual acuity, success of subsequent keratoplasties and preoperative risk factors were studied. Eighteen of 25 eyes (72%) developed a stable ocular surface. Fifteen eyes (60%) demonstrated a significant improvement in visual acuity. Preoperative persistent epithelial defects and symblephara were successfully managed with this procedure. Six of 13 (46%) subsequent penetrating or lamellar keratoplasties were successful. Patients with limbal deficiency due to SJS had a significantly worse outcome. Patients wit preoperative conjunctival keratinization also had a significant worse outcome. The median follow-up time was 20 months with a range of 6 to 63 months. These results compare favorable with other published studies except for patients with SJS who appear to have better results with a living related conjunctival limbal allograft.

Based on our results, as well as the results of other published studies of epithelial transplantation procedures, the following recommendations are made. For patients with unilateral limbal deficiency, a conjunctival limbal autograft is the procedure of choice. For patients with bilateral disease, a keratolimbal allograft or a living related conjunctival limbal allograft should be considered. However, patients with SIS may have a better prognosis with a living related conjunctival limbal allograft. The importance of HLA and ABO typing as well as the protocol for immunosuppression in the allograft procedures for limbal deficiency need further study.

WHICH FACTORS AFFECT SUTURES-OUT ASTIGMATISM?

Perry S. Binder

Vision Surgery and Laser Center; San Diego, California

Purpose: To determine the factor(s) responsible for sutures-out astigmatism following corneal transplantation (PKP). **Setting:** Data was obtained by technicians and the author in condensed refraction lanes. **Methods:** Keratometry (Bausch and Lomb and manifest refractions were used. Data was entered into computer database weekly. Indications for PKP: Keratoconus (KG), Pseudophalmic Bullous Keratopathy (PBK), All leucomas (LEU). **Results:** Of a total of 1141 eyes, 504 (sutures-out) operated by the author between 1978 and 1995 were in the database.

	N	MeanCyl	Std.Dev	Range	Mean K	Range
KC	134	3.7	2.5	0–16	45.7	39.4–53.5
Donor recipient disparity, suture, and trephine technique made no difference						
PBK	89	4.3	2.5	0–9	46.2	42.6–50.9
Donor recipient disparity, suture, and trephine technique made no difference						
LEU	144	4.1	2.4	0–12	46.2	41.9–53.5
Donor recipient disparity, suture, and trephine technique made no difference						
All 8/8 D/R	18	3.6	1.9	1.1–7.6	44.6	40.9–50.1
All 8.2518	103	3.9	2.6	0–16	45.2	39.4–52.0
All 8.5/8	160	4.3	2.6	0–12	46.3	41.9–51.6
All 8.7518	130	4.0	2.3	0–10	46.0	*41.9–53.5*

Host Dx V. Astigmatism	KC (134)	ABK (38)	LEU (163)	FFF(60)	PBK (89)
<1.25 D (n=60)	22	5	16	5	12
>7D (n=68)	16	8	25	7	12
D/R Disparity V Astigmatism	8/8 (18)	825/8 (103)	8.5/8 (160)	8.75/8 (130)	
<1.25 D (n=60)	2	14	19	18	
>7D (n=68)	2	11	26	14	

138 eyes (27%) required rigid contact lens (CL)wear for anisometropia and/or irregular astigmatism; 14.5% KG, *3%* PBK, 6.2% LEU

Conclusions: In spite of advances in suture techniques and trephine systems with early visual rehabilitation through suture manipulation techniques, analysis of sutures out cases performed by the same surgeon, and controlling surgical factors only minimally reduces astigmatism compared to results 10 years ago. Unmeasured and uncontrollable factors still play a major role in the distribution of postoperative corneal power affecting IOL calculations, anisometropia, and contact lens fitting. Anterior/posterior wound coaptation, donor hydration and topography, donor and host wound creation, and variable host wound healing need to be controlled to further improve results.

INCIDENCE OF HSV-1 DNA IN CULTURE MEDIA FROM HUMAN CORNEAL DONOR TISSUE

Justus Garweg and Matthias Böhnke

Dept. Ophthalmology, University of Bern, Inselspital, CH-3010 Bern

Background: Depending on the investigator, herpes virus isolation was successful in up to 25% of corneal buttons in herpetic eye disease. However, viral DNA was also found in normal corneal epithelium and in the corneal stroma post mortem. In this study, the incidence of herpes simplex DNA in culture media of healthy corneal transplant tissue was examined to define: 1. the incidence of detectable primary graft contamination with HSV-l; 2. the influence of storage conditions; and 3. the correlation of viral DNA to the endothelial cell loss in organ culture in order to calculate the risk of possible virus transmission by corneal transplantation.

Material and Methods: 391 corneal organ culture fluid samples were investigated for the presence of HSV-l DNA. For this, electro-separation of the samples, DNA amplification for fragments of the glycoprotein D and the thymidine kinase encoding genes and Southern blot analysis using Digoxigenin-labeled probes for DNA hybridisation and detection were performed. 116 of the culture media were worked up immediately after the end of culture (group 1), 90 after strorage at -8ºC for 30 - 60 days (group 2a), 100 after storage at room temperature for 6 - 60 weeks, and 85 after storage for 6 - 30 weeks at -20ºC (group 3). Endothelial cell counts before and after organ culture of herpes DNA negative and positive cultures were compared.

Results: In 2/391 corneal organ culture fluid samples, HSV-l DNA was detected. A correlation between the incidence of herpetic DNA in the culture fluid and the endothelial cell loss in organ culture thus was not calculated. However, DNA from the human betaglobin gene was amplified only from the samples of goups 1 and 3. In the samples of group 2, the degradation of DNA prohibited a detection of human genomic DNA. Consequently, a conclusion regarding the presence of HSV-l DNA in these media cannot be drawn.

Conclusion: An early degradation of DNA may be responsible for false negative results. However, the detection of herpetic DNA in less than 1% of culture media after elution prior to a degradation of the DNA fails to demonstrate an influence of HSV-1 on the biological quality of corneal tissue for transplantation during culture.

DETECTION OF PRK ON CADAVERIC GLOBES BY VIDEOKERATOGRAPHY

J.M. Williams, R. Chuck, R. Lim-Bon-Siong, and J.S. Pepose

Department of Ophthalmology and Visual Sciences, Washington University, St. Louis, MO

Purpose: In contrast to incisional keratotomy, refractive techniques such as auto-mated lamellar keratectomy (ALK) and excimer photorefractive keratectomy (PRK) are difficult to detect. Cadaveric corneas with high refractive myopic correction may result in substantial post-operative hyperopic correction if used for corneal transplants. Displace-ment of the treated optical zone within the graft could also result in induced astigmatism and distortion. This study examined the potential of videokeratographic (VKG) analysis of cadaveric whole globes to determine if topography may be a useful screening strategy for detecting PRK. **Methods:** A vertically mounted videokeratoscope from "EyeSys Tech-nologies" mapped the corneal topography of cadaveric corneas of whole globes and enu-cleated rabbit globes that had undergone PRK. A horizontal "EyeSys" keratoscope recorded topography on patient eyes pre- and post PRK correction. A Summit excimer system performed both 5 mm and 6 nim PRK ablation zones. **Results:** The vertically mounted VKG could reliably detect PRK on cadaveric corneas at all tested myopic correc-tions (6D, 5D, 4D, 3D, 2D, and 1.5 D). Low myopic PRK corrections (1.5 - 2.0 diopters), in patients, were more readily detected 6 months to 1 year post surgery using tangential maps as opposed to conventional color maps. Data processed in the tangential map mode yielded a "bullseye" topography pattern. Profile maps of the 0–180 and 90–270 axes were also useful in analyzing results and assessing excimer centration. **Conclusions:** VKG may be a useful method to screen donor globes for PRK; however, it is not amenable to screen donor corneal scleral rims and is therefore limited to whole globes. Studies of excimer treated rabbit corneas confirm PRK is detectable on enucleated globes 6 weeks post sur-gery. Low myopic PRK corrections are easily detected by VKG in patients 6 months to 1 year post surgery. Tangential and profile maps provide superior visual representations of low PRK corrections compared to the standard color maps. (Financial Support: EyeSys Technologies; Core Grant EY 02687, and RPB).

CLOSED-SYSTEM APPROACH FOR CORNEAL TRIPLE PROCEDURES: A REVIEW OF SURGICAL COMPLICATIONS IN 31 CONSECUTIVE CASES

Enrique S. Malbran, Enrique Malbran Jr., and Jorge Halbran

As have been described by the authors, in corneal triple procedure phacoemulsifica-tion, PCL and penetrating graft is the ideal method when no stromal opacities are present, and a good visualization of the anterior chamber is possible, once the epithelium has been removed. The latter, is the most frequent situation as in Fuchs' dystrophy and other simi-lar situations. Since the major advantage of this technique is based in a pressurized con-trolled system, that tends to avoid most of the complications that can occur with the open-sky approach during surgery, 31 consecutive cases are reviewed, specifically concerning the intraoperative complication observed. In 4 instances a posterior capsule rupture occurred. This complication appeared during the closed-system step in 2 cases, and in the open sky phase in the remaining two. The reasons for these events will be discussed, as well as demonstrated with videos and how they were solved without further difficulties.

RESULTS OF PERIPHERAL GRAFTS IN PERIPHERAL THINNING DISORDERS OF CORNEA

Aashish K. Bansal, Madhukar K. Reddy, and Gullapalli N.Rao

L.V. Prasad Eye Institute, Hyderabad, India

Purpose: To study the therapeutic and tectonic results of peripheral grafts in peripheral corneal thinning disorders. **Methods:** Results of eleven consecutive peripheral grafts done over past three years were reviewed. Eight grafts were full thickness while three were lamellar. Six grafts were annular, four oval while one was a crown graft. Indications included perforation or impending perforation of peripheral cornea due to various etiologies (Mooren's ulcer 2, Terrien's degeneration 1, Pellucid degeneration 2, Peripheral ulcerative keratitis 3 and others 2). The crown graft was done in a case of keratoglobus. **Results:** Progression of disease stopped and graft healed with vascularisation in ten (91%) cases though the graft remained edematous in six cases. Pre operative vision ranged from 20/50 to finger counting at one meter. In nine (82%) cases best corrected visual acuity improved and post operative vision ranged from 20/30 to hand movements. One case showed recurrence of Mooren's ulcer with melting of graft. **Conclusion:** Peripheral corneal grafts give good therapeutic and tectonic results in cases of peripheral corneal thinning disorders.

TOPOPLASTY

We describe a new surgical technique to correct anisometropia (myopia and astigmatism) after corneal transplants. The technique consist of deep marginal keratomy, keratectomy using a dentist drill, reapposition of the surgical margins and resuturing of the incision. The analysis of the results in 29 eyes is presented follow up of 2 to 5 years. Myopia was reduced from a mean of 6.32D. preop. to 1.88D. post op. and astigmatism was reduced from a mean of 6.43D. preop. to 3.15 diopters post. op. demonstrating the efficacy of the method.

METABOLIC CHANGES OF HUMAN CORNEAS STORED IN MODIFIED MEM OR OPTISOL

C. Redbrake, S. Salla, A. Frantz, and M. Reim

Department of Ophthalmology, Technical University of Aachen, Germany

Background: While in the USA mainly storage media like Optisol are used at 4°C for a maximum of 7 days, European Banks prefer storage in a modified minimal essential medium (MEM) at 31 °C. It was therefore the purpose of this study to compare both systems from the metabolic point of view. **Materials and Methods:** 12 human corneas were stored for 7 days in Optisol medium. To compare these corneas directly to MEM, 11 human corneas were stored for 7 days in a modified MEM with a subsequent deswelling period of 1 day in MEM containing 5 % dextran 500. Because the mean storage period in European Banks are 13 days, we also evaluated corneas after this time (12±1 day of deswelling). At the end of the storage period the endothelial cells were counted Glucose, lactate, ATP, ADP and AMP levels were determined in the corneas (μmol/g dryweight).

Results:

Storage	Glucose	Lactate	ATP	ADP	AMP	AEC
Optisol	3,438	16,316	0,646	0,529	0,031	0,498
MEM 7+1	4,968	7,545	0,119	0,112	0,021	0,538
MEM 12+1	0,746	15,569	0,093	0,082	0,016	0,539

Values in μmol/g dryweight

Endothelial cell count did not differ significantly in all three groups. **Conclusion**: From our data we conclude that Optisol and MEM medium for 7 days do not show statistically significant differences from the metabolic point of view. Organ culture in MEM medium offers the opportunity to store corneas beyond this point without worsening of the metabolic status of the human cornea which is especially reflected by the adenylate energy charge.

EFFECT ON RABBIT CORNEAL ENDOTHELIAL CELLS OF CORNEAL STORAGE MEDIA WITH TREHALOSE

Toshiyuki Takano, Angelico Alejo, Michifumi Watanabe, Kiyoo Nakayasu, and Atsushi Kanai

Department of Ophthalmology, Juntendo University, Japan

Purpose: Trehalose (I - α - D - glucopyranosyl - α - D - glucopyranoside) is detected in many kinds of fungi, yeasts and plants. This disaccharide can stabilize cell membranes under various stressful condition. In this study we examined the effects of trehalose on rabbit corneal endothelial cells of corneal storage media.

Material & Methods: The storage media were EP - II and Optisol. Albino rabbits eyes were stored in group I: EP - II (storage medium for whole eye ball), for group II: EP II +3.5 % Trehalose, group III: Optisol and group W : Optisol +3.5 % Trehalose. Pachymetric measurements were taken to measure corneal thickness every 2 days in the preservations. Scanning electron microscopy and light microscopy studies were done to assess the endothelial cell morphology of the stored rabbits cornea on day 5 and day 10.

Results: The thickness of the stored rabbit corneas on day 10 were 1.085mm in group I, 0.644mm in group 11, 0.632mm in group III and 0.516mm in group I. Trehalose added corneal storage media showed thinner cornea. Endothelial cells were more damaged and cell borders were more irregular with prominent interdigitations on day 10 in storage media without Trehalose.

Conclusion: Trehalose may play a role in providing better corneas on the preservation of donor rabbit cornea.

VIABILITY OF HUMAN CORNEAL KERATOCYTES DURING ORGAN CULTURE

Torben Møller-Pedersen

Department of Ophthalmology, Århus University Hospital, Denmark

Background. A stromal graft containing viable keratocytes will regain clarity more rapidly, than an implant containing dead keratocytes; however, the impact of preservation techniques on these cells is not well described. **Purpose.** To assess the viability of human corneal keratocytes during four weeks of "closed system" organ culture (European technique). **Methods.** 46 normal human donor corneas were cultured in MEM etc. at 31°C for 0–4 weeks. The keratocyte viability was quantified by monitoring the RNA-synthesis level using ^{3}H-uridine incorporation and subsequent autoradiography and digital image analysis. Similarly, the number of keratocyte mitoses were assessed after ^{3}H-thymidine incorporation. The medium was analyzed for changes in pH, pO_2, pCO_2, glucose, and lactate, as well as for the content of immunogenic keratan sulphate using the antibody 5D4 in an ELISA. **Results.** After 28 days of culturing, the entire keratocyte population was still alive and viable since all cells incorporated uridine. During the first 14 days, mitoses were found in the anterior half of the stroma (0.23% mitoses per 48 h), while only few keratocytes were able to divide at day 28 (0.01% mitoses per 48 h). Metabolic parameters revealed a progressing acidosis in the medium with oxygen and glucose depletion. Immunological measurements of keratan sulphate suggested that approximately 1% of the total content was lost during the period. **Conclusions.** The European organ culture technique can maintain a viable keratocyte population for four weeks; a viable stroma can be grafted within this period.

PREDICTION OF CORNEAL ENDOTHELIAL CELL LOSS IN ORGAN CULTURE

A. Kloss,[1] M. Hagenah,[1] M. Böhnke,[2] and R. Winter[3]

[1]Augenklinik, Medizinische Hochschule Hannover, 30623 Hannover, Germany;
[2]Augenklinik, Inselspital, Bern, Switzerland

Purpose: Corneal endothelial cell loss is a normal finding in organ culture preservation. However, there is hardly anything known about the extent of cell loss during culture. The purpose of this study was to develop a formula to predict corneal endothelial cell density at given periods of storage. **Materials and methods.** 1348 corneas were included in the study. All corneas were stored in MEM medium containing 2% fetal calf serum for a range between 1 and 99 days at 370 C. 71,3% of the corneas were preserved for at least 1 day in MEM-medium with 6% dextran at the end of storage. Variables investigated were donor age, post-mortem-time, duration of storage in dextran and dextran-free medium, endothelial cell density at the time of preparation, and cell density at the end of storage. Calculation was performed by multiple regression analysis. **Results:** Average endothelial cell density was 2688 cells/mm^2 at the initial count showing a significant decrease with increasing donor age (r=0,40, p<0,000 1), an observation, that was also found at the end of storage (r=0,37, p<0,0001). No impact on corneal endothelial cell density at the end of culture was found for post-mortem-time (r=0,03, p=0, 12) and storage in dextran-containing medium for less than 5 days (r=0,007, p=0,79).

The regression formula calculated by these results (y=(-2,73 x donor age)-(9,28 x days of culture)+(0,66 x cell count at dissection) +929) predicts endothelial cell density at the end of storage of up to 40 days at any given time period. It shows the expected average cell density and the lower 95% confidence interval for predicted individuals and takes the different variables, that have an impact on corneal endothelial loss in organ culture, into consideration **Conclusion:** Based on our raw data, we developed a regression formula to predict corneal endothelial cell density at the time of evaluation before transplantation for organ culture preserved corneas. Although it may currently have some disadvantages, it rationalizes the decision whether an organ cultured cornea is feasible for transplantation.

SCARRED CONJUNCTIVAL SURFACE REPLACED BY FRESH CORNEAL DONOR

A. Mieth and E. Arenas

Fundación Santa Fe de Bogotá, Bogotá, Colombia

Purpose: To treat eyes with severe damaged conjunctival and scleral tissue in cases with necrotic post-beta therapy ulcers, dellen and some vernal conjunctivitis plaques with a lamellar keratoplasty technique, which includes transplantation of the donor corneal epithelium.

Methods: The damaged tissue is marked with a corneal trephine at a deepness of 300 up to 400 microns of a select size (range 7 to 10 mm) and them is dissected in block leaving a smooth subscleral surface with clean conjunctival borders. A very fresh donor eye is utilized and a lamellar button 0.5 mm larger than the receptor bed is dissected. The donor tissue is placed carefully in the cruent zone, protecting all the time the epithelium surface. A border to border single suture 9.-0 nylon is placed and the patient is unpatched the next day and observed for graft reaction. **Results:** With this procedure, we have treated 6 cases with excellent results. The lacrimal film is recovered next day with immediate alleviation of signs and symptoms. The corneal epithelium is slowly replaced by conjunctival epithelium and the stroma slowly suffer differentiation changes to become scleral tissue. In rabbits we showed how the cornea suffers a paulatine change when transplanted in a scleral bed. Electro microscopic studies are shown in case followed 2 years. **Conclusions:** This technique provides a better solution for this type of cases, based on the necessity of replacing these distorted areas for a clean lacrimal film surface as soon as possible. Embryologically corneal tissue is a nonvascularized scleral tissue that becomes opaque as soon as it gets vessels.

A SYSTEMATIC APPROACH FOR ESTABLISHING AN INTERNATIONAL NETWORK OF EYE BANKS

Mahmoud Farazdaghi and James Leimkuhler

Tissue Banks International, International Federation of Eye Banks, Baltimore, Maryland

Corneal blindness continues throughout much of the world. Twenty-five percent of all blindness is due to corneal disease, defect or trauma. Waiting lists for corneal transplantation exist in developed and developing countries.

The systematic approach used by the International Federation of Eye Banks (IFEB) reduces corneal blindness in areas of the world where no effective eye banking program exists. It does this by establishing and maintaining a federation of eye banks in cooperation with local resources that makes available donor material for corneal transplantation on all equitable basis.

Initial Project Assessment includes the evaluation of Laws and Regulations; Religious and Social Norms; Ministry of Health and Ophthalmic Community support; Demographics; Feasibility of Financial Self-Sufficiency. Training of the Medical Director and Technical Staff involves an intensive program at one of our four training centers and continues at the project site until technical proficiency is certified. The work includes providing designs and floor plans; consultation on equipment selection; establishment of coroner and hospital development programs; on-going training and administrative services. Maintaining quality assurance and frequent site inspections are important components of a systematic approach. Tissue is distributed on an equitable basis without regard to race, religion, nationality or institution. If surplus tissue cannot be distributed in the country of origin, it will be placed through the IFEB/TBI International Tissue Distribution System.

Results: Trained 137 Eye Bank Personnel, established a cooperative, global Federation of 25 member Eye Banks and distributed 13,449 PKP quality corneas 1990–1995.

Conclusion: The number of surgical quality corneas can be significantly increased by a systematic approach to establishing successful eye banking programs with international networking through a cooperative global federation. The results of 'FEB programs are promising and strongly suggest that this methodology is working in varied locations throughout the world. However, the need for additional PKP continues to be overwhelming.

CLINICAL AND OPERATIVE FACTORS INFLUENCING CORNEAL GRAFT OUTCOME

D.L. Easty,[1] S.M. Gore,[2] B.A. Bradley,[3] C.A. Rogers,[4] and W.J. Armitage[1]

[1]Department of Ophthalmology, University of Bristol; [2]Medical Research Council Biostatistics Department, University of Leeds; [3]Department of Transplantation Sciences, University of Bristol; [4]United Kingdom Transplant Support Service Authority, Bristol (UK)

Purpose: To quantify clinical and operative factors influencing corneal graft outcome. **Methods:** Multifactorial analysis of 2242 grafts registered by United Kingdom Transplant Service from July 1987 to 1990.

Results: Increased risk of graft failure with: preoperative stromal oedema; small trephine size; difference in donor and recipient sizes greater than 0.25 mm and mixed continuous and interrupted sutures. Poorer 3 month visual acuity with: glaucoma and low visual acuity preoperatively; small trephine size; and combined vitreous surgery. Higher 3 month astigmatism with interrupted sutures. **Conclusions:** Effects of factors were generally in the same direction for each outcome measure. Only large scale, randomised, controlled trials will provide definitive answers to preferred operative techniques.

INFLUENCE OF DONOR AND STORAGE FACTORS ON QUALITY OF CORNEAS STORED BY ORGAN CULTURE

D.L. Easty,[1] W.J. Armitage,[1] R. Bawden,[2] and P. Bowerman[2]

[1]Department of Ophthalmology, University of Bristol (UK); [2]UKTSSA, Bristol (UK)

Logistic regression methods were used to analyse the influence of donor and storage factors on the quality of corneas stored by organ culture in the Bristol eye bank in 1991. Average donor age was 57 years (sd 22, n=2770) and time from death to enucleation was 8 hours (sd 7, n=2762). Corneas were placed into organ culture within 27 hours (sd 10, n=2550) of donor death and were stored for 22 days (sd 7, n-2716). Preliminary results showed that 126 of 2744 corneas (4.5%) were discarded through contamination. The risk of contamination increased with increasing death to enucleation time ($p<0.037$) but corneas from CVA donors were less likely to be contaminated ($p<0.003$). Overall, 27% of corneas were not suitable for PKP because of endothelial defects. Corneas stored for more than 4 weeks or corneas from donors over 80 years old were less likely to be suitable for PKP (both $p<0.0001$). But the likelihood of corneas having high endothelial cell densities (>2500 cells/mm²) was reduced with donors over 20 years old ($p<0.001$) with storage times more than 2 weeks ($p<0.004$) or when corneas came from donors that died of cancer ($p<0.04$) or respiratory disease ($p<0.020$). Corneas from CVA donors, however, were more likely to be suitable for PKP ($P<0.005$). Analyses such as this are important for monitoring donor procurement practices and the efficacy of eye banking techniques.

PENETRATING KERATOPLASTY IN PSEUDOPHAKIC CORNEAL EDEMA

Ritu Arora, L. D. Sota, Maneesh Kumar, and Lalit Sanga

Purpose: Pseudophakic corneal oedema (PCO) is one of the common indications for penetrating keratoplasty in the present era. The present study was undertaken to comprehensively analyze the results of PK in patients of PCO.

Method: We did penetrating keratoplasty in 50 eyes with PCO. The interval between cataract extraction with IOL implantation and PK ranged from 6 months to 5 years. The IOL was explanted in 18 (36%; Gr I), left in situ in 26 (52%; Gi II) and exchanged in 6 (12%; Gr III) cases respectively.

Conclusion: The commonest IOL associated with PCO was iris-claw, pupil supported lens. The visual results (BCVA) obtained after PK were encouraging in gr II and III (60% achieving >6/12) while only 20% achieved >6/36 in gr 1. Graft clarity at (14–24 months) follow up was obtained in 82% of cases in gr II and III and 50% of cases in gr 1. Ocular comfort was achieved in all patients with clear corneal grafts. Our results show that graft clarity is achieved in majority of patients, but the frequency of visual gain is not to the desired level.

INDICATIONS FOR PENETRATING KERATOPLASTIES, 1986–1995

Eugene Liu and Allan Slomovic

University of Toronto

Purpose: To determine leading indications for penetrating keratoplasty (PKP) and to observe trends over a ten year period. **Methods:** We reviewed 927 consecutive penetrating keratoplasties performed over a ten year period (1986–1995) by a single ophthalmologist (A.S.) at The Toronto Hospital. The charts for 904 cases were identified and classified according to the diagnostic categories described by the Wilmer Eye Institute (Arentsen et al, 1976). Where possible, the clinical indication was corroborated by the pathological report. **Results:** There were 456 female and 448 males; 454 left eyes and 450 right eyes. The number of PKP's performed rose from 37 in 1986 to a peak of 121 in 1989, and fell to 83 cases in 1995. Leading indications included pseudophakic bullous keratopathy (PBK) (28.5%), regraft (22.4%), Keratoconus (10.0%), Fuch's dystrophy (7.6%), aphakic bullous keratopathy (ABK) 6.1%), herpetic keratopathy (4.2%), bacterial infection (4.2%), physical trauma (4%), interstitial keratitis (3.7%), and corneal scarring (2.8%). These ten indications accounted for 94% of all PKP's performed. PBK remained the leading indication every year for the past ten years with the exception of 1992 and 1995 when it was surpassed by regraft. The most common type of intraocular lens found in PBK patients was the anterior chamber lens (AC IOL 71.6%, PC IOL 16%. IP IOL 12.5%). In our series, we noted a decrease in the incidence of aphakic bullous keratopathy (p<0.001), and an increase in the incidence of regraft (p<0.017). Our data does not show a statistically significant change in the incidence of Fuch's endothelial dystrophy, keratoconus, or PBK, however, the data does suggest a decreasing trend for PBK. Gender differences in the indications was statistically significant only for Fuch's dystrophy being more common in women by a 3:1 ratio over men. **Conclusions:** In our series, the leading indications for penetrating keratoplasty was found to be generally in agreement with the data reported in recent literature. The failure of the many authors to agree precisely on the leading indications reflects the wide variations in practice and referral patients.

NEEDLELESS ANESTHESIA FOR PENETRATING KERATOPLASTY SURGERY

Jayne S. Weiss

Kresge Eye Institute, Wayne State University, Detroit, Michigan 48201

Greenbaum has described the technique of subtenons anesthetic irrigation through a cannula to achieve a retrobulbar block without the risk of globe perforation by the retrobulbar needle. The technique is used successfully for cataract surgery and extra ocular procedures.

In order to determine if this mode of anesthetic delivery was equally effective for penetrating keratoplasty surgery, ten eyes undergoing penetrating keratoplasty had an incision made through the inferior temporal conjunctiva and tenons. A nineteen gauge cannula was placed under tenon's capsule and advanced posteriorly to irrigate I to 5 cc's of 2% xylocaine, 1% marcaine, and 1:10 xydase in the retrobulbar space.

All patients underwent uneventful penetrating keratoplasty surgery. One of ten patients experienced conjunctival chemosis and needed supplementation of the anesthetic during surgery. There were no other complications.

We recommend consideration of this needleless technique for anesthetic placement in the penetrating keratoplasty patient. The technique avoids the potential complications of inadvertent perforation of the globe and allows ease of supplementation of anesthetic even after the cornea is removed.

RESULTS OF PENETRATING KERATOPLASTY IN CASES OF SIGNIFICANT LOSS OF VISION AFTER RADIAL KERATOTOMY

D. Cuevas-Cancino, A.L. Perez-Balbuena, and E. Angel

Asociacion para Evitar la Queçuera en México, México, D.F.

Purpose: To evaluate the results of penetrating keratoplasty in cases of significant loss of vision after radial keratotomy. **Methods:** 10 cases with a significant loss of vision after aggressive and repeated incisional refractive attempts to correct astigmatism hyperopic overcorrection, residual myopia, and refractive errors associated with keratoconus were followed after they had a penetrating keratoplasty for a period between 8 and 16 months. Wound healing, graft transparency, corneal topography control were determined each month. Most of them (80%) were able to wear contact lenses and wear them successfully within 5 months after surgery; 80% reached more than 20/60. **Conclusion:** We consider penetrating keratoplasty in cases with significant loss of vision after repeated incisional attempts a good option.

CORNEAL TRANSPLANT IN CHILDREN: BRAZILIAN EXPERIENCE

Elcio H. Sato, Juliana M. Ferraz Sallum, Seiji Hayashi, and Rubens Belfort, Jr.

Sao Paulo Federal University - Paulista School of Medicine, Sao Paulo, Brazil

This is a retrospective study of 114 children, 16 years old or younger, who had 145 penetrating corneal transplants in 132 eyes, with an average follow-up of 27 months. The probability of obtaining a clear graft was 50% in 28 eyes in the congenital opacities, 87.5% in ~O eyes with acquired nontraumatic opacities and 75% in 24 eyes with opacities from trauma. Respectively, the visual acuity was better than 20/200 in 6.6% (1/15), 81.5% (62/76), and 40% (8/20). Corneal transplant in children is limited by the difficulty of the surgical procedure and the complicated postoperative care, but it seems to have its place.

PULSED METHYLPREDNISOLONE THERAPY IN THE MANAGEMENT OF CORNEAL GRAFT REJECTION

Ritu Arora, L. D. Sota, Maneesh Kumar, and Lalit Sanga

Purpose: Role of topical and systemic steroids in the management of corneal graft rejection is well known: There is a moderately high degree of nonresponsiveness to these steroid regimens. Our aim during the present study was to try and develop an effective alternative to the routine management of corneal graft rejection.

Method: We used 250–500 mg of parenteral methylprednisolone in the management of corneal graft rejections in 13 patients in the last 2 years. The onset of graft rejection in these patients varied from 3 months to 10 months after surgery. The patients presented between 48–96 hours of the onset of diminution of earlier achieved vision. They received pulsed methylprednisolone treatment, the dose of steroid depending upon the severity of graft rejection.

Conclusion: Ten of the patients showed complete recovery from the rejection episode while one patient showed delayed response and no response was obtained in two patients. Our results show that pulsed corticosteroid therapy may be beneficial in the management of severe corneal graft rejection with the advantage of avoiding prolonged topical and oral corticosteroid therapy.

MANAGEMENT OF PETERS' ANOMALY ASSOCIATED WITH CORNEAL PSEUDOSTAPHYLOMA

Gerald W. Zaidman and Kenneth Juechter

Department of Ophthalmology, Westchester County Medical Center Our Lady of Mercy Hospital, New York Medical College, Valhalla, New York

Peters' anomaly is an uncommon congenital corneal opacity. The morphologic characteristics vary but usually consist of a central corneal leukoma with adherent iris strands. Some patients may have involvement of the lens, and other ocular anomalies such as sclerocornea, microphthalmos, and glaucoma. Pathologically Descemet's membrane and the corneal endothelium are absent at the site of leukoma.

Recently I managed four infants with an unusual form of Peters' anomaly. One eye of each patient had a scarred cornea, mimicking a corneal staphyloma, protruding anteriorly from the corneal plane. The other eye in each patient ranged from normal to severe ocular anomalies (including microphthalmos and a retinal detachment).

A corneal transplant was performed in each case. In 3 eyes an anterior segment reconstruction, lensectomy and vitrectomy were also performed. Follow up has ranged from 1–3 years. Three eyes maintained graft clarity for at least one year. Each of these eyes developed vision. Two of the three eyes with clear grafts developed glaucoma. The eye with graft failure eventually developed an inoperable total retinal detachment. Histopathology of each corneal button was consistent with Peters' anomaly and a protruding corneal pseudo-staphyloma. No uveal tissue was seen on the posterior aspect of the specimens and therefore the diagnosis of congenital anterior staphyloma was not tenable. Despite the severe corneal anomalies surgical management successfully restored a more normal cosmetic appearance in all four eyes and vision in 3 of the eyes.

HYDROGEL CORE-AND-SKIRT KERATOPROSTHESES IN PIGS

Celia R. Hicks, Geoffrey J. Crawford, Jan J. Constable, Paul D. Dalton, and Traian V. Chirila

C. I. Lions Eye Institute, Nedlands, Western Australia

Methods: We have developed a core-and-skirt PHEMA keratoprosthesis (KPro) and assessed it as a full-thickness implant in the pig. Each KPro was made by sequential polymerization within a mould. The opaque sponge skirt was made first, then the transparent core was formed within the centre, such that the two components were permanently joined by means of an interpenetrating polymer network. The KPro was cryolathed to the required dimensions and curvature. Four animals were used in this study. Surgery was carried out under halothane anaesthesia. KPros were implanted full thickness by means of sutures placed in the sponge skirt, with conjunctival flap coverage. A tarsorrhaphy was created, and opened after I week. The conjunctival flap was opened over the optical core after 2 months.

Results: One animal was euthanased at 16 weeks because of conjunctival injection and partial retraction of the conjunctival flap from the KPro skirt. Although the eye was otherwise quiet with a formed AC and normal IOP, it was felt to represent a risk of leakage or loosening for which the pig's size (100 kg) precluded adequate daily examination. in the other 3 pigs, follow-up ranges from 6–16 weeks. There have been no cases of infection, leakage or extrusion and all eyes remain quiet with normal IOP (tonopen measurements), clear media and absence of afferent defects. However there is a tendency for the conjunctival flap to regrow towards the centre of the optic.

Conclusions: Full-thickness implantation of our KPro has been achieved in the pig. Histological findings confirm that fibrovascular ingrowth into the skirt allows biointegration between host and KPro; the conjunctival flap appears to promote this process. The surface of the optic requires modification to inhibit overgrowth by conjunctiva.

KERATOPROSTHESIS UPDATE

Claes H. Dohlman, Peter A. Netland, Wai-Ching Fung, Stephen Waller, and Hisao Terada

Massachusetts Eye and Ear Infirmary, Boston, Massachusetts

Purpose: To reduce complications, establish prognostic categories and simplify surgical procedures. **Methods:** A prosthesis of PMMA has been implanted in 48 cases during 1990–1995 (and compared with 36 earlier cases). **Results:** Postoperative necrosis has been reduced by temporary coverage with conjunctiva or lid skin, followed by topical enzyme inhibitors. In 44 patients the prosthesis is well retained. Postoperative uveitis has been markedly reduced by aggressive anti-inflammatory treatment. Retroprosthesis membranes are amenable to YAG laser opening. Vision has been much improved in two-thirds of the patients. 29 drainage shunts have also been implanted, minimizing the glaucoma problem. **Conclusion:** We feel that the prognosis for keratoprosthesis is markedly improving.

WARMING TIME AND RATE OF DONOR CULTURE POSITIVITY

Jerry Ford

Objective: To determine if the warming time (interval of time between removal of the donor corneoscleral material from refrigeration and donor trephination) has an impact on the rate of donor culture positivity.

Methods: Aerobic, anaerobic, and fungal cultures were obtained on 129 donor corneas stored in Optisol GS at the time of penetrating keratoplasty. The time the donor cornea was removed from refrigeration and the time of donor cornea trephination and culturing were recorded. The warming times were then divided arbitrarily into two groups: < 60 minutes and > 60 minutes. The rate of culture positivity between the two groups was then compared.

Results: The overall rate of culture positivity for the donor corneoscleral material was 40.31%. The average warming time was 62.46 minutes (range 10 to 205 minutes). For the < 60 minute group (n = 67), the rate of positivity was 40.30%, and for the >60 minute group (n = 62), it was 40.32%. Further breakdown of warming times into groups of < 40 minutes, 40 to 49 minutes, 50 to 59 minutes, etc., revealed no statistical significance between these groups' rate of positivity Propionibacterium, Staph, and Strep species predominated.

Conclusion: The positive culture rate of the donor corneoscleral material in our study was 40.31%. Using the donor material shortly after removal from refrigeration (warming time < 60 minutes) had no effect on the rate of positivity.

Session III

Corneal Stroma and Endothelium

24

AN UPDATE ON CORNEAL HYDRATION CONTROL

Jorge Fischbarg[1] and David M. Maurice[2]

[1]Department of Ophthalmology
[2]Department of Physiology and Cellular Biophysicis
College of Physicians and Surgeons
Columbia University
New York, New York 10032

ABSTRACT

This paper provides an account of recent developments in the understanding of the mechanism of corneal hydration control, particularly as regards the possibility of an active system for its regulation. Emphasis is given to issues that are contentious, such as the role of bicarbonate in the endothelial pump and the significance of water channels in both corneal limiting cell layers.

INTRODUCTION

This article reports developments that have taken place in the understanding of the mechanism that maintains the normal thickness of the cornea. In spite of a considerable amount of research activity, the picture is mixed. There is a convergence of opinion in some areas, but in others the central issues remain unclear, and even the experimental results presented by different workers appear to be contradictory. The basic model of water balance between the cornea and aqueous humor still accepted is the pump-leak hypothesis. In its original formulation[1] the swelling pressure of the stroma was assumed to be balanced by an excess of ions in the aqueous humor. The ionic excess was maintained by the active transfer of one of the major ions Na, K, Cl, or HCO_3, which created a difference in electrical potential across the endothelium that allowed ions of the opposite charge to be in electrochemical equilibrium across the layer. The two principal elements of the hypothesis are the leak of aqueous fluid into the stroma, which is driven by the stromal swelling pressure and controlled by the ionic permeability of the endothelium, and the pump that moves fluid out of the stroma and which is also located in the endothelium.

There has long been a question as to whether the corneal thickness is passively or actively regulated. In the former case, the pump continually operates at its maximum capacity and the swelling pressure and hence the leak increases as the cornea thins until the pump is balanced. In the latter, a sensing mechanism reduces the pump activity as the cornea approaches its physiologically normal value. Recently, receptor systems have been identified in the endothelium that could have a role in regulating the pump activity and these constitute a third element that will receive separate consideration.

Leak

Swelling Pressure. The existence of a swelling pressure in a charged gel resulting from the ionic imbalances it creates, the Donnan effect, has long been established. It was suggested as the cause of stromal swelling by Davson[2] and has been calculated to produce about one half of the swelling pressure by Hedbys, Mishima and Maurice.[3] Hodson and his group[4] more recently have established a good correlation between the magnitude of the swelling pressure and the fixed charge density in the stroma over a wide range of hydration and were able to account for the entire pressure on the basis of Donnan effect. The ratio of the concentrations of Cl between the stromal tissue water and the aqueous humor was different from that found for added lactate or acetate or expected from the Na ratio, and this they attributed to transient Cl binding by an unidentified ligand.[5] Ionic concentrations are determined by the amount of tissue water accessible to the ion, and they neglected to account for the water in the keratocytes, from which most ions other than Cl are excluded. It is not clear how the conclusions would be affected if this was considered, as it has been by previous workers.

The fixed negative charges in the stroma are principally located on its glycosaminoglycan molecules which are divided into keratan/chondroitin sulfates and dermatan sulfate on the basis of small differences in their chemical structure. Scott and Bosworth[6] have shown that these molecules are functionally equivalent; which ones are synthesized in a particular species is determined by the oxygen level in the tissue, and this is a function of its thickness. In accordance with this, enzymatic digestion of the individual glycosaminoglycans reduced the swelling pressure proportionally to their concentration.[7]

Before the pump-leak hypothesis was established, the possibility was raised that the thickness could be controlled by regulating the swelling pressure of the tissue.[2] This possibility has been suggested anew by Doughty[8] who observed large changes in the thickness of isolated corneas when different bicarbonate concentrations were applied to the base epithelial surface of the stroma. It would be very unexpected that a monovalent ion such as bicarbonate should have a direct effect on the swelling and the associated change in pH would be a more probable cause. Previous workers[9] had not noted a change in swelling of the stroma over the pH range 5–8, and the phenomenon deserves further examination.

Endothelial Permeability

The thickness of corneal grafts does not seem to depend on the density of endothelial cells over a wide range.[10] This suggests either that the corneal thickness is actively regulated or that the pump and the leak change in direct proportion to each other when the cell density alters. This might indicate that both occupy the same geometrical site, for example, the cell perimeter or the apical cell membrane.

Direct permeability comparisons by double labeling indicate that small solvents diffuse through the paracellular spaces.[11,12] Their permeabilities are generally in proportion to their free diffusion ratio, suggesting that steric hindrance is the main controlling factor.

Water flow across the endothelium under pressure was shown some time ago[13] to be proportional to its viscosity suggesting that this flow passes through the paracellular spaces as well. If these considerations are valid, they would suggest that the pump is located at the paracellular spaces. However, this is not in accord with the finding of water channels in the endothelial cell membranes noted below.

A suggestion has been made recently[14] that the resistance to water flow is increased by stromal acidosis in the physiological range, which might form the basis for a thickness control mechanism.

Pump

Since earlier investigators[15,16] implicated the bicarbonate ion as the prime mover in the endothelial fluid pump, the transport of this ion has been the focus of attention of recent studies. Clearly the presence of the bicarbonate ion would be essential if this mechanism was correct and this was found to be the case in early studies of the temperature reversal of thickness in swollen isolated cornea. The addition of bicarbonate to the perfusion medium was needed to return the tissue to normal. However, this conclusion was challenged by Doughty and Maurice,[17] who measured fluid transport across endothelium-stroma preparations bathed identically on either surface with large volumes of unstirred solution, the pH of which was controlled with a 50 mM concentration of organic buffer. Maximal pump rates were sustained with solutions that contained from 0 to 50 mM bicarbonate, and this led them to question whether the pump was dependent on this ion.

These experimental results were essentially confirmed by Kuang et al.[18] who found excellent pumping in rabbit endothelium-stroma preparations perfused with solutions that had no added bicarbonate and had its pH stabilized with 20 mM HEPES, or better, 10 mM phosphate. These researchers noted, however, that the pump was blocked by carbonic anhydrase inhibitors, indicating that bicarbonate was fueling the pump. These researchers calculated that enough CO_2 was generated by metabolism in the endothelium to supply the bicarbonate the pump required.

On the other hand, by observing pH changes in cultured bovine endothelial cells and how they were affected by metabolic inhibitors, Bonanno came to the conclusion[19] that the source of bicarbonate was not the cellular metabolism but the low level of CO_2 present in solutions that are in equilibrium with the air.

Riley et al.,[20] however, did not concede that the endothelial pump can function at a bicarbonate level less than 20mM. This conclusion was based on measurements of the stromal thickness of corneas observed under the specular microscope when they are bathed in bicarbonate free medium buffered with 10 mM phosphate. Apart from the nature of the buffer there are a number of differences in the conditions of these experiments and those of Doughty and Maurice: the volume of medium in contact with the surfaces, stirring in the chambers either forced or from small thermal gradients, and in some cases the presence of the epithelium. It is not evident whether one of these or yet another difference is the cause of the discrepancy in the results.

Doughty[8] has further confused the picture by claiming considerable differences in pumping behavior according to whether the bicarbonate concentration was varied on the anterior or posterior face of the endothelium. He insists that these are not the result of osmotic imbalances, and this phenomenon (as well as many other aspects of bicarbonate transport) deserves further study.

Such studies are best pursued in the course of testing an integrated model of endothelial transport. Such a model has been assembled to take account of recent and prior experimental data by Fischbarg.[21] In this, fluid transport is considered to essentially constitute a particular case of cell volume regulatory activity. The cell volume would vary in a cyclical manner as a result from the sequential inflow of osmolytes and water into the endothelial cells across the basolateral membrane, followed by their outflow from the cells via their apical membranes; this would cause a fluid movement directed across the cell layer. The basolateral entry of fluid and osmolytes would depend on the cellular elements that are involved in the regulation of cell volume increase, while the apical outflow would depend on the cellular elements involved in the regulation of cell volume decrease.

Thickness Regulation

The characterization of an active system controlling the thickness of the stroma requires the identification of a set of receptors that can sense the hydration of the tissue, another set of receptors that modulate the activity of the endothelial pump, and a mechanism linking the two sets. No system for sensing hydration changes in the cornea has yet been identified, but a number of receptors which could alter the pump rate have been found. A graphical depiction of some of the possible signaling pathways and endothelial receptors is given in Figs. 1 and 2.

The recent identification of several key membrane receptors in the endothelium has directed attention to the possible cellular processes that may depend on them. A case in point is the adenosine receptor. The work of Walkenbach and colleagues[22,23] described specific adenosine receptors that that stimulate adenyl cyclase in cultured bovine endothelium. That work was confirmed and extended recently by Riley et al.,[24] who described how endothelial adenyl cyclase is stimulated by a G-protein coupled to an adenosine receptor, and how the resulting increase in cAMP increases net endothelial fluid transport. Such results appear consistent with an adenosine-triggered cascade leading to protein kinase A (PKA) activation.

Another possibly important endothelial receptor that has been characterized and located recently is a muscarinic acetylcholine receptor (by Lind and Cavanagh[25]). Its presence is suggestive because there is an abundance of acetylcholine in the cornea, especially in the epithelium, whose purpose has never been satisfactorily explained. An acetylcholine receptor in the endothelium constitutes a potential target, and acetylcholine stimulation of

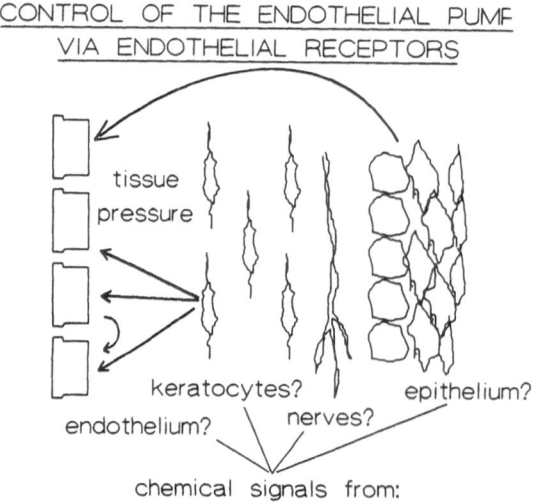

CONTROL OF THE ENDOTHELIAL PUMP
VIA ENDOTHELIAL RECEPTORS

tissue
pressure

keratocytes?   epithelium?
endothelium?   nerves?

chemical signals from:

Figure 1. Several possible origins for chemical signals that might affect endothelial function are depicted. The short arrow signifying signals from other endothelial cells is present because adenosine is a local signal in other systems.

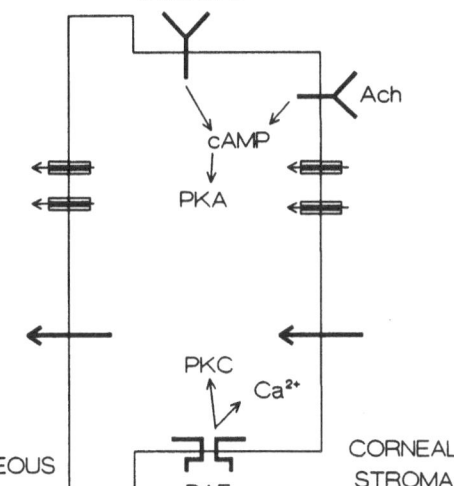

Figure 2. A corneal endothelial cell depicting some receptors discussed in the text, the signaling cascades they may be connected with, and membrane transporters and channels that may be activated by such cascades. Arrows signify transmembrane water movement across water channels.

transendothelial electrical potential difference and fluid transport has been recently observed.[26] In this connection, acetylcholine has been linked to the stimulation of fluid transport in other systems, the best known being in the avian salt gland where acetylcholine stimulates fluid transport via a cyclic cascade.[27]

Next, evidence for an endothelial receptor for platelet activating factor (PAF; a very potent phospholipid activating factor) has been recently reported from our laboratories.[28] PAF inhibits fluid transport in a dose-dependent, saturable manner, and such inhibition is countered by a specific antagonist of PAF, pointing to a PAF receptor. Although there are exceptions, PAF has been generally linked[29] to the stimulation of a cellular signaling cascade that leads to Ca_2+ mobilization and the activation of protein kinase C (PKC).

The fact that PAF leads to inhibition rather than stimulation suggests that the control of fluid transport in the endothelium is a complex matter. It supports the belief that PKA and PKC are separately involved in the modulation of two different stages of the endothelial fluid transport mechanism. For instance, the two cascades may activate or inhibit different sets of cell membrane transporters or channels. The inhibition of fluid transport by PAF does not contradict the presumed stimulatory activity of the PAF receptor and ensuing PKC cascade; rather, the inhibition observed might be due to excessive or uncoordinated stimulation of key elements, leading to eventual depletion of cellular components required for fluid transport.

In addition, the identification and cloning of cell membrane water channel proteins[30] and their location in the corneal endothelium[31–33] supplies a key element. It is becoming evident that not all cells have water channels and their presence denotes that a cell requires rapid water passage through its membrane. For example, in the kidney, it has been observed that water channels are found in all segments of the nephron involved in water passage, but only in those segments.[34] The presence of water channels in corneal endothelium and the further observation that they appear present over the entire surface of the endothelial cell membrane[35] suggest that there is an extensive water flux through these membranes. This would be in accordance with the fluid transfer operated by the endothelial pump taking place through the endothelial cells themselves rather than through the paracellular spaces.

In the recent Fischbarg model referred to above, it is envisaged that PKA activation is connected with the regulatory cell volume increase mechanism and PKC with the regulatory cell volume decrease. For functional reasons, optimal cell behavior would ensue if these two activation/deactivation cascades would operate alternately; in fact, it might well be that such a mechanism can only result in coordinated, vectoral fluid transport if the cascades succeed each other cyclically rather than operate simultaneously.[21]

Finally, it can be noted that not only the corneal endothelium but its epithelium has been observed to be endowed with a rich complement of membrane transporters and channels usually found in fluid secretory epithelia. It is a mystery why this layer is supplied with water channels[36–38] when previous studies have shown that it plays only a minor passive role in the regulation of corneal hydration. This must be added to many other points of contention, noted above, and to others not mentioned, such as the role of lactic acid and unstirred boundary layers, that call out for more intensive exploration.

ACKNOWLEDGMENTS

Supported by USPHS Grants EY00431, EY06178, and Research to Prevent Blindness, Inc. DMM is a Research to Prevent Blindness Senior Scientific Investigator.

REFERENCES

1. D.M. Maurice, The permeability to sodium ions of the living rabbits cornea. *J. Physiol. (London)* 112:367 (1951).
2. H. Davson, Some considerations on the salt content of fresh and old ox cornea. *Brit. J. Ophthalmol* 33:175 (1949).
3. B.O. Hedbys, Mishima,S., and Maurice, D.M., The imbibition pressure of the corneal stroma. *Exp. Eye Res.* 2:99 (1963).
4. S.A. Hodson, and Earlam, R., The incorporation of gel pressure into the irreversible thermodynamic equation of fluid flow in order to explain biological tissue swelling. *J. Theor. Biol.* 163:173 (1993).
5. S.A. Hodson, Hammond, S., Rebello, G., and Al-Omari, Y., Transient chloride binding as a contributory factor to corneal stromal swelling in the ox. *J. Physiol. (London)* 450:89 (1992).
6. J.E. Scott, and Bosworth,T.R., A comparative biochemical and ultrastructural study of proteoglycan-collagen interactions in corneal stroma. *Biochem. J.* 270:491 (1990).
7. D.M. Maurice, and Monroe, F., The role of polysaccharides in corneal swelling. *Invest. Ophthalmol. Vis. Sci. (Suppl., ARVO Abstrs.)* 31:1982 (1990).
8. M.J. Doughty, Evidence for a direct effect of bicarbonate on the rabbit corneal stroma. *Optom. Vis. Sci.* 32:687 (1991).
9. N. Ehlers, Variations in hydration properties of the cornea. *Acta Ophthalmol.* 44:461 (1966).
10. M. Sawa, Araie, M., and Tanishima, T., Permeability of the corneal endothelium to fluorescein - a follow-up of kerastoplasty cases. *Jpn. J. Ophthalmol.* 26:326 (1982).
11. D.M. Maurice, Passive ion fluxes across the corneal endothelium. *Current. Eye. Research* 4:339 (1985).
12. C. Wigham, and Hodson, S.: The movement of sodium across short-circuited rabbit corneal endothelium. *Curr. Eye Res.* 4:1241 (1985).
13. J. Baum, Maurice, D.M., and McCarey, B.E., The active and passive transport of water across the corneal endothelium. *Exp. Eye Res.* 39:335 (1984).
14. N.A. McNamara, Polse, K.A., and Bonanno, J.A., Stromal acidosis modulates corneal swelling. *Invest. Ophthalmol. Vis. Sci.* 35(Mar):846 (1994)-850.
15. S. Hodson, and Miller, F., The bicarbonate ion pump in the endothelium which regulates the hydration of the rabbit cornea. 263:563 (1976).
16. D.S. Hull, Green, K., Boyd, M., and Wynn, H.R., Corneal endothelial bicarbonate transport and the effect of carbonic anhydrase inhibitors on endothelial permeability, fluxes and thickness. *Invest. Ophthalmol. Vis. Sci.* 16:883 (1977).
17. M.J. Doughty, and Maurice, D.M., Bicarbonate sensitivity of rabbit corneal endothelium fluid pump *in vitro. Invest. Ophthalmol. Vis. Sci.* 29:216 (1988)-223.
18. K. Kuang, Xu, M., Koniarek, J.P., and Fischbarg, J., Effects of ambient bicarbonate, phosphate and carbonic anhydrase inhibitors on fluid transport across rabbit corneal endothelium. *Exp. Eye Res.* 50:487 (1990).

19. J.A. Bonanno, Bicarbonate transport under nominally bicarbonate-free conditions in bovine corneal endothelium. *Exp. Eye Res.* 58:415 (1994).

20. M.V. Riley, Winkler, B.S., Czajkowski, C.A., and Peters, M.I., The roles of bicarbonate and CO_2 in transendotheial fluid movement and control of corneal thickness. *Invest. Ophthalmol. Vis. Sci.* 36:103 (1995).

21. J. Fischbarg, A model for corneal endothelial fluid transport based on cyclic changes of cell volume. *Brit. J. Ophthalmol.* 81:1 (1997).

22. R.J. Walkenbach, and LeGrand, R.D., Adenylate cyclase activity in bovine and human corneal endothelium. *Invest. Ophthalmol. Vis. Sci.* 22:120 (1982).

23. R.J. Walkenbach, and Chao, W-Th., Adenosine regulation of cyclic AMP in corneal endothelium. *J. Ocul. Pharmacol.* 1:337 (1985).

24. M.V. Riley, Winkler, B.S., Starnes, C.A., and Peters, M.I., Adenosine promotes regulation of corneal hydration through cyclic adenosine monophosphate. *Invest. Ophthalmol. Vis. Sci.* 37:1 (1996).

25. G.J. Lind, and Cavanagh, H.D., Identification and subcellular distribution of muscarinic acetylcholine receptor-related proteins in rabbit corneal and Chinese hamster ovary cells. *Invest. Ophthalmol. Vis. Sci.* 36:1492 (1995).

26. R. Akiyama, Kuang, K., Koniarek, J.P., et al., Solutions containing mitotic agents: effects on corneal transendothelial electrical potential difference. *Graefe's Archive*, In press (1997).

27. M.R. Hokin, and Hokin, L.E., The formation and continuous turnover of a fraction of phosphatidic acid on stimulation of NaCl secretion by acetylcholine in the salt gland. *J. Gen. Physiol.* 50:793 (1967).

28. Z. Zhu, Kuang, K., Kang, F., et al., Platelet activating factor inhibits fluid transport by corneal endothelium. *Invest. Ophthalmol. Vis. Sci.* 37:1899 (1996).

29. W. Chao, Liu, H., Hanahan, D. J., and Olson, M.S., Platelet-activating factor-stimulated protein tyrosine phosphorylation and eicosanoid synthesis in rat Kupffer cells. *J. Biol. Chem.* 267:6725 (1992).

30. G.M. Preston, Carroll, W.B., Guggino, W.B., and Agre, P., Appearance of water channels in Xenopus oocytes expressing red cell CHIP28 protein. *Science* 256:385 (1992).

31. S. Nielsen, Smith, B.L., Christensen, E.I., and Agre, P., Distribution of the aquaporin CHIP in secretory and resorptive epithelia and capillary endothelia. *Proc. Natl. Acad. Sci.* 90:7275 (1993)

32. H. Hasegawa, Zhang, R., Dohrman, A., and Verkman, A.S., Tissue-specific expression of mRNA encoding rat kidney water channel CHIP28k by *in situ* hybridization. *Am. J. Physiol. Cell Physiol.* 33:264, C237 (1993).

33. Echevarria, M., Kuang, K., Iserovich, P., et al.: Cultured bovine corneal endothelial cells express CHJP28 water channels. *Am. J. Physiol., Cell. Biol.* 34:265, C1349 (1993).

34. S. Nielsen, Smith, B.L., Christensen, E.I., et al., CHIP28 water channels are localized in constitutively water-permeable segments of the nephron. *J. Cell Biol.* 120:371 (1993).

35. J. Li, Kuang, K., Nielsen, S., and Fischbarg, J., Molecular identification and localization of the water channel aquaporin 1 in cultured bovine corneal endothelial cells. In preparation (1997).

36. Raina, S., Preston, G.M., Guggino, W.P., and Agre, P., Molecular cloning and characterization of an aquaporin cDNA from salivary, lacrimal and respiratory tissues. *J. Biol. Chem.* 270:1908 (1995).

37. T. Horwich, Ybarra, C., Ford, P., et al., VMRNA from frog corneal epithelium increases water permeability in Xenopus oocytes. *Invest. Ophthalmol. Vis. Sci.* 36:2772 (1995).

38. F. Kang, Kuang, K., Li, J., and Fischbarg, J., Cultured bovine corneal epithelial cells express a functional water channel. *Invest. Ophthalmol. Vis. Sci (Suppl., ARVO Abstrs.)* 37:S1105 (1996).

25

CORNEAL VISCOELASTICITY SPECTRA AS A RESULT OF DYNAMIC MECHANICAL ANALYSIS

Fritz Soergel,[1] Sylvia Muecke,[2] and Wolfgang Pechhold[1,2]

[1]Institute for Dynamic Materials Testing
Science Park
University of Ulm
Germany
[2]Department of Applied Physics
University of Ulm
Germany

ABSTRACT

In this study, dynamic mechanical analysis (DMA) was utilized for the measurement of the viscoelastic properties of human cornea. The complex shear compliance J (reciprocal shear modulus G), Young's compliance D (reciprocal Young's modulus E), and the "indenter compliance" C were recorded as a function of frequency (spectrum), of time, of hydration and of temperature.

The viscoelasticity spectra revealed three different relaxation processes within the frequency range of twelve decades (0.1 mHz to 100 MHz). The parameters of these relaxation processes (relaxation frequency, relaxation strength, width-parameter) are affected by hydration, temperature (thermal softening, thermal coagulation, freezing), post mortem-interval, and pathological changes. Comparing Young's modulus $E_\perp$ (perpendicular to the corneal surface) and its correlated shear modulus G, we found $E_\perp \approx 100G$ (at 1 Hz). This reflects the cornea's structural anisotropy and the experience that a cornea is easy to shear but hard to compress.

The spectra of indenter compliance $C(f)$ were similar to the shear compliance spectra $J(f)$, i.e., indentation (like induced by an applanation tonometer) causes a shear deformation rather than a compression of the cornea.

Newly developed DMA set-ups for non-destructive characterization of eye bank eyes and for diagnosing non-physiological and pathological changes of the cornea in vivo, are in the experimental stage now.

INTRODUCTION

Regular cornea has a well-defined tissue architecture. To obtain transparency, the collagen fibrils have a nearly uniform diameter of 30.8 nm and (within a lamellar sheet) they are in a quasihexagonal arrangement with an average periodicity of 61.9 nm.[1] The fibrils are positioned by the ground substance's proteoglycan molecules, whose polysaccharide side chains imbibe water and build up the corneal swelling pressure. In addition to intralamellar cohesion, there is also interlamellar cohesion[2] connecting the lamellae, which are stacked with thin and flattened keratocytes between them.

Each disorder in the tissue's molecular structure and each surgical procedure coincides with a change in the tissue's biomechanical properties.[3–5] Corneal biomechanics is of interest, for example, for questions related to myopia, keratoconus, refractive surgery, corneal grafting, and corneal storage. Therefore, a novel measuring method that yields both a qualitative and a quantitative biomechanical characterization of the cornea would be advantageous.

Unfortunately, stationary measuring methods like viscosimetry and static measuring methods like stress strain measurements[6,7] yield only a static view of the biomechanical properties. Beyond that, dynamic mechanical analysis (DMA) yields information about how the viscoelastic properties depend upon frequency (viscoelasticity spectrum). Viscoelasticity spectra reflect molecular relaxation processes within the tissue and reveal their dependence on hydration, temperature, storage time, storage conditions, pathological changes, and other parameters.

MATERIALS AND METHODS

Materials

Explanted eye bank eyes, discarded for transplantation because of endothelial defects or small scars in the optic center of the cornea, were received from The Netherlands Ophthalmic Research Institute (NORI), Amsterdam and from the University Eye Clinics, Berlin and Tübingen. The eyes were stored cooled in a moist chamber. Preparing an eye for a measurement, it was brought to room temperature in its moist chamber.

For measurements with an **intact globe**, an eye was placed in an eye holder and the intraocular pressure was kept constant with sodium chloride solution (infusion solution 0,9 %). Those parts of the eye shell which were not covered by the measuring set-up, were prevented from drying by covering them with a wetted piece of wipes.

For measurements with **corneal buttons**, epithelium and endothelium were removed from the cornea. Cylindrical samples with a diameter of 3 mm were prepared and attached to the sample holder with our "two-step bonding method": In its first step, Bowman's and Descemet's layer were covered with a thin (0.03 mm-0.10 mm) solid state coating of tissue adhesive.[8] In the second step, six cylindrical buttons lying on a ring (7 mm in diameter, drawn with a pen) were punched out with a 3mm trepan. They were attached to the sample holder (with their marks aligned parallel) using only a very small drop of cyanoacrylate adhesive[9] (for further details cf.[10,11]).

Methods

DMA was made accessible for measurements of the viscoeleastic properties of the eye shell at the University of Ulm by Hanus and Pechhold in close cooperation with oph-

Table 1. Various DMA measuring modes at lower, medium and higher frequencies

Set-up (frequency range)	Viscoelasticity spectrometer (0.1 mHz–100 Hz)	Torsional/bending resonator (10 Hz–100 kHz)	Double resonator device (1 kHz)	Shear quartz resonator set-up (1 mHz–100 MHz)
Shear compliance	$J(f, d, T, pmi, \mu)$ of corneal buttons	$J(f, t, pmi)$ of intact globes	$J(d)$ of corneal buttons	$J(f, t, T, pmi)$ of intact globes
Young's compliance	$D(f, d)$ of corneal buttons			
Indenter compliance	$C(f, t)$ of intact globes	relaxation after flattening monitored in $J(t)$ of intact globes		relaxation after flattening monitored in $J(t)$ of intact globes

mHz = 10^{-3}Hz, kHz = 10^{3}Hz, MHz = 10^{6}Hz
Frequency f; measuring time t; hydration (sample thickness d); temperature T; postmortem-interval pmi; myopia μ.

thalmologists in 1985.[5] Special DMA set-ups and preparation methods were developed for measurements of human corneal tissue.[10,11]

Subjecting a sample to deformations with very small amplitudes (0.001 μm-100 μm), DMA provides the sample's complex shear compliance $J = J'$-i $\cdot$ J'' (i.e., the reciprocal value of its complex shear modulus G), Young's compliance $D = D'$-i $\cdot$ D'' (reciprocal Young's modulus E) or the so called "indenter compliance" $C = C'$-i $\cdot$ C''.

The real part of a viscoelasticity spectrum (index: prime) is called storage compliance or storage modulus, resp. This is a measure of the energy stored and recovered in the sample. Higher compliance values indicate softer samples, lower ones indicate harder samples. The imaginary part (index: double-prime) is called loss compliance or loss modulus. This is a measure of the energy dissipated or lost as heat.[12] A relative maximum in the imaginary part indicates a maximum in damping within a relaxation process (see below).

Table 1 gives a summary of the measurements performed *in vitro*. In order to make such a wide frequency range accessible (0.1 mHz-100 MHz, i.e., 12 decades), different set-ups had to be used. Only those set-ups that allow investigation of an intact globe can, in principle, be used *in vivo*. This was the motivation for the development of a new torsional/bending resonator set-up that allows measurement of intact globes at frequencies between 100 Hz and 100 kHz.

Besides developing *in vivo* usable set-ups, there was interest in gaining grounding in corneal biomechanics. The dependence of the viscoelastic data on frequency f was investigated measuring time t, hydration (given as sample thickness d), temperature T (this includes thermal softening, thermal coagulation and freezing), storage time (given as *post mortem*-interval *pmi*), and pathological changes (one pair of myopic eyes could be studied).

Viscoelasticity Spectrometer. The viscoelasticity spectrometer[13] can be equipped with various sample holders, depending on the sample's viscoelastic properties and depending on the desired deformation mode. Fig. 1 shows three sample holders developed for cornea measurements.[10] The spectrometer's oscillator generated a sinusoidal oscillation with frequency f, causing an up and down movement of the upper part of the sample holder, which is connected to the oscillator by a rigid rod. The samples were mounted between the sample holder's upper part and its lower part; they were deformed periodically

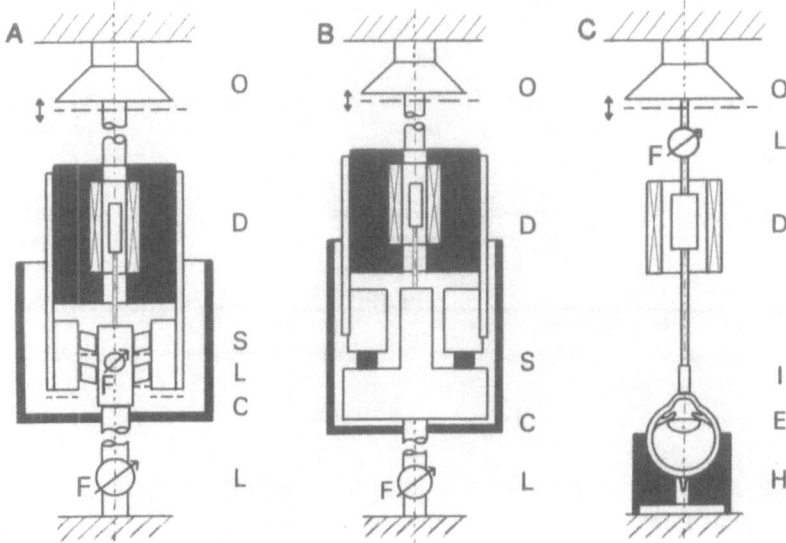

Figure 1. The viscoelasticity spectrometer can be equipped with different sample holders (schematic sketches). **A:** Double sandwich-sample holder (for shear compliance measurements), sample thickness adjustable. **B:** Sample holder for uniaxial deformation (Young's compliance), sample thickness adjustable. **C:** Arrangement for indenter measurements (indenter compliance). Abbreviations: O, oscillator (0.1 mHz-00 Hz); D, displacement tansducer: S, sample; L, load cell; C, container; I, Indenter; E, eye; H, eye holder.

with frequency f. The precision-displacement transducer (inductive) and the high-resolution load cell (strain gage) recorded periodic signals of displacement $x(t)$ and force $F(t)$, resp. From the amplitudes of x and F, and from the phase shift between these both signals, the sample's complex compliance (or complex modulus) was calculated, taking into account constants of the apparatus and of the sample's geometry.[14,10,11] The measurement uncertainty was the sum of the absolute and the relative uncertainty. The absolute uncertainty amounted to less than ± 25%, i.e., about ± *0.1* decades, covering the uncertainty in determining the constants of the apparatus and of the sample's geometry. The relative uncertainty was ascertained by measuring at f = 1 Hz as both the first and last measuring value of one spectrum.

In Fig. 1A there is a further load cell (strain gage) between the both sample gaps, allowing to measure the swelling pressure of the samples. The width of the sample gaps is adjustable, providing a corneal thickness d between 0.2 mm and 1.0 mm. The container surrounding the sample holder, is filled with sodium chloride solution (infusion solution 0.9 %) which is thermostated to a temperature of 29°C. Manufacturing the container from acrylic glass, allows to control the samples and their adhesive bonds during the measurements.

Resonator Set-Ups. To measure at medium and at higher frequencies, resonator-methods have been developed by Pechhold and co-workers.[15] When a resonator is unloaded, its resonance curve is narrow (low damping) with a high amplitude peak. Loading the resonator with a sample shifts the resonance frequency to lower values and makes the half-width of the resonance curve wider. From this decrease in frequency and increase in damping, the complex compliance (and modulus) of the sample can be calculated.

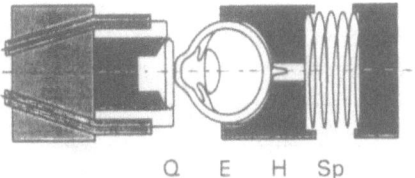

Q   E   H   Sp

Figure 2. Shear quartz resonator set-up. Abbreviations: Q, quartz resonator; E, eye; H, eye holder; Sp, Spring.

A laboratory device (Fig. 2) has been developed in which enucleated eyes with their corneal epithelium removed are positioned in an eye holder. The dried corneal surface is then mechanically coupled to the quartz resonator disc, by pressing it on with a weak spring. Measurements are carried out with this **shear quartz resonator set-up** at the resonance frequency of the quartz resonator and at its (uneven) higher harmonics.[15]

To measure the shear compliance of corneal buttons in the kHz-range, another setup, the **double resonator device,** consisting of two (identical) dumbbell shaped torsional resonators made of aluminum was used. The resonators were arranged one above the other with their front surfaces face to face, thus providing a disc-like sample gap between them.[10,14] The corneal buttons were placed within the horizontal sample gap and attached to the resonators with the two-step bonding method, described above. Then the sample gap was filled with sodium chloride solution and the double resonator device was thermostated to 35°C. Analogous to coupled pendula, the double resonator device revealed two resonance frequencies when a resonance curve was recorded. When the resonators oscillated in their parallel resonance mode (f_p), the samples were just taken along without being sheared, whereas they were sheared in the antiparallel resonance (f_a). The sample caused an increased damping D_a in the antiparallel resonance, compared to the damping of the parallel resonance D_p. The compliance of the sample (or its modulus) was calculated from $\Delta f = f_a - f_p$ and Symbol"D55D $= D_a$ Symbol"-55 D_p. (For details cf.[14,10])

As previously published, these measurements revealed that at medium frequencies, J' and J'' were affected significantly by several parameters.[10,11] Furthermore the medium relaxation process was located around 100 Hz (see f_{max} in case n = 2 in Tables 2, 3). The parameters determining this process were affected by biomechanical and biochemical changes within the corneal tissue. Our results indicated that the medium frequency range was very promising for a non-destructive characterization of eye bank eyes and for clinical studies to diagnose non-physiological and pathological changes of corneal tissue *in vivo*. A **torsional resonator** and a **bending resonator** have been developed by Muecke and Pechhold and are currently in the experimental stage.

Table 2. Parameters of the three relaxation processes at lower (n = 1), medium (n = 2) and higher (n = 3) frequencies, from Fig. 4

	$\lg(\Delta J/\text{Pa}^{-1})$			$\lg(f_{max}/\text{Hz})$			b_{cc}		
d/mm	n = 1	n = 2	n = 3	n = 1	n = 2	n = 3	n = 1	n = 2	n = 3
0.68	-3.37	-4.29	-5.67	-3.90	2.00	7.50	0.40	0.52	1.00
0.52	-3.66	-4.61	-5.77	-3.80	2.10	7.40	0.40	0.55	1.00
0.44	-3.90	-4.98	-5.87	-3.70	2.25	7.30	0.40	0.58	1.00
0.37	-4.35	-5.43	-5.97	-3.30	2.35	7.20	0.40	0.62	1.00

Relaxation strength ΔJ (logarithmic); relaxation frequency f_{max} (logarithmic); width-parameter b_{cc}.

Table 3. Parameters of the three relaxation processes at lower (n = 1), medium (n = 2) and higher (n = 3) frequencies, from Fig. 6

	$\lg(\Delta J/\mathrm{Pa}^{-1})$			$\lg(f_{max}/\mathrm{Hz})$			b_{cc}		
d/mm	n = 1	n = 2	n= 3	n = 1	n = 2	n = 3	n = 1	n = 2	n = 3
1.00	−2.49	−3.13	−4.75	−4.16	1.15	6.98	0.35	0.60	0.91
0.49	−2.60	−3.87	−5.05	−4.00	1.70	6.85	0.49	0.60	0.91
0.31	−3.75	−5.08	−5.83	−3.55	2.54	6.75	0.43	0.60	0.91
0.20	−5.00	−6.71	−6.30	−2.96	2.98	6.65	0.35	0.60	0.91

Relaxation strength ΔJ (logarithmic); relaxation frequency f_{max} (logarithmic); width-parameter b_{cc}.

RESULTS

Hydration

The hydration of corneal buttons was varied by changing the corneal thickness d (Figs. 3–6, 10–12), where d equals sample gap width minus adhesive thickness. Fig. 3 shows a double logarithmic plot of swelling curves $J(d)$, measured with the double resonator device at 1.2 kHz. As a check for reproducibility, the plot contains measuring points of two different corneas, which were prepared and measured independently of one another.

A small but systematic difference was found between the compliance values measured when increasing d (yielding higher values) and those measured when decreasing d (yielding lower values). This difference amounted to about 0.1 decades for *pmi*s of 30 h-90 h and to about 0.3 decades for *pmi*s of 350 h-700 h.[10] This means that the tissue needed a certain time to reach its swelling equilibrium (cf. also[16]), and that this time increased with increasing *pmi*. Therefore, Figs. 3–5 contain only values measured when d was increased.

Changing the corneal thickness from 0.2 mm to 1.0 mm (i.e., 5-fold) increases the shear compliance at 1.2 kHz by 1.8 decades, i.e., about 60-fold. An even higher increase was obtained for lower frequencies: for the same increase (0.2 mm-1.0 mm), Fig. 6 reveals an increase in the shear compliance by a factor of 600 at a frequency of 1 Hz. Such a significant effect has never been described for any technical polymer.[17]

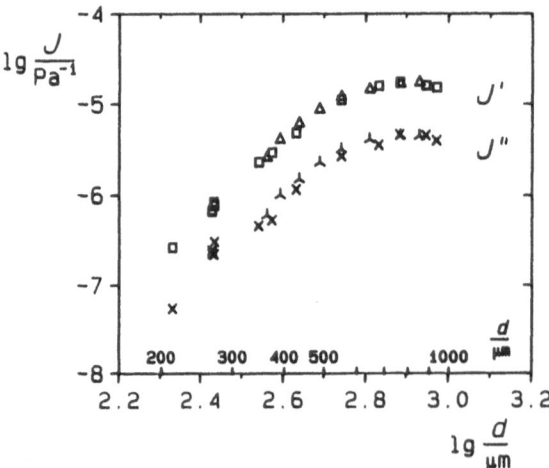

Figure 3. Swelling curves of two different pairs of corneas, measured with the double resonator device (f = 1.2 kHz; T = 35°C; *pmi* = 30 h-200 h; deformation amplitudes ≤1 μm, age unknown) Cornea 1 (△,Y), Cornea 2 (□, x).

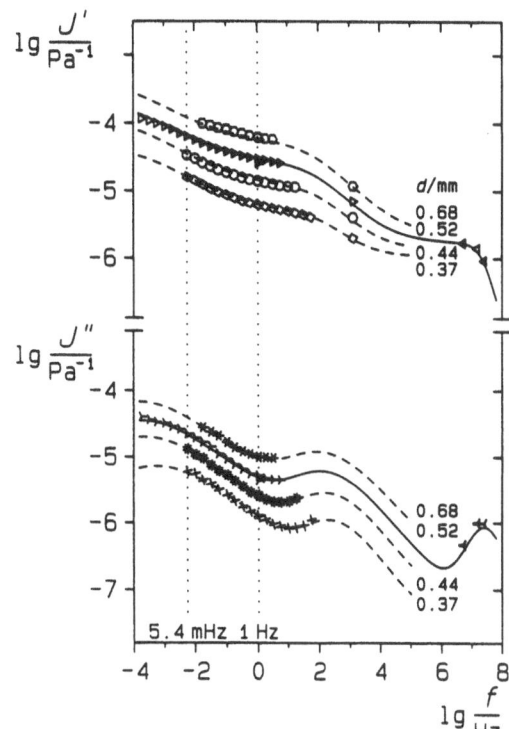

Figure 4. Shear compliance spectra measured at sample thicknesses d = 0.37 mm–0.68 mm (*pmi* = 49 h-77 h; deformation amplitudes 0.5 µm-50 µm, age 81 years).

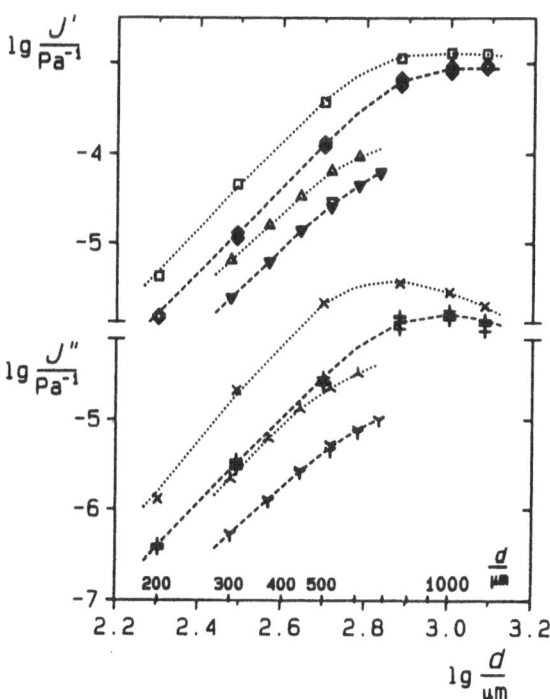

Figure 5. Swelling curves of two corneas with different *pmis*. This measuring values were selected from Fig. 4 ($\triangle$,**Y** and ∇,**Y**) as well as from Fig. 6 ($\square$, x and $\diamondsuit$,+) at 5.4 mHz and at 1 Hz, resp.

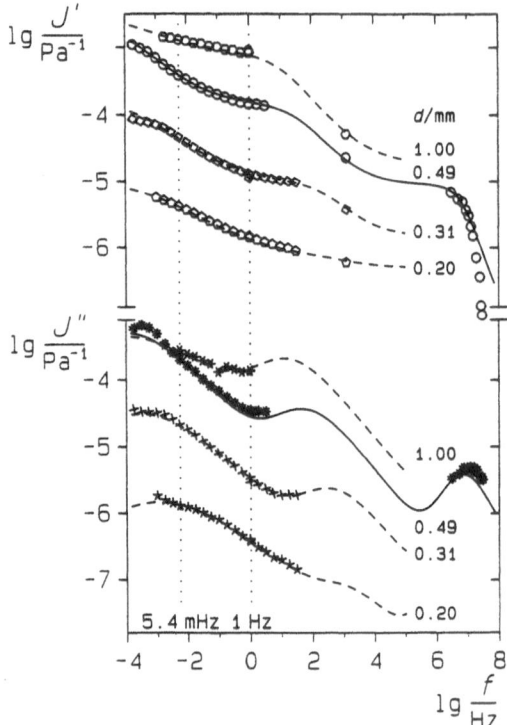

Figure 6. Shear compliance spectra measured at sample thicknesses d = 0.20 mm–1.00 mm (*pmi* = 698 h–718 h; age 70 years).

Hence, DMA was revealed to be very sensitive for all changes in corneal tissue that affect corneal hydration.

Relaxation Processes

Fig. 4 shows measurements of a cornea recorded with two different set-ups. First, the shear quartz resonator set-up was used to measure in the MHz range (intact globe). Then corneal buttons were prepared and measured from lower up to medium frequencies with the viscoelasticity spectrometer. As the samples could not be removed from the sample holder without damage, the shear compliance values at 1.2 kHz had to be taken from measurements of another cornea. In order to transfer kHz values from Fig. 3 into Fig. 4, the better comparable measurement was selected (squares in Fig. 3) and necessary corrections (*pmi*, sample thickness) were made, yielding a decrease of 0.1 decades for each J'-value. The J'' values were not transferred, because changes in the *pmi* are affecting the difference $\lg J'' - \lg J' = \lg(J''/J') = \lg(\tan \delta)$, i.e., the logarithm of the loss angle $\tan \delta$ (cf. Fig. 7).

When fitting a theoretical curve to the measuring points further conditions have to be observed, $J'(f)$ is a steadily decreasing function. In addition, J' and J'' are correlated according to Kramers-Kronig-relation, implying that a step in the real part is correlated with a local maximum in the imaginary part, thus indicating a relaxation processes. The theoretical curve is given by the following equation.[18]

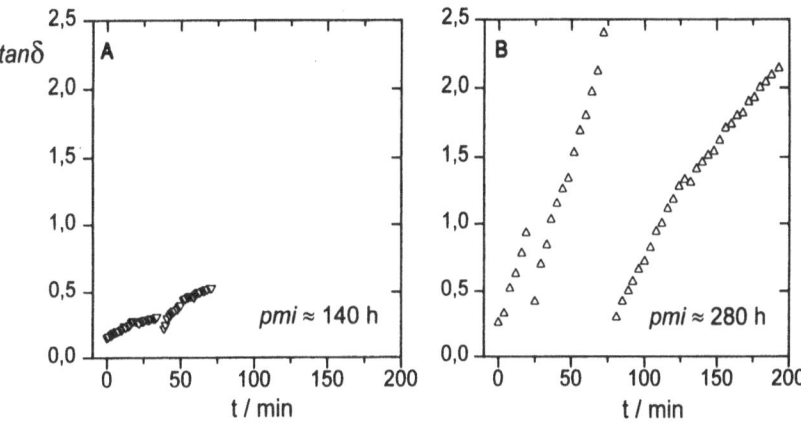

Figure 7. Loss angle *tan* δ as a function of measuring time *t* for different *pmis*. (**A**) *pmi* ≈140 hours; (**B**) *pmi* ≈280 hours (*f* = 5 MHz).

$$J(\omega) = J'_{\infty} + \sum_{n=1}^{3} \frac{\Delta J_n}{1 + (i \cdot \omega \cdot \tau_n)^{b_{CC,n}}}$$

Usually several relaxation processes overlap in the spectrum, although they can be separated by fitting the curve given by this equation to the measuring points. This kind of computer analysis yields three characterizing values for each relaxation process: relaxation frequency f_{max}, relaxation strength ΔJ and width-parameter b_{CC}. The index CC is indicating a relaxation time distribution according to Cole-Cole.[18] The average relaxation time τ corresponds to the frequency $f_{max} = 1/(2 \cdot \pi \cdot \tau)$, which is due to a relative maximum in $J''(f)$. For J'_{∞} (i.e., J' in case of f → ∞) a value which different polymers have in common, was used: $J'_{\infty} = 0.8 \cdot 10^{-9}$ Pa^{-1}.[17,18]

As the corneal architecture exhibits different structural levels with a high degree of organization, different relaxation times or - in the shear compliance spectrum - different relaxation frequencies should be detectable. The viscoelasticity spectra of corneal tissue revealed three relaxation processes within the accessible frequency range (Tables 2, 3). The frequencies f_{max} as well as the strengthens ΔJ of the relaxation processes are affected by changes of corneal hydration at lower (n = 1) as well as at medium frequencies (n = 2).

Post Mortem-Interval

After the enucleation, the globes were stored cold. The biochemical changes during storage, caused two significantly different effects for shorter *pmis* and for longer *pmis*.

For shorter *pmis*, an increase from *pmi* ≈ 60 h to *pmi* ≈80 h decreased the shear compliance values (i.e., stiffening) only at medium frequencies by a factor of 0.7.[10,11]

In order to demonstrate the effect for longer *pmis*, the swelling curves of a cornea with *pmi* ≈70 h and a cornea with *pmi* ≈700 h are plotted in Fig. 5, using the 5.4 mHz and 1 Hz measuring points from Figs. 4 and 6, resp. The shear compliance values of the cornea with the longer *pmi* are higher (i.e., softer) than the values for shorter *pmis* (harder) - for lower frequencies as well as for medium frequencies.

The measuring points of Fig. 6 were obtained as described above for Fig. 4 – with the difference that the kHz values were increased by 0.49 decades, according to the longer *pmi* of about 700 h. The parameters of the relaxation processes of Fig. 6 are listed in Table 3.

The manner in which autolytical decomposition during storage affects the shear compliance values gives hints for the discussion of which structural level might be related to which relaxation process. The short-term effect measured at medium frequencies was probably due to the decomposition of proteoglycans, whereas the long-term increase within a broader frequency range was probably due to the decomposition of collagen fibrils.

The relaxation process at higher frequencies (n = 3) showed the typical behavior of a glass relaxation process in polymers.[18] At frequencies above the glass relaxation none of the structural elements were able to follow the deformation.

The penetration depth of a transversal shear wave depended on measuring frequency f, the cornea's shear compliance J, and corneal density $\rho = 1076$ kg/m^3.[19] The shear waves were subjected to an exponential decrease within the sample, requiring about 15 periods of wavelength to be damped to negligible amplitude.

$$\lambda = \frac{1}{f} \cdot \sqrt{\frac{1}{J \cdot \rho}}$$

Figure 6 illustrates an explanation of why, at the highest frequencies, the measuring points of J' have lower values than the theoretical curve has: At 1 MHz the shear wave penetrates some hundred microns of the anterior stroma, where Bowman's layer, which is harder than the stroma, plays a negligible role. At 30 MHz, however, mainly Bowman's layer is measured.

In order to measure the *pmi*-dependence of the shear compliance of intact globes, the quartz resonator set-up (Fig. 2) was used. When coupling the quartz disc to the cornea, the central cornea was flattened. Its shear compliance revealed the tissue's response to flattening as a function of measuring time t. A time-dependent curve $J(t)$ occurred; this curve can be reproduced, but is not fully understood yet. Instead of plotting J' and J'' separately, their ratio $J''/J' = tan\,\delta$ (loss angle) can be plotted (Fig. 7). The slope of the loss angle curve $tan\,\delta\,(t)$ became steeper with increasing *pmi*. Improvement of this method allow its use as a non-destructive cornea control for eye bank eyes.

Temperature

The shear compliance of human cornea has been measured within the temperature range from -20°C to 80°C. The temperature was increased step by step, on the one hand recording shear compliance spectra $J(f)$ at fixed temperatures and, on the other hand, measuring the shear compliance as a function of temperature $J(T)$. In addition shear compliance spectra were taken before freezing, after freezing once and after freezing twice (Fig. 9).

As we have previously published,[10,11] the temperature curve $J(T)$ revealed thermal softening between 0°C and 48°C with increasing temperature. Looking at the 48°C spectrum, a first effect of thermal coagulation was found in $J(f)$ as an irreversible decrease (0.8-fold) in the relaxation strength of the lower frequency relaxation (corneal stiffening). Increasing the temperature further on, led to spectra with lower compliance values. $J(f)$ as

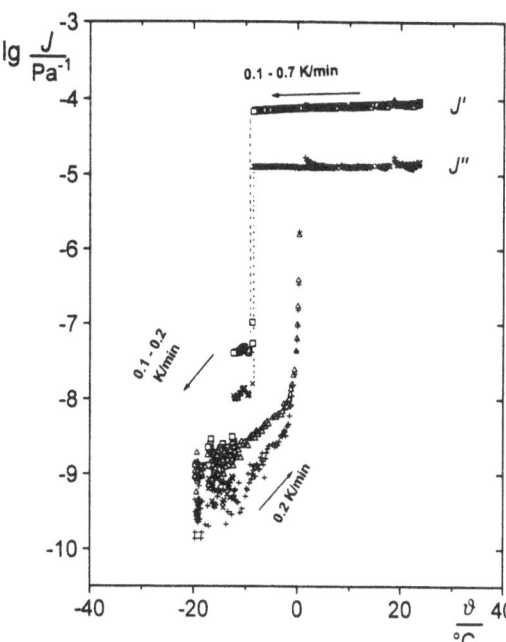

Figure 8. Temperature curves of cooling (□, x) and heating (△, ▲) of corneal tissue (f = 3 Hz; d = 0.62 mm; pmi = 610 h-747 h, age 69 years).

well as $J(T)$ showed their compliance minimum at 64°C. So far, $J'(f)$ has been decreased by 1 decade (factor 0.1) at lower frequencies and by 0.7 decades (factor 0.2) at medium frequencies. A further rise in temperature lead to thermal softening but failed to reproduce the shear compliance spectra recorded before the onset of thermal coagulation. This reflects the irreversibility of thermal coagulation[10,11]

The changes in the shear compliance during cooling and heating were recorded at a constant measuring frequency (3 Hz) as a function of temperature (Fig. 8). At the beginning of the cooling run, the container was filled with infusion solution. Then the solution

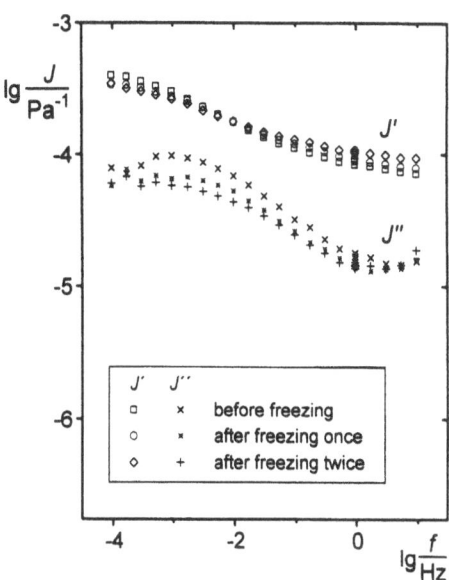

Figure 9. Shear compliance spectra of corneal tissue before freezing (□, x), after freezing once (o, S) and after freezing twice (◇, +) (T = 25°C; d = 0.62 mm; pmi = 610 h-747 h; age 69 years).

was removed and freezing was carried out in nitrogen gas atmosphere. Corneal tissue shows supercooling, i.e., a temperature difference between cooling and heating (here: 10°C). Cornea freezes in two steps, the first decrease (3 decades) probably related to the freezing of free water and the second decrease (1.5 decades) probably related to the freezing of bound water.

Figure 9 compares three shear compliance spectra $J(f)$ of the same cornea as in Fig. 8. These spectra were measured before freezing, after freezing once and after freezing twice. Each freezing caused a change in the shear compliance spectrum: The height of the step in $J'(f)$ was reduced and (according to Kramers-Kronig-relation) the height of the maximum in $J''(f)$ was decreased at the same time. Hence, DMA can be used to improve methods for corneal preservation.

Pathological Changes

The viscoleasticity spectra were believed to be affected by pathological changes. Usually the ophthalmologic results (e.g., refraction analysis) were not known from eye bank eyes. There were only two cases for which the ophthalmologic results were known: An emmetropic eye and a myopic eye (-3 D). Their spectra $J(f)$ were measured at physiological sample thickness $d = 0.5$ mm. The spectrum was higher for the myopic cornea than for the emmetropic one, by a factor of 7 at lower frequencies and by a factor of 4 at higher frequencies.[10,11] In Fig. 10 the swelling curves $J(d)$ of the emmetropic cornea and of the myopic cornea were plotted (measuring frequency 1 Hz) for different sample thicknesses. For medium sample thicknesses, the slope of the swelling curve of the myopic cornea is steeper than of the emmetropic one. For higher sample thicknesses the myopic shear compliance is higher than the emmetropic one. This first measurement should be cross-checked by further measurements with myopic eyes, in order to ascertain the method's significance concerning myopia and probably other pathological changes (e.g., keratoconus).

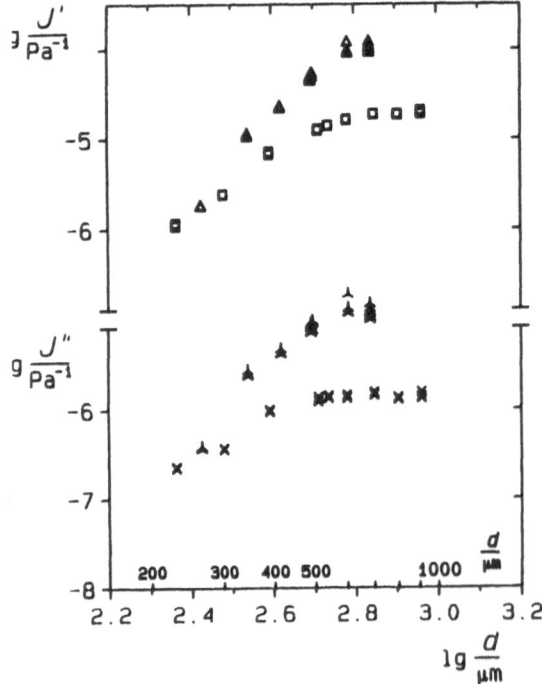

Figure 10. Swelling curve of cornea from an emmetropic eye ($\square$, x; $\geq$ *pmi* 53 h; age 36 years) and a myopic eye ($\triangle$; $\blacktriangle$; $\geq$ *pmi* 70 h; age 41 years; myopia -3 D) ($f = 1$ Hz; $T = 29$°C).

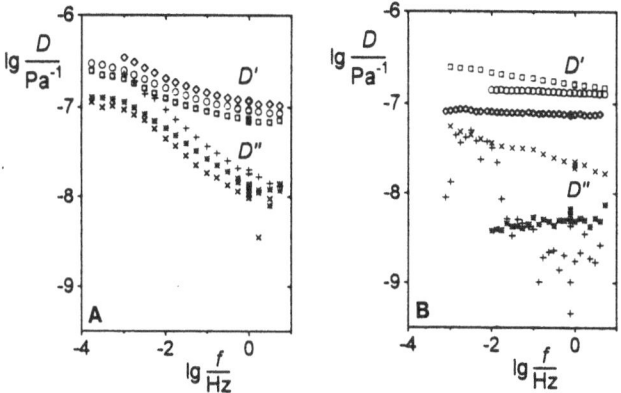

Figure 11. Spectra of Young's compliance $D\perp$ for different corneal thicknesses d: **(A)** 0,40 mm ($\square$, x), 0,41 mm (o, S), 0,44 mm ($\diamond$, +); **(B)** 0,53 mm ($\square$, x), 0,64 mm (o, $*$), 0,71 mm ($\diamond$, +) (T = 29°C; *pmi* = 113 h-206 h; age 78 years).

Young's Compliance D

Fig. 1B shows, how cylindrical buttons of cornea were arranged in the viscoelasticity spectrometer's sample holder, in order to perform uniaxial deformation (perpendicular to the corneal surface). After having adjusted a certain sample thickness d, the dynamic deformation was performed with an amplitude of 0.2 μm-1.2 μm (Remark: This small amplitude was the reason why the J' values were scattering) (Figs. 11, 12).

For sample thicknesses d smaller than the physiological value of 0.5 mm, the Young's compliance spectra $D(f)$ revealed an obvious low frequency relaxation process (Fig. 11A), while the spectra $D(f)$ for higher thicknesses were less structured (Fig. 11B). This finding corresponded to the maximum in the swelling curve $D(d)$ (Fig 12), which was found for a thickness of 0.5 mm when using a measuring frequency of 1 Hz.

The physiological values of corneal parameters were distinguished by the thickness of the cornea, as well as by its swelling pressure: Increasing the dynamic deformation amplitude beyond the amplitude described above, revealed the spectra $D(f)$ to be consistent as long as the "dynamic pressure amplitude" (see below) was lower than the cornea's

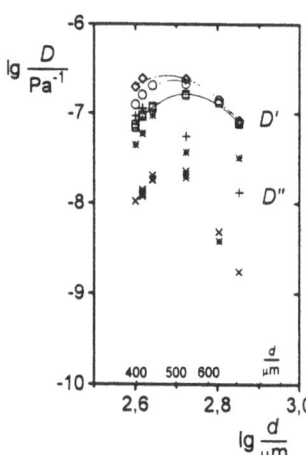

Figure 12. Swelling curves of Young's compliance $D\perp$. This measuring values were selected from Fig. 10 for different frequencies: 1 mHz ($\diamond$, +), 10 mHz (o, $*$), and 1 Hz ($\square$, x).

physiological swelling pressure, whereas the spectra became amplitude-dependent for amplitudes higher than the cornea's physiological swelling pressure (i.e. 60 mm Hg = 8.0 kPa.[16,21]). The "dynamic pressure amplitude" was calculated by dividing the force amplitude by the total sample area.[10]

$$E_\perp \approx 100G$$

Because of the corneal anisotropy, it was expected $E = 3\ G$, which is valid for isotropic substances, would not to be valid for the cornea. In order to compare Young's modulus $E_\perp$ (perpendicular to the corneal surface) and its correlated shear modulus G, measuring curves (Fig. 4, 11) with short *pmi*s were evaluated at physiological sample thickness and at a frequency of 1 Hz. We found $E_\perp \approx 100G$, which agrees with the findings of Pinsky and co-workers.[22] This reflects the cornea's structural anisotropy and the experience that a cornea is easy to shear but hard to compress.

Indenter Compliance *C*

Neither the sample holder for pure shear deformation (Fig. 1A) nor the sample holder for uniaxial deformation (Fig. 1B) can be used for *in vivo* measurements of the viscoelastic properties of cornea. Therefore, the upper part of the so called "penetrometer"[13] was combined with an eye holder (Fig. 1C). As usual, the intraocular pressure was maintained by infusion solution.

Analogous to an applanation tonometer, the central cornea was flattened by the entire front surface of the cylindrical indenter. Then a dynamic deformation was performed at room temperature with deformation amplitudes of 1 μm-40μm. One can assume, that the measuring effect on the one hand is due to a bending deformation along the edge of the indenter's front surface, and on the other hand to the deformation of an elastic shell which is filled with a liquid.

At first, the indenter compliance spectra $C(f)$ were decreasing with increasing measuring time t because the cornea was drying during the comparatively long lasting lower frequency measurements. This could be reduced when covering the cornea outside the indenter surface with a wetted piece of wipes. The recording of the spectra plotted in Fig. 13, took nearly 25 hours. The spectra $C(f)$ are given in arbitrary units (a.u.). The measuring values around $f = 30$ Hz could not be used, as there was an interference with a bending vibration of the set-up at that frequency. Nevertheless this first indenter compliance spectra $C(f)$ seem to be promising for measurements of a viscoelastic curve with an advanced indenter set-up.

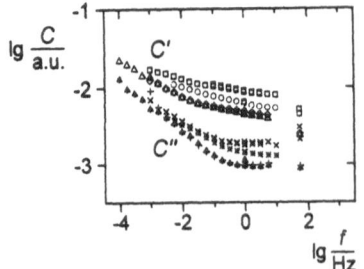

Figure 13. Spectra of the indenter compliance *C* for different periods of time 0 min-150 min (□, x); 150 min–290 min (o, *); 290 min-445 min (◇, +); 475 min-1490 min (△, ↑) (*T* = 20°C; *pmi* = 343 h–369 h, age 78 years).

DISCUSSION

It could be shown *in vitro* that this spectroscopic method (DMA), which is using periodical deformation with extremely small amplitudes, responds very sensitive to changes in corneal tissue. The viscoelasticity spectra revealed three different relaxation processes within the frequency range of twelve decades (0.1 mHz-100 MHz). The parameters of these relaxation processes (relaxation frequency, relaxation strength and width-parameter) were affected in different ways by hydration, temperature (thermal softening, thermal coagulation, freezing), *post mortem*-interval, and pathological changes.

The **lower frequency relaxation process** was affected by hydration, by (beginning) coagulation, by freezing, by long-term *pmi* and by myopia. Hence, it would be a very promising frequency range for *in situ* and *in vivo* measurements. However, the lower the measuring frequency selected, the longer the measuring time. Therefore, the limiting factor for measurements at lower frequencies would be the patient's tolerance (only several minutes).

The **relaxation process at higher frequencies** allowed detection of long-term *pmis* in the *tan δ (t)* curves, but was less sensitive to other corneal changes than the relaxation processes at lower and medium frequencies. The shear quartz resonator method could be used for measurements *in vivo*, but the corneal epithelium had to be removed beforehand. Therefore, measurements in the higher frequency range might be an appropriate means for a non-destructive test for corneas (with their epithelium removed) before grafting. In this frequency range, the penetration depth could be selected by the choice of the frequency. An advanced mathematical analysis would allow to measure depth selective.

The **relaxation process at medium frequencies** was the most sensitive process in case of a short-term increase of the *pmi;* it was also affected by hydration, coagulation, freezing, and myopia. Therefore, this relaxation process is very promising for *in situ* and *in vivo* measurements. The newly- developed DMA set-ups for this frequency range are in the experimental stage now. With such set-ups DMA might become a non-destructive dynamic measuring method, capable of characterizing eye bank eyes and of diagnosing non-physiological and pathological changes of the cornea *in vivo*.

ACKNOWLEDGMENTS

We gratefully acknowledge the support given by The Netherlands Ophthalmic Research Institute (NORI), Amsterdam and the University Eye Clinics, Berlin and Tübingen. Acknowledgments are also due to the Deutsche Forschungsgemeinschaft, who partly supported this investigations (grant Se534/1–1).

REFERENCES

1. D.W. Leonard, Meek, K.M., and Huang, Y., X-ray diffraction from the corneal stroma: Implications for light scattering. *Proceedings of the World Congress on the Cornea IV, Orlando, USA, 1996.*
2. D.M. Maurice, and Monroe, F., Cohesive strength of corneal lamellae. *Exp. Eye Res.* 50:59 (1990).
3. M. Reim, Chirurgische Anatomie, Physiologie, Biochemie sowie Fragen der Jnlay-Technik. *Ophthalmologe* 89:109 (1992).
4. J. Wollensak and Buddecke, E., Biochemical studies on human corneal proteoglycans - a comparison of normal and keratoconic eyes. *Graefe's Arch. Clin. Exp. Ophthalmol.* 228: 517 (1990).
5. J. Wollensak, Ihme, A., and Seiler, T., Neue Befunde bei Keratokonus. *Fortschr. Ophthalmol.* 84:28 (1987).

6. D.M. Maurice, Mechanics of the cornea. In, *The Cornea: Transactions of the World Congress on the Cornea III, Washington, D.C., USA, 1987,* H.D. Cavanagh, ed., Raven Press, New York (1988).

7. D.A. Hoeltzel, Altman, P., Buzard K., and Choe, K-I., Strip extensiometry for comparison of the mechanical response of bovine, rabbit and human corneas. *J. Biomech. Eng.* 114:202 (1992).

8. Braun-Dexon, *Histoacryl blau Gewebekleber* (Data sheet B. 02.05.92/2) B. Braun-Dexon GmbH, D-34286 Spangenberg, Germany (1992).

9. UHU, UHU sekunden alleskleber gel (Data sheet 04/94–2000). UHU GmbH, d-77813 Bühl, Germany (1994).

10. F. Soergel, Biomechanische Charakterisierung der menschlichen Augenhornhaut mit dynamisch-mechanischer Spektroskopie. PhD Thesis, University of Ulm, D-89069 Ulm (1994).

11. F. Soergel, Jean, B., Seiler, T., et al., Dynamic mechanical spectroscopy of the cornea for measurements of its viscoelaastic properties in vitro. *German J. Ophthalmol.* 4:151 (1995).

12. J.D. Ferry, *Viscoelastic properties of polymers,* Wiley & Sons, New York (1961).

13. IDM. Dynamic mechanical wide range spectrometer - principle of measurement and applications (data sheet 5/95) Institute for Dynamic Materials Testing, University of Ulm, D-89081, Ulm, Germany, 1995).

14. K-H. Hanus, Pechhold, W., Soergel, F., et al., Phase behavior and elastic properties of a slightly crosslinked liquid crystalline main-chain polymer. *Colloid Polym. Sci.* 268:222 (1990).

15. W. Pechhold, and Schwarzenberger, P., Phasediagram, superstructure and properties of poly(diethylsiloxane). In *Frontiers of High Pressure Research,* H.D. Hochheimer and Etters, R.D., eds., Plenum Press, New York (1991).

16. D.M. Maurice, The cornea and sclera. In, *The Eye. Vegetative Physiology and Biochemistry (Vol. 1b).* H. Davson, ed., Academic Press, Orlando (1984).

17. M. Boehm, Grassl, O., Pechhold, W., and Soden, W. von, Dynamic shear compliance of swollen networks and its dependence on crosslinking density. *Progr. Colloid Polym. Sci.* 75:62 (1987).

18. W Pechhold, Grassl, O., and doen W. von, Dynamic shear compliance of polymer melts and networks in dependence of crosslinking density. *Colloid Polym. Sci.,* 268:1089 (1990).

19. F.A. Duck, ed., *Physical Properties of Tissue: A Comprehensive Reference Book.* Academic Press, London (1990).

20. J. Chang, Soedeberg, P.G., Denham, D., et al., Quantification of temperature-induced corneal shrinkage. *Invest. Ophthalmol. Vis. Sci.,* 37:S65 (1996).

21. T. Seiler, Laserchirurgie der Kornea. Habilitationsschrift (Postdoctoral thesis required for qualification as a university lecturer), FU Berlin 91987).

22. S.S. Chang, Pinsky, P.M., and Datye, D.V., Inverse estimation of the in vivo mechanical properties of the cornea modeled as a transversely isotropic material. *Invest. Ophthalmol. Vis. Sci.* 36:S38 (1995).

26

MORPHOLOGIC AND FUNCTIONAL EVALUATION OF THE HUMAN CORNEAL ENDOTHELIUM

William M. Bourne

Department of Ophthalmology
Mayo Clinic and Mayo Foundation
Rochester, Minnesota

ABSTRACT

The corneal endothelium maintains corneal deturgescence, apparently by a pump-leak mechanism in which the cellular monolayer constitutes a leaky barrier to fluid movement into the cornea and actively pumps ions out of the cornea. The clinical status of these functions can be estimated by measuring the endothelial permeability to fluorescein (proportional to the leak) and the rate of stromal deswelling after hypoxia-induced edema (proportional to the pump minus the leak). The test is conducted by measuring stromal and aqueous humor fluorescence and corneal thickness at intervals over a 7-hour period after first instilling topical fluorescein and inserting an aphakic soft contact lens for 2 hours. Morphologic evaluation is obtained from endothelial photographs by measuring the cell density, cell size distribution, and percentage of hexagonal cells. Functional abnormalities often reflect morphologic abnormalities. The rate of stromal deswelling is decreased in the eyes of individuals with diabetes mellitus, Fuchs' dystrophy, penetrating keratoplasty, and contact lens wear. Morphologic abnormalities have been demonstrated in the corneal endothelial cells of patients with all these conditions.

INTRODUCTION

Morphologic evaluation of corneal endothelial cells *in vivo* is obtained by endothelial photomicroscopy with the clinical specular microscope.[1,2] Functional evaluation requires additional tests. The corneal endothelium functions to maintain corneal deturgescence by a pump-leak mechanism in which the cellular monolayer constitutes a leaky barrier to fluid movement into the cornea and actively pumps ions out of the cornea.[3] To estimate the status of these functions, two clinical tests have been devised. First, the barrier function is estimated by measurement of the permeability of the cellular mono-

Advances in Corneal Research, edited by Lass
Plenum Press, New York, 1997

layer to fluorescein.[4-6] Second, the combined barrier and pump mechanism in nonsteady-state is estimated by measuring the rate of deswelling of the corneal stroma from edema induced by the wearing of a hypoxic contact lens.[7] These two tests can be administered simultaneously in a combined measurement of corneal hydration control.[8] At the present time, these three procedures to measure endothelial morphology, permeability, and deswelling provide the most complete evaluation of the status of the corneal endothelial cells of an individual.

MORPHOLOGIC EVALUATION

Because the corneal endothelium is a monolayer of flat cells, the cellular outlines can be viewed and photographed with a specular microscope.[9] We use this instrument to record images of the central endothelial cells. The individual areas of at least 50 cells[10] are measured by digitizing their apices. With appropriate calibration of magnification, the mean cell area (and its reciprocal, the cell density), coefficient of variation (standard deviation/mean), and percentage of hexagonal cells can then be calculated.

ENDOTHELIAL PERMEABILITY

Passive fluid movement across the endothelial monolayer is governed by its permeability to ions and small molecules. To estimate this endothelial permeability, we measure the permeability to the small molecule, fluorescein was measured. After its deposition in the corneal stroma, fluorescein diffuses across the endothelium into the aqueous humor, which is constantly renewed. The gradual disappearance of fluorescein from the eye obeys first-order pharmacokinetics as modeled by Jones and Maurice and others.[4-6] The concentration of fluorescein in the cornea and anterior chamber can be measured noninvasively with a fluorophotometer.[11] Data from repeated measurements over several hours allow the calculation of the endothelial permeability to fluorescein and the aqueous humor flow rate. If the corneal thickness changes substantially during the measurement period, then the values obtained must be corrected for the focal diamond effect of the fluorophotometer and for the change in fluorescein binding.[8]

When endothelial permeability is measured simultaneously with the deswelling rate (see below), measurements must be made at least 50 minutes after removal of the contact lens. Before this time, stromal pH is decreased,[12] which decreases the fluorescence efficiency of fluorescein[13] and thus causes an underestimate of fluorescein concentration.

CORNEAL DESWELLING

As a test of corneal hydration control, Polse et al.,[7] devised a procedure to measure the ability of the endothelial cells to restore a swollen cornea to its normal thickness. Approximately 10% stromal swelling is induced by two hours of aphakic soft contact lens wear with the eyes closed. Corneal thickness is then measured at frequent intervals for several hours, and the data fit to a first-order exponential deswelling curve with the rate of deswelling expressed as the percent recovery per hour (PRPH). Although it is not known if corneal deswelling is a first-order process, the data seem to fit the exponential model reasonably well. The asymptote of the curve is the open eye steady state (OESS) thickness

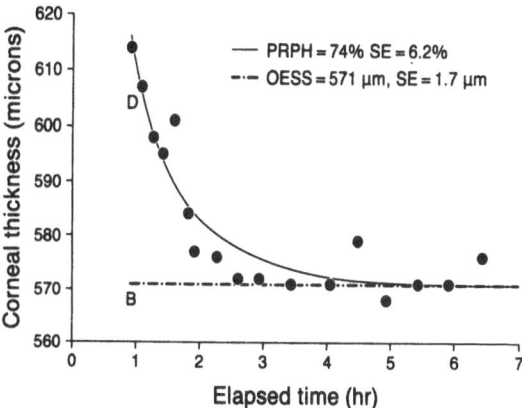

Figure 1. Typical deswelling curve for normal subject with calcalated results for percent recovery per hour (PRPH) and open eye steady state (OESS) thickness (SE = standard error). The deswelling rate constant (D) and OESS thickness (13) are estimated from The following relationship (8): $qt = B + (q_0 - B)e^{-Dt}$, where qt = corneal thickness at time t, q_0 = corneal thickness at time 0 (calculated), and t = time in minutes.

(Figure 1). The pH in the corneal stroma is decreased for up to 50 minutes after contact lens removal.[12] Because the rate of deswelling appears to be retarded during this period,[12] thickness data from the first 50 minutes after contact lens removal cannot be used to measure the deswelling rate. The deswelling rate in normal individuals decreases substantially with age[7,8] so that age-matched control subjects are necessary.

An early study indicated that stromal pH returned to normal within 30 minutes after contact lens wear.[14] For this reason, in the first two studies performed with the combined permeability and deswelling tests,[8,15] we used both thickness and fluorescence data starting 30 minutes after contact lens removal. The functional values published for these studies, therefore, are incorrect because subsequent data indicate that stromal pH does not return to normal for 50 minutes after contact lens wear.[12] Fortunately, the conclusions of these two studies[8,15] were unchanged after the results were recalculated omitting the measurements from the first 50 minutes after contact lens removal (Table 1). The results of correlations were also unchanged except that endothelial cell density and PRPH were no longer significantly correlated in the long-term corneal transplants (r=0.47, p=0. 13).

Table 1. Corneal function in diabetes mellitus and in corneal transplants – corrected values

	20 Patients with diabetes		21 Controls			12 Long-term corneal transplants		
	Mean	S.D.	Mean	S.D.	P*	Mean	S.D.	P**
Percent recovery per hour,	67.9	13.3	63.9	7.5	0.23	46.4	15.4	<0.001
PRPH (%/hr)	(64.0)[1]	(11.7)	(62.5)	(7.6)	(0.63)	(43.9)	(11.7)	(<.001)
Endothelial permeability,	3.49	0.80	3.94	0.67	0.05	2.73	1.14	0.001
AM (x 10^{-4} c/min)	(3.55)	(0.83)	(4.14)	(0.68)	(0.02)	(2.79)	(1.34)	(0.001)
Endothelial permeability,	3.98	0.56	4.27	0.50	0.09	3.37	0.97	0.001
PM (x 10^{-4} c/min)	(3.85)	(0.60)	(4.03)	(0.53)	(0.31)	(3.33)	(0.99)	(0.01)

*20 Patients with diabetes vs. 21 controls (two-tailed Student t-test for means).

**12 corneal transplants vs. 21 controls (two-tailed Student t-test for means).

[1]Values in parentheses are published results(8,15) calculated from sequential measurements starting 30 minutes after removal of the contact lens. The corrected data in the table were calculated after eliminating measurements made during the initial 50 minutes after contact lens removal.

RESULTS OF CLINICAL EVALUATIONS

Morphologic and functional evaluations of human corneal endotheliurn have been conducted to date in four conditions: diabetes mellitus, penetrating keratoplasty, Fuchs' dystrophy, and contact lens wear.

The corneal deswelling rate in insulin-dependent diabetes mellitus has been measured in three investigations,[8,16,17] two of which found it to be significantly decreased.[16,17] The endothelial permeability to fluorescein was measured simultaneously in two of these studies[8,17] and found to be normal, confirming earlier work. [18,19] If the endothelial permeability (and thus the barrier function or leak) is normal, and the deswelling rate is low, a plausible explanation is that the pumping action of the endothelial cells is decreased. This possibility is consistent with the known inhibition by polyols of Na/K ATP-ase activity.[20]

In penetrating corneal transplants, the corneal deswelling rate has been found to be markedly decreased.[15] The endothelial permeability to fluorescein., measured simultaneously, was also decreased, confirming previous results.[21] If the endothelial barrier is intact and increased (decreased leak), and the deswelling rate remains very low, a possible explanation is a markedly decreased endothelial pump rate in these long-term corneal transplants.

Corneas with Fuchs' dystrophy also have decreased deswelling rates, as measured by Mandell, et al.[21,22] The permeability to fluorescein in Fuchs' dystrophy was found to be normal by Wilson, et al.[23] As in diabetes mellitus, a plausible explanation for decreased deswelling with normal baffler function is a decrease in the pumping action of the endothelial cells.

Corneal deswelling in contact lens wearers has been measured by Nieuwendaal, et al.,[24] who found the PRPH in 21 long-term contact lens wearers to be significantly less than that in 18 control subjects of similar age. Carlson et al.[25] found normal endothelial permeability in long-term contact lens wearers.

In all four conditions in which measurements have been attempted, therefore, a decreased deswelling rate has been found in the presence of normal or increased barrier function (no increase in leak). A possible explanation for this finding is that the pumping action of the endothelial cells is decreased in each of these conditions. According to the pump-leak hypothesis,[3] one would expect an increase in the steady-state corneal thickness if the pump is decreased and the leak is not. Indeed, the OESS thickness was increased in diabetes mellitus,[8,16, 17,19,26] long-term penetrating keratoplasty,[15] and Fuchs' dystrophy.[22,23] Although the thickness in contact lens wear was not different from controls in the studies by Holden et al.,[27] Carlson et al.,[25] and Nieuwendaal et al.[24] the former investigation found that the thickness was significantly decreased 7 days after cessation of lens wear. If chronic contact lens wear causes corneal thinning, then the thickness recorded in these studies may represent an increase over the OESS thickness for the lens-wearing cornea, consistent with a decreased endothelial pump.

In all four of these conditions with abnormal corneal endothelial function, morphologic endothelial abnormalities have also been found. The endothelial cell density is decreased in penetrating keratoplasty[15,28] and Fuchs' dystrophy.[23] Polymegethism (increased coefficient of variation of cell area) and pleomorphism (decreased hexagonal cells) are present in diabetes mellitus[17–19] and contact lens wear.[24,25,27]

SUMMARY

Specular microscopy, fluorophotometry, and pachometry can be used to measure the morphologic and functional status of the corneal endothelium in living humans. In the four conditions studied to date in which abnormal endothelial function has been found, morphologic abnormalities have also been present.

ACKNOWLEDGMENTS

This study was supported in part by research grant Ey 02037 from the National Institutes of Health, an unrestricted grant from Research to Prevent Blindness, Inc.; New York NY, and the Mayo Foundation; Rochester, MN. Dr. Bourne is a Research to Prevent Blindness Senior Scientific Investigator.

REFERENCES

1. R.A. Laing, Sandstrom, M.M., Berrospi, A.R., and Leibowitz, H.M., Changes in the corneal endothelium as a function of age. *Exp. Eye Res.* 22:587 (1976).
2. W.M. Bourne, and Kaufman, H.E., Specular microscopy of human corneal endothelium *in vivo. Am. J. Ophthalmol.* 81:319 (1976).
3. D.M. Maurice, The cornea and sclera. In, *The Eye, Vol. IB, Third Edition*, H. Davson, ed., Academic Press, New York (1984).
4. R.F. Jones, and D.M. Maurice, New methods of measuring the rate of aqueous flow in man with fluorescein. *Exp. Eye Res.* 5:208 (1966).
5. K.H. Carlson, Bourne, W.M., McLaren, J.W., and Brubaker, R.F., Variations in human corneal endothelial cell morphology and permeability to fluorescein with age. *Exp. Eye Res.* 47:27 (1988).
6. R.F. Brubaker, Maurice, D.M., and McLaren, J.W., Fluorometry of the anterior segment. In, *Noninvasive Diagnostic Techniques in Ophthalmology*, B.R. Masters, ed., Springer-Verlag, New York (1990).
7. K.A. Polse, Mandell, R., Vastine, D., et al., Age differences in corenal hydration control. *Invest. Ophthalmol. Vis. Sci.* 30:392 (1989).
8. B.C. Weston, Bourne, W.M., Polse, K.A., and Hodge, D.O., Corneal hydration control in diabetes mellitus. *Invest. Ophthalmol. Vis. Sci.* 36:586 (1995).
9. D.M. Maurice, Cellular membrane activity in the corneal endothelium of the intact eye. *Experientia* 24:1094 (1968).
10. W.M. Bourne, Morphologic and functional evaluation of the endothelium of transplanted human cornea. *Trans. Am. Ophthalmol. Soc.* 81:403 (1983).
11. J.W. McLaren, and R.F. Brubaker, Two-dimensional scanning ocular fluorophotometer. *Invest. Ophthalmol. Vis. Sci* 26:144 (1985).
12. S.R. Cohen, Polse, K.A., Brand, R.J., and Bonanno, J.A., The association between pH level and corneal recovery from induced edema. *Current Eye Res.* 14:349 (1995).
13. J.V. Thomas, Brimijoin, M.R., Neault, T.R., and Brubaker, R.F., The fluorescent indicator pyranine is suitable for measuring stromal and cameral pH *in vivo. Exp. Eye Res.* 50:241 (1990).
14. J.A. Bonanno, and Polse, K.A., Corneal acidosis during contact lens wear: effects of hypoxia and CO_2. *Invest. Ophthalmol. Vis. Sci* 28:1514 (1987).
15. W.M. Bourne, Functional measurements on the enlarged endothelial cells of corneal transplants. *Trans. Am. Ophthalmol. Soc.*, 93:66 (1995).
16. P. Herse, and Hooker, B., Corneal edema recovery dynamics in diabetes: is the alloxan-induced diabetic rabbit a useful model? *Invest. Ophthalmol. Vis. Sci.* 35:310 (1994).
17. N.A. McNamara, Brand, R.J., Bourne, W.M., et al., Hyperglycemic effects on corneal function. *ARVO Abstract. Invest. Ophthalmol. Vis. Sci.* 37:S315 (1996).
18. G.M. Keoleian, Pach, J.M., Hodge, D.O., et al., Structural and functional studies of the corneal endothelium in diabetes mellitus. *Am. J. Ophthalmol.* 113:64 (1992)
19. L-I. Larson, Bourne, W.M., Pach, J.M., and Brubaker, R.F., Structure and function of the corneal endothelium in diabetes mellitus type 1 and type 2. *Arch. Ophthalmol.* 114:9 (1996).
20. D.R. Whikehart, The inhibition of sodium, potassium-stimulated ATPase and corneal swelling: the role played by polyols. *J. Am. Optom. Assoc.*, 66:331 (1995).
21. W.M. Bourne, and Brubaker, R.F., Decreased endothelial permeability in transplanted corneas. *Am. J. Ophthalmol.* 96:362, (1983).

22. R.B. Mandell, Polse, K.A., Brand, R.J., et al., Corneal hydration control in Fuchs' dystrophy. *Invest. Ophthalmol. Vis. Sci.* 30:845 (1989).

23. S.E. Wilson, Bourne, W.M., O'Brien, P.C., and Brubaker, R.F., Endothelial function and aqueous humor flow rate in patients with Fuchs' dystrophy. *Am. J. Ophthalmol.* 106:270 (1988).

24. C.P. Nieuwendaal, Odenthal, M.T.P., Kok, J.H.C., et al., Morphology and function of the corneal endothelium after long-term contact lens wear. *Invest. Ophthalmol. Vis. Sci.* 35:3071 (1994).

25. K.H. Carlson, Bourne, W.M., Brubaker, R.F., Effect of long-term contact lens wear on corneal endothelial cell morphology and function. *Invest. Ophthalmol. Vis. Sci.* 29:185, 1988.

26. N. Busted, Olsen, T., and Schmitz, O., Clinical observations on the corneal thickness and the corneal endothelium in diabetes mellitus. *Br. J. Ophthalmol.* 65:687 (1981).

27. B.A. Holden, Sweeney, D. F., Vannas, A., et al., Effects of long-term extended contact lens wear on the human cornea. *Invest. Ophthalmol. Vis. Sci.* 26:1489 (1985).

28. W.M. Bourne, Hodge, D.O., and Nelson, L.R., Corneal endothelium five years after transplantation. *Am. J. Ophthalmol.* 118:185 (1994).

SESSION III: CORNEAL STROMA AND ENDOTHELIUM

Abstracts of Other Conference Presentations and Posters

MACROMOLECULAR MORPHOGENESIS OF CORNEAL STROMA

C. Cintron

Schepens Eye Research Institute/Harvard Medical School, Boston, MA

Purpose: The function, development and pathobiology of the corneal stroma are intimately associated with and dependent on the biochemical components of this tissue, their macromolecular interactions, and the regulation of corneal matrix morphogenesis. Since the major function of the corneal stroma is to serve as a strong and transparent structure for vision, a long-term objective is to determine the molecular basis of corneal transparency and its loss during wound healing. **Methods:** To this end, analyses of the physical, molecular and biochemical structure of normal developing and healing adult cornea have been conducted to elucidate the critical components necessary for transparency. **Results:** The temporal and spatial organization of cell migration, differentiation, and extracellular matrix deposition are significantly different in fetal and adult healing cornea. The increased average spacing between collagen fibrils is believed to be responsible for the loss of transparency in scar tissue. The interfibrillar region is composed of several macromolecules including type VI collagen type XII collagen, and the proteoglycans decorin and lumican. We have discovered that type VI collagen is associated with some of these components and with a novel extracellular matrix protein, excellin. **Conclusion:** This has led us to conclude that Type VI collagen plays an important role in maintaining proper fibril spacing during corneal morphogenesis by interacting with fibrillar collagens, proteoglycans and other collagens in the interfibrillar space. The highly evolutionarily conserved amino add sequence homology of excellin, its ubiquitous distribution in connective tissues, and the temporal expression of excellin message suggest that this protein plays a role in normal and pathological morphogenesis of extracellular matrix.

(Supported by NIH Grant EY01199.)

CORNEAL KERATOCYTE ACTIVATION AND MYOFIBROBLAST TRANSDIFFERENTIATION IN STROMAL WOUND HEALING

James V. Jester, Patricia A. Barry-Lane, W. Matthew Petroll, Jiying Huang, Partha Roy, Penny Marr, and H.P. Dwight Cavanaugh

University of Texas, Southwestern Medical Center, Dallas, Texas

Purpose: Myofibroblasts, which have been identified in a variety of corneal wounds, are muscle-like cells which express smooth muscle specific actin (α-SM). Recent studies suggest that myofibroblasts play a critical role in matrix deposition and organization following corneal injury and are responsible for incisional wound contraction following radial keratotomy (RK) and the development of corneal haze following excimer photorefractive keratectomy (PRK). Both of these effects tend to negate the desired refractive effect and thus represent the major obstacle to effective and predictable refractive surgical procedures. Identifying the cellular and molecular events involved in myofibroblast transdifferentiation is fundamental to our understanding of the corneal wound healing process. **Methods:** Studies have been performed using tissues from primates, cats, and rabbits under *in vivo, in situ,* and *in vitro* conditions. Various types of injuries including radial keratotomy, lamellar keratectomy, and full thickness corneal lacerations have been evaluated by *in vivo* confocal microscopy (CM) as well as conventional and laser confocal microscopic techniques. **Results and Conclusions:** The normal corneal stroma is populated by broad, flat cells that are inter-connected through the cornea by branching processes containing functional gap injunctions (connexin 43). Injury leads to activation of keratocytes, synthesis of fibronectin, expression of $\alpha5\beta1$ integrin and migration of activated and functionally inter-connected keratocytes. Once inside the wound, activated keratocytes express α-SM actin, and develop a contractile apparatus composed of intracellular microfilament bundles containing α-SM actin, myosin and α-actinin, membrane receptor, $\alpha5\beta1$ integrin, and extracellular fibronectin fibrils. Three-dimensional and temporal studies indicate that myofibroblasts establish a "shoestring-like" structure that contracts the wound by tightening the interwoven network of cells. Recent studies indicate that the keratocyte to myofibroblast transdifferentiation process is mediated, in part, by transforming growth factor-β (TGF$_\beta$): TGF$_\beta$ is a potent chemotactic factor for keratocytes; induces the expression α-SM actin, fibronectin, and $\alpha5\beta1$ integrin; and neutralizing antibodies to TGF$_\beta$ block development of corneal fibrosis. The effect of TGFb appears to be mediated by its initial effects on extracellular matrix and formation of focal contacts and tyrosine phosphorylation of pp125[FAK] and p130 leading downstream to cell proliferation, α-SM actin expression and myofibroblast formation. Further study of this process may lead to potential therapeutic interventions to control myofibroblast-mediated corneal fibrosis and wound contraction. (Supported by NEI EY07348 and a Senior Scientist Award and unrestricted grant from Research to Prevent Blindness, Inc.)

RECEPTOR-MEDIATED REGULATION OF THE ENDOTHELIAL FLUID PUMP

Michael V. Riley

Eye Research Institute, Oakland University, Rochester, MI

The transparency of the cornea is determined largely by the degree of hydration of the stromal matrix. This, in turn, is governed by the balance between the rate of movement of fluid across the endothelium into the stroma (leak) and its rate of removal (pump) by the active transport mechanism of this cell layer. Corneal thickness increases when leak increases or pump activity decreases and corneal deturgescence ensues when leak is reduced or pump activity is stimulated.

Adenosine is known to prolong the maintenance of normal hydration of isolated corneas during perfusion and to promote the deturgescence of swollen corneas. Our studies show that this effect is due to a signalling system within the endothelial cells that stimulates the fluid pump. Adenosine binds to a specific receptor on the plasma membrane and, via the action of G-proteins, increases the production of cyclic adenosine monophosphate (cAMP) in the cells. The effect of adenosine is abolished in the presence of ouabain or absence of bicarbonate ions and is impaired in the absence of chloride ions, suggesting that the net increase in fluid extrusion from the tissue is the result of cAMP causing either an alteration of the transmembrane fluxes of these ions or an increase in the activity of the primary driving force for fluid movement, the Na^+-K^+ ATPase.

PHYSIOLOGICAL AND PHARMACOLOGICAL MECHANISMS OF CORNEAL ENDOTHELIAL POLYMEGATHISM

Henry F. Edelhauser

Department of Ophthalmology, Emory University, Atlanta, GA

Corneal endothelial cell polymegathism can occur from age, intraocular surgery, inflammation, diabetes and contact lens wear. Age-related and surgery-induced endothelial cell changes result from a loss of cells associated with endothelial remodeling. Diabetic and contact lens-induced polymegathism results from a physiological and/or pharmacological change induced within the endothelial cells or by affecting the metabolic pump. The purpose of this presentation is to compare the mechanism of corneal endothelial cell changes that occur in diabetics and contact lens wearers in order to focus on the etiology of the observed polymegathism.

Diabetic endothelial cells contain increased levels of polyolys, which can lead to progressive osmotic stress and changes in endothelial cell volume regulation. The aldose reductase pathway is important in regulating polyoly levels and the observed polymegathism. In contrast, contact lens induced polymegathism may be related to the metabolism of arachidonic acid in the corneal epithelium and the production of 12(R)HETE via the epithelial cytochrome P-450 pathway. 12(R)HETE has been shown to diffuse across the corneal stroma from the epithelium and cause corneal swelling by inhibiting the endothelial metabolic pump. With continued pump inhibition, the endothelial cells are under stress and their physiological volume regulation may become altered. Therefore, in both diabetics and contact lens wearers, endothelial cell pump inhibition and time-related volume regulation stress results in endothelial cell cytoskeletal alterations and may be the prime factor causing the polymegathism.

ACCURACY AND ERRORS IN ENDOTHELIAL CELL ANALYSIS

Ronald A. Laing

Departments of Ophthalmology and Physiology
Boston University School of Medicine, Boston, MA

Endothelial cell analysis provides methods for calculating values for parameters such as endothelial cell density, pleomorphism, polymegathism, etc. that are useful in evaluating the function of the corneal endothelium. Although the errors associated with the experimental procedures have generally been addressed in the literature, the systematic and random errors inherent in the methods and procedures used has not generally been considered. All instruments used to make measurements have errors associated with them; all experimental measurements have errors associated with them; all experimental and analytical methods have errors associated with them; all computer algorithms used to calculate numeric values have errors associated with them. In order to be sure that values calculated from experimental measurements represent valid representations of the parameters being measured, it is necessary that these errors be understood and that an error analysis be performed using standard methods to determine the accuracy of the calculated values. Known systematic errors can generally be minimized to an acceptably small value by calibrating against a suitable secondary standard, and this should be done, as appropriate. Random errors should be minimized by proper choice of the method, procedures used, and analysis performed. The precision of the experimental measurements and the various errors inherent in the analytical methods should be understood and analyzed using standard procedures. The method chosen for use should have an inherent precision less than the difference in value expected between the controls and the test samples. If this is not the case, and providing that the errors associated with the methods used can be determined to be random rather than systematic, a sufficiently large data sample 'mast be used and statistical methods used to reduce the effect of random errors. Statistical analysis provides methods for determining the statistical significance of a set of numbers and is often used in endothelial cell analysis. However, statistical analysis assumes that the numbers used as input are valid measures of the parameters being investigated. If this is not the case, then the statistical analysis performed generates numbers that are scientifically invalid and do not represent the true values associated with the calculated parameters. The number given for the calculated values associated with an experimental measurement should reflect the accuracy of the number rather than be given with some arbitrary number of decimal places. (Supported in part by Research to Prevent Blindness.)

MINERALS IN THE CORNEA, NEW ANALYTICAL APPROACHES

N.F. Schrage, S. Flick, C. Redbrake, and M. Reim

Introduction: Reported are the results of a new method to measure mineral contents in volumes of about 3 femtoliters in the cornea. We present measurements on a collective of 70 apparently normal human corneas. **Methods, materials:** Samples of these were examined by energy dispersive x-ray analysis (EDXA) under calibrated conditions in a scanning electron microscope (SEM). The method allows the simultaneous quantitative analysis of elements with atomic number higher than 11 as for example sodium (Na), sulfur (S), chloride (Cl), phosphorus (P), calcium (Ca) and potassium (K). The results are related to the dry weight of the analyzed samples. All distinct layers of the cornea were analysed for all measurable elements in each cornea. **Results:** In the middle stroma we found concentrations of sodium: 0.609±0. 13 , chloride 0.557±0. 115, sulfur 0.257±0.35 potassium 0.058±0.02 and phosphorus 0.038±0.01 in mmol/kg dry weight. **Discussion:** The collation of normal minerals concentrations provides reference values for future studies on changes of the corneal mineral composition in diseased or injured eyes and gives new hints for galenic formulations in ophthalmic drugs. Supported by a Grant of the "Deutsche Forschungsgemeinschaft Az: Re 152/27-1."

FISH EYE DISEASE

Gabriel van Rij, Eveline J.G.M. van Voorst tot Voorst, and Jan Albert Kuivenhoven

Department of Ophthalmology, University of Groningen; Department of Clinical Chemistry, De weezenlanden, Zwolle; and Department of Haemostasis, Thrombosis, Atherosclerosis and Inflammation Research University of Amsterdam, The Netherlands

Two brothers, 58 and 64 yrs of age, and two sisters, 55 and 57 yrs of age, of a kindred with eleven siblings presented with bilateral corneal opacities. The corneal cloudiness was observed in all layers of the cornea, except the epithelium, and was more opaque in the periphery. In the superficial corneal stroma of the two brothers vacuoles were clearly visible. Visual acuity of the brothers ranged between 0.9 and 1.25 and of the sisters between 0.7 and 1.0. The male index patient presented with corneal opacification, HDL deficiency, a near total loss of plasma lecithin: cholesterol acyltransferase (LCAT) activity and premature coronary artery disease. Sequencing of the LCAT gene revealed homozygosity for a novel missense mutation resulting in an Aspl3l-Asn (N131D) substitution*.
(*J. Clin. Invest. 1995,96:2783–2791.)

SCHNYDER'S CRYSTALLINE DYSTROPHY: A New Definition for an Old Disease

Jayne S. Weiss

Kresge Eye Institute; Wayne State University

Schnyder's crystalline dystrophy of the cornea is a rare autosomal dominantly inherited disease in which there is abnormal bilateral deposition of cholesterol and lipid in the cornea. Thirty- three patients with Schnyder's crystalline dystrophy were identified by the author since 1987. Each patient had a complete ophthalmic evaluation including slit lamp examination by the author.

Only 51% of patients with Schnyder's crystalline dystrophy actually had clinical evidence of corneal crystalline deposits. The majority of patients had predictable corneal changes based on age at examination. Patients less than twenty-three years had only subepithelial crystal and deposits or central disc-like opacity. Patients older than twenty-three years of age had arcus lipoides. Those patients thirty-nine years or older also demonstrated panstromal peripheral haze.

The non-crystalline form of Schnyder's crystalline dystrophy has been poorly recognized to date but is equally common to the crystalline form.

MACULAR CORNEAL DYSTROPHY PROTEOGLYCANS CONTAIN A 4.6Å PERIODIC REPEAT: X-RAY DIFFRACTION EVIDENCE

Andrew J. Quantock,[1] Gordon K. Klintworth,[2] David J. Schanzlin,[1] Malcolm S. Capel,[3] Mary Ellen Lenz,[4] and Eugene J-M.A. Thonar[4]

[1]Anheuser-Busch Eye Institute, Saint Louis University School of Medicine, St. Louis, MO; [2]Duke University Eye Center, Durham, NC; [3]Nadonal Synchrotron Light Source, Upton, NY; [4]Rush-Presbyterian-St. Luke's Medical Center, Chicago, IL

Background: Normal human corneas contain two main proteoglycans (PGs) - lumican with its keratan sulphate (KS) side chains, and decorin with its glycosaminoglycan (GAG) chain which is a mix of chondroitin sulphate (CS) and dermatan sulphate (DS). Both PGs play important, although not fully understood, roles governing stromal architecture. An affliction whose pathogenesis has been linked to an erroneous GAG metabolism is macular corneal dystrophy (MCD). Wide-angle, X-ray diffraction patterns from M.D. corneas contain an unusual reflection due to an ultrastructure with a periodic repeat in the region of 4.6Å. In previous work, we postulated that PGs or GAGs could be the origin of this 4.6Å reflection. Presently, we attempt to test this hypothesis. **Methods:** Wide-angle, synchrotron X-ray diffraction patterns were obtained from 4 normal human corneas and 4 M.D. corneas (2 type I and 2 type H). Portions of two of the M.D. corneas were incubated in either chondroitinase ABC (M.D. type I) or N-glycanase (M.D. type II). Following X-ray diffraction analysis the tissue content of sulphated GAG was measured. **Results:** None of the normal corneas produced an X-ray reflection in the region of 4.6Å, whereas all four of the M.D. corneas did (M.D. type I at 4.65Å and 4.63Å: M.D. type II at 4.63Å and 4.67Å). The 4.6Å reflection was diminished following incubation with chondroidnase ABC, a process that removed more than 90% of the sulphated GAG from the tissue. The 4.6Å reflection was also diminished following incubation in N-glycanase (an enzyme that separates intact KS chains from the core protein of lumican), however, subsequent immunochemistry revealed no loss of antigenic KS from the tissue. **Conclusions:** Our results imply that, in M.D., periodic 4.6Å ultrastructures reside in intact, unsulphated lumican molecules and in regions of the CS/DS-containing molecules, or else they reside in a region of a hybrid macromolecular aggregate formed by the interaction of the two molecules.

REGULATION OF CORNEAL ENDOTHELIAL DIFFERENTIATION DURING WOUND HEALING

W.M. Petroll, P.A. Barry-Lane, J. Huang, H.D. Cavanagh, and J.V. Jester

Department of Ophthalmology, University of Texas Southwestern Medical Center, Dallas, TX

Purpose. To identify phenotypic changes expressed by corneal endothelium during wound healing, and to evaluate the role of specific wound-related factors in regulating these changes. **Methods.** *In Vivo* studies: Healing following *in vivo* mechanical scrape injury (MS, 20 eyes) was compared to transcorneal freeze injury (FI, 22 eyes) in a cat model. At various times nines eyes were enucleated, stained *en bloc* with phalloidin, anti-ZO-1, anti-fibronectin and anti-α-smooth muscle (SM) actin, and analyzed using laser confocal microscopy. *Ex Vivo* Studies: The effects of serum, basic fibroblast growth factor (bFGF) and transforming growth factor-ß1 (TGF-ß1) on f-actin and ZO-1 organization were evaluated using an organ culture SI model (22 eyes). **Results.** *In Vivo* studies: Resurfacing following MS was characterized by conservation of apical staining of endothelial cell borders by phalloidin and anti-ZO-1, suggesting maintenance of cell connectivity and apical-basal polarity. Quantitative analysis showed that there was a significant decrease in the intensity of phalloidin-FITC staining at the leading edge of the wound (R=0.98, p<0.01), suggesting a decrease in f-actin. By contrast FI was characterized by the loss of apical staining by phalloidin and anti-ZO-1, and an apparent increase in total phalloidin staining localized to basal f-actin bundles. In addition, detachment and migration of individual cells was observed at the leading edge, and a retrocorneal fibrous membrane (RCFM) developed as healing progressed. The RCFM stained positively for α-SM-actin and fibronectin, features consistent with transdifferentiation of endothelial cells to a mesenchymal phenotype. *Ex Vivo* Studies: Evaluation of SI in cat corneal buttons under serum-free conditions showed maintenance of normal endothelial differentiation, similar to *in vivo* SI. However, addition of TGF-ß1 (10 ng/ml) resulted in a dramatic endothelial transformation to a fibroblastic-like phenotype, similar to that seen after *in vivo* FI. bFGF and serum had much less pronounced effects on f-actin and ZO-1 organization. **Discussion.** Corneal endothelial wound healing following scrape injury (SI) in the cat is characterized by cell spreading and maintenance of endothelial differentiation. In contrast, freeze injury (FI), which is more severe, heals by transformation of endothelial cells to a fibroblastic phenotype. The data suggests that TGF-ß1 may play a critical role in regulating this transdifferentiation. Recent studies by others have demonstrated that ZO-1 is a member of the MAGUK (membrane-associated guanylate kinase homologs) family of proteins, which may be involved in functional signal transduction at the plasma membrane. TGF-ß is known to act through a serine-threonine receptor kinase, and ZO-1 is phosphorylated on serine residues. Together, these findings suggest the hypothesis that regulation of endothelial differentiation by TGF-ß1 may be mediated through a down-stream, ZO-1-associated signaling cascade.

(Supported by NIH EY09667, Senior Scientist Awards (NJ, HDC) and Unrestricted Grants from Research to Prevent Blindness Inc. and the Eleanor Dana Charitable Trust.)

CAPABILITIES, APPLICATIONS, AND LIMITATIONS OF CONFOCAL MICROSCOPY, *In Vivo*

Charles J. Koester and James D. Auran

Columbia University, New York, NY

Details of corneal nerve structure, location, and growth have been documented by high numerical aperture, scanning slit confocal microscopy. Fungus hyphae and Acanthamoeba cysts are readily observed and identified, permitting early diagnosis and treatment. Keratocytes are observed with high resolution at all depths in the stroma.

With confocal microscopy, in vivo, details are visible only when they scatter or reflect light, or in some situations when they absorb light. The basis for visualization is therefore very similar to that of the slit lamp, but with higher resolution, thinner optical sections, and greatly enhanced ability to image weakly scattering details such as cell membranes, basal epithelial nerves, and stromal lamina structure. A limitation is that histological staining is not available for identification of cells or tissue components. Furthermore, resolution is one micron or slightly less, which is not competitive with electron microscopy.

The compensating advantages are first that the subject can be examined immediately, without biopsy or tissue preparation, and in some cases a diagnosis can be reached before a patient leaves the office. Second, the effects of treatment can be followed over time, and in many cases it is possible to return to exactly the same area in the cornea for follow-up examination.

Measurement possibilities include epithelial layer thickness (particularly changes with time), variations in nerve density with time or disease, distribution of epithelial cell size, basal epithelial nerve growth rate, and pigment migration.

ALAMAR BLUE (alamarBlue™ ASSAY): A NEW SIMPLE NON-RADIOACTIVE, NON-TOXIC IN-VITRO ASSAY TO MONITOR CORNEAL PROLIFERATION AND VIABILITY

D.J. Doughman, E.M. Larson, and W.F. Obritsch

Department of Ophthalmology
University of Minnesota Medical School, Minneapolis, Minnesota

Purpose. To compare alamar Blue TM Assay with (3H) thymidine uptake in evaluating corneal endothelial density & viability. **Methods.** Alamar Blue incorporates a proprietary oxidation-reduction (Redox) indicator that both fluoresces and changes color in response to growth and metabolic activity. Rabbit endothelial cells were cultured from 10 days to two months and plated onto micro well plates at concentrations ranging from 1250 to 40,000 cells per well. After 9 to 24 hours incubation, 10 uL Alamar Blue was added to each well and absorbance measured hourly from 1 to 13.5 hrs and at 19, 24, & 48 hr. (3H) thymidine was added to the same wells containing Alamar Blue and radioactivity measured at 14 and 19 hours. Sodium azide was used to create a negative control. **Results.** At 4 hours Alamar Blue absorbance was significantly different ($P < 0.05$) at all cell concentrations. except 1250 cells per well. From 1 to 13.5 hours, absorbance of Alamar Blue varies linearly ($r > 0.97$) with time at all cell concentrations. At 19 and 24 hours, there was a relationship between mean cell concentration and absorbance. At 48 hours, Alamar Blue absorbance was complete at all cell concentrations. (3H) thymidine uptake on non-confluent cultures demonstrated a linear relationship between cell absorbance and (3H) thymidine incorporation. The simultaneous Alamar Blue assay showed linear absorbance for both confluent and non-confluent cell cultures. **Conclusion.** In this study Alamar Blue absorbance is related to cell concentration and demonstrates several advantages over (3H) thymidine: 1) It is as accurate as (3H)thymidine in assaying proliferation of endothelial cells. 2) As opposed to (3H) thymidine, it can assay non-proliferating endothelial cell metabolism. 3) Allows rapid assessment of large numbers of samples. 4) Is non-toxic to cells or technician. 5) Is non-radioactive. 6) Is less costly. 7) Is non-labor intensive. 8) Allows for continuous monitoring of endothelial cell viability.

IN VIVO EPITHELIAL AND CORNEAL THICKNESS MEASUREMENTS BY 3-D CONFOCAL IMAGING

H. Li, W.M. Petroll, I. Maurer,[1] H.D. Cavanagh, and J.V. Jester

Department of Ophthalmology, University of Texas Southwestern Medical Center at Dallas, Texas; [1]Procter & Gamble, Ohio

Purpose: We studied the feasibility and accuracy of measuring epithelial and corneal thickness using in vivo confocal microscopy (CM) through-focusing (CTF). **Methods:** Six normal rabbit eyes and five normal human eyes were studied. Corneas were scanned using *in vivo* CTF from epithelium to endothelium at a constant lens speed (80 μm/s). CTF z-series were digitized and image intensity curves were generated by averaging pixel intensity in the central 180x180 region of the image as a function of z-depth. Peak intensities corresponded to major reflections emanating from epithelium, basal lamina, and endothelium. Based on the z-positions of the corresponding peaks, epithelial and corneal thicknesses were determined. The repeatability and accuracy of CTF measurement were assessed using the standard deviation of three repeated measures, and comparison to ultrasonic pachemetry (UP). **Results:** Distinct epithelial, basal laminar, and endothelial peaks were identified for all 6 rabbit eyes. The mean corneal thickness of rabbit eyes was 357.7+6.9 μm by CTF and 363.5+6.3 μm by UP. The mean difference of corneal thickness by CTF and Up for rabbit eyes was -5.8±9.8 μm; epithelial thickness measured by CTF was 48.2+1.7 μm; the standard deviations for successive measures were 1.1+0.5 μm for epithelial and 2.8±1.7μm for corneal thicknesses. Intensity curves for human corneas also showed strong epithelial and endothelial peaks, as well as smaller peaks corresponding to the basal epithelial nerve plexus and anterior stromal layers. The mean corneal thickness of human eyes was 563.9+29.7 μm by UP and 543.3±39.8 μm by CTF; epithelial thickness measured by CTF was 53.9+2.4 μm with a standard deviation of 2.3+3.09 μm for repeated measures. **Conclusions:** CTF of *in vivo* cornea provides accurate and repeatable epithelial and corneal thickness measurements for both rabbit and human. More importantly, this novel methodology may also provide an accurate and quantitative technique for evaluating corneal structural and functional c hang es related to ocular toxicity, contact lens wear, refractive surgery, corneal infection, and other pathologies. (Supported by a grant from Procter & Gamble, and an unrestricted grant from RPB, Inc.)

MEASUREMENT OF TENSILE FORCES GENERATED BY SINGLE CORNEAL FIBROBLASTS ON COLLAGEN GELS

P. Roy,[1,2] W.M. Petroll,[1,2] H.D. Cavanagh,[1] C.J. Chuong,[2] and J.V. Jester[1]

[1]Dept. of Ophthalmology, Univ. of Texas Southwestern Medical Center, Dallas, TX; [2]Joint Program in Biomedical Engineering, UT Southwestern Medical Center & UT Arlington

Purpose: As an in vitro model of wound healing, a force measurement assay has been developed to quantify the tension exerted by isolated corneal fibroblasts during early reorganization of collagen matrix. **Methods:** Fine glass microneedles were calibrated by measuring the bending stiffness in cantilever-construct experiments. Collagen lattice was prepared by polymerizing 50 μl of bovine dermal collagen mixed with fibronectin conjugated latex beads on a scored 12 mm circular area. The material stiffness of the collagen matrix was characterized by pulling the lattice at 8–10 random locations with the calibrated microneedle using a micromanipulator, and recording the bead movement and needle tip bending. Fibroblasts were derived from early passage subconfluent or confluent culture of rabbit corneal keratocytes m serum-supplemented medium (10% FCS), These cells were sparsely plated on the top of the lattice and viability was maintained using a microincubator. The activity of a single cell was then imaged for 2 hours using phase contrast optics. Videomicroscopic images were digitally sampled at 3 minute intervals and were subsequently analyzed to determine the pattern of bead and cell movement. A force map was constructed based on the recorded displacement of the beads surrounding the cell. **Results:** The collagen lattices were found to be linearly elastic within the range of applied forces; the stiffness values of the lattices (n=6) ranged from 2. 18x10–8 to 3.2x10–8 N/µm with a mean of (2.58 ± 0.59)x10–8 N/µm. At the end of the 2 hour interval, the majority of the beads were displaced towards the cell indicating generation of a tensile stress field in the vicinity of the cell; a maximum tension of 5. 02x 1 0–7 N was developed. The pattern of bead movement in relation to the cell was complex, and could not be explained by simple tractional mechanism of force generation. **Conclusion:** This is the first attempt to measure the tension generating capability of single fibroblasts during early reorganization of collagen matrix. This force measurement assay should be useful for both qualitative and quantitative analyses of cell-matrix interactions during contraction.

Supported by NEI EY07348 (JVJ), Whitaker Foundation (WMP), Senior scientist awards (JVJ, HDC) and an unrestricted grant from Research to Prevent Blindness, Inc.

X-RAY DIFFRACTION FROM THE CORNEAL STROMA: IMPLICATIONS FOR LIGHT SCATTERING

D.W. Leonard, K.M. Meek, and Y. Huang

Open University, Oxford Research Unit, Oxford, UK

The corneal stromas of over forty animal species were examined at physiological hydration using X-ray diffraction. Ultrastructural parameters measured included the collagen fibril diameter, interfibrillar spacing, intermolecular spacing and the number density and volume fraction of hydrated fibrils in the stroma. The refractive indices of the fibrils and the ground substance (GS) were also estimated from the X-ray diffraction data. Although the refractive indices differed from previously published values, the X-ray derived data were shown to be compatible with two existing mathematical models of light transmission through the stroma. Four species were tested in the models, (human, cow, rabbit and trout), since there were cross-species ultrastructural variations, particularly between aquatic and non-aquatic species. Values for the most important parameters are summarised below:

Species	Fibril radius (nm)	Fibril spacing (nm)	Fibril number density ($\times 10^{-4}$ nm^{-2})	Refractive index of fibrils	Refractive index of GS
Rabbit	19.4	65.9	2.2	1.420	1.355
Cow	19.1	63.6	2.3	1.417	1.355
Human	15.4	61.9	2.2	1.415	1.364
Trout	12.4	50.8	3.8	1.422	1.363

The refractive indices of the fibrils and GS for the cow were confirmed using a second method based on the chemical composition of the bovine stroma. Our studies of the change in interfibrillar spacing with hydration suggest that 15% of the water in the stroma is contained in cells. The published chemical composition of bovine cornea was modified to account for this cellular water and for non-fibrillar collagen. Using the second method the refractive indices of the fibrils and GS were calculated to be 1.416 and 1.356, respectively, in good agreement with the tabulated figures.

RECIPIENT CORNEAL STROMA REMODELLING AFTER LAMELLAR KERATOPLASTY IN A RABBIT

E. Rakowska, P.J. Szczesny, and Z. Zagórski

Department of Ophthalmology, Lublin School of Medicine, Chmielna 1, 20–079 Lublin, Poland

The aim was to examine the pattern of corneal wound healing after lamellar keratoplasty in the rabbit using a full thickness allograft. Donor's Descemet's membrane was used as a topographical marker during stromal remodelling. **Materials and methods.** In 30 rabbits a homologous full thickness corneal transplants, 6mm in diameter, were sutured into the lamellar bed of 1/4 to 113 of the corneal thickness. Topical medication was stopped after suture removal 2 weeks after surgery. Clinical evaluation and histology was performed 3 and 5 days, 1, 3 and 6 weeks and 3 months after surgery. **Results.** Donor's endothelial cells disappeared within the first 3 days of surgery. Macrophages and inflammatory cells were numerous only in the early stages. The epithelial cells invaded the wound margins, occasionally ingrowing to the level of donor Descemet's membrane. The latter was, however, denuded of cells and fragmented by weeks. The fragments of donor Descemets membrane were displaced towards the superficial corneal layers at 3 months. Epithelial plugs marking the wound margins were observed initially, but later were replaced by scar tissue. At 3 months there was no scar tissue visible and the border between the donor and the recipient cornea was not identifiable. The thickness of the transplant gradually decreased and after 3 months the cornea had a uniform thickness and a normal histological appearance. Occasionally some small fragments of donor Descemet's membrane were present under the corneal epithelium. **Conclusions.** Our results indicate that during the healing process the recipient corneal stroma regenerates and gradually replaces the donor corneal button. It may be related to the following: 1) a healthy rabbit cornea seems to have strong tendency to repair. 2) there were enough keratocytes of the recipient left in the stromal bed to facilitate the reparative process 3) the immunological differences between the donor and the recipient could enhance the elimination of the donor tissue. Supported by the Lublin Medical School grant and Krwawicz Foundation grant.

NUMERICAL MODELLING OF THE CORNEAL ANISOTROPY

Jaroslaw W. Jaroński, Henryk T. Kasprzak, and Elżbieta B. Jankowska-Kuchta

Institute of Physics, Technical University, Wroclaw, Poland

Purpose. To find the influence of the corneal anisotropy on a ray tracing through the cornea. To compare an analytical model of the corneal anisotropy with experiential observations and to estimate some parameters of the corneal birefringence (retardation and azimuth).

Methods. A theoretical model of the corneal birefringence is considered. Ray tracing through such a model is calculated for different parameters of approximation: corneal topography, radius of curvature, thickness, direction of axis of anisotropy and refractive indices. Then polarisation properties of this model using the Jones calculus were examined in different optical systems. First, the plain linear and circular polariscope was used. In this case no precise results were obtained because of low sensitivity of this method. Therefore we proposed new advanced method which gives more precise measurement. Different states of polarization were projected on corneal model and then the retardation and tile azimuth were computed. Experimental measurements of corneal birefringence were compared with the theoretical model.

Results. There is no significant difference between retardation for different geometry of the cornea. We proposed a model which assumes that cornea behaves like uniaxial cristal with an axis of anisotropy perpendicular to the corneal surface. That model is in good agreement with polarisation patterns recorded on the human cornea in vivo.

Conclusion. Investigation of anisotropic properties of cornea offers new possibilities of testing the stromal optical anisotropy and the diagnosing process.

MITOTIC ACTIVITY IN THE CULTURED HUMAN CORNEA I. PCNA EXPRESSION AS EVIDENCE FOR ENDOTHELIAL CELL DIVISION

Per Fagerholm, Lisha Gan, and Gysbert van Setten

Kalrolinska Institutet, St. Eriks Eye Hospital, Stockholm, Sweden

Introduction: Recent studies have provided some evidence of corneal endothelial cell division in the human adults in vivo and in vitro. However, little is known about the proliferating potential of corneal endothelium and its regulation of wound repair. In the present study we have used for the first time the antibodies against PCNA (proliferating cell nuclear antigen) in the human cornea. The purpose of this study is to see the expression of proliferating cell nuclear antigen in cultured human cornea. The role of growth factors will be discussed. **Materials and Methods:** Twelve human corneas from donors (ages from 59–91) were cultured in the medium (MEM + 8 % FBS). The proliferating state of the endothelium were evaluated by immunostaining of PCNA in the cells. Four corneas of each time-point were fixed in paraformalin after 0 day 3 days, 3 weeks cultured in media. Paraffin embedded section ($4 \mu m$) were stained used antibody PC 10 against PCNA. The number of PCNA positive cells was counted under light microscope. **Result:** PCNA positive cell were seen in the corneas which cultured in medium for 3 days. The mean of PCNA positive endothelia is. 2.4% (SD :1: 2). **Conclusions:** 1. Expression of PCNA in cultured human corneal endothelium presents additional evidence of that cell division can occur in the adult human corneal endothelium in vitro. 2. The proliferation of the corneal endothelium under the tissue culture conditions may be induced by the growth factor in the medium. 3. PCNA can be used as a marker for evaluating the role of growth factors in the medium and monitor the condition of the culture medium.

Sessions IV and XII

Refractive Surgery

27

CORNEAL TATTOOING TO TREAT GLARE SYMPTOMS FOLLOWING RADIAL KERATOTOMY

George J. Florakis, Aaron M. Fay, Richard W. Darrell, and
B. Dobli Srinivasan

The Edward S. Harkness Eye Institute
Columbia University
New York, New York

ABSTRACT

Radial keratotomy (RK) may be complicated by postoperative glare and night vision may be compromised when parts of RK incisions fall within the boundary of the dilated pupil. Surgical pigmentation of the cornea has been used to treat glare symptoms caused by corneal trauma and iris loss. In this study, corneal tattooing was performed in a patient who had undergone 16-incision RK and 6-incision astigmatic keratotomy (AK) elsewhere. With one eye covered, the patient in this study was shown a white spot projected onto a visual acuity screen and asked to draw the image on a Night Vision Recording chart before and after tattooing. Sterile iron oxide powder was suspended in sterile saline to approximate the patient's iris color. Using a 69 Beaver blade, Sinskey hook, and 30-gauge needle, the wounds were reopened and pigment deposited. The procedure was repeated twice. The patient studied reported marked decrease in glare symptoms following tattooing. Postoperative drawings of the projected spot image showed significant regression of halation. Focal areas of pigment dispersion required retreatment, which improved symptoms to a lesser degree. From this result it is concluded that tattooing procedures can be used to pigment radial keratotomy scars in patients who complain of glare. The material best suited for this purpose has yet to be determined. Iron oxide suspensions have been successful, though pigment migration out of the scars seems to have contributed to recurrence of symptoms.

INTRODUCTION

Refractive surgery is an effective means of improving uncorrected Snellen visual acuity. Postoperatively, patients may have subjective complaints of glare or night vision

Advances in Corneal Research, edited by Lass
Plenum Press, New York, 1997

disturbances. Physiologic dilation of the pupil under scotopic conditions may permit the central limits of radial incisions to overlie the entrance pupil[1] and thereby cast irregularly refracted light onto the retina. Halation of bright objects on the retina may also result in subjective glare. Subjective symptoms may be barely noticeable or severely debilitating, and measurable visual performance may be compromised.[2]

Corneal tattoo can be achieved by chemical precipitation of pigments or by direct deposition of exogenous pigment into the corneal stroma. It has been used successfully to treat corneal scarring and glare symptoms caused by large iridectomies[3] and by traumatic iris loss.[4] In this study researchers treated the right eye in a patient with debilitating glare resulting from 16 incision radial keratotomy and six incision astigmatic keratotomy with corneal tattoo. A significant reduction of symptoms was observed. Symptoms recurred upon partial dispersion of the pigment, but were markedly improved over initial presentation.

CASE REPORT

A 34-year-old man complaining of debilitating glare in his right eye was referred for consideration of penetrating keratoplasty. He had undergone radial keratotomy eleven months prior to presentation. The surgery consisted of sixteen radial and six astigmatic incisions performed in three separate sessions over a two-month period. Visual acuity with rigid contact lenses was 20/30 in the right eye and 20/25 in the left unoperated eye. Manifest refraction of -4.50 -0.50 X 170 yielded 20/20 visual acuity in the right eye. The left eye, which had not undergone treatment, corrected to 20/20 visual acuity with a -5.25 -2.00 X 180 refraction.

The pupils were equal, round, and concentric with respect to the limbus. Biomicroscopy was remarkable for sixteen radial and six arcuate corneal incisions (Figure 1). The incisions were irregularly contoured and of variable depth and thickness. The arcuate incisions and radial incisions intersected at several points. The epithelium was intact, there was no corneal edema, and the cornea was otherwise clear. No neovascularization was

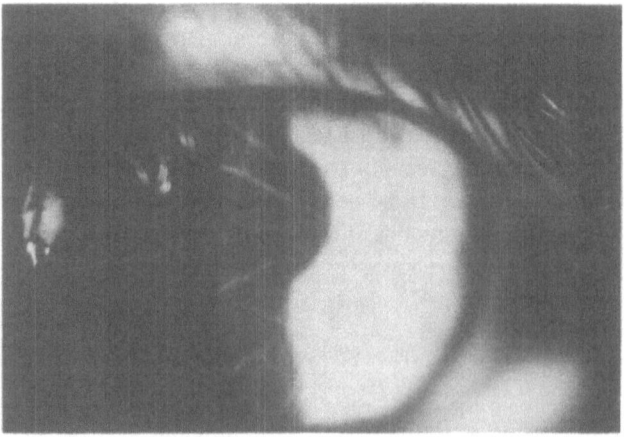

Figure 1. Pre-tattoo slit lamp photograph demonstrating multiple radial and astigmatic corneal incisions that partially involve the central cornea.

noted. The crystalline lens was clear. Indirect ophthalmoscopy demonstrated a normal appearing fundus.

Objective assessment of light scatter using the Night Vision Recording Chart[2] in a darkened room revealed significant image degradation in the involved eye. This technique is described elsewhere.[2] Rigid contact lenses did not relieve the symptoms.

After discussing risks and benefits of various treatment modalities, the patient consented to penetrating keratoplasty but wished to pursue less invasive techniques first. Corneal tattoo of the radial and astigmatic incisions was performed using a 69 Beaver blade; 1 30 gauge needle; and black, white, and brown iron oxides (Spaulding-Rogers Manufacturing, Inc.; Voorheesville, NY) suspended in balanced saline solution to approximate the patient's iris color. All incisions were uniformly pigmented. Ciprofloxacin and diclofenac drops were given postoperatively.

RESULTS

Preoperative Night Vision Recording Chart analysis revealed image degradation involving greater than 130 boxes on the image grid (and extending off the recording chart) (Figure 2A).

Four days after application of tattoo in the incisions, the corneal epithelium had healed and visual acuity was 20/25 with a contact lens in place. The patient reported a marked decrease in subjective glare symptoms. Image degradation had decreased to 26 boxes (Figure 2B).

Eight days after the initial tattoo, retreatment was applied to the inferior incisions due to partial pigment loss. One week later the visual acuity was 20/20. All incisions were uniformly pigmented (Figure 3). The patient reported a "90% improvement" in glare. The Night Vision Recording revealed nearly complete resolution of image degradation with only eight boxes involved (Figure 2C).

Seven weeks after the initial tattoo was applied, the patient reported recurring glare symptoms. He was examined and found to have dispersed pigment beyond the incision

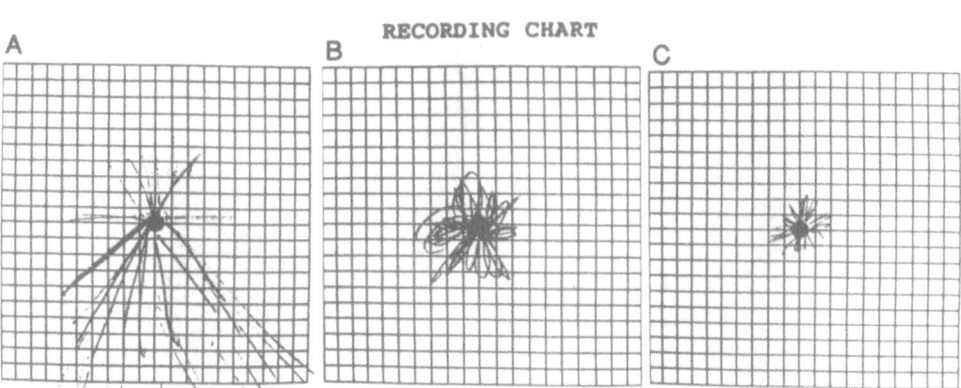

Figure 2. Night Vision Recording Chart demonstrating (A) severe image degradation prior to tattoo; (B) marked improvement following initial procedure; and (C) nearly complete resolution of image degradation following reapplication of pigment.

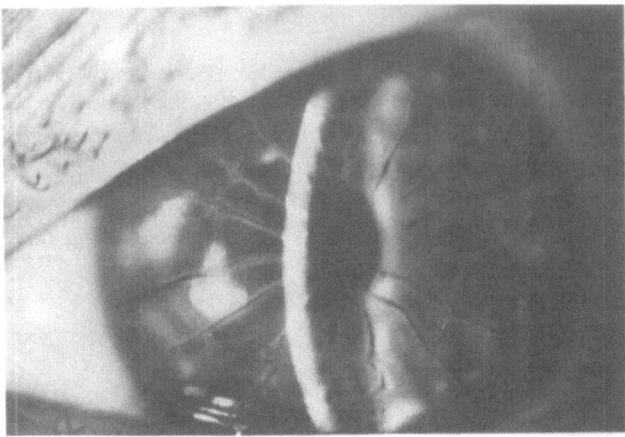

Figure 3. Slit lamp photograph demonstrates uniform pigmentation of corneal scars after initial application.

borders (Figure 4). Visual acuity was 20/30. A Sinskey hook was used to reopen the radial incisions and tattoo pigment was deposited in a deeper fashion. The patient reported persistent but significantly improved symptoms. Subjectively, night driving and other activities were improved.

DISCUSSION

Galen first described corneal tattooing to disguise corneal leukomas using copper sulfate. Wecker (1870), using India Ink, is credited with pioneering the modern day use of corneal pigmenting procedures. Others have described various methods of chemical precipitation and direct deposition of pigment for cosmesis.[5-7] Recently, Reed described corneal tattooing to reduce glare in patients with monocular diplopia from large iridectomies or in cases of traumatic iris loss.[3,4]

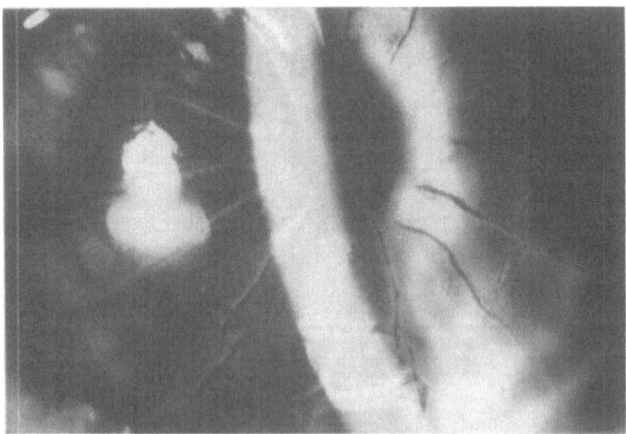

Figure 4. Migration of pigment and recurring symptoms required deeper application of pigment.

A number of studies have demonstrated glare or other night vision disturbances after refractive surgery. Some of these studies have relied on subjective questionnaires.[8] Others have been able to document glare or image degradation with a physiologically dilated pupil using the Night Vision Recording Chart.[2] When the pupil dilates larger than the optical zone (i.e., in scotopic conditions) or if the incisions are irregular with scars of varying thickness, patients may experience light scattering and image degradation. They may describe this image degradation as glare, halos around lights, or scattered light rays. Some may not notice significant problems or describe them poorly, while others will have severely debilitating symptoms. These issues are of particular concern with night driving and may represent a significant public health concern in the future as the refractive surgical population ages.[9]

Duke Elder noted that in addition to its cosmetic effect, corneal tattooing had "…a considerable optical value, inasmuch as, when a diffuse scar translucent nebula with irregular edges is converted into an opaque plaque with a well-defined margin, the annoying effect of irregular scattering of light is eliminated."[10] The case reported here clearly demonstrates this effect on image quality. Corneal tattooing procedures can be used to pigment radial keratotomy scars in patients who complain of glare and night vision disturbances.

The material best suited for this purpose has yet to be determined. Pigment dispersion may be minimized by using finer or coarser materials than the iron oxide suspension used here. In addition, iron oxide, available in many colors, allows one to approximate the natural iris color, which may be cosmetically desirable. However, it is not clear that non-black pigments will decrease glare as well as black pigments. Investigations into the most suitable tattooing material and color are ongoing.

In summary, corneal tattooing appears to be effective in decreasing image degradation that may result from incisional refractive surgery. Furthermore, a simple documentation of such disturbances by methods such as the Night Vision Recording Chart (rather than questionnaires) should be the standard for both pre-operative and post-operative evaluations.

ACKNOWLEDGMENTS

Supported in part by an unrestricted research grant from Research to Prevent Blindness.

REFERENCES

1. A.M. Fay, Trokel, S.L., and Myer J., Pupil diameter and the principal ray. *J. Cataract Refract. Surg.* 18:348 (1992).
2. G.J. Florakis, Jewelewicz, D., Michelsen, H., and Trokel, S.L., Evaluation of night vision disturbances. *J. Refract. Corneal Surg.* 10:333 (1994).
3. J.W. Reed, and Beran, R.F., Elimination of monocular diplopia by corneal tattooing. *Ophthalmic Surgery* 19:437 (1988).
4. J.W. Reed, Corneal tattooing to reduce glare in cases of traumatic iris loss. *Cornea* 13:401 (1994).
5. D.K. Pischel, Tattooing of the cornea with gold and platinum chloride. *Arch. Ophthalmol.* 3:176 (1930).
6. K.L. Pickrell, and Clark, E.H., Tattooing of corneal scars with insoluble pigments, *Plastic Reconstr. Surg.* 2:44 (1947).
7. S.R. Gifford, and Steinberg, A., gold and silver impregnation of cornea for cosmetic purposes. *Am. J. Ophthalmol.* 10:240 (1927).
8. G.O. Waring, Lynn, M.J., Nizan, A., and the PERK Study Group, Results of the Prospective Evaluation of Radial Keratectomy (PERK) Study. Five years after surgery for myopia. *Ophthalmology* 98:1164 (1991).
9. L.J. Maguire, Keratorefractive surgery, success, and the public health. *Am. J. Ophthalmol.* 117:394 (1994).
10. Sir Stewart Duke-Elder, *System of Ophthalmology, Volume VIII (2)*. C.V. Mosby Co., St. Louis (1965).

28

REFRACTIVE RESULTS FOR THE NIDEK EC-5000 EXCIMER LASER USING A NEW ALGORITHMIC CORRECTION IN 482 EYES

Anupam Chatterjee,[1] Sunil Shah,[1,2] and David A. R. Bessant[3]

[1]Optimax Laser Eye Clinic
Manchester, United Kingdom
[2]Royal Eye Hospital
Manchester, United Kingdom
[3]Institute of Ophthalmology
London, United Kingdom

ABSTRACT

The goals of this study are to assess the results of photorefractive keratectomy (PRK) using a new algorithmic correction for the Nidek EC-5000 excimer laser. A modified algorithm was obtained from the manufacturer after data previously presented indicated that the existing algorithm tended to overcorrect the spherical error and undercorrect the astigmatism. In the new algorithm the spherical component was undercorrected as the associated cylinder increased and the cylinder was overtreated by a similar amount. In this study, 482 consecutive patients undergoing PRK & photoastigmatic refractive keratectomy were evaluated. The spherical corrections performed were between 0.00 D and -10.75 D and the astigmatic corrections between -0.00 D and -3.50 D. Postoperative results at six months of follow-up showed a mean spherical equivalent of -0.05 ± 0.78 diopters, a mean spherical correction of +0.18 ± 0.77 D and mean astigmatism of -0.45 D ± 0.40 D. Vector analysis showed that mean surgically induced astigmatism was +0.29 D ± 1.02 D. When compared with results obtained using the original algorithm these patients achieved improved spherical corrections although their astigmatic results were similar. It is recommended that manufacturer's algorithms are regularly updated on the basis of the actual patient results.

INTRODUCTION

Excimer laser photorefractive keratectomy (PRK) and photoastigmatic keratectomy (PARK) have become popular surgical options for the treatment of ametropia,[1,2] and have

Advances in Corneal Research, edited by Lass
Plenum Press, New York, 1997

been used to treat 250,000 eyes world-wide.[3] In the experience of the authors, when used with the manufacturer's standard algorithm, PARK with the Nidek EC-5000 excimer laser, when used with the manufacturer's standard algorithm, tended to produce overcorrecting of the patient's spherical error and undercorrection of the astigmatism.[4] For example, a patients final mean spherical equivalent (MSE) could be 0.00 diopters (D), but his refraction might be +0.50 / -1.00 x 90.

This relationship was discussed with the manufacturer (Nidek), who provided a new algorithm for use with the Nidek EC-5000 excimer laser. The results of PRK and PARK were then studied using this new algorithm.

PATIENTS AND METHODS

In this study, 482 consecutive patients underwent PRK and PARK at Optimax Laser Eye Clinics. All patients were treated using a Nidek EC-5000 excimer laser. Patients with less than 6 months post-operative follow up were excluded. All data was entered by the treating doctors at the time of surgery or follow-up into a networked computer database and subsequently analyzed. Manual epithelial debridement was carried out under topical anaesthesia. Either Maxitrol or Chloramphenicol ointment was used for the first post-operative week at the surgeons discretion. Topical steroid drops were not used routinely. Postoperative follow up was performed routinely at one, six, twelve, and twenty four weeks in all patients, and then on an "as needed" basis. Patients treated with topical steroid drops were seen monthly. All patients had extensive preoperative screening and counseling. Careful fundal examination excluded any macular or other retinal pathology. No patients had pre-existing glaucoma but they were counseled that PRK and PARK affects

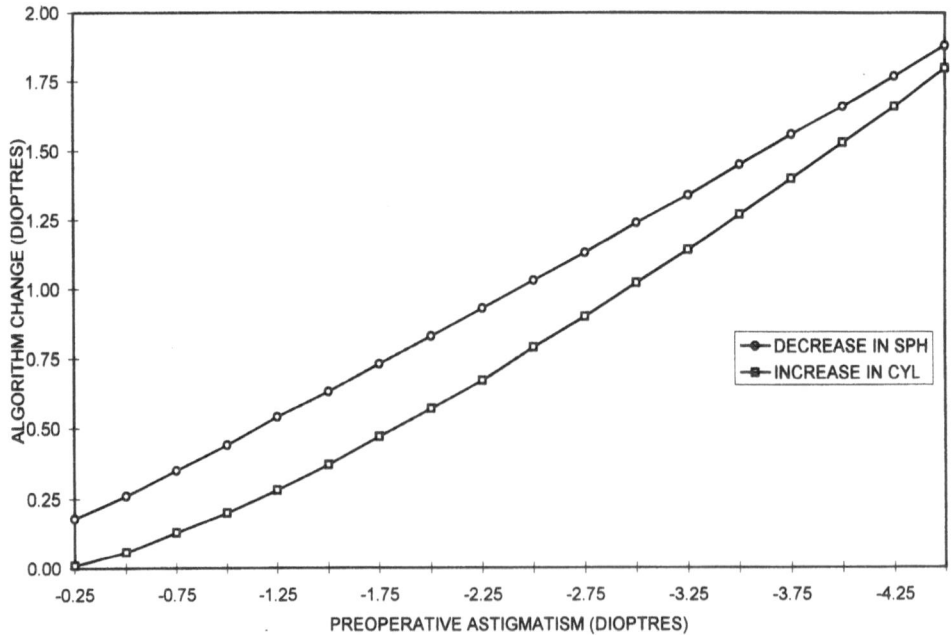

Figure 1. Modifications to Nidex algorithm.

Table 1. Pre- and post-algorithm modification results

Group	Preop. MSE	Preop. sphere	Preop. cyl.	Postop. MSE	Postop. sphere	Postop. cyl.	SIA
A	-4.48 ± 2.02	-4.04 ± 1.96	-0.87 ± 0.85	-0.07 ± 0.88	+0.28 ± 0.91	-0.42 ± 0.53	+0.29 ± 1.01
B	-4.77 ± 2.04	-4.15 ± 2.02	-1.24 ± .082	+0.14 ± 0.92	+0.42 ± 0.95	-0.56 ± 0.55	+0.49 ± 1.16
C	-4.54 ± 1.96	-4.10 ± 1.89	-0.87 ± 0.78	-0.05 ± 0.78	+0.18 ± 0.77	-0.45 ± 0.40	+0.29 ± 1.02
D	-4.76 ± 1.97	-4.12 ± 1.93	-1.27 ± 0.79	-0.01 ± 0.77	+0.25 ± 0.78	-0.52 ± 0.46	+0.56 ± 1.15

Group A: All patients (PRK & PARK) using the original algorithm (n=5378).
Group B: Patients with astigmatism (PARK only) using the original algorithm (n=3504).
Group C: All patients (PRK & PARK) using the new algorithm correction (n=482).
Group D: Patients with astigmatism (PARK only) using the new algorithm correction (n=325).

both applanation and non-contact tonometry, giving a falsely low reading[5] and this makes future screening difficult.

The choice of treatment zone size was at the discretion of individual surgeons, but was usually between 6.5 mm and 7.5 mm (transition zone values).

Modifications to the manufacturers standard algorithm were applied as shown in Fig. 1.

Statistical analysis was performed using the software package SPSS 6.0 for Windows.

RESULTS

The mean age of the 482 patients was 33.6 years. Mean follow-up was 28.6 weeks (range 26 to 35 weeks).

The final mean uncorrected visual acuity (Snellen fraction) was 0.85 ± 0.28 (range 0.10 to 1.5) and the final mean best corrected visual acuity was 1.04 ± 0.19 (range 0.40 to 1.50).

Pre- and postoperative results (at minimum six months of follow-up) are shown in Table 1 and Figs. 2 to 6. Data from all patients treated with the new algorithm correction was analyzed in two groups; all 482 patients (Group C) and those 325 who had PARK (Group D). Results are also given for patients treated using the original algorithm and divided into similar groups A and B.

For patients with astigmatism who were treated post algorithm modification (Group D), the postoperative. MSE was -0.01 D ± 0.77 D (range +3.75 to -4.50), postoperative. sphere was +0.25 D ± 0.78 D (range +4.00 to -4.00), postoperative. cylinder -0.52 D ± 0.46 D (range 0.00 to -3.75) and surgically induced astigmatism (SIA) (Alpin Method[6]) +0.56 D ± 1.15 D (range +4.75 to -3.50).

DISCUSSION

It has previously been reported that PARK performed using the Nidek EC5000 excimer laser tends to overcorrect the spherical error and undercorrect astigmatism.[4] Similar findings have also been obtained with other excimer lasers.[7] In the light of these findings we approached the manufacturer and obtained a modified algorithm which agreed closely with our accumulated clinical data. In the new algorithm, the spherical component was progressively undercorrected as the associated cylinder increased, and the cylinder over-treated by a similar amount (Fig. 1).

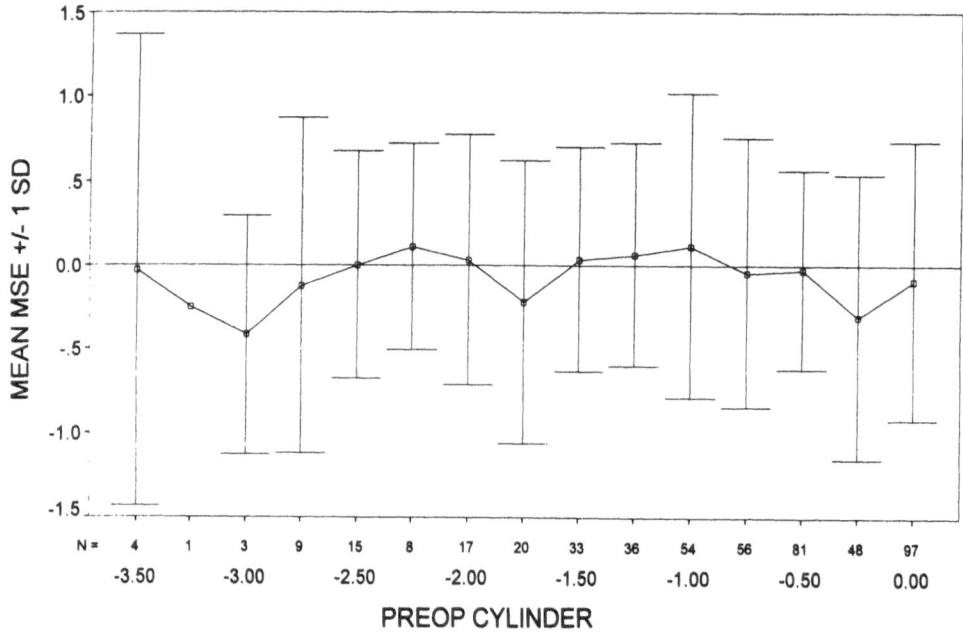

Figure 2.

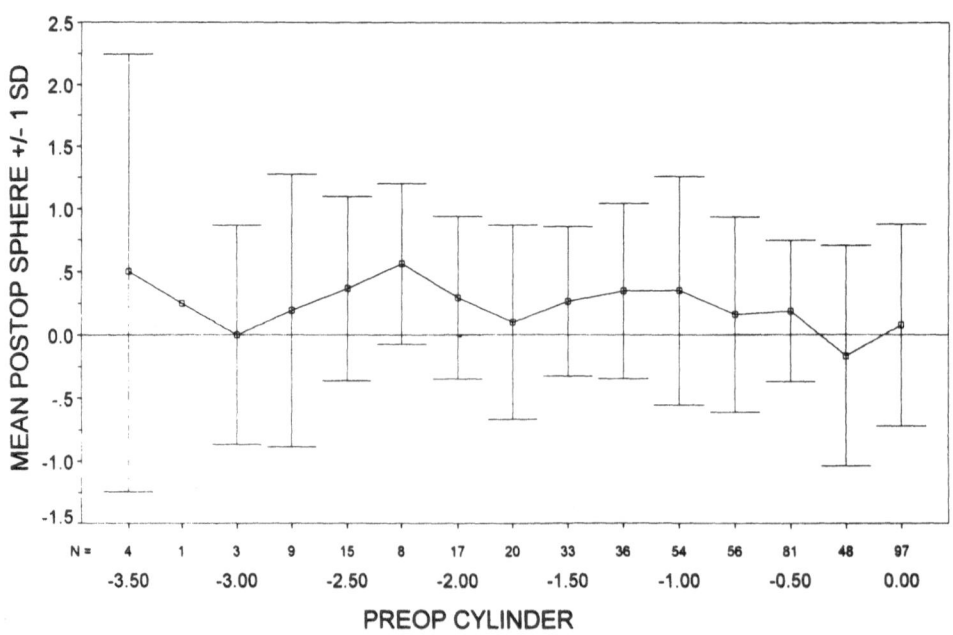

Figure 3.

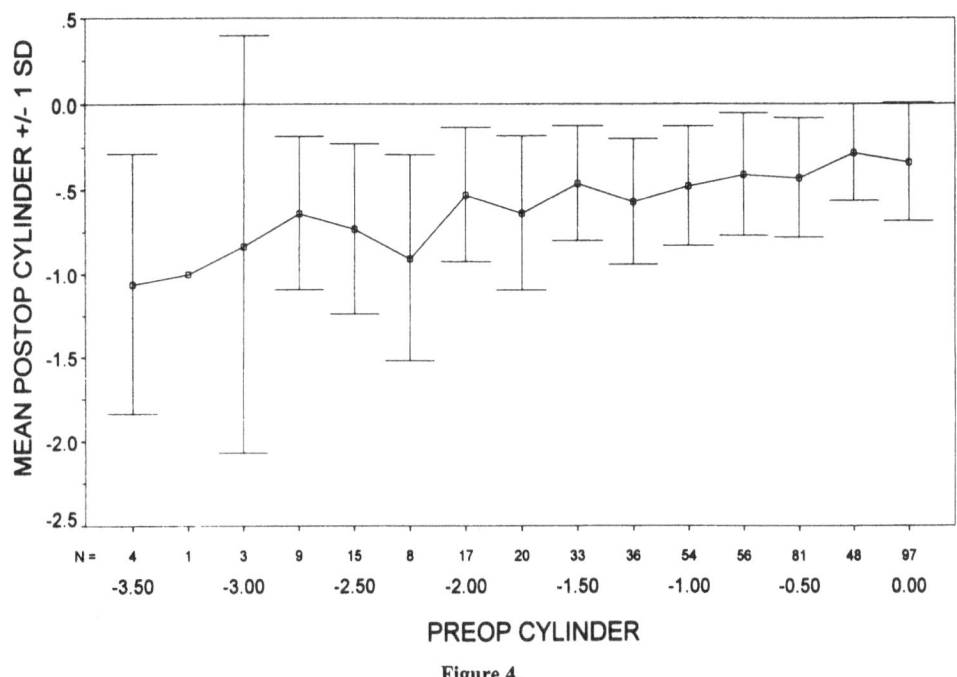

Figure 4.

Figure 5.

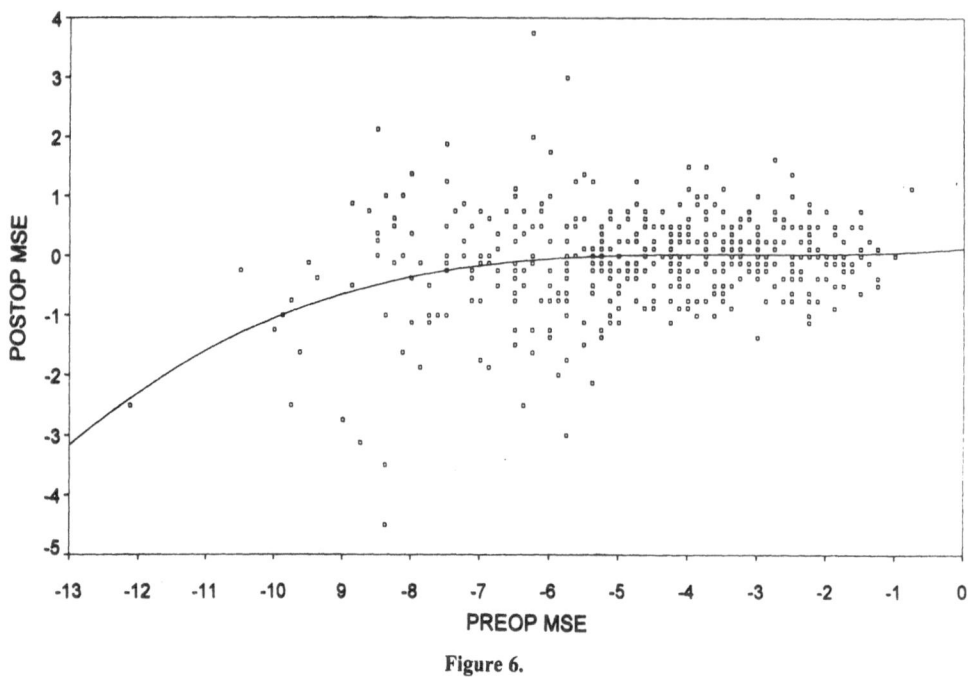

Figure 6.

Table 1 shows the data before (Groups A & B) and after (Groups C & D) the new algorithm correction. These results show that patients in Groups C & D achieved an improved spherical correction with a similar final astigmatic result. (Figs. 2 to 6).

To allow an accurate measure of the actual correction required in the given plane of original astigmatism attempted, correction factors need to be calculated from the achieved vector versus intended vector.

The authors recommend that excimer laser manufacturers need to update their algorithms on the basis of these results and continue regular updates as new clinical data become available in order to get the best refractive outcome for the patient.

ACKNOWLEDGMENTS

We would like to acknowledge the following doctors & optometrists working in the Optimax Clinics who let us use their patients for this study: V. Brogan, C.C. Cory, R. Dingley, S.J. Doyle, H. Flayeh, R Hameed, A.A. Hashim, E.F. Hynes, N.W. Marshall, A.G.E. Nylander, S. Ramanathan, B.E.B. Williams, M. Begum, I. Kara, A. Jarosz, and B. Shah.

Part of this data has been presented at the Int. Ophthalmic Excimer Laser Cong., Tring, Oxford, UK. April 1996.

REFERENCES

1. A. Gartry, Treating myopia with the excimer laser: the present position. *Br. Med. J.* 310:979 (1995).
2. T. Seiler., and P.J. McDonnell. Excimer laser photorefractive keratectomy. *Surv. Ophthalmol.* 40:89 (1995)

3. C.N.J. McGhee, Bryce, I.G., Weed, K.H., Surgical correction of myopia and myopic astigmatism. *Eye News* 2:7 (1995).

4. S. Shah, Doyle, S., Cory, C., Astigmatic corrections using the Nidek EC-5000 excimer laser - 6 months follow up in 2320 patients. *European Society of Cataract and Refract. Surg., Amsterdam* (1995).

5. A. Chatterjee, Shah, S., Doyle, S.J. et al., Intralocular pressure drop following excimer laser photorefractive keratectomy. *Poster, JERMOV congress, Montpelier 16–18 Oct 1995. Ophthalmology.* In Press.

6. N.A. Alpins. A new method of analyzing vectors for changes in astigmatism. *J. Cataract Refract. Surg.* 19:524 (1993).

7. S. Verma, Corbett, M.C., O'Brart, D.P., and Marshall ., Preliminary results using the Summit Apogee system. *UK & Ireland Society of Cataract and Refract. Surg., Dublin,* Sept (1995).

29

PATIENT MOTIVATION IN PRK AND CONTACT LENSES

Is PRK Only for Contact Lens Failures?

Shehzad A. Naroo,[1,2] Sunil Shah,[1,3] Anupam Chatterjee,[1] Philip Morgan,[2] Rakesh Kapoor,[4] and Paul Rigby[5]

[1]Optimax Laser Eye Clinic, Manchester
[2]Department of Optometry and Vision Sciences
 University of Manchester Institute of Science and Technology
[3]Royal Eye Hospital, Manchester
[4]Specsavers Opticians, London
[5]Manchester

ABSTRACT

The purpose of this study was to compare the motives of patients presenting for photorefractive keratectomy (PRK) compared to those for contact lenses (CL). This study included 102 consecutive patients undergoing PRK and 85 consecutive patients attending a local optometric clinic for CL. These patients were asked to complete a questionnaire that covered demographic features, refraction, and reasons for choosing PRK or CL and not choosing alternative options. Results indicated that the mean age was 36 years (PRK) and 25 years (CL) ($p<0.0001$). Mean spherical equivalent was -4.6D (PRK) and -2.9D (CL). Among PRK patients, 83% were previous CL wearers, most of whom had given up CL due to ophthalmic complications. For new CL patients their main reason not to have PRK was cost. Few patients in either group were swayed by advice from their contact lens practitioner. The results led to the conclusion that the main patient group for PRK appears to be CL failures in their thirties developing CL intolerance and having a higher degree of refractive error, many of whom could have continued successfully with CL if wear problems had been better managed.

INTRODUCTION

World-wide, 250,000 patients have undergone photorefractive keratectomy[1] (PRK) and following Food and Drug Administration (FDA) approval in the USA, numbers are set to rise dramatically. Knowledge of demographic features and motives for patients under-going PRK compared to those wearing contact lenses (CL) is essential for future planning of these services.

Issues of direct relevance to optometrists are whether PRK will reduce the number of patients choosing CL and if PRK will become the correction of choice for most myopes. This study set out to compare patients attending for PRK and CL, and the reasons for seeking their respective correction modality.

METHODS

A group of 102 consecutive patients presenting at a High Street clinic for the treat-ment of myopia and myopic astigmatism by excimer laser PRK were compared to 85 pa-tients presenting for contact lenses. Only patients presenting for their first PRK consultation were included, eliminating bias from patients already treated, as this group could be influenced by the result of their treatment. The second group were patients pre-senting for their first CL consultation. Previous CL wearers were excluded eliminating bias from previous CL wear.

A simple questionnaire was presented to the patient at the time of their visit, and completed by the practitioner asking the patient questions on the day of the appointment, ensuring a 100% completion rate. All patients were seen between June and August 1995.

The questionnaire included demographic questions on age, sex, and occupation. In-formation about the refractive error was obtained from the patients records. Previous CL type worn was noted in patients giving up CL in favor of PRK.

PRK patients were asked about reasons for choosing PRK in preference to CL, prior contact lens problems. If they had not worn CL previously they were asked reasons for not choosing CL. Similarly, patients presenting for CL were asked about reasons for choosing CL and why they had not chosen PRK. All responses were limited to Yes/No options to aid interpretation of answers. Patients were also asked for any other comments in the questionnaire.

RESULTS

The PRK group consisted of 102 patients, 51 male and 51 female, compared to the CL group, which consisted of 52 female and 22 male. Thus there was a greater number of females seeking CL correction, although this was not statistically significant. (X^2=3.45, p=0.0637. Patients for PRK (35.5 ± 10.5 years) were older than those choosing CL (25.3 ± 7.4 years) (ANOVA; F=56.4, p=0.0001). Eighty-three percent of PRK patients were pre-vious CL wearers.

Table 1. Prior CL use in PRK patients

CL Type	Number ($n=102$)
Soft	59 (57.8%)
Gas Permeable	24 (23.5%)
Hard	1 (1.0%)
None	18 (17.6%)

Table 2. Refractive results

	PRK Patients	CL Patients
Mean sphere	-4.25D ± 1.90	-2.63D ± 2.96
Mean cylinder	-0.90D ± 0.08	-0.62D ± 0.83
Mean MSE	-4.56D ± 1.94	-2.88D ± 3.02

Tables 1–6 and Figs. 1–4 present the results of the questionnaire.

DISCUSSION

The results of this study showed that the average age of patients presenting for PRK is 10 years higher than that for CL, agreeing with previous papers.[2] 83% of PRK patients had already tried CL, which may explain some of the age difference between the two groups. There was an equal male to female ratio for the PRK patients but a 1:2.5 ratio for CL patients. Although this was not statistically significant, the trend indicated that more females are likely to try CL. PRK patients had 1.68D greater myopia (mean MSE) for average refractive errors in each group. Patients occupation was a factor (X^2=30.4, p<0.0001) with the main reasons being the increased numbers of clerical and semi-skilled

Table 3. Social background

Occupation	% PRK Patients	% CL Patients
Professional	18.6	15.3
Management	11.8	8.2
Semi-skilled	5.9	0
Clerical & Administration	14.7	3.5
Unskilled	32.4	34.1
Retired	2.9	24.7
Student	8.8	5.9
Unemployed	4.9	8.2

Table 4. Factors influencing treatment modality

Factor	% PRK Patients	% CL Patients
Inconvenience: Glasses (CL patients) / CL (PRK patients)	96.1	82.4
Cosmetic	57.8	70.6
Cost of PRK	52.0	69.4
Sport	58.8	43.5
Work	38.2	37.6
Advice of friends/relatives	29.4	38.8
Advertising	36.3	12.9
Cost of CL	33.3	9.4
Professional advice	10.8	3.5
Medical / Disease	6.9	5.9

Table 5. Factors for choosing PRK
(for previous CL wearers)

Factor	% Patients
Costs	39.3
Dry eye	39.2
Intolerance to CL	32.1
Overwear	31.0
Red eye	28.6
Intolerance to solutions	13.2
Professional advice	10.7
Advice of friends / relatives	1.2

Table 6. Factors for choosing CL rather than PRK

Factor	% Patients
Adverse effects	63.5
Long-term effects	58.8
Lack of information	57.6
Scared of surgery	49.4
Bad publicity	27.1
Advice of friends/relatives	11.8
Professional advice	1.2

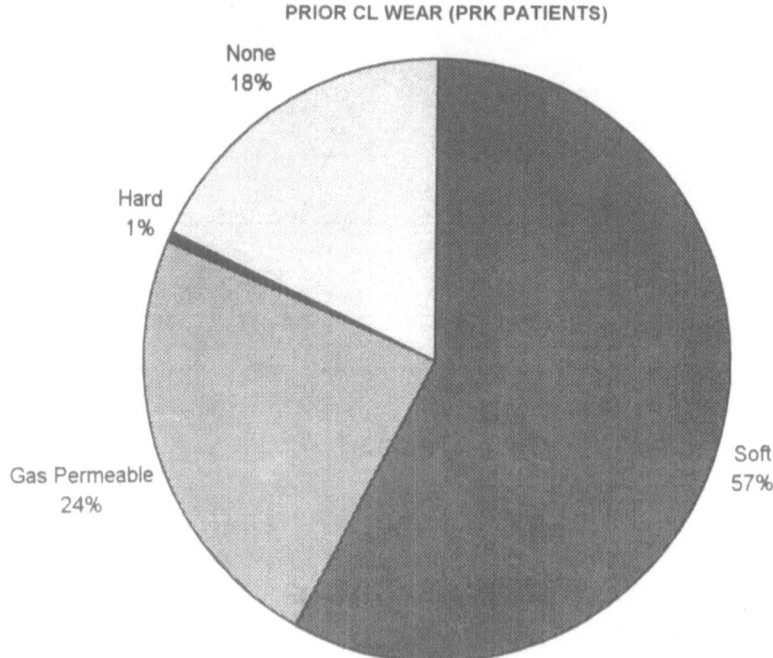

Figure 1. Prior CL wear (PRK patients).

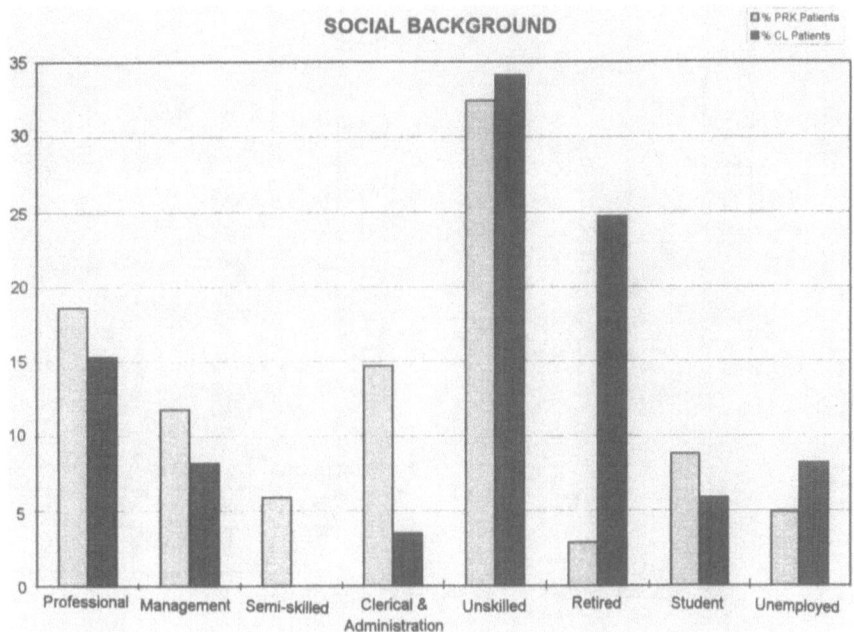

Figure 2. Social background.

for PRK (11.2% greater with PRK patients), and retired patients for CL (21.8% greater with CL patients).

Reasons for choosing CL rather than PRK include concerns over potential problems (63.5%) such as stromal haze, loss of acuity or contrast sensitivity. Although improvements with PRK techniques continue, these problems still persist.[3-5] However, better control of post-operative results and long-term effects will help pave a future for PRK[6-10] (58.8% of CL patients were concerned about the long-term effects of PRK). Many clinics now offer treatment of astigmatism (outside the USA), increasing the number of patients suitable for PRK. Many patients choose CL for temporary social or sports use only because CL are suitable for occasional use unlike the irreversibility of PRK. However 15.3% more PRK than CL patients favored PRK because of sport. Younger patients may choose CL because of the availability of colored CL and therefore not present for PRK; 12.8% more CL than PRK patients were concerned about cosmesis.

Reasons for choosing PRK among the 83% of prior CL wearers included prior CL wear problems such as dry eye (39.2%), CL intolerance (32.1%), or red eye (28.6%). PRK patients tended to be older as they have a more stable refraction (a stable refraction being one of the requirements for PRK) and will probably be more able to meet the costs of PRK. Costs influenced both groups of patients, the higher initial cost of PRK discouraging younger patients. The long term costs of PRK are lower and as they continue to fall more patients will favor PRK. However younger patients tend to have a more short term outlook preferring CL as demonstrated by 17.4% more CL than PRK patients concerned about the cost of PRK.

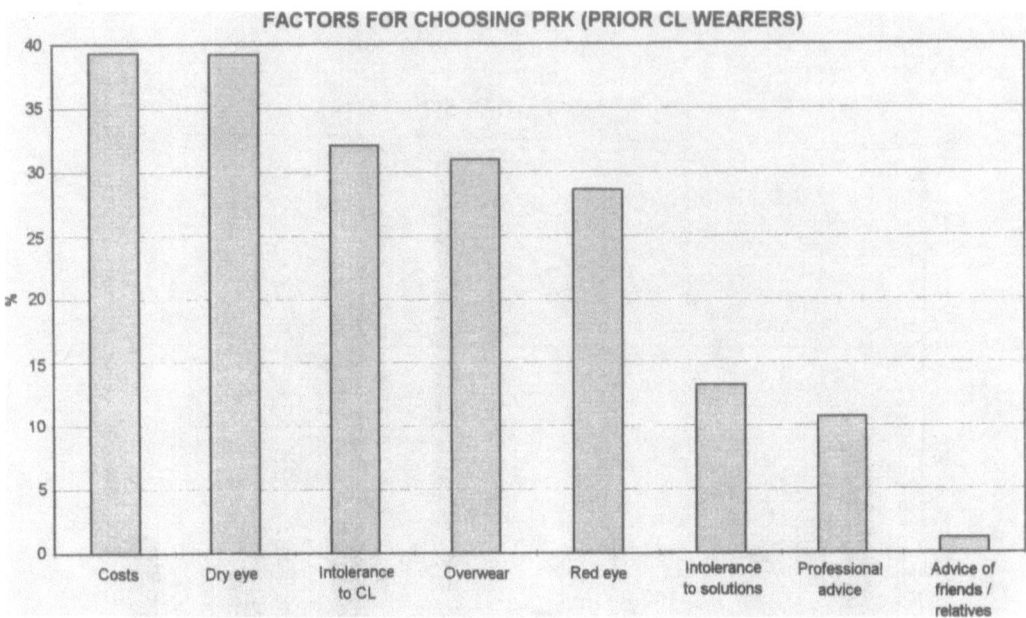

Figure 3. Factors for choosing PRK (prior CL wearers).

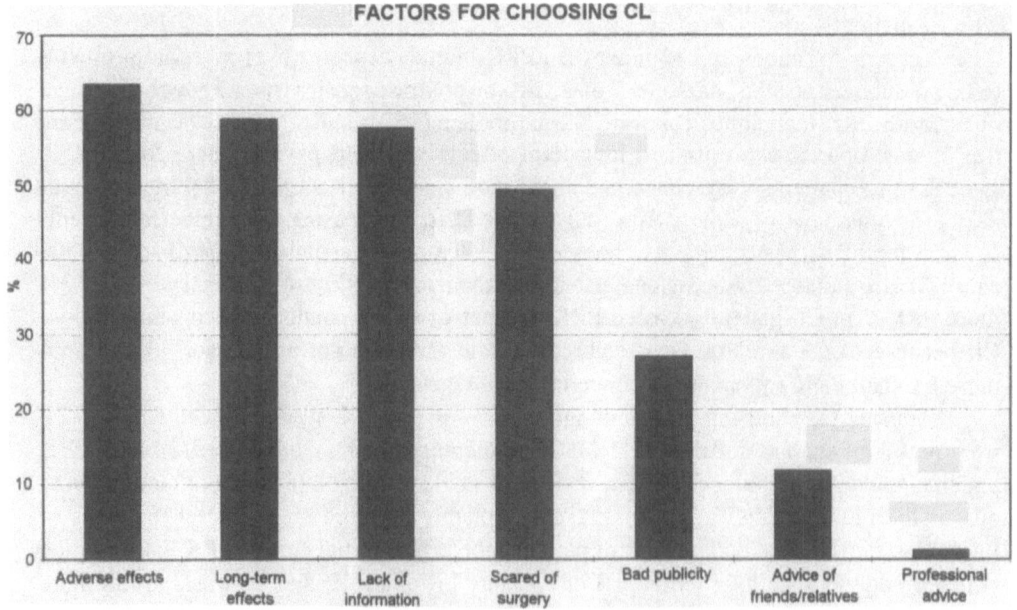

Figure 4. Factors for choosing CL.

PRK patients often travel further for their appointments than the CL group due to the smaller number of PRK clinics and incur a larger initial cost. This may result in these patients being more motivated. The CL group will usually be from the population in the locality of the CL practice.

It would appear that aggressive marketing by laser clinics is influencing large numbers of patients into PRK—in this study, 23.4% more PRK than CL patients had been influenced. Strong advertising, however, is also an effective ploy by CL companies, together with special offers by opticians on CL.

Patients presenting for PRK were more likely to seek professional advice but both groups would appear to be more inclined to seek the advice of their friends and relatives. As more patients have PRK and results improve, this factor will be even more significant.

Patients were also asked for any other comments in the questionnaire. PRK patients who were ceasing CL use remarked on being unhappy with their CL practitioner, ill-fitting CL, presbyopia, and astigmatism as reasons to stop CL use. These patients could have continued CL wear if they were better managed. Problems such as overwear, dry eyes, red eyes, allergies to solutions could also be helped by better patient compliance coupled with improved management. Many patients stated how PRK was their first choice and had not wished to try CL as they were fearful of touching their eyes, or worried about the long-term effects of CL, especially following bad publicity. Equally, many of the CL patients complained of bad publicity and also the lack of information about PRK. Some younger patients in the CL group stated that they would consider PRK in the future. One CL patient was deemed unsuitable for PRK by a laser clinic and another CL patient stated that he had never even heard of PRK.

CONCLUSION

This study set out to determine which groups of patients are most likely to present for CL and PRK and reasons for their choice. The number of patients choosing PRK due to becoming CL failures could be reduced by better management of problems by their CL practitioner. Although PRK is becoming increasingly popular, patients choosing CL are worried about the adverse effects and long-term outcome of PRK. It is therefore unlikely that PRK will become the treatment of first choice for myopia at the present time.

ACKNOWLEDGMENTS

Part of this data has been presented at the Int. Ophthalmic Excimer Laser Cong., Tring, Oxford, UK. April 1996.

REFERENCES

1. C.N.J. McGhee, Bryce, I.G., and Weed, K.H., Surgical correction of myopia and myopic astigmatism. *Eye News* 2:7 (1995).
2. G. Kahle, and Seiler, T., Report on psychosocial findings and satisfaction amongst patients 1 year after excimer laser photorefractive keratectomy. *Refract. Corneal Surg.* 8:286 (1992).
3. E. Caubet, Cause of subepithelial corneal haze over 18 months after photorefractive keratectomy for myopia. *Refract. Corneal Surg.* 9:565 (1993).

4. D.S. Gartry, Kerr Muir, M.G., and Marshall, J., Excimer laser photorefractive keratectomy. *Ophthalmol.* 99(8)1209 (1992).

5. T. Seiler, and McDonnell, P.J., Excimer laser photorefractive keratectomy: major review. *Surv. Ophthalmol.* 40(2):89 (1995).

6. S. Shah, Doyle, S.J., Chatterjee, A., et al., Debridement following excimer laser PRK. *Eur. Soc. Cataract & Refract. Surg. Amsterdam* Oct 1995.

7. B. MacInnis, Excimer laser photorefractive keratectomy. *Can. J. Ophthalmol.* 30(1):51 (1995).

8. S. Shah, Doyle, S.J., and Cory, C., Photorefractive surgery using the Nidek EC-5000 Excimer: laser requirement for a new nomogram. *United Kingdom & Ireland Soc. Cat. Refract. Surg., Dublin,* Sept. 1995

9. S. Shah, Brahma, A., Doyle, S.J., et al., Topical non-steroidal therapy for pain following excimer PRK. *Br. Excimer Keratorefract. Laser Soc. 2nd Ann. Cong.,* Harrogate, UK. Feb. (1995).

10. J.A. Vanwestenbrugge, Our experience with 5 excimer lasers. *Review of Ophthalmol.* March:61 (1995).

30

EXCIMER LASER FOR CORRECTION OF MYOPIC ASTIGMATISM AFTER PENETRATING KERATOPLASTY

Rita A. Yee Chan, Tito Ramirez Luquin, Enrique Grane Wiechers, Lourdes
Moreno, Raul Suarez, Alejandro Climent, and Roberto I. Yee Chan

Instituto de Oftamologia
Universidad Nacional Autonoma de Mexico
Mexico City

ABSTRACT

The purpose of this study was evaluate effectiveness and safety of excimer laser for
the treatment of myopic astigmatism post-penetrating keratoplasty (PKP) with keratoconus. *Methods*: Three patients (four eyes) who could not tolerate the use of contact lenses
received photorefractive keratectomy (PRK) with the Meditec Aesculap Excimer Laser. In
these patients, the mean age was 34 years old, previous PKP ranged from 4 to 9 years, uncorrected visual acuity ranged from 20/80 to 20/400, preoperative myopia range from -
0.50 to -6.50 diopters (D), and astigmatism range from -0.50 to -5.00 D. Evaluation
occurred preoperatively, as well as at 2 weeks, and 1, 3, and six months postoperatively.
Included in each evaluation were clinical examination, specular microscopy, contrast sensitivity test and corneal topography measurement.

Results indicate that all patients improved at least three lines on the Snellen Chart.
Uncorrected visual acuity range from 20/20 to 20/60. No graft rejections were observed
and one patient developed haze at the second month. Specular microscopy did not show
any statistically significant changes. Contrast sensitivity showed a decrease for the low
and middle spatial frequencies. These results suggest that PRK could be a solution for patients with significant myopic astigmatism after PKP, who cannot tolerate the use of contact lenses; and may even be a solution for those who can tolerate them.

BACKGROUND

High postoperative astigmatism is a problem primarily seen following penetrating
keratoplasty, with estimates of approximately 10% of penetrating grafts resulting in at
least 5–6 diopters of keratometric astigmatism. In keratoconic eyes this percentage may be

as high as 27%.[1,2] A number of treatment modalities, both non-surgical and surgical, may be applied in these cases and contact lenses can correct moderate corneal astigmatism. However, in cases of intolerance, additional correction in the form of spectacles or corrective surgery may be needed.[1-3]

Many surgical procedures, including relaxing incisions (e.g, radial, transverse, and arcuate), trapezoidal astigmatic keratotomy (Ruiz procedure), and wedge resection, have been described for the correction of postoperative astigmatism. Unfortunately, the results of such procedures tend to be relatively unpredictable, with large standard deviations reported in most series.[4-6]

PURPOSE

Because of the prevalence of myopic astigmatism post-penetrating keratoplasty (PKP) with keratoconus this study was undertaken to evaluate the effectiveness and safety of the excimer laser in these cases.

METHODS

Three patients (four eyes) with previous penetrating keratoplasty (PKP) who could not tolerate the use of contact lenses received photorefractive keratectomy (PRK) with the Meditec Aesculap Excimer Laser (mel 60) (Table 1).

EXCIMER LASER

1. Tetracaine was used to anesthetize the cornea.
2. Visual axis was determined with the microscope light, and the corneal epithelium was marked in the center of its reflection.
3. Epithelium was removed with methanol 18% for 30 seconds with the KIMURA spatula.
4. The suction ring (MASK for Myopia I or Myopia II) was applied on the cornea and the photoablation performed.
5. Postoperative treatment consisted of therapeutic contact lenses, topic antibiotics, analgesics and patch until the epithelium healed.

Effectiveness and safety of the procedure was evaluated with clinical examination, specular microscopy, contrast sensitivity testing, and corneal topography, which were measured preoperatively, and at two weeks, one month, three and five months postoperatively.

Table 1. Refraction before and after PRK with diameters of visual axis and ablation zone

Case	Preop Rx	Optic zone	Ablation	Postop Rx
1	-0.50 = -5.00 x 94	5.5 mm	48 μM	-1.75 x 90
2	-6.50 = -5.75 x 170	5.5 mm	90 μM	-3.00 x 3
3	-4.50 = -0.50 x 100	6.0 mm	59 μM	-0.50 x 90
4	-3.00 = -5.50 x 90	5.5 mm	51 μM	-3.75 x 74

Table 2. Visual acuity preoperative, postoperative and
best corrected visual acuity (p=0.0099)

Case	Preop VA	BCVA	6 m. Postop VA
1	20/80	20/25	20/30
2	11/200	20/50	20/60
3	20/80	20/20	20/20
4	20/180	20/30	20/40

Statistical analyses were performed with small samples and frequencies, chi squared, and student T testing.

RESULTS

1. All patients improved at least three lines on the Snellen Chart. Mean uncorrected visual acuity improved to 20/40 (range from 20/20 to 20/60) (Table 2).
2. Mean residual astigmatism was -1.50 D (Figure 1).
3. Haze was graded on a scale of 0 to 4. (O=No haze; 4=severe haze) One eye developed haze 2 (Figure 2).
4. No graft rejection was observed (Figure 3).
5. Specular microscopy did not showed any statistically changes (Figure 4 and Graphic I).
6. Contrast sensitivity test showed a decrease for the low and middle spatial frequencies.

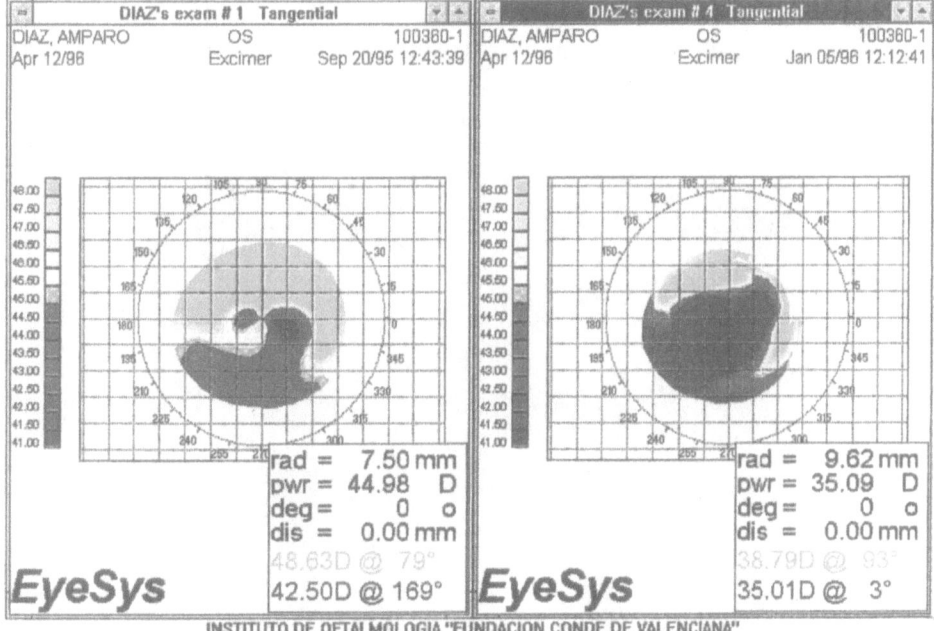

Figure 1. Tangential topography (case 2). Left = preop; right =6 months postop.

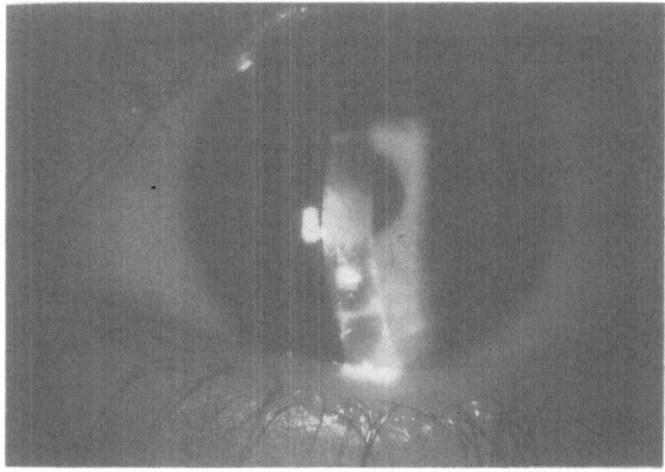

Figure 2. Case 1 developed haze.

DISCUSSION

A large number of patients and a long term follow up is needed to evaluate the resolution of the subepithelial opacity (haze) in those patients who develop it.

CONCLUSIONS

Our results suggest that the photorefractive keratectomy could be a safe and effective procedure for patients with significant myopic astigmatism after penetrating keratoplasty who cannot tolerate the use of contact lenses.

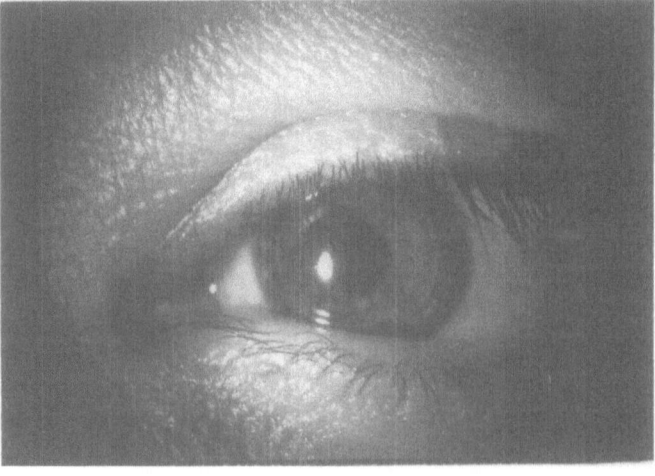

Figure 3. No corneal graft rejection was observed.

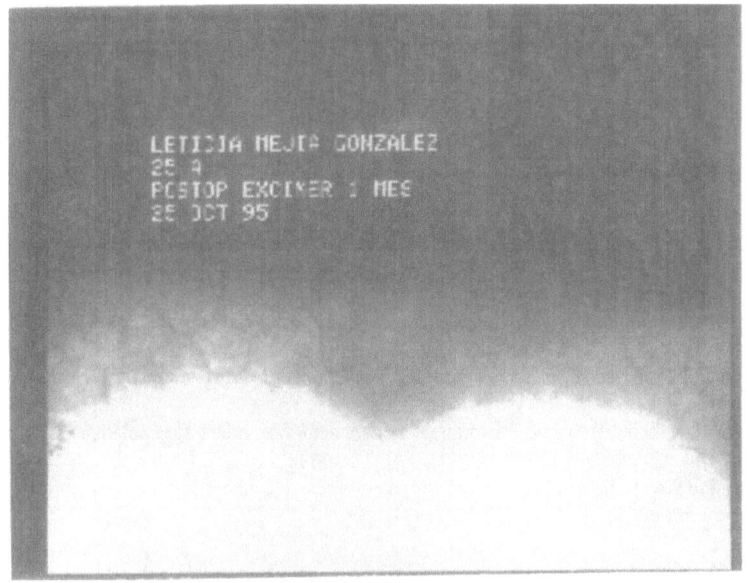

Figure 4. Specular microscopy (case 1). Left = preop; right = postop.

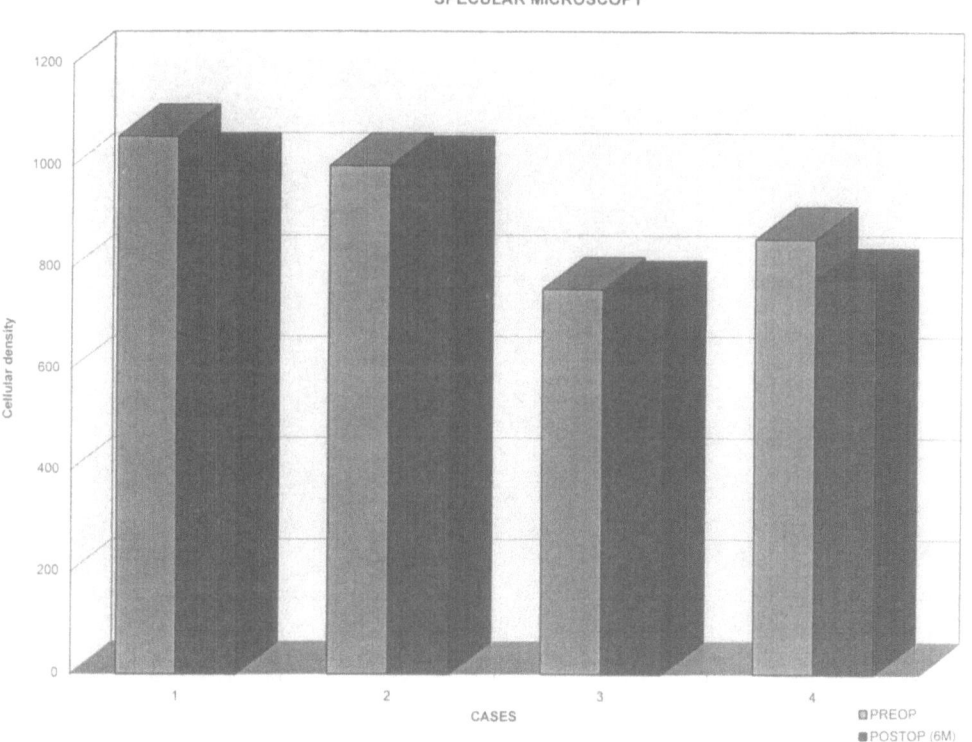

Graphic 1. Specular microscopy. No statistical difference in cellular density was observed preop and postoperatively.

ACKNOWLEDGMENTS

Partially supported by CONACYT Grant F082-I-91 10.

REFERENCES

1. C.A. Swinger, Postoperative astigmatism. *Surv. Ophtalmol*. 31(4):219 (1987).
2. J.H. Krachmer, and Fenzl, R.E., Surgical correction of high postkeratoplasty astigmatism. *Arch. Ophthalmol.* Aug. 98:1400 (1980) .
3. R.L. Lindstrom, and Lindquist, T.D., Surgical correction of postoperative astigmatism. *Cornea* 7 (2):138 (1988).
4. P.J. Mc Donnell, Moreira, H., et al., Photorefractive keratectomy for astigmatism. *Arch. Ophthalmol.* 109:1370 (1991).
5. P.J. Mc Donnell, Moreira, H., et al., Photorefractive keratectomy to create tone ablations for correction of astigmatism. *Arch. Ophthalmol.* 109:710 (1991).
6. Jae Ho Kim, Tae Won Hahn, et al., Excimer laser photorefractive keratectomy for myopia: two year follow up. *J. Cataract. Refract.* Surg. 20(Suppl.):229 (1994).

31

PHOTOTHERAPEUTIC KERATECTOMY FOR THE TREATMENT OF PERSISTENT EPITHELIAL DEFECT

Man Soo Kim, Sang Wroul Song, Tae Won Hahn, Woo Jin Sah, and
Jae Ho Kim

Catholic University Medical College
Department of Ophthalmology
Kangnam Street, St. Mary's Hospital
505 Banpo-dong, Seochu-gu
Seoul, 137-040 Korea

ABSTRACT

Persistent epithelial defect (PED) is an important ocular surface disorder. These defects can be frustrating in chronic diseases, as in the case of inflammation, chemical burn, denervated cornea, tear deficiency, and radiation keratitis. Therapeutic modalities that have been utilized in the treatment of PED include topical steroid, patching, bandage soft contact lenses, superficial keratectomy, and anterior stromal puncture. This report evaluates the use of 193 nm excimer laser (PTK) for the treatment of indolent and persistent epithelial defect as a new therapeutic device for PED.

Twelve eyes diagnosed with PED were treated with Summit excimer laser phototherapeutic keratectomy. All cases had failed to cover the epithelium with the use of therapeutic contact lenses. Laser treatment was delivered to sites surrounding the epithelial defect area to promote epithelial ingrowth.

All eyes receiving PTK were covered with new epithelium in two or three days as shown by photo refractive keratectomy and remained completely healed for at least three months of follow-up.

This study finds PTK with the 193 nm excimer laser to be a safe, effective treatment for PED that is unresponsive to conventional therapy.

INTRODUCTION

Epithelium normally regrows over the surface of an abraded cornea in a relatively rapid and predictable manner. However, there are numerous conditions and events that might either interfere with, or create non-healing epithelial defects. This persistent epithelial defect might be associated with tear film abnormalities, intrinsic epithelial disorders, basement membrane disorders, lid abnormalities, metabolic disturbances, infections, inflammation, trauma, and immune disease.[1–7] If it is not treated appropriately, this condition often leads to severe stromal melting, secondary infection, or rapid disease progression.[8,9] Conventional treatments that have been utilized in the treatment of PED include topical steroids, fibronectin, chondroitin sulfate eyedrop, patching, soft contact lens wear, and, in some cases, debridement of the diseased epithelial cells.[3,9–13] The 193 nm excimer laser has been used for such diseased epithelial and/or stromal debridement.[10,14–18] However, the 193 nm excimer laser phototherapeutic keratectomy of the entire PED lesion in active ulcer might involve the risk of perforation and aggravate the disease process. Thus the excimer laser was used to remove the heaped up margin surrounding the wound to encourage epithelial migration for achieving the therapeutic goal. This study reports on the use of 193 nm excimer laser (PTK) for the treatment of indolent and persistent epithelial defect.

MATERIALS AND METHODS

Patient Selection

Twelve eyes previously diagnosed with PED caused by chemical burn (three cases), fungal ulcer (two cases), bacterial ulcer (five cases), and metaherpetic keratitis (two cases) were treated as excimer laser phototherapeutic keratectomy. Informed consent was obtained from each patient after extensive discussion. Patients with recently developed corneal ulcer (less than 1 week) were excluded.

Instrumentation

The laser used was the Summit Excimed UV 200 (Summit Technology; Waltham, MA). The excimer laser produced 193 nm ultraviolet light with a fluence of 180 mJ/CM2 and a pulse rate of 10 Hz. To assure uniform operation, the laser was calibrated before each patient was treated. The energy transmitted through a 1.0 mm diameter therapeutic ablation setting was measured by a joulemeter built into the delivery arm. The laser system computer program was used to record parameters such as patient identification and ablation depth, rate, and diameter.

Preoperative Examination

All patients underwent complete ophthalmologic examinations, including slit-lamp corneoscopy, corneal topography, ultrasonic pachymetry, digital keratoscopy, and endothelial cell counts. Visual acuity was evaluated without correction and with manifest refraction. The defect area was measured and examined with fluorescein dye. Symptoms and PED period were recorded.

Surgical Procedure

Several drops of 1% proparacaine hydrochloride were instilled in the operative eye. The lids were prepared and draped in a sterile manner, and a wire lid speculum was inserted. The nonoperative eye was taped closed. Sometimes the pupil was restricted with pilocarpine. The patient was then asked to fixate on the coaxial blinking red light in the microscope objective and was repositioned until the image of the lesion was centered within the ablating laser beam. Before treatment, the plane of the corneal surface was determined by focusing the microscope at a magnification of x18, and treatment was performed at a magnification of x12. Visualizing the patient's eyes through the microscope and video monitors, the surgeon aligned the corneal lesion to the laser plane by adjusting table travel in the x, y, and z directions. The eye was fixated with a forceps or Thornton ring (Storz, U.S.A) to stabilize the position of the eye during the laser exposure. The laser delivered a series of pulses at each setting, according to the preoperative specifications entered into the computer, to sites surrounding the epithelial defect for promotion of epithelial ingrowth. The ablation was carried out and the process repeated until a smoother corneal ablative bed was achieved.

Postoperative Regimen

Before epithelial healing, the eye drops (which were determined by the individual underlying disease) were instilled continuously. The 0.1% fluorometholone was added after epithelial healing had occurred. Postoperative complications were defined as the presence of recurrent epithelial defect, reactivation of corneal ulcer, aggravation of disease and graft rejection. Postoperative evaluations were performed at one, two, three, and seven days; two weeks; and one, three, and six months.

RESULTS

Twelve eyes in 12 patients underwent PTK for persistent epithelial defect between July 1995 and November 1995. Preoperative etiologies for the persistent epithelial defect included bacterial ulcer in five eyes, metaherpetic keratitis in two eyes, fungal ulcer in two eyes, and chemical burn in three eyes (Table 1). Before excimer laser treatment, patients had received the conventional treatments for PED. All patients had failed therapy

Table 1. Clinical data of phototherapeutic keratectomy for the treatment of persistent epithelial defect

Patient	Preoperative diagnosis	Duration Pulse of PED	Healing period*	Follow up duration**	Past history
1. OS F/82	B. ulcer	29 - 300	6	5	
2. OS M/45	B. ulcer	21 - 500	3	5	PPKP
3. OD F/71	B. ulcer	23 - 500	7	2	DM
4. OD F/61	B. ulcer	55 - 850	7	6	NVG
5. OS F/22	B. ulcer	15 - 500	7	3	Uveitis, Phlyctenulosis
6. OS F/57	F. ulcer	120 - 800	11	6	Foreign body
7. OS F/64	F. ulcer	34 - 400	5	3	
8. OS M/47	Herpes	59 - 1000	7	5	
9. OD F/55	Herpes	43 - 200	5	4	
10. OD M/28	Chemical Burn	137- 500	7	5	PPKP
11. OD M/47	Chemical Burn	271 - 500	4	3	PPKP
12. OS F/51	Chemical Burn	20 - 800	7	4	

*Days; **Months; PED: Persistent Epithelial Defect; B: Bacterial Ulcer; F: Fungus; PPKP: Partial penetrating Keratoplasty; DM: Diabetes mellitus; NVG: Neovascular glaucoma.

with any eyedrop, patching, and bandage soft contact lens treatment. Mean duration of PED was 69 days. Postoperatively, patients were followed for from three months to six months. The goal of treatment of the patients was to cover the epithelial defect. All cases receiving PTK were covered with new epithelium. Reepithelialization usually occurred within two or three days following PTK as expected in photorefractive keratectomy, and was completed within seven days. PED remained completely healed throughout the follow up. One case (patient 10) developed epithelial defect in a different site on the cornea. Patients in this study did not experience any complication like perforation, graft rejection experienced by postkeratoplasty patients, and the recurrence in the herpetic patients in the follow up period.

CASE REPORT (PATIENT 8)

A 47-year old male had a geographic ulcer in May, 1995. Although the treatment with bandage soft contact lens was performed for 59 days, the epithelial defect was not improved (Figure 1). A 50 um, 1,000 pulse, 193 nm excimer laser ablation was performed to the site of the surrounding epithelial defect, heaped up margin. Seven days following PTK, no epithelial defect was found (Figure 2). No further corneal erosion developed and visual acuity was 4/20.

DISCUSSION

The use of UV radiation at 193 nm wavelength to remove a precise amount of tissue from the anterior cornea was first suggested by Trokel et al.[19] Since the early 1980s, the 193 nm ArF excimer laser has undergone rapid development in the clinical field of ophthalmology. The excimer laser emits pulses of ultraviolet light that ablate the cornea with

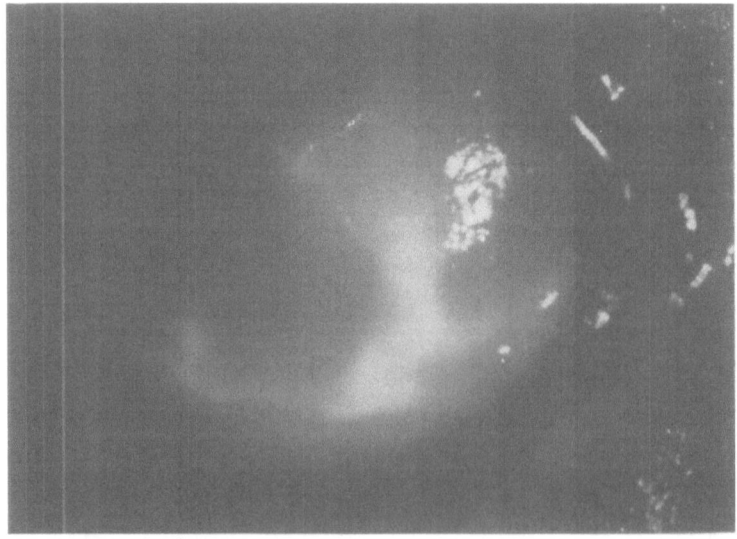

Figure 1. Before excimer laser ablation, persistent epithelial defect was showed in a metaherpetic ulcer.

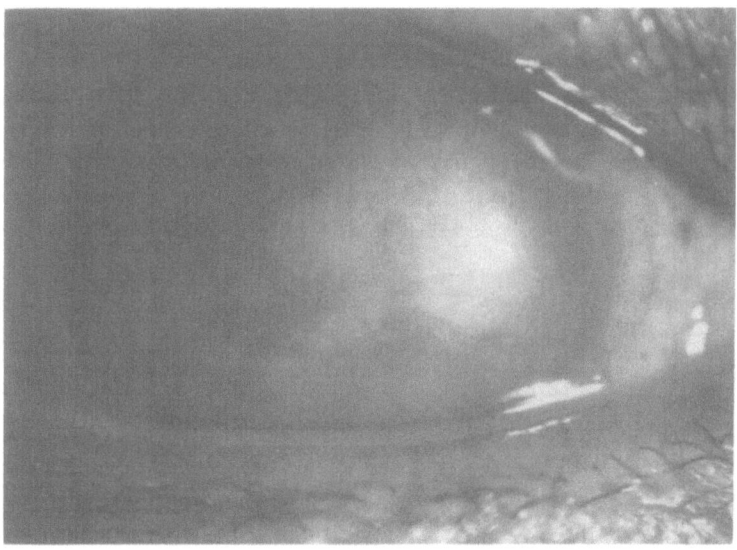

Figure 2. After excimer laser ablation, no epithelial defect was shown.

submicron precision and minimal distortion to adjacent tissue.[18,19] It has been demonstrated that the procedure of removing precise amounts of superficial corneal epithelium and stroma offers a potentially beneficial effect by leaving an optically smooth surface, reformation of basement membrane complexes, and minimal corneal scarring.[19-22] The 193 nm excimer laser has been used for phototherapeutic keratectomy in the treatment of recurrent corneal erosion syndrome, anterior stromal and superficial scarring from postinfectious and posttraumatic causes, including inactive HSV keratitis, anterior corneal dystrophies, granular dystrophy, and band keratopathy.[14-18] The capability of the excimer laser to remove small amounts of corneal tissue precisely and leave the surface of the cornea smooth, with subsequent regeneration of corneal epithelium and adhesion complexes,[15,20-22] might offer a therapeutic benefit to patients with PED. Thus, patients in this study were treated with the excimer laser for PED.

Epithelial defect in recalcitrant cases persist despite treatment with numerous therapeutic regimens on the especially denervated cornea, diabetic cornea, and actively inflamed cornea.[1-7,10] Pathobiology of PED has not yet been clarified. One explanation for the pathobiology of PED is that the basement membrane was damaged during the course of diabetes and herpes infection, and corneal epithelial cells could not attach.[10,23] PED with rolled-up epithelium at the ulcer edge is presumably caused by weak adhesion of epithelial cells to Bowman's membrane. Other factors include drug toxicity, eyelid dysfunction, tear deficiency, autoimmune disease, ocular inflammation, and perilimbal epithelial loss.[1,7,24,25] In this study, factors associated with PED, including dry eye, inflammation, denervated cornea, diabetes, and PPKP, were found. All the eyes had previously failed treatment with conventional medical therapy. All cases were completely covered with new epithelium after excimer laser photokeratectomy. These findings, namely, the flattening of rolled-up epithelium at the PED margin, the subsided area of epithelial defect, and the absence of fluorescent staining, show that PTK, removing the heaped up margin surrounding the wound, only facilitates reepithelialization. It was also found that once epithelialization was completed, epithelial defects did not recur and remained covered with new epithelium without graft rejection, reactivation of ulcer, or perforation in the follow-up period. The mechanism of this therapeutic modality also encourages the new epithelial cell to cover the defective area for removing the barrier. This new technique has several advantages, as follows: There is less risk of perforation, no refractive change, relief of symptoms, and rapid epithelial healing. It is believed that this procedure can offer a significant number of selected patients relief for PED. The long term effects of excimer laser photokeratectomy for PED must be observed carefully and the suitability of the procedure for various conditions must be evaluated critically.

CONCLUSION

Although the follow up period was short, PTK with the 193 nm excimer laser was found to be a safe and effective treatment for indolent and persistent epithelial defect patients unresponsive to conventional medical therapy. Therefore excimer laser phototherapeutic methods might be promising for promotion of epithelial healing on the compromised cornea.

REFERENCES

1. R. R. Pfister, Clinical measures to promote corneal epithelial healing. *Acta. Ophtalmologica* 70: 73 (1992).
2. R.R. Pfister, and Burstein N., The effects of ophthalmic drugs, vehicles, and preservatives on corneal epithelium: a scanning electron microscope study. *Invest. Ophthalmol.* 15: 246 (1976).
3. L.T. Groden, White, W., and Updegraff, S., Porcine collagen corneal shield treatment of persistent epithelial defects following penetrating keratoplasty. *Invest. Ophthalmol. Vis. Sci.* 30(Suppl): 340 (1989).
4. W.D. Mathers, Shields, B.S., Sachdev, M.S., et al., Meibomian gland dysfunction in chronic blepharitis. *Cornea* 10: 286 (1991).
5. R. R. Pfister and Murphy, G.E., Corneal ulceration and perforation associated with Sjögrens syndrome. *Arch. Ophthalmol.* 98: 89 (1980).
6. H.R. Taylor and Kinsey, R.A., Corneal epithelial basement membrane changes in diabetes. *Invest. Ophthalmol. Vis. Sci.* 20: 458 (1981).
7. M.D. Wagoner, Kenyon, K.R., Gipson, I.K., et al. Polymorphonuclear neutrophils delay corneal epithelial wound healing *in vitro. Invest. Ophthalmol. Vis. Sci.* 25: 1217 (1984).
8. M. Grayson., Viral diseases. In: K. Kimberly, editor, *Diseases of the Cornea*, Third Edition, Mosby Co., St. Louis (1991).
9. Teruo Nishida, Ohashi, Y., Awata, T., et al., Fibronectin. *Arch. Ophthalmol.* 101: 1046 (1983)
10. R.T. Audrey, Neal, A.S., Donald, D.D., et al., Phototherapeutic keratectomy for the treatment of recurrent corneal erosion. In *Medical Cornea - Corneal and Refractive Surgery,* R.E. Selser, ed., Kugler Publication, New York (1994).
11. E.N. McLean, MacRae, S.M., and Rich, L.J., Recurrent erosion: treatment by anterior stromal puncture. *Ophthalmol.* 93: 784 (1986).
12. S.I. Brown, and Bondino, B.J., Therapy of Mooren's ulcer. *Am. J. Ophthalmol.* 98: 1 (1984).
13. R.S. Rubinfeld, Laibson P.R., Cohen, E.J., et al., Anterior stromal puncture for recurrent erosion: further experience and new instrumentation. *Ophthalmic Surg.* 21: 318 (1990).
14. A.S. Neal, Richard A.B., Ralph, W.Z., et al., Clinical use of the 193 nm excimer laser in the treatment of corneal scars. *Arch. Ophthalmol.* 109: 491 (1991).
15. J.S. Walter, Wallace, C., Mary T.K., et al., Clinical follow up of 193 nm ArF excimer laser photokeratectomy. *Ophthalmol.* 99: 805 (1991).
16. S.S. Harry., Successful treatment of recurrent corneal erosion with Nd:YAG anterior stromal puncture. *Am. J. Ophthalmol.* 110: 404 (1990).
17. M.T. Daniel., Francis, A.L., Jr., L'esperance, J., et al., Human excimer laser lamellar keratectomy: a clinical study. *Ophthalmol.* 96: 654 (1989).

18. C.S. Wilson, Walter, J.S., and Green, W.R., Corneal wound healing after 193 nm excimer laser keratectomy. *Arch. Ophthalmol.* 109: 1429 (1991).

19. S.L. Trokel, Srinivasan R., and Braren, B.A., Excimer laser surgery of the cornea. *Am. J. Ophthalmol.* 96: 710 (1983).

20. J. Marshall, Trokel, S.L., Rothery S., and Krueger, R.R., Long term healing of the central cornea after photorefractive keratectomy using an excimer laser. *Ophthalmol.* 95: 1411 (1988).

21. G.L. Goodman, Trolkel, S.L., Stark, W.J., et al., Corneal healing following laser refractive keratectomy. *Arch. Ophthalmol.* 107: 1799 (1989).

22. A.L. Michael, Corneal wound healing after excimer laser photokeratectomy. In: *Medical Cornea-Corneal and Refractive Surgery* Selser, R.E., Jr., ed., Kugler Publication, New York (1994).

23. T. Nishida, Nakagawa, S., and Manabe, R., Clinical evaluation of fibronectin eyedrops on epithelial disorders after herpes keratitis. *Ophthalmol.* 92: 213 (1985).

24. T. Nishida, Yagi., J., Fukuda, M., et al., Spontaneous persistent epithelial defects after cataract surgery. *Cornea* 6: 32 (1987).

25. R.R. Pfister, Haddox, K.D., Dodson, R.W., and Deshazo, W.J., Polymorphonuclear leucutic inhibition by citrate, other metal chelators, and trifluoperazine. *Invest. Ophthalmol. Vis. Sci.* 25: 955 (1984).

32

CORNEAL ENDOTHELIAL MORPHOLOGY AND BARRIER FUNCTION FOLLOWING EXCIMER LASER PHOTOREFRACTIVE KERATECTOMY

Ki-San Kim,[1] Sae-Jin Jeon,[1] and Henry F. Edelhauser[2]

[1]Department of Ophthalmology
Dongsan Medical Center
Keimyung University, Korea
[2]Department of Ophthalmology
Emory University Eye Center
Atlanta, Georgia

ABSTRACT

To investigate the effect of deep stromal excimer laser ablation on corneal endothelial morphology and barrier function, excimer laser photorefractive keratectomy (PRK) was performed to obtain residual corneal thickness between 90–250 µm in NZW rabbit corneas (N=50). Corneal endothelium was stained with Alizarin red S for 2 minutes three days after excimer laser ablation, and analyzed morphometrically. Five groups of PRK were performed to obtain three residual corneal thicknesses of 150, 175, and 200 µm in one eye of NZW rabbits (N=30), and also to ablate -6 D and -12 D of correction (N=10). The paired corneas were used as control. Three days after PRK, corneal endothelial permeability was measured according to the method of Watsky et al. and compared to control. Corneas with residual thickness of 90–130 µm showed severe corneal endothelial damage. In 130–200 µm of residual thickness, the damage was inversely proportional to the residual corneal thickness (p<0.05). In corneas of residual thickness over 200 µm, endothelial damages were rarely seen. Corneal endothelial Pac (mean ± SD) three days following -6 and -12 diopter of PRK were 3.21 ± 0.76, and 3.25 ± 1.16 x 10^{-4} cm/min which were similar to control (p>0.1). Three days following PRK, corneal endothelial Pac with residual corneal thickness of 200 µm was 3.28 ± 0.55 x 10^{-4} cm/min which was also similar to control, whereas Pac with residual thickness of 175 µm and 150 µm were 3.68 ± 0.82, and 3.97 ± 0.58 x 10^{-4} cm/min, which were significantly different from control (p<0.05). EM showed an intact monolayer of hexagonal endothelial cells, intact intercellular junctions, and normal subcellular organelles, but amorphous granular material ap-

Advances in Corneal Research, edited by Lass
Plenum Press, New York, 1997

peared within posterior Descemet's membrane in all excimer laser treated corneas suggesting that the endothelial cells were stimulated to secrete. The results of this study showed that corneal endothelial morphology and barrier function were maintained if ablation level did not go beyond 200 μm of residual corneal thickness. Deeper stromal ablation caused both a morphologic changes and impaired barrier function.

INTRODUCTION

Photorefractive keratectomy (PRK) offers good predictability, efficacy, and safety.[1-3] However, its potential risk to the corneal endothelium is still unknown. Many studies have been undertaken to assess the effect of excimer laser ablation on the corneal endothelium.[4-11] Previous animal studies have shown that excimer laser incision could cause endothelial damage if the ablation incision depth was within 40 μm of Descemet's membrane.[4] Other authors[5] have demonstrated that excimer laser keratotomies performed in rabbits could induce endothelial changes such as cellular edema and formation of an incisional ridge, but did not affect the endothelial cell density. Clinically, it has been demonstrated that PRK caused no damage to the corneal endothelium.[12-15]

Corneal endothelial cells may be affected in various ways by excimer laser ablation. Fluorescence from and scattering of the incident laser beam can result in long wavelength radiation which can be absorbed by deep corneal layers. In addition, acoustic and shock waves are generated by the ultrashort energy pulses and by target recoil as tissue is ablated from the corneal surface. Pulse repetition may result in resonance at the posterior corneal surface.[12] Thus high repetition rates (over 80 Hz) used during excimer laser corneal surgery may cause irreversible damage to the corneal endothelium.[11]

Shallow excimer laser ablation appears to be free of corneal endothelial damage. However, deeper ablation is needed to correct higher myopia. In particular, in excimer laser assisted *in situ* keratomileusis (LASIK), laser ablation is closer to the corneal endothelium. Endothelial cells close to the photoablative process may be directly or indirectly damaged by the laser beam. Therefore, it is important to quantify the maximal ablation depth at PRK without causing endothelial damage. The purpose of this study was to investigate if deep stromal excimer laser ablation can affect the corneal endothelial cells morphometrically and functionally, and to establish the depth of excimer laser ablation that will not cause the endothelial damage.

MATERIALS AND METHODS

Endothelial Morphology

Fifty New Zealand white rabbits (2–3 kg) were anethetized intramuscularly with ketamine chloride (5 mg/kg) and xylazine hydrochloride (95 mg/kg). Topical 0.5% proparacaine hydrochloride was instilled and the eyelids were held open with a wire speculum. Central corneal thickness was measured using an ultrasonic pachymeter, and the depth to be ablated was calculated. 193 nm excimer laser (ExciMed UV 200LA, Summit Technology, Inc.; Waltham, MA, USA) photorefractive keratectomy (PRK) was performed randomly to obtain various residual central corneal thicknesses calculated within a range of 90–250 μm. The corneal epithelium was not removed before PRK. The repetition rate was 10 Hz, and the pulse energy density was 180 mJ/Cm^2. The ablation zone diameter was 5 mm. Colistin-erythromycin eye ointment and tobramycin eye solution were instilled four times a day for three days after PRK. Rabbits were euthanized with overdose of sodium pentobarbital IV (80 mg/kg) at three days postoperative. Eyeballs were enucleated, and the corneas were excised. The corneal endothelium was stained with Alizarin red S (0.2%, pH 4.2)(Sigma Chemical Co.; St. Louis, MO, USA) for two minutes, and photographs were taken and developed. Cells were observed and analyzed morphometrically using a computer-assisted digitizer and compared to normal controls (N=6).

Endothelial Permeability Measurement

For the endothelial permeability study, different groups of rabbits were included. Five groups of excimer laser PRK were performed to obtain three residual corneal thicknesses of 150, 175, and 200 μm in one eye of rabbits (N=30), and also to ablate -6 D and -12 D of correction (N=10). The paired corneas were used as a control. Corneal endothelial permeability (Pac) was measured according to the method of Watsky et al.[16] and compared to control. Three days after PRK, rabbits were euthanized and the corneal epithelium was removed by scraping with a corneal Gill knife. Corneas with a 1 to 2 mm corneoscleral rim were mounted in a thermostatically controlled (34°C) dual chambered perfusion *in vitro* specular microscope.[17,18] Silicone oil (Dow Chemical Co.; Midland, MI) was applied to the anterior stromal surface to prevent desiccation and to optically couple the objective of the microscope to the tissue. The endothelium was perfused with GBR (Glutathione-Bicarbonate-Ringer solution) at a rate of 100 μl/minute (pH 7.2 $\pm$ 0.1, mOsmol= 302). Temperature and hydrostatic pressure were maintained at 34°C and between 15 to 20 mmHg respectively. Stromal thickness was measured at 15-minute intervals using a calibrated digital counter coupled to the fine-focus adjustment of the specular microscope.

Corneas were mounted in the specular microscope and the endothelium perfused for a one-hour stabilization period. The silicone oil was then removed from the anterior stromal surface with a disposable plastic pipette, and the surface was blotted free of oil with cellulose sponges (Weckcel; Research Triangle Park, NC). Then, 0.3 ml of a 2.6 x 10^{-4} M CF solution (Eastman Kodak; Rochester, NY) was applied to this oil-free surface for 30 seconds. The CF solution was removed, the anterior stromal surface was blotted free of residual CF solution, and silicone oil was reapplied. Immediately thereafter, an air bubble was injected at the origin of the outflow tubing in order to accurately determine the location of the dye within the outflow and minimize dead space perfusate. Upon passage of the bubble through the distal end of the outflow tube, the perfusate was collected in a preweighed test tube for 30 minutes during which three corneal thickness readings were taken. At this time, the perfusion pump was stopped, the outflow tube was placed in a different preweighed plastic tube, and the perfusate remaining under the cornea and in the outflow tubing was collected by injecting a large bolus of air through a valve located at the junction of the inflow tubing and the perfusion chamber. The weights of fluid in each of the test tubes were determined and expressed as milliliters of fluid (specific gravity assumed to be 1 ml/g). The perfusion block was disassembled, the cornea was removed and the peripheral scleral rim was excised. The cornea was blotted dry with a cellulose sponge, and was eluted in 20 ml BSS (Alcon Laboratories; Fort Worth, TX) at 4°C for 48 hr to allow for equilibration of the free dye in the stroma with the BSS and to measure stromal dye mass (Ms). The mass of CF in the perfusate (Mp) and eluate (Ms) were determined fluorometrically.

The cornea-aqueous transfer coefficient (kc.ca) and endothelial permeability (Pac) were calculated as: kc.ca = { ln (Mp + Ms) - ln Ms }/t , Pac = kc.ca x Rca x q where t is the time following dye application (30 minutes), Rca is the steady-state distribution ratio (a rabbit value of 1.07 was used), and q is the average stromal thickness from the three final thickness readings of each perfusion.

Electron Microscopy

In the same way as in the permeability study, for ultrastructural studies, three days after PRK the corneas (N=20) were mounted in the specular microscope and the endothelium was perfused with GBR for one hour. The corneas were then fixed in 2.5% glutaraldehyde containing phosphate buffer. After fixation, each cornea was bisected. One half of each cornea was processed for scanning electron microscopy (SEM) and the other half for transmission electron microscopy (TEM). The corneas were postfixed in 2% osmium tetroxide for two hours, dehydrated, and embedded in LX-112 resin (Ladd Research Industries, Inc.; Burlington, VT). They were thin sectioned, stained with uranyl acetate and lead citrate, and viewed with a JEOL 100 CX transmission electron microscope. The other half of the cornea was prepared for scanning electron microscopy by postfixation in 3% osmium tetroxide dehydration (Ted Pella, Inc.; Redding, CA) using Paldri II as a substitute for critical point drying. The tissue was glued to stubs, sputter-coated with gold-palladium, and viewed with a JEOL 35 CF scanning electron microscope.

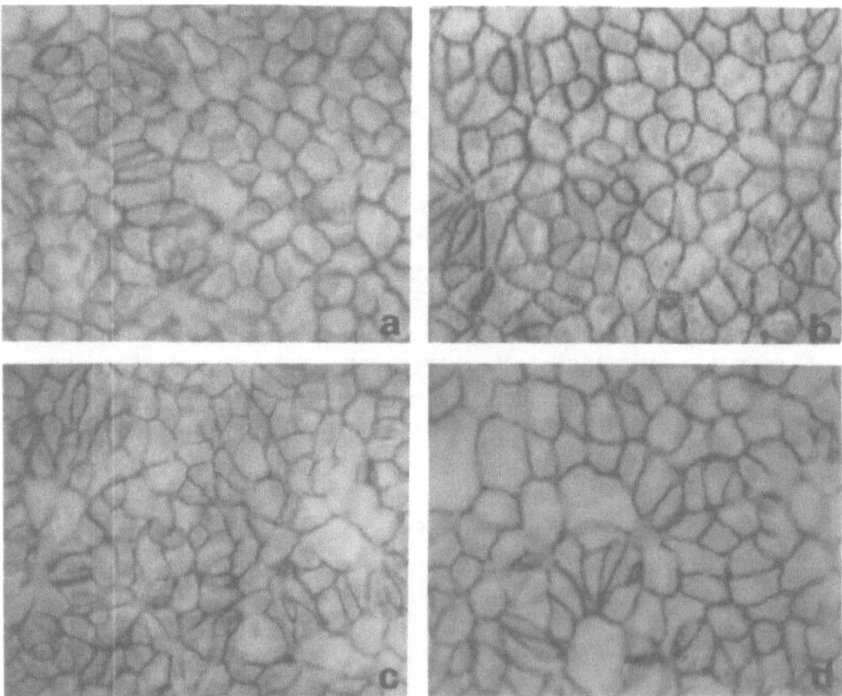

Figure 1. Photographs of rabbit corneal endothelium three days following excimer laser ablation. Residual corneal thickness of 141 μm (a), 130 μm (b), 115 μm (c), and 92 μm (d). Hexagonal shaped cells were rarely observed. Many elongated or round and small or rosette-like cells were found (Alizarin Red S stain, x100).

RESULTS

Average corneal thickness of rabbits was 334.82 ± 23.55 μm (range; 295–404 μm), average ablation depth was 173.13 ± 51.11 μm (range; 62–248 μm), and average residual thickness was 161.18 ± 47.75 μm (range; 95–255 μm). Corneal endothelial damage occurred in corneas with a residual corneal thickness of 90–130μm. Hexagonal shaped cells were rarely observed; most intercellular junctions remained separated; and many elongated, or round and small, or rosette-like cells were found. In corneas of residual thickness between 130 and 150 μm, the cells were pleomorphic, and there were some areas of missing cells (Fig. 1). Between 150 and 200 μm of residual thickness, the endothelium had large endothelial cells and pleomorphic areas were found (Fig. 2). These changes were inversely proportional to the residual corneal thickness ($p<.01$). In corneas of residual thickness over 200 μm, endothelial changes were rarely seen (Fig. 3). There were no significant changes in endothelial cell density or area, while percentage of hexagonal cells (pleomorphism), coefficient of variation of the cell area (polymegathism), and shape factor correlated significantly with the decrease of the residual corneal thickness ($P<.01$)(Fig. 4).

Corneal endothelial Pac (mean $\pm$ SD) three days following -6 and -12 diopter of PRK were 3.21 ± 0.76, and 3.25 ± 1.16 x 10^{-4} cm/min and were not statistically different from controls (3.08 ± 1.25, 3.32 ± 0.94 x 10^{-4} cm/min, respectively)($p>0.1$). Three days following PRK, corneal endothelial Pac with residual corneal thickness of 200 μm was

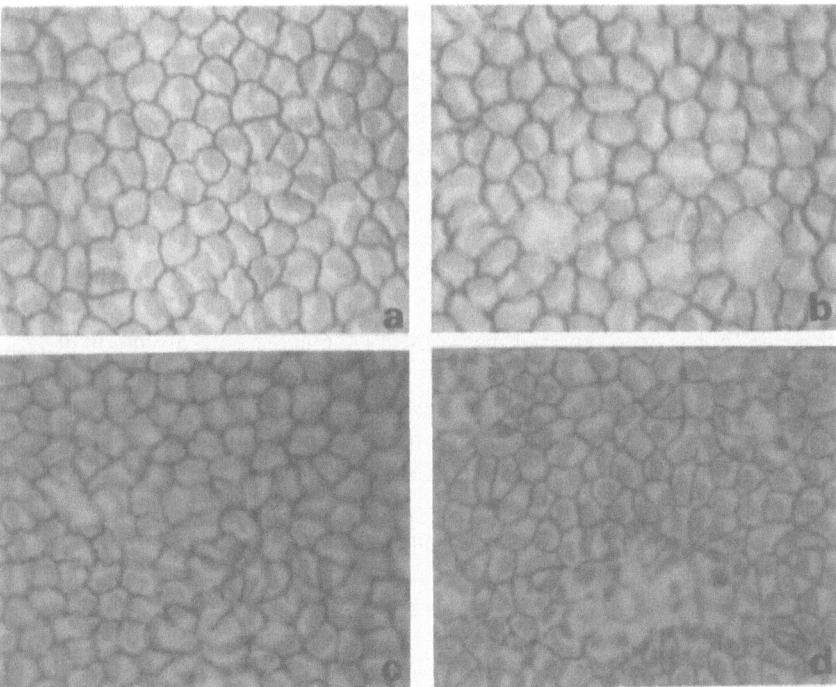

Figure 2. Photographs of rabbit corneal endothelium three days following excimer laser ablation. Residual corneal thickness of 190 μm (a), 180 μm (b), 162 μm (c), and 150 μm (d). Large cells and abnormal shaped cells became less with residual corneal thickness (Alizarin Red S stain, x100).

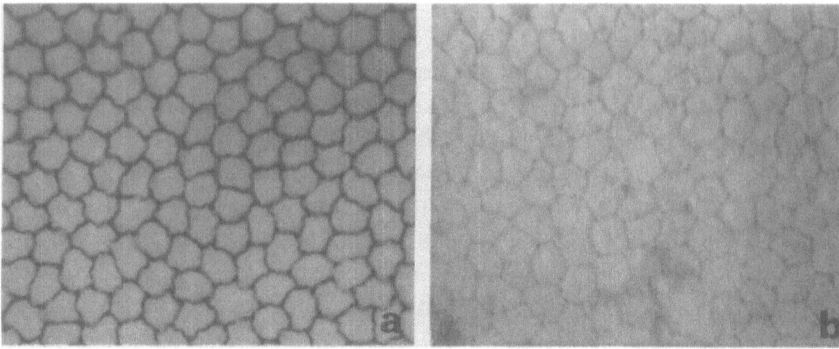

Figure 3. Photographs of normal rabbit corneal endothelium (a). Rabbit corneal endothelium three days following excimer laser ablation. Residual corneal thickness of 210 µm (b). Normal hexagonal shaped corneal endothelium was observed (Alizarin Red S stain, x100).

$3.28 \pm 0.55 \times 10^{-4}$ cm/min, which was also similar to control results ($3.11 \pm 0.54 \times 10^{-4}$), while Pac with residual thickness of 175 µm and 150 µm were 3.68 ± 0.82, and $3.97 \pm 0.53 \times 10^{-4}$ cm/min, which were significantly increased compared to control (3.02 ± 0.48, $3.10 \pm 0.54 \times 10^{-4}$ cm/min, respectively)($p<0.05$)(Fig. 5).

Electronmicrography obtained three days after excimer laser ablation showed a regular hexagonal cell pattern, normal cellular organelles, and intact intercellular junction in corneas with 6 and 12 diopter of correction (Figs. 6–8) and 200, 175, and 150 µm of residual corneal thickness (Figs. 9–11). Corneas with 175 and 150µm of residual corneal thickness showed endothelial shape changes. There was the presence of an amorphous fibrillogranular material deposited in posterior Descemet's membrane in all excimer laser treated corneas. Higher magnification of TEM showed many electron dense amorphous material at outer surface of basal plasma membrane close to Descemet's membrane suggesting lipofuscin pigments secreted from stressed endothelial cell (Fig. 12).

DISCUSSION

It generally has been reported that corneal endothelial cells are not damaged by excimer laser ablation. In clinical studies,[12–15] there were no endothelial changes reported even with a -17.00 diopter correction. However, experimental studies have shown that excimer laser ablation can affect the adjacent tissue. In particular, deeper ablation can alter the corneal endothelial cells. One previous study[7] reported no endothelial changes after non-perforating excimer laser keratectomies. These investigators stated that there were mild cell contact alterations and discrete single cell damage even with the 90% deep excimer laser incisions. Marshall et al.[4] found endothelial cell loss in rabbit corneas beneath the line of excimer laser irradiation in non-perforating incisions with ablation within 40 µm of Descemet's membrane. Dehm et al.[5] observed that 193 nm excimer laser incisions to 90% of corneal depth in rabbit corneas also produced endothelial changes, although endothelial cell loss was not observed. In this study, however, in corneas with residual corneal thickness of 90–130µm, endothelial cell changes were difficult to analyze with a digitizer, and there was marked polymegathism. In corneas with a residual thickness over 130 µm, there was a significant correlation between thickness and coefficient of variation

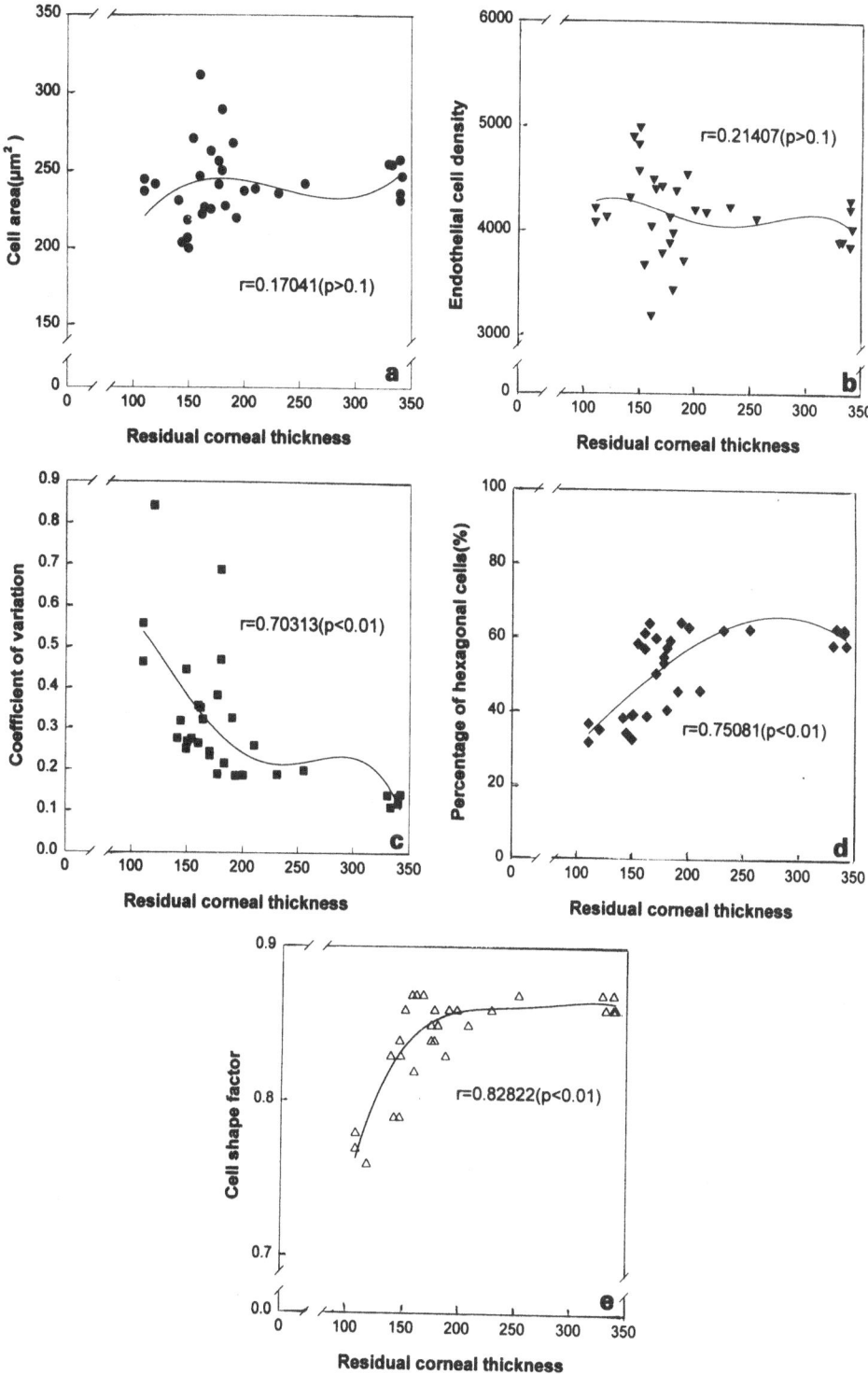

Figure 4. Scattergrams of endothelial cell morphometry with different residual corneal thickness. Endothelial cell area (a) and density (b) showed no significant changes with the decrease of the residual corneal thickness while coefficient of variation of the cell area (c), percentage of hexagonal cell (d), and endothelial cell shape factor (e) showed significant changes.

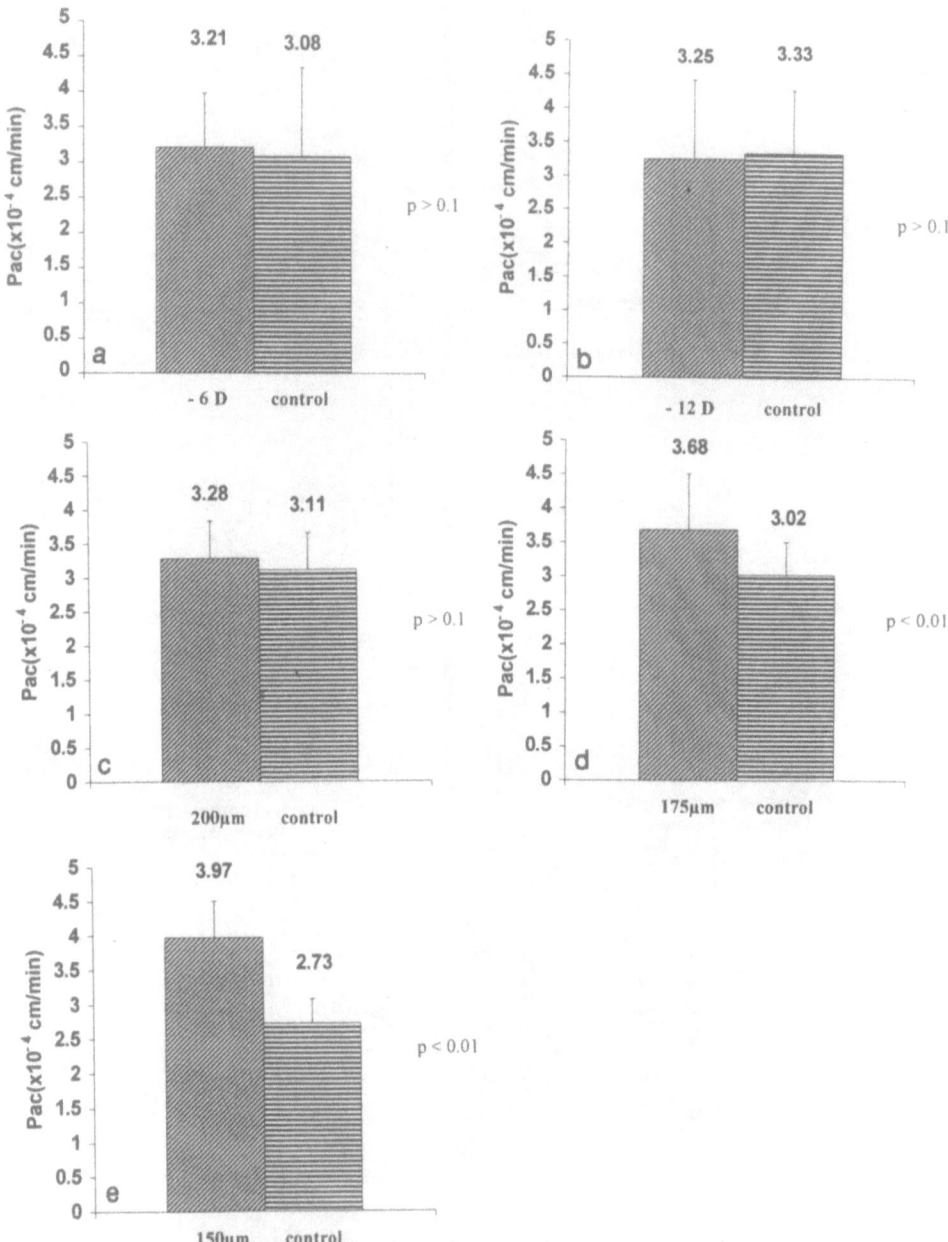

Figure 5. Corneal endothelial Pac in rabbit corneas (N=40) three days following -6 diopter (a) and -12 diopter(b) of photorefractive keratectomy showed no significant difference from control corneas. In corneas with the residual corneal thickness of 200 μm (c) following excimer laser ablation, endothelial Pac was similar to control. Residual corneal thickness of 175 (d) and 150 μm (e) showed significant increase of endothelial Pac compared to control.

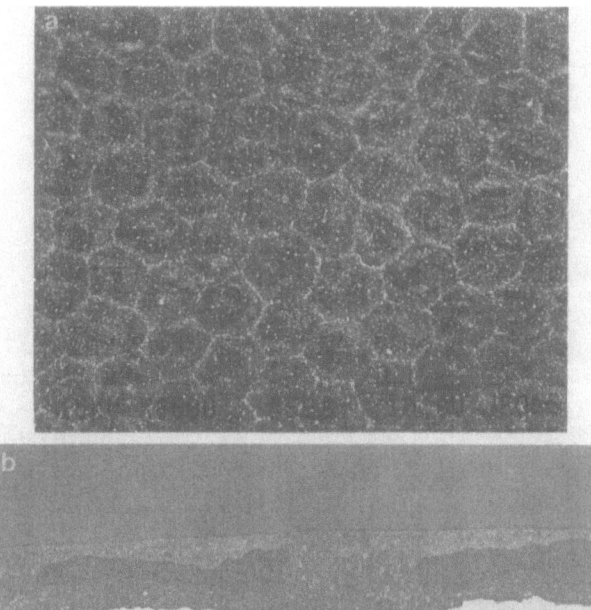

Figure 6. Scanning (a, x1000) and transmission (b, x4640) electron micrographs of control rabbit corneas perfused with glutathione-bicarbonate-Ringer solution for one hour showing intact mosaic pattern of endothelial cells.

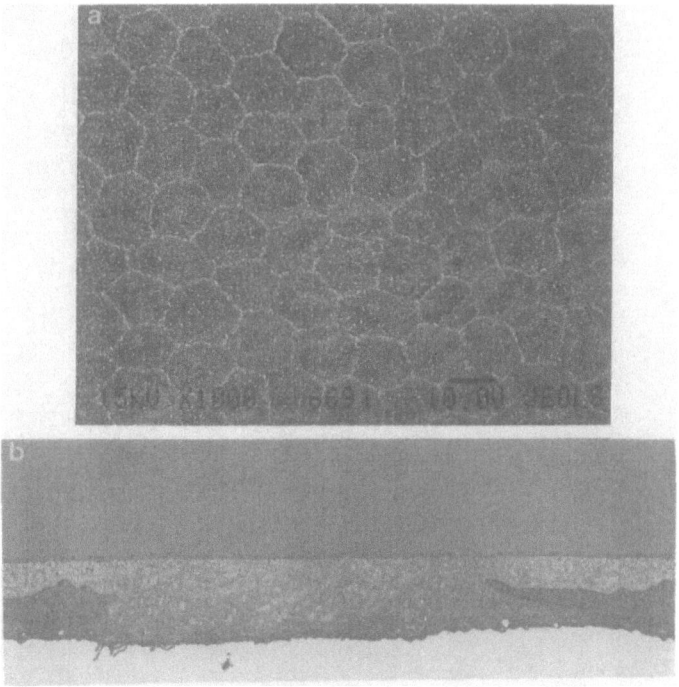

Figure 7. Scanning and transmission electron micrographs of rabbit corneas (perfused with GBR) three days after -6 D of excimer laser PRK. SEM (a) shows an intact monolayer of hexagonal endothelial cells (x1000). TEM (b) shows intact intercellular junctions, normal subcellular organelles, but a sheet of dark amorphous material in Descemet's membrane adjacent endothelial cell l(x4640).

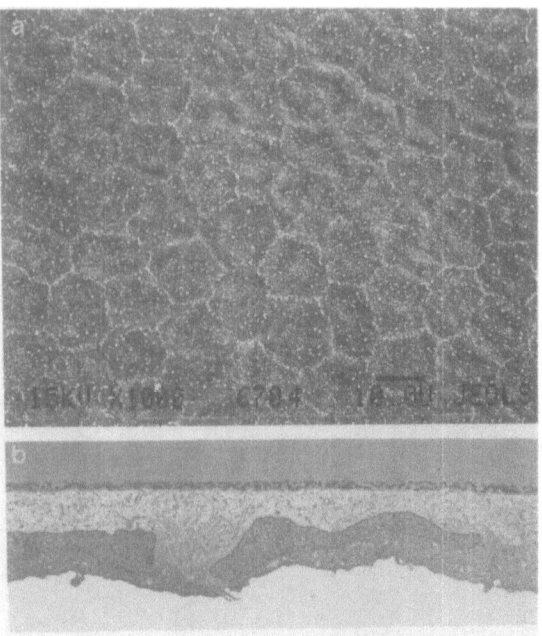

Figure 8. Scanning (a, x1000) and transmission (b, x4640) electron micrographs of rabbit corneas (perfused with GBR) three days after -12 D of excimer laser PRK. Normal hexagonal cells and intact intercellular junctions are seen. Dark amorphous material in Descemet's membrane are prominent.

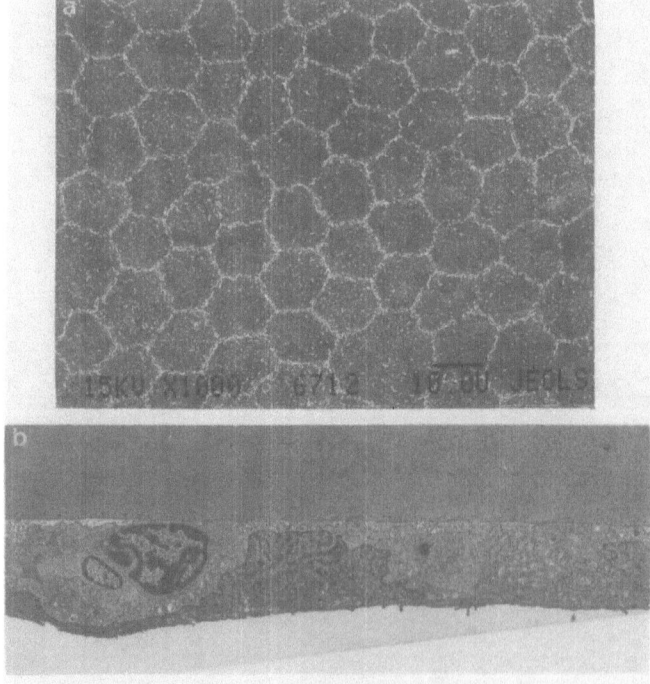

Figure 9. Scanning and transmission electron micrographs of rabbit corneas (perfused with GBR) with residual corneal thickness of 200 μm three days after excimer laser ablation. SEM (a) shows an intact monolayer of hexagonal endothelial cells showing some floppy borders (x1000). TEM (b) shows intact intercellular junctions, normal subcellular organelles with deposition of dark amorphous material in Descemet's membrane (x4640).

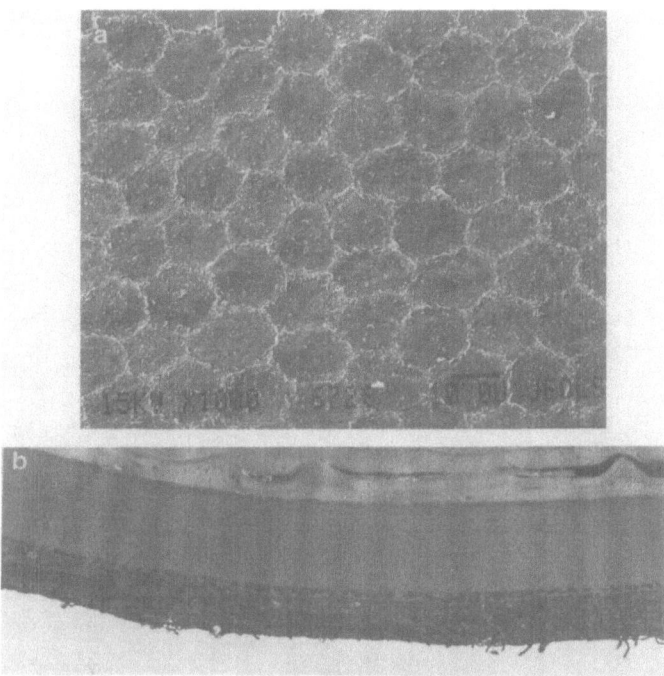

Figure 10. Scanning and transmission electron micrographs of rabbit corneas (perfused with GBR) with residual corneal thickness of 175 µm three days after excimer laser ablation. SEM (a) shows an normal mosaic pattern of endothelial cells (x1000). TEM (b) shows intact intercellular junctions, normal subcellular organelles with dark amorphous material in Descemet's membrane adjacent endothelial cell (x4640).

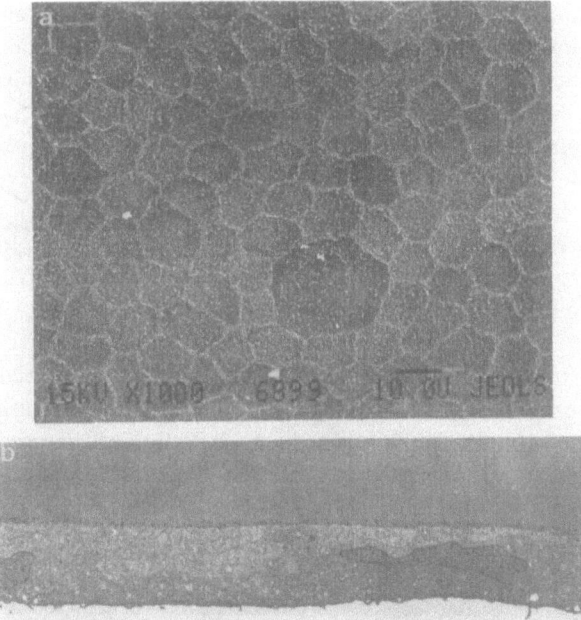

Figure 11. Scanning and transmission electron micrographs of rabbit corneas (perfused with GBR) with residual corneal thickness of 150 µm three days after excimer laser ablation. SEM(a) shows an intact monolayer of hexagonal endothelial cells (x1000). TEM (b) shows intact intercellular junctions, normal subcellular organelles with a sheet of dark amorphous material in Descemet's membrane adjacent endothelial cell (x4640).

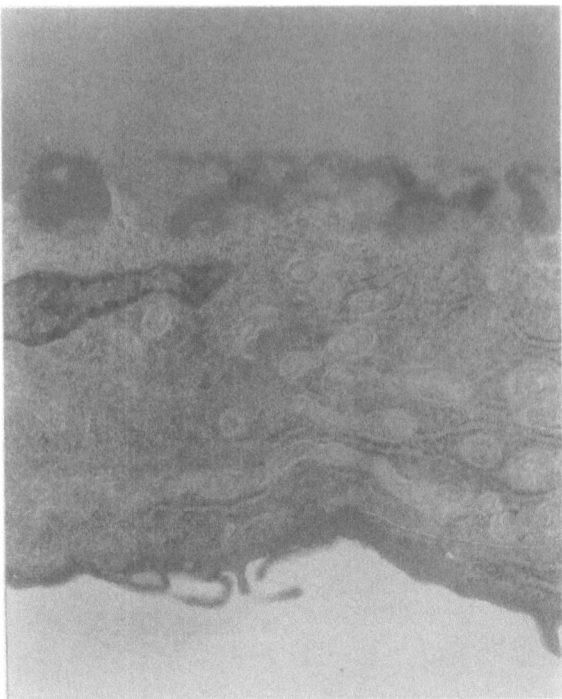

Figure 12. Higher magnification (x12000) of trasmission electron micrograph of rabbit corneas (perfused with GBR) with residual corneal thickness of 222μm three days after excimer laser ablation. Electron dense amorphous material at outer surface of basal plasma membrane close to Descemet's membrane suggesting lipofuscin pigments secreted from stressed endothelial cell.

of the cell area, shape factor, and percentage of hexagonal cells (p<.01). This damage was inversely proportional to the residual corneal thickness. In corneas with a residual thickness over 200 μm, endothelial damage were rarely observed.

In permeability experiments, corneas with 175 or 150 μm of residual thickness had an increased permeability compared to controls, while corneas with 200 μm were similar to controls. Following excimer laser ablation, however, the steady state distribution ratio (Rca) of carboxyfluorescein between the cornea(c) and the aqueous(a) may change because excimer laser ablates part of corneal stroma. In the current experiments, it was assumed that Rca did not change. Corneal thickness was corrected and adjusted to the change of the paired control cornea.

The SEM showed relatively normal endothelial cells, which was somewhat different from the alizarin red S stained cells. Fixation of the cornea for EM may stabilize the membrane more than the alizarin red S performed on fresh endothelium. The TEM showed an intact intercellular junctions. Carboxyfluorescein used in permeability measurement has a 5Å radius so small changes in the junctions may reflect the measure of increased permeability in this study. The increase in permeability was small, but statistically significant. Deposition of the amorphous granular material within posterior Descemet's membrane adjacent to endothelium was also noted in the corneas after excimer laser ablation, which suggests that the corneal endothelium was affected metabolically by excimer laser. Based on these results, the effects of excimer laser (193 nm) may not be confined to a few microns at the surface of the cornea. Other investigators[19] have reported a similar finding in rabbit corneas in which the amorphous material appears six hours after excimer laser ablation and migrates anteriorly in Descemet's membrane with time. Immunohistochemical staining showed the presence of type IV collagen, laminin, fibronectin and proteoglycans for this amorphous material. Although the amorphous materials may represent these molecules, it has yet to be proved and it may be due to UV damage or the acoustic shock waves that are affecting the endothelial cells to lay new Descemet's membrane material. Zabel et al.[6] measured the pressure produced by shock or acoustic waves near the posterior surface of a bovine cornea during 193 nm excimer laser ablation of the surface. The pressure was approximately 100 atm during ablation of the superficial stroma. Endothelial disruption and junctional separation ocurred only when 85% to 90% of the corneal thickness had been ablated. Thus, it is possible that acoustic damage may be responsible for the endothelial cells to secrete the amorphous granular materials.

In summary, excimer laser ablation can cause alterations in the corneal endothelial morphology and barrier if the corneal stroma is ablated to below a residual corneal thickness of 200μm. Excimer laser ablation also stimulates the corneal endothelial cells to secrete an amorphous granular material which is deposited in Descemet's membrane. The amorphous granular material even occur with minimal diopter correction (-6 D). The results of this study emphasize that special care should be used in patients with high myopia correction since endothelial changes in the barrier function and morphology may occur following deep stromal ablation, particularly in LASIK.

ACKNOWLEDGMENTS

Supported in part by a special grant from Dongsan Medical Center, Institute of Medical Science of Keimyung University, National Institutes of Health grants EY 00933, P30EY06360. H.F.Edelhauser is an RPB senior scientist awarder.

REFERENCES

1. S.L. Trokel SL, Srinivasan, R., and Braren, B., Excimer laser surgery of the cornea. *Am. J. Ophthalmol.* 96:710 (1983).
2. M.B. McDonald, Frantz, J.M., Klyce, S.O., et al., One year refractive results of central photorefractive keratectomy for myopia in the non-human primate cornea. *Arch. Ophthalmol.* 108:40 (1990).
3. N.A. Sher, and Chen, V., The use of the 193nm excimer laser for myopic photorefractive keratectomy in sighted eyes. *Arch. Ophthalmol.* 109:1525 (1990).
4. J. Marshall, Trokel, S., Rothery, S., and Krueger, R.R., A comparative study of corneal incisions induced by diamond and steel knives and two ultraviolet radiations from an excimer laser. *Br. J. Ophthalmol.* 70:482 (1986).
5. E.J. Dehm, Puliafito, C.A., Adler, C.M., and Steinert, F.S., Corneal endothelial injury in rabbits following excimer laser ablation at 193 and 248 nm. *Arch. Ophthalmol.* 104:1364 (1986).
6. R. Zabel, Tuft, S., and Marshall, J., Excimer laser photorefractive keratectomy: endothelial morphology following area ablation of the cornea. *Invest. Ophthalmol. Vis. Sci.* 29(suppl):390 (1988).
7. J.W. Koch, Lang, G.K., and Naumann, G.O.H., Endothelial reaction to perforating and non-perforating excimer laser excisions in rabbits. *J. Refract. Corneal Surg.* 7:214 (1991).
8. R.A. Del Pero, Gigstad, J.E., Roberts, A.D., et al., A refractive and histopathologic study of excimer laser keratectomy in primates. *Am. J. Ophthalmol.* 109:419 (1990).
9. F.E. Fantes, Hann, D.D., and Waring, G.O. III, Wound healing after excimer laser keratomileusis in monkeys. *Arch. Ophthalmol.* 108:665 (1990).

10. G.L. Goodman, Trokel, S.L., Stark, W.I., et al., Corneal healing following laser refractive keratectomy. *Arch. Ophthalmol.* 107:1799 (1989).

11. Ozler S.A., Liaw, L.L., Neev, J., et al., Acute ultrastructural changes of cornea after excimer laser ablation. *Invest. Ophthalmol. Vis. Sci.* 33:540 (1992).

12. G. Cennamo, Rosa, N., Guida, E., et al., Evaluation of corneal thickness and endothelial cells before and after excimer laser photorefractive keratectomy. *J. Refract. Corneal Surg.* 10:137 (1994).

13. J.J. Perez-Santonja, Meza, J., Moreno, E., et al., Short-term corneal endothelial changes after photorefractive keratectomy. *J. Refract. Corneal Surg.* 10(suppl):194 (1994).

14. S. Amano, and Shimizu, K., Corneal endothelial changes after excimer laser photorefractive keratectomy. *Am. J. Ophthalmol.* 116:692 (1993).

15. F. Carones, Brancato, R., Venturi, E., and Morico, A.. The corneal endothelium after myopic excimer laser photorefractive keratectomy. *Arch. Ophthalmol.* 112:920 (1994).

16. M.A. Watsky, McDermott, M.L., and Edelhauser, H.F., *In vitro* corneal endothelial permeability in rabbit and human. The effect of age, cataract surgery and diabetes. *Exp. Eye. Res.* 49:751 (1989).

17. S. Dikstein, and Maurice, D.M., The metabolic basis to the fluid pump in the cornea. *Physiol.* 221:29 (19972).

18. H.F. Edelhauser, Gonnering, R., and Van Horn, D.L., Intraocular irrigating solutions. A comparative study of BSS plus and lactated Ringer's solution. *Arch. Ophthalmol.* 96:516 (1978).

19. K.D.Hanna, Pouliqeun, Y., Waring, G.O. III, et al., Corneal stromal wound healing in rabbits after 193-nm excimer laser surface ablation. *Arch. Ophthalmol.* 107:895 (1989).

SESSIONS IV AND XII: REFRACTIVE SURGERY

Abstracts of Other Conference Presentations and Posters

WOUND HEALING AND CORNEAL TRANSPARENCY

John Marshall

UMDS Department of Ophthalmology, St. Thomas' Hospital, University of London

Subsequent to photorefractive keratectomy (PRK) all corneas experience some change in transparency. An initial phase within the first couple of days relates to epithelial change. Over the next three months changes result from keratocyte activity. Persistent loss of corneal transparency seems to he a function of epithelial keratocyte interaction and subsequent deposition of subepithelial material. The time course, cellular interactions, and consequences for vision will be discussed using objective analytical techniques.

REFRACTIVE KERATOTOMY IN THE LASER ERA: MINI RK AND Arc-T

Rachel Lindstrom

Philips Eye Institute, Minneapolis, Minnesota

Radial keratotomy (RK) is a common surgical technique for correcting myopia. The RK incisions, like any corneal incisions, permanently weaken the cornea and this structural weakening can cause several complications and side effects, including diurnal fluctuation, progressive hyperopic shift, and the potential for traumatic rupture of the keratotomy scars. I describe a new technique—minimally invasive RK (mini-RK)—that reduces the millimeters of cornea incised and present preliminary laboratory and clinical results. In a cadaver eye study, eight short, deep incisions extending from the 3.0 mm optical zone to the 7.0 mm optical zone produced 92% of the efficacy of full-length incisions to the 11.0 mm optical zone. This finding was confirmed by intraoperative surgical keratometry in six patients in whom a 1 % increase in central corneal flattening was achieved when incisions were extended from the mini-RK configurations to full length. In a retrospective evaluation of 100 patients with -1.0 to -6.0 diopters (D) of myopia, 92% of eyes were within 1.0 D of ametropia and 94% had 20/40 or better uncorrected visual acuity. No significant complications were encountered. Mini-RK may be a useful alternative to reduce the invasiveness of RK but retain its efficacy in eyes with low to moderate myopia. (Key words: mini-RK, myopia, radial keratotomy)

INCREASE OF AQUEOUS FLARE INTENSITY AFTER RADIAL KERATOTOMY AND EXCIMER LASER KERATECTOMY IN HUMANS

R. C. A. Plut, M. Campos, and E. Il Paiva

Department of Ophthalmology, Paulista School of Medicine, Federal University of São Paulo, Brazil

Purpose: Laser flare meter (LFM) was used to assess alterations of the blood-aqueous barrier following radial keratotomy (RK), photorefractive keratectomy (PRK), excimer laser intrastromal keratomileusis (LASIK) and phototherapeutic keratectomy (PTK). **Methods:** Aqueous flare was evaluated using the LFM Kowa FM 500 in 87 eyes from 82 consecutive patients. Measurements were obtained in 51 eyes from 51 RK operated patients preoperatively, at the end of surgery, one day and one week postoperatively. These patients were randomized (double masked), to receive topical 0.1% Dexamethasone, Polimixin B and Neomicin qid during one week after surgery; or just antibiotics for the same period. Measurements were also obtained in 36 eyes from 31 excimer laser operated patients preoperatively, one day, one and two weeks postoperatively. All patients in this group received postoperative topical 0.1% Dexamethasone and Polymixin B and Neomixin qid during fifteen days after surgery. **Results:** Uneventful RK induced significant elevation on flare immediately after the surgery returning to baseline 1 day postoperative (Friedman Test). Measurements obtained up to 7 days postoperatively were similar in both steroid treated and untreated groups, Limbal bleeding did not induce significant increase flare when compared to uneventful RK. Microperforations induced intense inflammation that persisted for more than 1 day, however it returned to preoperative levels at the 7th postoperative day. PRK and LASIK did not induce significant increase inflammation after surgery. PRK induced elevation of flare measurements after surgery that did not restore to normal levels at the 15th postoperative day (Friedman test). **Conclusion:** Uneventful RK appears to induce short lasting elevations on aqueous flare on steroid treated or untreated patients. Microperforation induced significant postoperative inflammation. PTK appears to induce significant elevations on aqueous flare. Localized anterior stromal melting over epithelial cells retained in the corneal interface after automated lamellar keratoplasty.

COMPRESSION KERATOPLASTY

Richard J. Fugo

Compression Keratoplasty or CK is a new keratorefractive system which provides the Ophthalmologist with a modality to improve the reliability and precision of most present day

RK protocols. Preoperatively, the overall goal of CK is to arrive at a diamond blade setting that more accurately reflects a true corneal thickness. This is achieved largely through the scientific application of Mode Pachymetry and Data Ganging. Postoperatively, CK teaches how to use the normal healing processes of the cornea to stimulate a progressively titrated production of additional corneal connective tissue into the RK incision. CK teaches how this may be performed in a slow progressive fashion at the slit lamp in the exam room until patient vision is satisfactorily improved. The initial RK incision produces an exudation of healing connective tissue into the original RK incision cavity. As additional healing tissue is stimulated and secreted into the original cavity, this new tissue is added to the original microwedge of corneal healing tissue. In this way, CK teaches to progressively titrate the thickness of the original microwedge of healing tissue in the cornea and thereby progressively increase the separation of the original RK/AK corneal incision walls. Minute increases in the thickness of the corneal microwedges and subsequent separation of the original incision walls creates a dramatic flattening of the central cornea. Residual myopia as well as residual astigmatism may be corrected in this way with resultant improvement in vision. This technique teaches away from violation of virgin cornea tissue during vision enhancement. CK is the missing link in present day standard RK enhancement protocols...the step between topical medical enhancement and incisional surgical enhancement. CK also allows keratorefractive surgeons to further improve the vision of uncorrected 20/30 and 20/40 residual myopia in a safe effective fashion. This group of patients has been to date the refractive surgeons "no man's land". CK microwedge thickening has been documented and demonstrated with high magnification photography.

BIPOKERATOPLASTY: USING CAUTERY TO ADVANTAGE

Richard J. Fugo

Bipokeratoplasty is a method to neutralize astigmatism at the time of cataract surgery. This procedure provides an effective, simple and cost effective method of reducing postoperative astigmatism. No additional equipment purchases are needed. As opposed to astigmatic keratotomy, Bipokeratoplasty is a method by which the low K meridian is tightened in order to minimize astigmatism. For years it has been known that cautery may induce astigmatism. Bipokeratoplasty harnesses the energy of bipolar cautery in order to alter corneal topography in such a way that corneal astigmatism is reduced. The corneal topography is evaluated through the operating room microscope with a qualitative keratoscope. This qualitative analysis is correlated with preoperative keratometric values. In the operating room, arcs of bipolar cautery are placed along the corneal limbal stroma along the low K meridian. Moderate intensity of energy levels are applied with the cautery tip.. Epithelial cells are removed from the bipokeratoplasty arc sites. The effect of the bipolar cautery on the corneal stroma and subsequent alteration in corneal topography is followed with a qualitative keratoscope intraoperatively. Maximum efficacy is obtained by utilizing a normotensive eye. The goal of intraoperative bipokeratoplasty is to overcorrect the low K axis and convert this K axis into the higher K axis by approximately 1.5 to 2 diopters. This overcorrection will account for post operative regression. Bipokeratoplasty is performed on astigmatism of 1 diopter or more. There is a moderate learning curve with this technique. The bipokeratoplasty arcs re-epithelialize and are invisible to slit lamp observation 3 to 5 days postoperatively. The effective stabilization of K readings occurs within 2 to 3 weeks post operatively in small incision, self sealing wound cataract surgery. Bipokeratoplasty arcs are not placed over the self sealing wounds. The most prominent side effect in Bipokeratoplasty even with topical anesthesia is post operative foreign body sensation for 1 to 2 days: It takes approximately 30 seconds to perform bipokeratoplasty. The tools needed for bipokeratoplasty include standard bipolar cautery, any qualitative keratoscope, and surgical skill. Bipokeratoplasty has been performed in over 500 patients with minimal complications and excellent results. Regression in bipokeratoplasty is similar to that in keratorefractive surgery with the greater amount of regression noted in more compliant corneas.

POSITIVE ELLIPSE FOR THE CORRECTION OF COMPOUND HYPEROPIC ASTIGMATISM

Cesar Carriazo

Purpose: To define a unique geometric figure that will not antagonize with the corneal thickness law, and that will help us in the steepening of both corneal meridians in order to correct hyperopic astigmatism. **Methods:** Pre- and post-operative topographical studies of 13 eyes with simple hyperopia, 7 with compound hyperopic astigmatism (CHA) of less than 1 diopter (D) and 22 with CHA greater than 1 D. All of them had correction of the spherical hyperopia done with excimer laser hyperopic intrastromal keratomileusis. Different topographical optical patterns were analyzed. For each patient we performed a computerized differential analysis substracting the topographical pattern from the pre-operative one and produced a topographical arrangement in order to determine the ideal topographical figure for the correction of CHA. **Results:** Three topographical patterns were found: 52.6% were circular, 42.1% an oval oriented vertically, and 5.3% had an irregular pattern due to a hinge effect. We found no horizontally oriented oval pattern. A circular pattern on patients with simple hyperopia and with CHA less than 1 D was found, compared to the vertically oriented oval found in patients with CHA greater than 1D. A final figure shown by the topograph when the differential analysis was made, by substracting the ideal final spherical result (circular optical zone) from a sphero-cilindrical pattern as the one found in CHA, was an oval pattern with its major axis oriented towards the flatest pre-operative meridian. **Conclusions:** In order to obtain a final positive and spherical surface from a sphero-cylindrical one (CHA), a positive ellipse should be made (peripherical ablation with a greater OZ in one meridian) with the mayor axis over the flattest meridian.

LOCALIZED ANTERIOR STROMAL MELTING OVER EPITHELIAL CELLS RETAINED IN THE CORNEAL INTERFACE AFTER AUTOMATED LAMELLAR KERATOPLASTY

John S. Berestka,[1,2] David R. Hardten,[1,2,3] and Richard L. Lindstrom[1,3]

[1,2]Phillips Eye Institute, Minneapolis, Minnesota; St. Paul Ramsey Medical St. Paul, Minnesota [3]University of Minnesota, Minneapolis, Minnesota

Automated lamellar keratoplasty (ALK) and laser in situ keratomileusis (LASIK) are lamellar keratorefractive procedures in which epithelial cells may occasionally be retained in the corneal interface. We present a case of stromal melting anterior to a nest of retained epithelial cells following ALK.

A 25-year-old man with significant blepharitis underwent ALK for myopia and was noted to have epithelial cell inclusions in the mid-peripheral lamellar interface at his two week postoperative appointment. Because this nest of cells later enlarged and the patient's vision was limited by irregular astigmatism, the epithelium was debrided three months postoperatively by lifting the flap and removing the cells with a metal blade. Three months after debridement, the patients uncorrected acuity improved to 20/30, but a 1.2 x 1.5 mm epithelial plaque was noted in the mid-peripheral lamellar interface. He was examined three months later and was noted to have a well-demarcated depression in the anterior stroma down to the level of the lamellar interface in the same mid-peripheral location. The epithelium was intact over this stromal depression, and the epithelial cells were no longer present in the interface. The patient was asymptomatic prior to this visit.

We postulate that this stromal ulceration represents a localized aseptic melting of the stroma anterior to epithelial cells with intact tight junctions. As lamellar keratorefractive procedures become more common with the advent of LASIK, the incidence of anterior stromal melts following epithelial inclusions may become more common.

ONE YEAR FOLLOW-UP ON PRK FOR MYOPIA

Hugh R. Taylor, Mary Liew, and Cathy McCarty

Melbourne Excimer Laser Group

We have prospectively examined the efficacy and safety of photorefractive keratectomy (PRK) and photoastigmatic refractive keratectomy (PARK) for high (-5.01D to -10.00D spherical equivalent) and extreme (>-10.00D SEQ) myopia and compared this with the twelve month results of low myopia (≤ -5.00 D SEQ).

1177 eyes (752 patients) were treated with a VisX Twenty/Twenty excimer laser and followed prospectively for 12 months. Low myopia was treated in one ablation zone (6.0mm), high myopia in two ablation zones (5.0mm and 6.0mm) and extreme myopia in three ablation zones (4.5mm, 5.0mm, and 6.0mm) with a maximum treatment of 15.00D. Up to 6 D of astigmatism were corrected.

988 (84%) of treated eyes were available for 12 month follow-up. The retreatment rate at 12 months was 4% for low myopes, 11% for high myopes and 17% for extreme myopes. The percent of low myopes within 1 and 2D of ametropia at 12 months was 85% and 98% respectively, while the corresponding percentages for high myopes were 63% and 88%, and for extreme myopes 44% and 63%. At 12 months uncorrected vision of 20/20 and 20/40 or better was achieved in 48% and 87% of the low myopes, 24% and 69% of the high myopes and 3% and 33% of the extreme myopes, respectively. Sixteen (3%) of the low myopes, 24 (7%) of the high myopes, and 14 (18%) of the extreme myopes had lost two or more LogMAR lines of best corrected visual acuity at 12 months.

Our data show that although excimer laser surgery is highly predictable for low and high myopia, it is somewhat more variable for extreme myopia. More data are needed to determine the factors associated with losing best corrected visual acuity in extreme myopes.

OPTIMIZING THE ABLATION PROFILE

M. McDonald

Refractive Surgery Center, South, Eye, Ear, Nose & Throat Hospital, New Orleans, LA

As excimer laser technology evolves, the primary goal has become clear: to make the smoothest ablation possible. Much anecdotal evidence exists, as well as published comparative data, indicating that a smoother ablation leads to less haze and regression and better maintenance of best corrected visual acuity. Modern lasers are designed to provide smooth ablations with sophisticated aspheric algorithms. In this fashion, larger myopic and astigmatic corrections are possible without increasing the sagittal depth of the ablation or the surface roughness. In the future, exceedingly smooth ablations will be produced by small beams scanning and tracking systems which utilize real time topographic feedback to deliver customized ablations.

ADVANTAGES AND DISADVANTAGES OF EYE TRACKING SYSTEMS

Daniel Durrie and Timothy Cavanaugh

Eye Center, Kansas City, Missouri

As laser vision correction becomes a more and more popular alternative to incision procedures in the correction of myopia, Eye Tracking Systems' roles must be defined. In "Advantages and Disadvantages of Eye Tracking Systems" the surgeons's role will be defined. Alignment and tracking will also be defined, and their relative importance specified. Ablation patterns using present and future laser systems will be discussed. Types of correction will be discussed, including simple myopia, myopia/astigmatism, hyperopia and hyperopia/astigmatism. The value of tracking systems with different types of correction will be discussed.

PHOTOREFRACTIVE KERATECTOMY FOR MYOPIA OF 6 TO 12 DIOPTERS

Wing-Kwong Chan, Peter Tseng, Donald Tan, and Cze Hong Low

Singapore National Eye Centre, Singapore

PURPOSE: A prospective, open ended, non-randomized clinical trial was conducted to assess the efficacy, stability and safety of the use of excimer laser photorefractive keratectomy (PRK) to correct myopia of greater than 6 diopters (D).
PATIENTS & METHODS: Two hundred and fifty six eyes of 200 patients with a mean pre-operative spherical equivalent of -8.5 +/- 2 D (range -6.00 D to -18.13 D) underwent PRK with a 193nm ArF excimer laser (ExciMed® UV200LA, Summit Technology NC., Waltham,MA) for attempted corrections of between -6.0 D to -11.9 D with an abla-

tion zone of 5mm. The first 117 of 256 eyes that had reached one year or more of post-operative follow-up were examined.

RESULTS: After a mean follow-up period of 17 months (range 12 to 37 months), the mean manifest spherical equivalent refraction was -0.9 +/- 1.6 D (range -5.50 D to +4.50 D); 49% of eyes were within +1–1.00 D of the attempted correction; uncorrected visual acuity was 6/12 or better in 71% of eyes. Two eyes lost 2 or more Snellen lines of best corrected visual acuity. Central corneal haze was mild in 41% of eyes and moderate in 3% of eyes.

CONCLUSION: Excimer laser PRK is reasonably effective and safe in the treatment of - 6 D to -12 D of myopia. However, it is less accurate compared to PRK in eyes with low to moderate myopia and is more likely to result in significant corneal haze.

SINGLE-PASS MULTIZONE PHOTOREFRACTIVE KERATECTOMY FOR HIGH MYOPIA

P.D. Rodrigues, W. Chamon, and M. Campos

Department of Ophthalmology, Paulista School of Medicine

Purpose: To evaluate safety and effectiveness of excimer laser photorefractive keratectomy in high myopes using a single-pass multizone technique with the Summit Omni-Med Excimer Laser.

Methods: The procedure was performed in 20 eyes of 17 patients (8 males, age ranging from 21 to 46 years), using the Summit OmniMed Excimer laser with built-in multizone single-pass software. A variety of optical zones combination was utilized with a minimum of 4.5 mm. Stromal depth of treatment ranged from 75 to 107 µm (300 to 428 pulses). Follow-up was at least 3 months. Results are presented as average ± standard deviation, at most recent visit. Longer follow-up will be available at the time of presentation.

Results: Three eyes presented lattice retinal dystrophy and two needed photocoagulation prior excimer laser surgery. Preoperative spherical equivalent ranged from -6.00 to - 15.25 D (-10.93 ± 3.15D), and changed to -0.04 1 3.6D. Postoperatively, 9 eyes presented uncorrected visual acuity of 20/40 or better. Six eyes decreased, and 3 eyes improved at least 2 Snellen lines of spectacle-corrected visual acuity after the treatment. Moderate to severe corneal haze was present in 3 eyes between the 3rd and 6th postoperative month. Four eyes developed corneal infiltrates due to epidemic keratoconjunctivitis during the follow-up period.

Conclusions: Although multizone single-pass approach is not a definite solution for high myopes, this small series results are encouraging. A longer follow-up is needed to better analyze this procedure.

SINGLE PASS-MULTIZONE PHOTOREFRACTIVE KERATECTOMY FOR HIGH MYOPIA

Hyo-Myung Kim and Hai Run Jung

Department of Ophthalmol, KUMC, Seoul, Korea

Conical haze and myopic regression are not uncommon complications following photorefractive keratectomy(PRK), especially for high myopia. To avoid these problems, multipass-multizone technique has been introduced. However, it is quite difficult to coincide the center of the each ablation zone during the procedure and needs to take longer operation time. Single pass-multizone technique may override them The current study evaluates the clinical results of single pass-multizone PRK for high myopia.

Sixty-five eyes of 61 patients underwent single pass-multizone PRK using new software released by Summit Technology, USA. Average preoperative myopia was -9.45 diopters (D), ranged from -8.25 D t -16.00 D. Mean postoperative refraction was +1.21 D at one month, +0.16 D at 3 months, and -0.26 D at 6 months postoperatively. In terms of predictability, 50 eyes (76.9%) were within 2.00 D of the desired correction at postoperative 1 month, 58 eyes (89.2%) at postoperative 3 months, and 57 eyes(87.7%) at postoperative 6 months. There was no serious complications. Increased intraocular pressure was developed on 9 eyes, but controlled after cessation of the steroid drops. Night halo or glare was reported in 4 patients. All patients were satisfied. These results show that single pass-multizone PRK would be safe, predictable, and effective to correct high myopia.

LASERSIGHT COMPAK-200 MINI-EXCIMER INITIAL PHASE 2A RESULTS

Michael W. Belin

Lions Eye Institute, Albany Medical College, Albany, New York

The LaserSight Compak-200 Mini-Excimer utilizes a scanning technology and a small (approximately 1.0 mm) spot laser. While the fluence at the cornea is comparable to other broad beam lasers (160–200 mJ/cm^2), the power requirements are substantially less because of the total coverage area is small. The lower energy requirements and small spot size obviates the need for extensive beam homogenization and allows for ablations zone diameters to 7.0 mm. The scanning technology incorporates a multi-zone ablation profile. The U.S. Phase 2a trial commenced on May 25,1995 and finished recruitment in December. The Phase 2a protocol allows for 50 patients at 5 investigational sites with a myopia range of -1.50 to -10.00 diopters. Each center is allowed to enroll two patients (total ten) in the high myopia group (>6.0 diopters).

To date 25 of 50 patients have obtained a minimum of 3 month data. In the low to moderate myopia group (-1.50 to -6.00 diopters) 94% of patients obtained UCVA of 20/40 or better with 41 % 20/20 or better. In the high myopia group (-6.25 to -10.00 diopters) 75% achieved UCVA of 20/40 or better, with 38% 20/20 or better.

The LaserSight Compak-200 Mini-Excimer is a small, relatively low cost laser with initial results comparable to current broad beams lasers.

CENTRAL AND PARA-CENTRAL CORNEAL TOPOGRAPHY IN 2000 PROSPECTIVE PRK PATIENTS

Cyprian S. Asota,[2] Chris O. Imafidon,[1] Charles C. Cory,[3] Bernice K. Glover, and Joe E. Imafidon[2]

[1]Biomedical Sciences Division, East Road, Anglia P. University, Cambridge, UK; [2]Ife Eye Center, PMB 11, Obafemi Awolowo University, Ile-Ife, Nigeria; [3]Optirnax Laser Clinic, London, UK

Purpose: To investigate the distribution and relation between different types of central and paracentral topography of the human cornea in each eye and the fellow eye. **Method:** A Placido-based keratoscope was used for the assessment of the right and left corneas of normal subjects who were prospective PRK/PARK/PTK candidates. Study population were tested for normality and data obtained subject to student t test. **Results:** This keratoscopic study revealed a strong correlation between the central curvatures of each eye of the same subject. No correlation was found when the right and left para-central topographies were compared. This was also true of the rate of cornea flattening from the central cornea to the limbus of each eye of the same subject. **Conclusion:** The central corneal curvature values of an eye are independent of the para-central curvatures. Thus, counting eyes instead of subjects will lead to sample size overestimation if each eye is regarded as a data point when studying central topography. The reverse is the case if paracentral topography is being studied.

EVALUATION OF MULTIFACTORIAL FACTORS INFLUENCING REGRESSION AFTER PHOTOREFRACTIVE KERATECTOMY

M.S. Kim, C.K. Park, W.J. Sah, Y.C. Lee, C.K. Joo, and J.H. Kim

Department of Ophthalmology, Catholic University Medical College, Seoul, Korea

Purpose. We evaluated the possible factors influencing the myopic regression of patients following photorefractive keratectomy performed from April 2, 1991 to May 2, 1993. **Methods.** For this study we selected the special grouped 30 (60 eyes) patients who had -6.0D, all female, the range of age from 25 to 30, and both eye were treated. The parameters of Summit excimer Laser were set in the same conditions (frequency, repetition, diameter of abrasion, depth of abrasion). We performed excimer laser in the same technique. We followed up the patients more than one year. We evaluated epithelial wound healing time, IOP, K-readings, corneal thickness, occupation, surgeon, steroid responder vs non-responder, hyperpic peak after PRK and tophographic analysis between regressed and non-regressed group. **Results.** We didn't find any difference in the individual parameters we checked in this study except the corneal haziness between two group. In case where one eye experienced regression, following PRK, the incidence of the regression of the other eye following PRK is statistically significant (P=0.05) and the increased likelihood of the other eye experiencing corneal haziness, too (P=0.01 2). **Conclusions.** We suggest corneal haziness is likely related to cause the myopic regression following PRK. We recommend that if one eye showed regression after PRK, the surgeon must keep in mind that the other eye has an increased likelihood of regression. Therefore, the surgeon should particularly try to prevent this regression by preventing corneal haziness following PRK.

CORNEAL TEMPERATURE CHANGE FOLLOWING EXCIMER LASER PHOTOREFRACTIVE KERATECTOMY

S. Betney,[1,2] P.B. Morgan,[1] S.J. Doyle,[2] N. Efron,[1] A. Chatterjee,[2] and S Shah[2]

[1]University of Manchester Institute of Science & Technology; [2]Optimax Laser Eye Clinics, Manchester

Purpose: Corneal temperature changes in photorefractive keratectomy (PRK) have been implicated in the aetiology of subepithelial haze. This study was undertaken in order to quantify the temperature change during this surgical procedure.

Methods: Non-contact, colour coded ocular thermography was performed using a 6T62 Thermo Tracer infrared detector (NEC San-el Instruments, Japan). During PRK OD the Nidek EC5O()C excimer laser (Nidek Instruments, Japan) on a group of 13 subjects of refraction between -1.75 D and -6.25 D.

Results: Mean (+1- SD) central ocular surface temperature (OST) following epithelial debridement was 29.15 +/- 0.39°C. Mean peak OST was 37.73 +/- 0.65 °C. Maximum peak OST was 38.70 oC and minimum peak OST was 36.70°C. Most of the rise in temperature occurred in the first 15 seconds. Factors such as ablation depth optical correction and procedure duration were not demonstrated as having a significant effect on corneal temperature during the procedure.

Conclusions: Previous work has suggested that corneal collagen denatures at 36–39 °C. At 38.2°C, 25% denaturation occurs compared with 50% at 38.7 °C. It has been demonstrated that corneal temperature may be elevated to this level during routine PRK. Future modifications to PRK procedure could include a pause in the treatment during the last 10 seconds of treatment to minimize any collateral heat damage to the ablation bed.

Supported by the Corneal Research Fund of Manchester Royal Eye Hospital.

THE EFFECT OF EXCIMER LASER PRK ON CORRECTION OF HYPEROPIA IN RABBIT

H. Mori, T. Suzuki, Y. Sonoda, R. Muramatsu, and M. Usui

Department of Ophthalmology, Tokyo Medical College, Hospital, Japan

Purpose. To investigate the effect of excimer laser photorefractive keratectomy (PRK) in correcting hyperopia in rabbits. **Methods.** Four JW rabbits underwent +8.00D, 7.0mm diameter ablation bilaterally. Ablation was performed using the Aesculap Meditec Excimer laser (Mel60). Special-designed rotating mask was used to create a ring-shaped ablation. Corneal epithelium was removed mechanically prior to ablation. Slit lamp and corneal topography examinations were performed pre-operatively and at 3 days, 1 and 2 weeks, and 1, 3 and 6 months post-PRK. The rabbits were sacrificed postoperatively, and eyes were enucleated and processed for histological examination. **Results.** The corneal epithelium recovered during the first week without subsequent defects. Haze was peaked at 2 weeks and disappeared by 3 months. Corneal topography showed a central steepening. The steep area was round and showed a relatively homogenous curvature. On transmission electron microscopy (TEM), a densely staining material in Descemet's membrane appeared under the entire ablated zone by the end of the first week. This change was especially intense at the periphery of ablated zone. TEM indicated that the reaction in Descemet's membrane was correlated with the depth of ablation. **Conclusion.** Corneal topography showed that this treatment was effective in correction of hyperopia in rabbits, and the corneal epithelium recovered quickly and corneal wound healing was not delayed in this PRK.

CORRECTION OF HYPEROPIA USING THE VISX STAR EXCIMER LASER

W. B. Jackson, G. Mintsioulis, P.J. Agapitos, and E.J. Casson

University of Ottawa Eye Institute, Ottawa General Hospital, Ottawa, Canada

PURPOSE: To evaluate the safety, efficacy, predictability and stability of surface PRK for the correction of low hyperopia in normally sighted eyes using the VISX STAR.

METHOD: Twenty-five patients with cycloplegic refractions SE +1.00 to +4.00 with +1.00 D or less of astigmatism, BCVA of 20/40 or better and a stable refraction for at least a year in both eyes were enrolled in this 2-year study. There were 10 males and 15 females treated, with a mean age of 50 years (39–62) and mean preoperative SE of +2:50 D (+1.00 to +4.00). Mechanical epithelial removal out to 9 mm was accomplished using either a Paton spatula alone or combined with the Amoills rotary epithelial brush. Patient self fixation was used during the procedure. Post-operatively all eyes were patched with an antibiotic/steroid ointment and examined daily until reepithelialization was achieved. FML were used t.i.d. for I week followed by frequent use of non-preserved artificial tears for 5 months.

RESULTS: Epithelial healing occurred in 3.6 (3–6) days. Patients at one week had a mild myopic refractive shift mean -0.52 +0.83 D, at one month -0.41+0.43 D and at 2 months -0.31 +0.63 D with marked improvement in their uncorrected near visual acuity. At one month 64% had achieved 20/25 UCVA and 93% 20/40 or better. One, three and six month results of uncorrected and best corrected visual acuities at distance and near, manifest and cycloplegic refraction, corneal haze, and topography will be presented.

CONCLUSIONS: Hyperopic eyes from +1.00 to +4.00 D can be treated using the VISX STAR excimer laser. Current results will be discussed with an emphasis on 1, 3 and 6 month follow-up data for the determination of efficacy and stability.

THE ANALGESIC EFFICACY AND SAFETY OF KETOROLAC OPHTHALMIC SOLUTION IN PATIENTS UNDERGOING PHOTOREFRACTIVE KERATECTOMY (PRK) WITH THE ExciMed® UV2OOLA/OmniMed® EXCIMER LASER

R.K. Rajpal,[1,2] M. Bejanian,[3] J.K. Cheetham,[3] R. DeGryse,[3] and B.L. Reis[3]

[1]Georgetown University Medical Center, Washington DC; [2]George Washington University Medical Center, Washington DC; [3]Allergan, Inc., Irvine California

Purpose: Ketorolac tromethamine (ketorolac) is a NSAID whose analgesic and anti-inflammatory effects are mediated primarily by inhibition of cyclo-oxygenase activity which blocks prostaglandin synthesis. This study tested the analgesic efficacy and safety of ketorolac 0.5% ophthalmic solution (Acular®) following PRK. **Methods:** Two hundred patients enrolled into a double-masked study were randomized to receive one drop of ketorolac or vehicle (both are BAK preserved) QID beginning immediately after PRK and for three days following the procedure. Each installation of ketorolac or vehicle was preceded 5 minutes earlier by instillation of one drop of Ocuflox. Patients were instructed to take one capsule of Mepergan F9rtj5® every six hours as escape medication for intolerable pain. Patients returned for daily visits until day 3 or until re-epithelialization was complete (days 4–8). Pain intensity and pain relief were recorded by patients in daily diaries. Use of escape medication, symptoms of ocular discomfort and functional activity measurements were included in post-operative daily visit assessments. **Results:** The ketorolac group had a significant reduction in pain intensity during the first 12 hours after PRK ($p = 0.001$). In addition, pain relief was significantly greater in the ketorolac group at 6 and 12 hours ($p = 0.001$), and, 36 and 48 hours ($p < 0.05$) after PRK when compared to the vehicle group. The first use of escape medication after PRK was significantly delayed from a mean of 3.9 hours in the vehicle group to 8.4 hours in the ketorolac group ($p = 0.001$). Ketorolac-treated patients had a significantly reduced incidence of sleep difficulties (awakened by pain; trouble falling asleep; took additional medication to fall asleep) for up to 2 days after PRK ($p < 0.05$). The ketorolac-treated patients also had significantly less difficulty in opening their surgical eye during the 3 days after PRK and had reduced incidence of symptoms of ocular discomfort such as foreign body sensation and photophobia during the first 4 hours after the surgery ($p < 0.05$). Incidence of functional impairment such as difficulty watching television and difficulty spending time in a well-lighted room was significantly decreased ($p < 0.05$) in the ketorolac group during the first 2 days after PRK. However, a statistically significant modest delay in re-epithelialization was observed ($p = 0.001$) from 2.7 days in the vehicle group to 3.2 days in the ketorolac group. The clinical importance of this finding is unknown. **Conclusion:** Ketorolac, when used four times daily, is effective in relieving pain and other related discomfort symptoms for up to three days following PRK.

CYCLOOXYGENASE INHIBITORS IN OCULAR PAIN TREATMENT POST PRK

S.de Ita J. Graue E., Trapatsas C , Moreno L., Ramirez T., Suarez R., Climent A.

Instituto De Oftalmologia, Universidad Nacional Autonoma De Mexico, Mexico City

Purpose. To evaluate and compare the analgesic efficacy of topical ketorolac and diclofenac in postoperative patients with PRK and excimer laser for myopia. **Methods.** In this prospective study, 72 patients (64 eyes) were subject of PRK divided in 4 topical treatment groups. Group 1. Diclofenac 0.1% 24 hrs preoperative. Group 2. Diclofenac 0.1% postoperative. Group 3. Ketorolac 0.5% 24 hrs preoperative. Group 4. Ketorolac 9.5% postoperative. In all 4 groups, we used a therapeutic contact lens and topical treatment until epithelialization was completed . All patients were seen biomicroscopically at 24 and 48 hrs postoperative. We evaluated ocular pain, its maximum intensity and other associated ocular symptoms through a categorical scale (0=absent, 1=rnild, 2=moderate, 3=intense, 4=very intense) and a visual analogical scale. We also used a standardized scale of 1/2, 2, 4, 6, 8, 12 and 24 hrs postoperative. **Results.** At the first 8 hrs, both drugs had significative differences in ocular pain intensity when compared with the treatment application pre and postoperative. Groups 1 and 2 ($p=0.001$), Groups 3 and 4 ($p>0.01$). At

24 hrs we compared Groups 1 and 2 (p=0.001). groups 3 and 4 (p>0.05). We found increased ocular complaints as photophobia and foreign body sensation in Groups 2 and 4. The epithelization time decreased in Group 3 (32hrs) compared with Group 4 (44.6hrs).

Conclusions. Haring known that pain is more intense in the first hours of surgery, the start of treatment 24 hrs before surgery reduces significantly pain and associated ocular manifestations. Preoperative diclofenac (group 1) presents the highest analgesic efficacy after PRK and excimer laser for myopia. We did not find any relationship between application time of both drugs and epithelialization time. Supported by Conacyt Grant F082I9110.

COLLAGEN MODULATORS IN EXCIMER LASER SURGERY

Richard A. Eiferman and Dale DeVore

VA Medical Center, Louisville, KY and Autogenesis, Inc., Boston, MA

Excimer laser energy does not discriminate topographically and will reproduce corneal irregularities deeper within the stroma. In phototherapeutic keratectomy (PTK), the surgeon endeavors to remove elevations and protect the valleys to produce a uniform corneal surface. Modulators for corneal surgery have been developed which absorb ultraviolet radiation and protect the underlying stroma while allowing surface irregularities to be leveled. An optimal modulator would flow evenly across the cornea with little to no meniscus, resist rippling effects due to gas flow and maintain corneal hydration.

Many materials have been evaluated as potential modulators including dextrans, HPMC, saline and sodium hyaluronidate. However, liquids tend to form a meniscus and may splatter when struck by a laser beam whereas more viscous materials may prevent adequate treatment.

We have developed a solution of type I collagen that rapidly gels forming a firm surface on the cornea. Gellation occurs within 20 seconds after exposure to a buffer and adheres to the cornea.

We tested several collagen modulator on enuclated human and porcine eyes. A checkerboard grid pattern was formed by firing the excimer laser thru a fine mesh screen. Various concentrations of modulator were tested for their ability to fill the depressions and allow ablation of the elevated grid. 5mg/ml was optimal and this concentration appeared to ablate at the same rate as corneal collagen. Additional experiments indicate concentrations could be varied to provide different ablation rates. Collagen modulators may be useful in therapeutic excimer laser surgery and as a template for refractive laser surgery.

MORPHOLOGY OF HAZE WITH THE CONFOCAL MICROSCOPY

Lourdes Moreno, Enrique Graue, Tito Ramirez, Raul Suarez, Alejandro Climent, and Adriana Hernández

Instituto de Oftalmologia, Mexico, D.F.

After PRK, a series of events takes place: the epithelium is removed, Bowman's layer disappears, and the anterior stroma is remodeled. As a result, fibronectin is deposited In the anterior stroma, a new basal membrane is gradually formed, and a migration of fibroblasts takes place. In most cases, this response is observed clinically as a haze that assumes a patchy pattern and tends to disappear with time. In others, the haziness increases and persists with subsequent loss of vision. It has been noted that this response is related to the amount of the ablation, and to the steepening of the transition zone. However, there are patients who do not respond in the same manner. In this study we present 10 eyes of 10 patients who were submitted to PRK for correction of different levels of myopia and astigmatism, and were evaluated with the confocal microscopy, monthly during the first year post op trying to elucidate the nature of the response, that could help us to better understand the corneal behaviors after PRK. (Supported by Conacyt Grant F08219110.)

HYALURONAN, WATER, AND WOUND HEALING IN RABBIT CORNEAS AFTER PIANO AND PHOTOREFRACTIVE KERATECTOMY

Beat Weber[1] and Per Fagerholm[2]

[1,2]St. Eriks Eye Hospital; Karolinska Institute; Stockholm, Sweden, Augenklinik Kantonspital Luzern; Luzern, Switzerland[1]

The purpose was to localize hyaluronan and water in rabbit corneas and to compare the extension of the subepithelial low dry mass areas after plano and refractive keratectomy, respectively.

Twenty rabbits assigned into two groups were treated on one eye each with plano and refractive keratectomy, respectively.

In a first study, quantitative microradiography and specific histochemical staining for hyaluronan were consecutively applied on the same freeze-dried corneal sections of the five rabbits sacrificed 4 weeks after photorefractive keratectomy. Of the treated eyes the mean quotient between the dry mass in the superficial stroma and in the basal epithelium was 0.66, whereas in the untreated eyes the corresponding value was 1.29. This means a considerable amount of water was accumulating in the superficial stroma 4 weeks after photorefractive keratectomy. Furthermore water was shown to accumulate where hyaluronan was found, i.e. in the subepithelial stroma of the wounded area.

In both treatment groups the water accumulation was further analysed by planimetry in order to follow the reactivity of corneal wound healing after plano and steep refractive treatment, respectively. Our results suggest that a flat surface causes less reactivity during the subsequent wound healing when compared to a steep curve refractive treatment. The difference was statistically significant alter 4 weeks.

APOPTOSIS IN THE RABBIT CORNEA AFTER PHOTOREFRACTIVE KERATECTOMY (PRK)

J. Gao, T. A. Gelber-Schwalb, and M. E. Stem

Biological Sciences, Allergan, Inc. Irvine, California

Purpose: PRK is currently used as a method in refractive conditions such as myopia an astigmatism. It has been well documented that there is a loss of keratocytes in the cornea after surgical or traumatic insult such as PRK. Recent study has suggested that apoptosis programmed cell death, might be involved in this disappearance of keratocytes. The goal this study is to evaluate the mechanisms and level of apoptosis in the cornea post PR.

Methods: Rabbits (Dutch-Cross, 2.5 kg) were anesthesized systemically with Ketamine HCI (20 mg/Kg) and Xylazine (4 mg/Kg) and topically with proparacaine (Ophthetic®). The corneal epithelium was removed using phototherapeutic keratectomy (PTK, 100 pulses PRK was then performed (-9.0D, 5.0mm optical zone). Rabbits were time sacrificed at four days and four weeks and the corneas were isolated and fixed (10% formalin) for TUNEL apoptosis assay. This assay detects DNA segmentation, the initial event in apoptosis. All procedures involving the use of rabbits in this study conformed to the ARVO resolution of the use of animals in research. **Results:** The TUNEL assay demonstrated that: (1) the normal cornea exhibited a limited level of apoptosis, primarily in the superficial epithelium, with very little in the basal epithelium, and none in the keratocytes and endothelium; (2) the entire epithelial layer was found to be apoptotic at four days as well as four weeks post PR and (3) an elevated level of apoptosis was also detected in both keratocytes an endothelial cells following PRK at the same time points. **Conclusions:** These finding suggest that apoptosis is involved in the natural turn-over of the superficial epithelial cell. Additionally, apoptosis also plays an important role in the corneal wound healing process. Following PRK, reepithelialization yields, initially, a totally apoptotic epithelium. The keratocytes as well as endothelial cells are also activated and turn-over rapidly via apoptosis. Potential mediators of this process in the post PRK cornea is currently under investigation.

CORNEAL NERVE DAMAGE AND REGENERATION AFTER LASIK

Timo Tervo,[1] C. Barraquer-Coll,[2] J.J. Perez-Santonja,[3] K. Tervo,[1] T. Latvala,[1] and J. Alio-Sanz[3]

Departments of Ophthalmology, University of Helsinki, Finland[1] and Alicante, Spain[3]; Clinique America Barraquer, Bolivia, Bogota[2]

Purpose. To investigate the changes in the corneal nerves after laser assisted keratomileusis (LASIK) performed on 3 human and 14 rabbit eyes, and to compare these alterations with those observed earlier by us after PRK.

Methods. The human LASIK operations were performed on blind eyes 8 days, 1.5 or 4 months prior to an enucleation for medical reasons. The hinged corneal flaps were made with an automated microkeratome and the photoablation of the stromal bed was done with a VisX 20/20 excimer laser. Similar operations (flap thickness about 120–130 μm, diameter 6 mm photoablation 6 D) were performed on the rabbit corneas. The nerves were demonstrated histochemically by their acetylcholinesterase (AchE) -activity. **Results.** In human corneas, the flap appeared thinner than planned and showed some epithelial downgrowth into the wound. In general, there was less healing response and scar tissue than after PRK. Deep stromal nerves were normal but cut profiles were found in the superficial stromal bed. Regenerating fibers emerged from them. The subepithelial plexus, epithelial fibers and some stromal profiles of the flap showed only relatively minor changes. Essentially similar observations were made with the rabbit corneas. Anastomizing fibers between the neighbouring stromal nerves and patterns suggesting regeneration via the existing but cut stromal nerve channels were also observed. **Conclusion.** LASIK seems to induce less striking and more completely and rapidly healing damage to corneal nerves than PRK.

AVOIDANCE AND MANAGEMENT OF SELECTED COMPLICATIONS OF EXCIMER PRK

Jonathan H. Talamo

Assistant Clinical Professor of Ophthalmology, Harvard Medical School, Cornea Consultants, Boston, Massachusetts

While surgical techniques for excimer PRK are usually straightforward, meticulous attention to preoperative and intraoperative details is important to avoid complications such as damage to Bowman's membrane or ablation decentration during surgery and persistent epithelial defects postoperatively. Strategies for preventing and treating such complications will be discussed.

REOPERATIONS AFTER PRK

U. Genth, I. Tersi, T. Seiler, and R. Krueger*

University Eye Clinic, TU Dresden, Dresden, Germany and *Department of Ophthalmology, Anheuser-Busch Eye Institute, St. Louis, MO

Purpose: Reoperations after PRK may be necessary because of overcorrection, undercorrection, scarring, central islands and small optical zones. **Methods:** During April 94 and March 95. 69 eyes were retreated at least 6 months after primary PRK In all reoperations the epithelium was removed with a centered Fm with diameters of 6 to 7.5 mm. This resulted in a hyperopic correction of 1.5 D, sufficient to correct small amounts of overcorrection. In cases of undercorrection, scarring, and enlargement of the optical zone the VTK was followed by a PRK with the attempted correction of "refractive error -1.5 D". In central island-cases also an additional PRK (ø 3 mm, attempted correction 100% of initial PRK) was performed. **Results:** Except in patients with scarring the reoperations were successful in resolving the patients' complaints (Table). **Conclusion:** Reoperations are safe and efficient in the management of complications after PRK.

Type of error	Number of eyes	Success rate
Overcorrection	12	10 (92%)
Undercorrection	18	16 (89%)
Scarring/undercorrection	10	6 (60%)
Central islands	8	8 (100%)
Small optical zone	8	8 (100%)

UNDERCORRECTION AFTER EXCIMER LASER REFRACTIVE SURGERY

Rasik B Vajpayee, Catherine A McCarty, Geoffrey F Aldred, and Hugh R Taylor

Melbourne Excimer Laser Group, The University of Melbourne Department of Ophthalmology, Melbourne, Australia

Purpose: Over a period of one year we studied the incidence, pattern and correlations of undercorrection in 645 patients who had undergone excimer laser refractive surgery. **Methods:** The cohort included a consecutive series of 645 patients who had undergone excimer PRK or PARK. All patients underwent an initial pre-laser ocular examination and follow-up ocular examinations at one, three, six and twelve months. The parameters evaluated were visual acuity, refraction and corneal clarity. **Results:** The incidence of undercorrection by $\geq$ -1.00D exhibited a gradual increase from 10% at one month to 40% at twelve months. The degree of pre-operative myopia showed a significant association with occurrence of undercorrection at 3 months (X^2 = 17.3, p <0.001), 6 months (X^2 = 53.6, p <0.001), and 12 months (X^2 = 64.8, p <0.001). After controlling for amplitude of attempted correction the odds of undercorrection in patients who had PRK as compared to those who had PARK were 0.40 (95% CL = 0.25, 0.60). At one year a loss of two or more lines of best corrected visual acuity was recorded in 38% of undercorrected patients. The multivariate odds ratio for loss of two or more lines of best corrected acuity for these undercorrected cases was 8.8 (95% CL = 5.4, 14.6). No relationship was seen between corneal haze and loss of best corrected visual acuity. No association of undercorrection was seen with age, gender, use of NSAID, bandage contact lens wear and corneal haze. At six months, 71 % of them were within ±0.5D of their one year refraction. Of the 17 cases with undercorrection treated with topical corticosteroids only one patient showed a permanent beneficial change. **Conclusion:** Occurrence of undercorrection is more common in higher myopes and when simultaneous astigmatic corrections are undertaken. Also people who exhibit a loss of best corrected visual acuity are more likely to be undercorrected. It seems that irregular epithelial hyperplasia is important for both undercorrection and loss of best corrected visual acuity.

A DECENTERED P.R.K

A.J.M. Geerards and W.H. Beekhuis

Eye Hospital Rotterdam, The Netherlands

A 38 year old male was treated for his myopia S -5.50=C-2.50 axis 20 on a Visx 20/20, zone 6 mm.. Poor fixation and inexperience caused a considerable decentration. After three months, a rigid gas permeable lens was fitted because of monocular diplopia (S -1.25=C -2.25 axis 130 J. B.C.V.A. was 20/20.

Nine months after the first treatment, retreatment was done with masking the area already treated. Refraction before treatment was S-3.50=C-2.50 axis 30, B.C.V.A. 20/24. Diplopia remained a major complaint, caused by the residual epithelial hyperplasia at the edge of the treatment, which necessitates retreatment after a year. Refraction before treatment S -0.5=C-1.50 axis 80, B.C.V.A. 20/20. Retreatment consisted of mechanical abrasion with slit lamp control, followed by phototherapeutic smoothing of the irregular area.

This case is illustrated with videokeratoscopy and photographies to explain the extreme difficulties encountered by this complication of photorefractive keratectomy.

PHOTOREFRACTIVE KERATECTOMY FOR ASTIGMATISM

Ramón Naranjo-Tackman, Karla Uribe, and Diego Cuevas-Cancino

Cornea Department, Asociación Para Evitar la Ceguera en México, México, D.F.

Purpose: To evaluate the efficacy, visual outcome and complications of PRK for astigmatism. **Methods:** A prospective evaluation of cases that underwent Photorefractive Keratectomy for astigmatism larger than -2.5 D up to -6.00 D of cylindrical defect, with less than -1.00 D of myopia, was done. A VISX 20/20 Excimer Laser was used. In all cases Visual Acuity (VA),Best Corrected Visual Acuity (BCVA), Cylinder and Sphere, as well as Keratometries were evaluated. Corneal topography was evaluated, using a TMS-1 Corneal Modeling System. Postoperative treatment was similar to the one used in myopic PRK. No bandage lens or non-steroidal anti-inflammatories, were used until epithelization or after. **Results:** Epithelization took 2 to 4 days, after the procedure. A total of 19 eyes-15 patients, were treated. % patients received simultaneous bilateral treatment.

	Mean VA	BCVA	Cylinder	Sphere
Preop:	20/200	20/25	-4.12 D	-0.50 D
Postop6/12	20/40	20/25	-0.75 D	+0.16 D
Postop12/12	20/30	20/25	-0.33 D	-0.25 D

74% of all cases had a VA of 20/40 or better at 12 months. 87% of cases had 20/40 or better BCVA. Topographic maps correlated well with VA and BCVA The more regular the pattern, the better VA and BCVA were obtained. One patient required retreatment after 8 months, because of regression. In 2 patients loss of one line of vision was reported, 2 patients gained 2 lines of vision. Haze was considered not significant, ranging from 0 to +. **Conclusions:** This series shows that PER for astigmatism, has a good result, that tend to be stable and with the risks reported for PER for myopia in low to moderate cases. Although some loss of effect was observed, the procedure tended to correct with more predictability moderate or high cases of astigmatism.

EFFECTS OF DICLOFENAC SODIUM AND FLUOROMETHOLONE DROPS IN POST-EXCIMER PHOTOREFRACTIVE KERATOTOMY THERAPY

A.L. Perez-Balbuena, N. Gudino, A. Figueroa, and D. Cuevas-Cancino

Associon para Evitar lad Ceguera en Mexico, Mexico, D.F.

Purpose: Compare the effects of (Diclofenac Sodium) and fluorometholone on the rate of re-epithelization and on refractive and visual results after photorefractive keratotomy.

Methods: Twenty subjects were submitted to diclofenac, fluorometholone, on control (cellufresh artificial tears). In each treatment, drops were instilled 4 times a day immediately after surgery, and taped over a 4 month period. The time of re-epithelization was definite by analysis of the epithelial defect in slit lamp examination, visual acuity, manifest refraction, and central corneal clarity were determined at one and three months. There were no significant differences between treatments in appearance or re-epithelization refractive outcome or clarity.

Conclusion: Neither Voltaren (Diclofenac Sodium) nor Fluorometholone retardes or stimlated re-epithelization after excimer laser photorefractive keratectomy therapy and there were practically no differences between them regarding refractive outcome during the phase of therapy.

PHOTOREFRACTIVE KERATECTOMY FOLLOWING PENETRATING KERATOPLASTY

Donald T.H. Tan, Li Lim, W.K. Chan, and V. Balakrishnan

Singapore National Eye Centre

Purpose: We conducted a study to investigate the safety and efficacy of performing PRK following penetrating keratoplasty in patients with significant postoperative astigmatism and myopia. **Methods:** Consecutive cases of post-graft myopia or astigmatism not correctable with spectacles or unsuccessful with contact lens wear underwent PRK with a 193 nm ArF excimer laser (VisX 20/20B, VisX Corporation, Santa Clara, CA). All cases had prelaser manifest refraction with fogging and/or cycloplegic refraction and EyeSys corneal topography. Postoperatively all patients were monitored with manifest and cycloplegic refractors and 6 cases had postlaser corneal topography performed Astigmatic change was analysed by computerised vector analysis. **Results:** PRK was performed in 11 eyes of 10 patients at a mean of 21.9 months postkeratoplasty. The mean age was 33.8 years (range 19–81). Mean follow-up period after PRK was 6.1 months. The pre-laser spherical error varied from +1.5D to -7.0D (mean -2.2 D), while the pre-laser cylindrical error varied from -3.0D to -10.0D (mean -6.8D). Attempted spherical and cylindrical correction with the laser in general closely followed the cycloplegic refraction. Assessment of postlaser refractive results at 1 month showed an overall improvement in spherical refraction to a mean of -0.5D (range +4.OD to -3.5D). At a mean follow-up of 6.1 months, minimal myopic regression had occurred, and the mean spherical refraction remained at -0.75D (range +3.7SD to -3.5D). Analysis of residual cylindrical error at 1 month revealed a mean cylinder of -2.2D (range plano to -4.5D). With the exception of one case in which significant astigmatic regression occurred, this remained stable at an average follow-up period of 6.1 months (mean of -2.5D, range plano to -7.0D). One month after PRK, the ratio of achieved refractive cylindrical change to intended correction was 0.78, and this remained constant at 6 months. No eye in this series lost best-corrected Snellen acuity, 2 eyes gained one line of acuity, and 1 eye gained 2 lines. Trace haze was encountered in 3 eyes, and 1 eye developed mild haze associated with significant astigmatic regression. **Conclusions:** Excimer laser PRK appears to be a safe and effective procedure to reduce myopia and astigmatism after penetrating keratoplasty. The achievement of 78% astigmatic correction suggests that a planned overcorrection of 20% should be considered in the treatment of postkeratoplasty astigmatism with the excimer laser.

PROSPECTIVE EVALUATION OF DIFFERENT TREATMENTS FOR MYOPIC ASTIGMATISM

I. Tersi, N. Alkara, H. Schmidt-Petersen, and T. Seiler

University Eye Clinic, TU Dresden, Dresden, Germany

Purpose. Two procedures to correct myopic astigmatism were studied prospectively: photoastigmatic refractive keratectomy (PARK) and standard PRK combined with arcuate incisions (PRK + AK). **Methods.** Twenty eyes of 20 patients were enrolled in each treatment group and followed for at least 6 months. The spherical equivalent ranged from -1.5 D to -7.0 D and the cylinder up to -5.0 D in each group (average: -2.5 D in PARK, -2.6 D in PRK + AK). The PARK procedure was performed with the Schwind Keratome providing an elliptical beam (short axis: 5.1 mm, long axis: 8.1 mm). In the PRK + AK group arcuate keratotomies were performed with a local depth of 80%, an optical zone of 7 mm, and variable length. One month later, the residual myopia was treated by a standard PRK (ø 6 mm). **Results.** At 6 months, in both groups astigmatic undercorrection was common (residual cylinder PARK: -1.02 D, PRK + AK: -0.97 D) whereas the spherical correction was satisfying (PARK: +0.38 D, PRK + AK: +0.45 D). These differences were not statistically significant. **Conclusion.** The two procedures are clinically equivalent. Long term data is necessary to study the stability of the results.

CORNEAL TOPOGRAPHY APPLIED TO LASER KERATOMILEUSIS

Angela Mana Gutiererrez

A review of the topographic studies performed on 106 patients submitted to Excimer laser is presented. Patients were divided into two groups: a first group of 34 patients submitted to superficial myopic keratomileusis (SMK) and a second group of 72 eyes submitted to intrastromal myopic keratomileusis (IMK). The relationship between the centering of the ablation and visual acuity, the configuration of the optic zone, the ablation's regularity, the optic zone's dimensions and the parametric indexes were analyzed. An association between pre-operative and post-op topographies was established.

No difference in the centering of the ablation was found among the two procedures. We found it easier to predict the optic zone with the intrastromal technique. A correlation between the Sim K arid Min K in both groups was found. Differential mapping between the pre-operative arid post-operative topographies and among the various post-operative exams comes forth as a new and valuable application of the topographic study.

CORNEAL SURFACE ABLATION USING A NEW SOLID STATE LASER (FIFTH HARMONIC ND:YAG AT 213 NM)

R.W. Snyder,[1] T.R. Kramer,[1] M.Yarborough,[2] G. Marcellino,[3] T.L. Rottler,[1] and C. Bindi[1]

[1]University of Arizona, Tucson, AZ; [2]Coherent Laser, Inc., Tucson, AZ; [3]Coherent, Inc., Palo Alto, CA

Purpose: To evaluate the surface ablation characteristics of a new solid state laser (fifth harmonic Nd:YAG at 213 nm) for use in photorefractive keratectomy (PRK) and compare it to a commercially available Summit excimer laser (193 nm). **Methods:** Six diopter PRKs were performed in PMMA discs with a Summit excimer laser and a fifth harmonic Nd:YAG laser; wavelength =213 nm, 3 mJ/ pulse, pulse duration approximately 3 ns (Coherent, Inc., Palo Alto, CA). Both ablations used a 6 mm optical zone. The Nd:YAG (213 nm) ablation was performed with a 1 mm beam diameter scanned with a computer generated raster pattern with 50 to 80% overlap. Hyperopic and astigmatic corrections were also performed with the Nd:YAG (213 nm) laser. The resultant ablation profiles were determined with a Coherent optical profilometer. Surface ablations of rabbit corneas were also performed with the Nd:YAG (213 inn) and Summit excimer laser following epithelial debridement. The rabbits were sacrificed and the cornea tissue was examined by scanning electron microscopy (SEM), transmission electron microscopy (TEM) and standard light microscopy (LM). **Results:** The surface heights of the myopic corrections on PMMA discs were determined and the deviation in height over the entire ablation zone was +A 3 μm when compared to a best lit sphere for both the excimer and Nd:YAG (213 nm) lasers. The hyperopic and astigmatic corrections with the Nd:YAG (213 nm) also approximated the expected surface profiles by within a few microns. The SEM of rabbit corneal ablations for both the excimer and Nd:YAG (213 nm) revealed smooth bases and no evidence of collagen shrinkage. There was no coagulative damage noted with the excimer or Nd:YAG (213 nm) lasers by LM or EM. **Conclusion:** The surface ablation patterns obtained with a scanning Nd:YAG (213 nm) laser compare favorably with the Summit excimer laser. We believe this laser warrants further evaluation for PRK (Supported in part by Coherent, Inc., Palo Alto, CA).

PHOTOTHERAPEUTIC KERATECTOMY

Christopher Requaro

The excimer laser has been undergoing rapid development for clinical use since the early 1980s. The authors report 5-year follow-up results from studies of 115 eyes to evaluate the excimer laser in performing phototherapeutic keratectomy. Patients were divided into two groups: 64 eyes (group 1) underwent phototherapeutic keratectomy for treatment of a dystrophy or scar, and 51 eyes group 2) underwent phototherapeutic keratectomy for refractive abnormalities. Visual function improved in 86% of cases in group 1 and 78% of cases in group 2. Complications were minimal and manageable. The authors describe a procedure to minimize induced hyperopia in phototherapeutic keratectomy patients, and, although not statistically significant, less induced hyperopia was noted in these patients. Photokeratectomy may be an alternative to penetrating or lamellar keratoplasty and more invasive refractive procedures, but the long-term effects must be carefully observed.

PHOTOTHERAPEUTIC KERATECTOMY FOR RECURRENT CORNEAL EROSIONS

G.R. Snibson, R. Vajapayee, T. Couper, and H.R. Taylor

University of Melbourne Department of Ophthalmology, Australia

Aim. To evaluate the use of the excimer laser in the treatment of recurrent epithelial erosions of the cornea.

Method. Thirty-one eyes of 29 patients with recurrent corneal erosions resistant to other forms of therapy were followed for 6–41 months after phototherapeutic keratectomy (PTK). In 14 eyes (45%) the erosions followed an episode of trauma, in 13 (42%) there were signs of epithelial basement membrane dystrophy, and two eyes of one patient were affected by Reis-Bücklers dystrophy. One eye developed recurrent epithelial erosions following HSV keratitis and another as a consequence of a chemical injury. The epithelium was easily removed by gentle mechanical debridement in all cases. Superficial (5–15 micron) ablations were performed using the VISX twenty/twenty excimer laser to remove residual basement membrane and the superficial part of Bowman's layer. Deeper ablations (25–89 microns) were performed where there was anterior stromal opacity (2 eyes) and when treatment of coexistent myopia or myopic astigmatism was requested (8 eyes). **Results.** No further erosions have occurred in 16 eyes (52%). This result was more likely in post-traumatic recurrent erosions (57%) than in eyes with basement membrane dystrophy (38%). Six patients (19%) reported minor symptoms consistent with corneal microerosions but were markedly improved and expressed a high degree of satisfaction with the procedure: In three eyes (10%) there was some improvement in either the frequency or severity of the symptoms but in six eyes (19%) there was no discernible benefit from PTK. Superficial (non-refractive) ablations were accompanied by only minor refractive changes and minimal haze. **Conclusions.** Phototherapeutic keratectomy would appear to be a safe and effective treatment for recurrent corneal erosion syndrome when more conservative measures have been unsuccessful.

SHORT AND LONG-TERM FOLLOW-UP OF EXCIMER LASER PHOTOTHERAPEUTIC KERATECTOMY FOR ANTERIOR CORNEAL PATHOLOGY

Christopher J. Rapuano

Cornea Service, Wills Eye Hospital, Thomas Jefferson University, Philadelphia, Pennsylvania

Purpose: To determine the safety and efficacy of excimer laser phototherapeutic keratectomy (PTK) for anterior corneal pathology . **Methods:** Excimer laser PTK was performed using the VISX, Inc. Model B system as part of the FDA phase III clinical trials on patients with anterior corneal pathology. Diagnostic, demographic as well as pre-operative and post-operative visual acuity with and without correction, keratometric readings, corneal clarity, corneal topography and patient symptom data were collected and evaluated. **Results:** 29 eyes of 25 patients underwent excimer laser PTK by the author. Pre-operative diagnoses included Salzmann's nodular degeneration (5), granular dystrophy (4), superficial variant of granular dystrophy (4), corneal scars (4), recurrent erosions (3), keratoconus nodules (2), anterior basement membrane dystrophy scarring (I), Schnyder's crystalline dystrophy (1) and Reis-Buckler's dystrophy (1). Mean follow-up was 20 months (range 1.5–40 months). Uncorrected and best corrected visual acuity improved in between 50–67% of eyes and deteriorated in only 5%. Complications included induced hyperopia, induced myopia, induced astigmatism, elective retreatment, lamellar keratoplasty and penetrating keratoplasty. There were no corneal ulcers. **Conclusions:** Excimer laser PTK appears to be a safe and effective modality to treat certain anterior corneal pathologies. In the author's experience, the smoothness of the cornea, the density and depth of the opacity, and whether the pathology is elevated or depressed are the best.

ONE YEAR FOLLOW-UP RESULTS OF PHOTOTHERAPEUTIC KERATECTOMY PATIENTS USING THE CHIRON-TECHNOLAS 116 EXCIMER LASER

C. Lee,[1] F. Brightbill,[1] N. Barney,[1] D. Durrie,[2] S. Johnson,[3] R. Lembach,[4] R. Lindstrom,[5] D. Hardten,[5] M. McDonald,[6] F. Price,[7] W. Whitson,[7] J. Robin,[8] K. Solomon,[9] M. Speaker,[10] A. Sugar,[11] and R. Meyer[11]

[1]Madison, [2]Kansas City, [3]DesMoines, [4]Columbus, [5]Minneapolis, [6]New Orleans, [7]Indianapolis, [8]Cleveland, [9]Charleston, [10]New York, [11]Ann Arbor

We have yet to identify the precise technique with which excimer laser is delivered to remove stromal pathology and concomitantly improve corneal clarity and visual acuity without leaving residual astigmatism and inducing hyperopia. In an effort to identify factors that influence the results of PTK, we reviewed the data of all patients who underwent PTK at 11 Chiron-Technolas laser sites in the United States.

As of 12/31/95, a total of 85 patients had been enrolled in this study. At the University of Wisconsin-Madison, 10 patients were treated for corneal opacities due to band keratopathy, anterior corneal dystrophies, nodular degeneration, or leukoma secondary to penetrating or chemical injuries. Two patients were lost to follow-up; one patient with preexisting corneal edema required penetrating keratoplasty and one patient died. At the time of this writing, charts reviewed had an average follow-up of 8.75 months (range: 1–12 months). All patients had re-epithelialized by post-operative day 7.

Preliminary results showed that a relative hyperopia had been induced in all patients with an average relative hyperopic shift of 1.5 Diopters (range: 0.35–5.00D). Two eyes demonstrated an initial hyperopic shift with subsequent myopic regression due to progression of cataract. Corneal clarity improved in all patients. 87.5% of patients showed an initial improvement in visual acuity. In those patients without improvement, visual acuity was limited by progressive cataract and age-related macular degeneration.

Despite visual improvement in most eyes, corneal topographic studies revealed residual irregular astigmatism in all patients. Interestingly, in those patients who had been followed for one year, an increase in peripheral corneal thickness was noted by the six month follow-up visit. Recurrent erosions, bacterial keratitis and iritis have not been documented in any patients.

The Chiron-Technolas excimer laser used for PTK has improved the corneal clarity and visual acuity in most eyes. The design of this laser allows for excellent surgeon control using "joy-stick" delivery of laser energy.

PROSPECTIVE TRIAL OF LASER *IN SITU* KERATOMILEUSIS (LASIK) FOR MYOPIA

George O. Waring III, Keith P. Thompson, and R. Doyle Stulting

Emory University, Atlanta, Georgia

We report the interim results of an ongoing prospective trial of laser *in situ* keratomileusis (LASIK) for myopia. To date, 546 eyes have entered the study, 18% with simultaneous arcuate transverse keratotomy for astigmatism. We present the three month results on ~318 eyes of 171 patients with a baseline refraction from -2.00 to -21.00 D. We used the Summit Omnimed excimer laser with either a 6 mm diameter single zone or a multizone (3 zones: 5.0, 6.01 6.5 mm) ablation and the Chiron automated corneal shaper microkeratome with a 160 um thick hinged corneal flap. Of 513 eyes at 24 hours after surgery, 52% saw 20/40 or better uncorrected. At 3 months after the primary LASIK procedure (no enhancements), 22% of eyes saw 20/20 or better and 67% saw 20/40 or better; 38% of eyes had a refractive error within ±0.50 D of desired outcome, 67% within ±1.00 D, and 93% within ±2.00 D. The mean refractive error at 3 months of -0.17 D (±1.5 D). Stability as determined by cycloplegic refraction demonstrated a mean refractive error at 24 hours of -0.21 D, a mean at 2 weeks of -0.14 D, and a mean at 3 months of -0.17 D, indicating good stability after 2 weeks on average. An overcorrection of +1.00 to +2.00 D occurred in 6 eyes (1.8%). A loss of 2 to 5 Snellen lines of spectacle corrected visual acuity occurred in 17 (5.4%) eyes, 2 seeing worse than 20/40.

The protocol contained two randomizations: simultaneous surgery on both eyes vs sequential surgery separated by two weeks and single zone vs multizone ablation pattern on the two eyes of each patient; results of these randomizations will be presented. Eighty four (15%) eyes received a second LASIK or transverse keratotomy (enhancement procedure) and the results after enhancements will also be reported.

We think LASIK is a safe and effective method of reducing or correcting a wide range of myopia. The algorithms for the refractive correction need improvement.

PROSPECTIVE EVALUATION OF CHIRON TECHNOLAS EXCIMER LASER *IN SITU* KERATOMILEUSIS (LASIK) FOR MODERATE TO HIGH MYOPIA

John S. Berestka, David R. Hardten, Paula J. Parker, and Richard L. Lindstrom

As part of a Phase II clinical trial, the Chiron Technolas Keracor 116 193nm excimer laser was used to perform LASIK on 28 patients with -4.00 to -10.00 D of myopia and less than 1 D of astigmatism. Preoperative refractive error (spherical equivalent) averaged -6.18 ± 1.20 D. At one month postoperatively, 95% of patients had uncorrected visual acuities of 20/40 or better. At six months, 93% of patients had uncorrected acuities of 20/40 or better. The mean spherical equivalent improved from +0.49 ± 0.67 D at one month to 0.00± 1.01 D at 3 months (p = 0.02). The mean spherical equivalent at 3 months and 6 months (+0.03 ± 0.68) were not statistically different (p =0.39). One patient developed a free cap during the procedure and lost 2 lines (20/16 to 20/25) of best corrected visual acuity (BCVA). Four patients (14%) lost one line of BCVA, seventeen patients (61%) had no change in BCVA, and six patients (21.4%) gained one line of BCVA. All patients had a BCVA of 20/25 or better. Laser *in situ* keratomileusis is safe and effective for the treatment of moderate and high myopia and may be superior to photorefractive keratectomy for treating this range of myopia. The refractive results regress by approximately 0.50 D over the first three months and then appear to stabilize.

LASIK VS. MULTI-ZONE PRK FOR TREATMENT OF MODERATE TO HIGH MYOPIA: CLINICAL ANALYSIS

M.F. Sartori, W. Chamon, E. Nascimento, W. Nosé, and M. Campos

Paulista School of Medicine, Federal University of São Paulo-Brazil

Background: Laser *in situ* Keratomileusis (LASIK) has been proposed as a method of reducing stromal scarring after photorefractive keratectomy (PRK). **Purpose:** To compare LASIK and Multi-zone PRK in treating moderate to high myopia. **Methods:** Ten eyes from five patients were randomized for multi-zone PRK (GI) in one eye and LASIK (GII) in the fellow eye. The preoperative mean cycloplegic spherical equivalent was -10.85 D ± 2.19 D in GI and -14.75 D ±2.36 D in GII. Mean postoperative follow-up was 8.8 months (range: 1–16) in LASIK treated eyes and 6.6 months (range: 3–18) in multi-zone PRK treated eyes. **Surgical Technique:** A clear corneal molder (Draeger modified microkeratome) was used to perform the lamellar dissection creating a hinged flap. Stromal ablation was performed using the Omnimed Summit Excimer Laser. Ablation zones were 5.0 mm since all treated eyes had spherical equivalent exceeding -9.00 D. For the multi-zone PRK operating eyes 3 different ablation zone diameters (5.5, 6.0 and 6.5 mm) were performed, using the same machine, after manual keratectomy. **Results:** Myopia was reduced from -10.85 (±2.19D) to -1.1 D(±2.07D) in GI and from -14.75 D (±2.36D) to -2.02D (± 2.72 D) in GII. Best uncorrected visual acuity improved in every patient, and 90% of the treated eyes had lost none or only one line of the best corrected vision. Longer follow-up will be presented. **Conclusion:** Both methods appear to be effective in treating moderate to high myopia.

LASIK IN HYPEROPIA

Klaus Ditzen

Method: Based on the LASIK-procedure of Pallikaris (Crete, Greece) we used the combination of the ALK from Chiron with the ArF 193 nm MEL from Aesculap Meditec.

We used the biggest flap diameter of 8,5 mm. The thickness was 160 µm. For the PRK-procedure we used the hyperopic iris-mask with a special section ring.

Results: There were 41 eyes, divided in two groups: Group I: 18 eyes till + 3,75 dpt, group II: 23 eyes till + B dpt. The follow-up post-op was 1 year. There were nearly no regression. There were as light undercorrection. No haze and less pain were seen. In the second group there was a regression in the first month post-op and after the first month there was only a small regression from about 0,75 dpt. There were nearly no haze and a better stability than in the normal hyperopic PRK.

Disadvantages of the method: No optical control with the keratome and a very bright suction ring of the keratome, probably dislocation or loss of the flap.

ENDOTHELIAL AND INFLAMMATORY REPERCUSSIONS OF LASIK

João Paulo Costa, Mesquita Marques, Paulo Torres, Rui Pinto, and Antanio Marinho

We evaluated the endothelial anatomic alterations and the blood-aqueous barrier functional disturbance in LASIK. Quantification of the flare in the anterior chamber with a Laser Flare Meter®. Computer assisted analysis of endothelium's specular micrographs, obtained with a contact microscope (Bio-Optics LSM 2000 C®) The exams were performed before, at the lst and 3rd days and 6 months after LASIK in 30 eyes with high myopia. The density and the size and shape variability of the endothelial cells didn't show any significant variation. The flare had a significant 2.3 times increase in the 1st and 3rd days. In our experience LASIK didn't have any measurable endothelial repercussions. It causes a mild and transient increase in the permeability of the blood-aqueous barrier.

THE TOPOGRAPHY OF LASIK, PRK, ALK, AND RK

S.D. Klyce

LSU Eye Center, New Orleans, Louisiana

Purpose: Videokeratography has been useful for the characterization, evaluation, and refinement of refractive surgical procedures. We have developed a series of algorithms design to evaluate qualifies of the refractive surgical treatment zone as well as qualities of the corn overlying the apparent entrance pupil of the eye. **Methods.** Corneal topography was evaluated with custom software to evaluate TMS-1 videokeratographs. The custom software required the operator to indicate the exam to be processed, to provide the post-operative time interval, and to indicate on the TMS video the size and position of the patient's pupil and subsequently the position of the treated area using a moveable, size-adjustable circular cursor. Irregular astigmatism was assessed with the Surface Regularity index (SRI), the Coefficient of Variation of corneal Power (CVP), and the Elevation Depression Magnitude (EDM) for preoperative refractive surgical patients (as controls), for an RK cohort at 10 years follow up, for a PRK group at two years, a LASIK cohort at 6 months, an ALK < 9 D subset, and an ALK group treated up to 30 D. **Results:** Mean SRI's were found in the following order of progressively increasing values: PRK <RK < LASIK* <ALK9* < ALK* (* The difference between the mean SRI for treated corneas and the SRI mean for preoperative corneas was statistically significant; $P < 0.05$). A similar progression was found for the average CVP and average EDM. Calculating the Potential Visual Acuity (PVA) from SRI, it was found that ALK reduced PVA by 1.5 to 2.0 lines on the average. **Discussion:** This approach is useful for objective comparisons of irregular astigmatism among alternative approaches to refractive surgery. (Supported by NIH EY 03311 and Computed Anatomy, Inc. Dr. KIyce is a paid consultant to Computed Anatomy, Inc.)

PHAKIC INTRAOCULAR LENSES FOR THE CORRECTION OF HIGH MYOPIA

Joseph Colin

The surgical treatment of high myopia remains a challenge for refractive surgeons. All the keratorefractive procedures share the inability to predict an accurate result for an individual patient and are irreversible. Intraocular procedures, either phakic intraocular lenses (IOLs) or clear lensectomy and implantation of low power posterior chamber IOLs give better refractive results but are more invasive phakic IOLs include all lenses located between the cornea and the anterior surface of the crystalline lens, which is left undisturbed inside the eye.

Three types of phakic IOLs are currently under evaluation:

Developer	Location	Attachment mechanism
Fyodorov	Post. chamber	supported by ant. surface of the lens
Worst-Fechner	Ant. chamber	iris`clip
Baikoff	Ant. chamber	angle supported by haptics

Endothelial cell damage may occur during surgery with the WorstFechner IOL. The first generation of the Baikoff's IOL induced a progressive cell loss in some patients because of an intermittent contact of the periphery of the implant and the corneal endothelium. The cell count decreased with time and was worse with higher implant powers. If endothelial cell losses exceeded 50%, the IOL was removed. Baikoff's IOL was therefore modified to reduce its height and increase the distance between the edge of the implant and the endothelium. After a three year evaluation, it appears that the central endothelial cell loss is statistically stable for all eyes at -5.5%; the loss is similar in the periphery.

CORNEAL PHOTODISRUPTION WITH A Nd:YLF PICOSECOND LASER FOR INTRASTROMAL REFRACTIVE SURGERY

Mitsutoshi Ito, Andrew J. Quantock, Ronald R. Krueger, and David J. Schanzlin

Anheuser-Busch Eye Institute, Department of Ophthalmology Saint Louis University School of Medicine, St. Louis, Missouri

Background. In recent years the concept of intrastromal refractive surgery has evolved along with the advent of neodymium-doped, yttrium-lithium-fluoride (Nd:YLF) lasers that are able to focus picosecond laser pulses inside the stroma. Each laser pulse forms a localized plasma within the stroma. The high temperatures associated with this plasma formation generate a shock wave, and cause a liquid-gas phase change to give rise to a gas bubble within the tissue. The gas bubble expands rapidly before collapsing, and in doing so disrupts the structural integrity of the surrounding tissue. Using cadaver human eyes, we have investigated the histology of the stroma following photodisruption with picosecond laser pulses, and qualitatively evaluated the merits of various types of refractive surgery. **Methods.** Firstly, we placed laser pulses, 30 picoseconds in duration with energies of 20–25 μJ per pulse, 15μm apart in the mid-stroma. The tissue was examined using SEM and TEM. We then went on to establish laser parameters that were suitable for forming an intrastromal incision. Finally, we investigated the feasibility of several types intrastromal refractive surgery in eyebank eyes. These surgeries included (i) the photodisruption of several layers of stroma parallel to the corneal surface, (ii) the generation of an intrastromal lenticule that was removed through a small peripheral incision, and (iii) the creation of an anterior corneal flap for LASIK. **Results.** There was no evidence of thermal damage following intrastromal photodisruption at the parameters used. Some tissue loss was evident when we placed layers of laser pulses in the mid-stroma, but the major photodisruptive effect seemed to be separation of collagen fibrils. A 5–10 nm thick pseudomembrane was occasionally observed. We found that 40 μJ laser pulses (1000Hz) placed 20 μm apart were suitable for creating intrastromal dissections parallel to the corneal surface that could be used to fashion an intrastromal lenticule or anterior corneal flap. **Conclusion.** With its potential to remove intrastromal tissue and make intrastromal dissections of various dimensions and orientations, the Nd:YLF laser offers considerable promise for intrastromal refractive surgery.

THE ICR

David J. Schanzlin, Penny A. Asbell, and Daniel S. Durrie

[1]Anheuser-Busch Eye Institute, Louis, MO; [2]Mount Sinai Medical Center, New York, NY; [3]Hunkeler Eye Clinic, Kansas City, MO

Background: As an alternative to existing vision correction techniques, the ICRS® (Intrastromal Corneal Ring Segments) corrects common vision problems by reshaping the anterior corneal curvature through implantation of two PMMA segments having an arc length of 150° each. One of the unique aspects of ICRS surgery is that it does not involve direct surgical intervention to the central visual axis. Changes in corneal curvature are achieved by varying the thickness of the device, with increased corneal flattening resulting from increased device thickness.

Preliminary data on the ICRS: In order to evaluate the safety and efficacy of the ICRS, a U.S. Phase II clinical trial was initiated in May 1995. Initial enrollment involved 75 patient eyes and three investigational sites. The patient population was divided into 15 patients per ICRS thickness. The five thicknesses being studied are: 0.25, 0.30, 0.35, 0.40, and 0.45 mm. Two segments were implanted into one eye of each patient. Data collected includes visual acuities, manifest and cycloplegic refraction, keratometry, computerized topography and contrast sensitivity. Available data at postoperative Month 3 (39 patients; all thicknesses) show that 92% (36/39) of the patients had uncorrected visual acuities of 20/40 or better. Cycloplegic refraction results at Month 3 indicate that 77% (30/39) of the patients were within +1.00 D of their intended correction. These patients have followed a normal postoperative course, with no significant complications. Data collection is ongoing and current results will be presented at the meeting. These preliminary data suggest that the ICRS design effectively decreases myopia, is well-tolerated by the human cornea and provides predictable refractive correction.

SOCIOECONOMIC ISSUES IN REFRACTIVE SURGERY

Jeffrey I. Robin

NuVista Refractive Surgery & Laser Centers; Cleveland, Ohio

Over the last 5 years, refractive surgery has enjoyed an explosive increase in professional and public acceptance. This has been largely the result of a renaissance of interest in incisional refractive procedures as well as the introduction of excimer laser photokeratectomy. Presently, around the world, excimer techniques have supplanted incisional procedures as the primary surgical method to correct ametropias.

The rapid ascendancy of the excimer laser has engendered several major changes in refractive surgery. First, it has enabled refractive surgery to move from the exclusive realm of corneal specialists into the purview of comprehensive ophthalmologists. Second, the laser has proven more attractive to non-ophthalmologist eye care providers and, more importantly, to the general public than did previous refractive surgical approaches, contributing greatly to the increased interest in and acceptance of refractive surgery. Third, the cost of the laser necessitates delivery of refractive surgery services routinely in higher volumes than with previous surgical technologies.

These factors have combined to create a unique and rapidly changing refractive surgery landscape. In 1996, refractive surgery's characteristics include: (1) it is the most rapidly growing area of eyecare: (2) nearly every ophthalmologist and optometrist wants to be involved, (3) an increasing public acceptance of the concept of surgical correction of refractive errors; (4) recognition of the fact that most refractive surgery patients do not have routine ophthalmic care and will not access refractive surgeons through "traditional" routes; (5) an increasing cooperation between ophthalmologists and optometrists for delivery of refractive care; (6) direct marketing of services to potential refractive surgery patients/consumers; (7) increasingly complex governmental, regulatory and medicolegal environments affecting refractive surgery practice; (8) recognition of the international nature of the field: and (9) development of several business strategies to allow for cost and risk sharing, as well as maximizing quality control and market share.

CORNEAL ASPHERICITY IN SIGHTED PATIENT EYES FOLLOWING ICR@ (INTRASTROMAL CORNEAL RING) IMPLANTATION

T.E. Burris, D.K. Holmes-Higgin, T.A Silvestrini, P.C. Baker, P.A. Ashell, D.S. Durrie, and D.J. Schanzlin

Purpose: Corneal asphericity was assessed with videokeratography and laser holographic interferometry following ICR implantation in patients participating in the U.S.

Phase II myopic eye clinical trials. **Methods:** ICR thickness sizes from 0.25 mm to 0.45 mm were implanted into 90 patient corneas. Asphericity profiles were created from videokeratographic data and corneal shape was examined preoperatively and up to 2 years postoperatively. The profiles were derived by calculating and plotting the difference in dioptric power between the central EyeSys optical zone and successive zones. Corneal asphericity was also evaluated using laser holographic interferometry and wave front analysis on selected patient eyes. **Results:** Both videokeratographic and laser holographic interferometer analyses demonstrated that preoperative positive corneal asphericity was maintained in patient eyes implanted with ICRs. **Conclusions:** Positive corneal asphericity was preserved after ICR insertion. Further investigation correlating postoperative positive corneal asphericity after ICR insertion with measures of visual outcome are being conducted.

INTRA CORNEAL IMPLANTS

Rubens Belfort, Jr.,[1] Walton Nose,[1] Renato Neves,[1] Terry E. Burris,[2] Thomas A. Silvestrini,[3] and David J. Schanzlin[4]

[1]Escola Paulista de Medicina - Sao Paulo Hospital, Sao Paulo Brazil; [2]Northwest Corneal Services, Portland, OR; [3]KeraVision, Inc., Fremont, CA; [4]Anheuser-Busch Eye Institute, St. Louis, MO

Background: ICR® (Intrastromal Corneal Ring) technology corrects common vision problems by reshaping the anterior corneal curvature through implantation of a ring or ring segments. The most significant principle of ICR surgery is that it allows for the introduction of an intrastromal refractive device without direct surgical intervention to the central visual axis. Changes in corneal curvature are achieved by varying the thickness of the device, with increased corneal flattening resulting from increased product thickness. The 360° ICR was designed to correct myopia, the technology's first indication. In a recent study, ring segments having an arc length of 45° each are being implanted to correct for astigmatism.

Myopia Study: To evaluate the safety and refractive effect of the 360° ICR, a study in myopic eyes was initiated in October 1991. Ten patients each received a 0.30 mm thick ICR in one eye. Preoperative refractive errors ranged from -2.50 D to -4.50 D, with uncorrected VAs between 20/200 and 20/400. At Month 36, the mean SE change in manifest refraction was -2.52 D ± 0.78 D, with UCVAs of 20/40 or better, for all patients. All BCVAs remained 20/20 or better throughout the study period. Data collection is ongoing, and Month 48 data will presented at the meeting. Results indicate that the ICR is a viable alternative for the correction of myopia with stable, long-term refractive results.

Astigmatism Study: In order to assess the viability of correcting astigmatism with the ICR Astigmatism Arcs, a study was initiated in August 1994. Eight sighted eye patients each received two 45° arcs. Seven received 0.30 mm thick arcs and one received 0.40 mm thick arcs. Preoperative uncorrected VAs ranged from 20/40 to 20/400, with preop cylinders ranging from -1.75 D to 4.75 D. At 3 to 12 months postop, 75% (6/8) had uncorrected VAs of 20/25 or better. All had uncorrected VAs of 20/40 or better. All BCVAs were 20/20 or better. The mean cylindrical correction achieved with the 0.30 mm thick arcs was -1.68 D. The 0.40 mm thick arcs imparted -4.00 D of correction. Corneal topography changes were also assessed by videokeratography (EyeSys). Data collection is ongoing and current results will be presented at the meeting. These preliminary results indicate that the ICR Astigmatism Arcs reduced astigmatic cylinder and improved visual acuity.

CLINICAL RESULTS OF INTRAOCULAR ANTERIOR CHAMBER IMPLANTS IN PHAKIC EYES FOR MYOPIC CORRECTION

L. L. Vanzella,[1] W. Nosé,[1,2] P. Schor,[2] N. Allemann,[2] R. M. Nosé,[1] and W. Chamon[2]

[1]Eye Clinic Day Hospital, São Paulo -SP, Brasil [2]UNIFESP-EPM

PURPOSE: To evaluate safety and efficacy of intraocular chamber implants in phakic eyes for myopic correction. **METHODS:** Spectacle-corrected and uncorrected visual acuity, refraction, central endothelium density, and incidence of pre- and post-operative complications were evaluated retrospectively in 15 eyes of 12 patients that had been followed for a minimum of 6 months (average 25.8 months) after surgery. **RESULTS:** There were no complications in this series. The average spherical equivalent reduced from -15.1 SD to 43.77 D after the surgery (p< 0.001). Average postoperative uncorrected visual acuity was 20/34, and was at least 20/40 in 11 of 13 eyes (85%) examined. No patients presented decrease in spectacle-corrected visual acuity, and it was improved in 8 of 15 eyes (53%). No endothelium cell loss was detected. Endothelium density averaged 2719.4 cells/mm^2 and 2774 cells/mm^2, before and after the surgery, respectively (p> 0.05). **CONCLUSIONS:** With the methodology used, the procedure was safe and effective in this small series. It is important to evaluate larger populations with longer follow-up to determine the definite clinical value of the procedure.

THE EYE FIXATION SPECULUM: A NEW INSTRUMENT FOR STABILIZATION OF THE EYE DURING REFRACTIVE SURGICAL PROCEDURES

Neal Sher

Alignment and fixation of the eye are essential to the achievement of a beneficial postoperative result after refractive surgery. Misalignment of the laser or movement of the eye during excimer PRK can result in a degraded optical result with glare, shadows, irregular astigmatism, undercorrection and reduced contrast sensitivity. Current methods of stabilizing the eye include patient self-fixation, forceps, hand-held vacuum rings or Thornton type rings. These methods all have significant drawbacks. An easy to use, disposable device has been developed which will immobilize the globe in a painless and nontraumatic manner. The disposable instrument consists of a low profile luminescent scleral vacuum fixation ring which is attached by a ball jointed arm to a lid speculum. Advantages of this device include safety, comfort, a uniform and predictable intraocular pressure, and the lack of corneal distortion from point fixation. Results will be presented from new clinical trials on PRK patients and on normal volunteers with data on saccadic eye movement, topography and changes in intraocular pressure with use of this instrument.

PRK CORRECTION OF PENETRATING KERATOPLASTY INDUCED MYOPIA

Rui Pinto, A. Mmiflho, J. Pauto Costa, M. Ceu, and Paulo Torres

As we know one of the biggest problems in the post op. of penetrating keratoplasty (PK) paste is the induction of high ametropias. With the wide spread use of excimer laser for myopia correction, the treatment for these situations was achievable by surgical means. 17 patients with induced myopia post-PK ranging from -3.00 to -16.00 were submitted to PRK using the Summit Excimer Laser; we used optical zones of 4.7 and 5 mm in a single or double optical zone delivery. With a mean follow-up of 13 months, in all the patients we obtain a reduction of their previous myopia and in some cases an increase in the best visual acuity; we don't report any case of graft failure, and only 2 cases of mild and transitory haze, and 1 case of severe haze. We think excimer laser is a good and safe option for treatment of induced myopia post-PK.

Session V

Molecular Biology, Cellular Biology, and Genetics

33

WOUND HEALING MODULATORS IN TEAR FLUID

Timo Tervo and Minna Vesaluoma

Helsinki University Central Hospital
Department of Ophthalmology
Eye Bank
Haartmaninkatu 4 C
FIN-00290 Helsinki, Finland

ABSTRACT

Unexpected variations in corneal wound healing affect the predictability of photorefractive keratectomy (PRK). Several modulators coming from tears, inflammatory cells, extracellular matrix, nerve cells, corneal epithelial cells, or stromal fibroblasts can regulate the complex wound healing process. This report evaluates the presence and release of these modulators in tear fluid following PRK. The release of plasmin, cellular fibronectin, tenascin and calcitonin gene-related peptide (CGRP) into tears following excimer laser keratectomy has been shown to be increased during the first postoperative days. Lately studies have focused on growth factors/cytokines. The release of hepatocyte growth factor (HGF), transforming growth factor-$\beta 1$ (TGF-$\beta 1$), vasoendothelial growth factor (VEGF), and tumor necrosis factor-α (TNF-α) in tear fluid is also significantly increased during the first two days after excimer laser-induced corneal wound. These healing modulators are likely to regulate epithelial differentiation, proliferation, and migration; cell-to-cell and cell-to-matrix interactions; stromal extracellular matrix production; and transition of keratocytes into contractile myofibroblast-like cells. They are possibly also involved in the formation of postoperative stromal scar.

INTRODUCTION

Correction of refractive errors by photorefractive keratectomy (PRK) is based on remodeling of corneal curvature by photoablation of the corneal stroma with Argon-Fluoride excimer laser.[1] Much of the predictability of PRK depends on the subsequent healing of the photoablated cornea. Epithelial healing is seldom a problem, but unexpected variations in stromal healing—probably regulated by the epithelium—may result in formation of haze or regression in refractive result. Perioperative corneal drying or elevation of corneal temperature, the patient's relative tear deficiency, the laser itself and the ablation depth can all influence the ablation rate or the smoothness of the surface.[2,3] Rough surface has been suggested to correlate with haze formation.

Cell migration, mitosis, and differentiation, as well as reconstitution of adhesive structures to stroma are important features of corneal epithelial wound healing.[4,5] After PRK, reconstitution of the epithelial surface over the ablated area usually lasts two to three days, but stromal regeneration, which is essential for the refractive result, continues for months. Only minimal ECM changes appear after laser-assisted keratomileusis (LASIK) at the center of the flap.[7] The recovery of the innervation is a very slow process, and the nerves apparently remain morphologically abnormal.[8] LASIK preserves the neural integrity better and allows more rapid neural recovery, although epithelial ingrowth is sometimes a problem.[7,9] Several modulators coming from tears, inflammatory cells, extracellular matrix, nerve cells, corneal epithelial cells, or stromal fibroblasts can regulate this complex biologic process of corneal wound healing. This review concentrates on those wound healing modulators that have been found in tear fluid.

METHODS

Tear Fluid Collection

For all these studies, tear fluid samples were collected with fire-polished microcapillary tubes. Tears were collected preoperatively (DAY 0), on the first (DAY 1) or second (DAY 2), and seventh (DAY 7) postoperative days. The tear fluid flow in the collection capillary (μl/min) was calculated by dividing the volume of the tear fluid sample by the tear fluid collection time. In the capillary method both the residual tears of the conjunctival fornix and the newly-secreted tears are collected. The tear fluid flow in the collection capillary is thus considerably higher than the actual tear fluid secretion rate. The parameter release is calculated by multiplying the protein concentration in the sample by the tear fluid flow in the collection capillary. PRK wound clearly induces considerable hypersecretion of tears during the first postoperative days, which sometimes makes the collection of all the tears difficult during this time. Thus, the capillary method is not quite accurate, but it does offer a simple and practical way to adjust for the very variable tear fluid flow rates that are typical during wound healing.

Extracellular Matrix (ECM)

Immediate epithelial healing is preceded by accumulation of fibronectin on the stromal wound surface followed by slow reassembly of the adhesion complex, consisting of hemidesmosomes, basement membrane components, and anchoring fibrils.[10] Both the corneal epithelial cells and activated keratocytes seem capable of synthesizing these adhesive elements.[11,12] Profound changes occur in the stromal ECM during 12 months after PRK.[6] Immediately after PRK keratocytes in the superficial stroma degenerate, and programmed cell death (apoptosis) regulated by inflammatory mediators such as IL-1α has been suggested.[13] Corneal photoablation trauma also results in infiltration of polymorphonuclear leukocytes.[14] In wounded cornea, the necrotic keratocytes and stromal and subepithelial nerves are removed by invading macrophage-like cells and other inflammatory cells during the first three days.[15] Later stromal keratocytes turn into activated myofibroblast-like contractile cells that disappear until six months postoperatively.[16] The activated keratocytes produce fibronectin and tenascin,[6,17] among other ECM components. Their synthesis is most abundant during first three months after wounding and gradually declines during the following nine months. Hyaluronic acid and water are also accumulated to the wounded area .[18]

Fibronectin is an adhesive extracellular glycoprotein consisting of two 200–220 kD subunits.[19] Cellular fibronectin is synthesized locally in developing or regenerating tissues, while soluble plasma fibronectin is a hepatocyte-produced component of plasma and body fluids.[19–21] An extradomain A (EDA) sequence is contained in cellular fibronectin, and distinguishes it from plasma fibronectin.[22] Fibronectin probably serves as a suitable adherent surface to the migrating epithelial cells during the early stages of healing.[22,23] Interleukins 1α, 1β, and 6, epidermal growth factor (EGF) as well as tumor necrosis factor-α (TNF-α) enhance the fibronectin-induced migration.[24,25] During the epithelial migration phase fibronectin first appears as a narrow zone between the stroma and epithelial cells, but is later found in the anterior stroma.[6, 17]

Tenascin, on the other hand, is a large ECM glycoprotein that consists of six disulfide-linked subunits (MW 150–240 kD).[26] It contains both fibronectin and epidermal growth factor-like repeats.[27] Tenascin is expressed during tissue repair; it is also present during embryogenesis and in diverse malignant tumors, which suggests that it has a modulatory role on cell growth.[28] Tenascin expression in the stroma following corneal wounding resembles that of fibronectin.[6,17] After LASIK the immunoreactions for cellular fibronectin and tenascin disappear faster than after PRK, except for the sites of epithelio-stromal contacts.[7] The biological role of tenascin in healing process is poorly understood, but it is presumed to be involved in cell migration, cell proliferation, or modulation of interactions between cell and fibronectin.[26,29,30] LASIK appears to induce growth of epithelial cells into the stroma, and in the margin of the wound, epithelial cells show immunoreaction for tenascin for some days.[31]

The release of both cellular fibronectin and tenascin in tear fluid is enhanced following PRK.[32,33] Their release in tears is highest when the epithelial defect is present. Consequently, the wounded corneal stroma probably releases both ECM proteins. However, there seems to be a difference in their release pattern. The release of cellular fibronectin reaches its maximum level already on the following day after PRK, while tenascin release further increases on the second postoperative day. The magnitude of increase in cellular fibronectin release is also more striking. In tissue sections from rabbit corneas exposed to PRK, cellular fibronectin also appeared earlier than tenascin.[17] The mean tear fluid flow in the collection capillary, cellular fibronectin and tenascin concentrations and their releases are shown in Figures 1–3. It has also been suggested that ocular surface damage followed by reflex tearing and dilation of conjunctival vessels leads to leakage of plasma fibronectin into tears.[34]

Hyaluronic acid is also present in human tears.[35] This study revealed that its concentration in patients with corneal diseases did not differ from that found in normal subjects. In this study, however, the flow of tears was not taken into account.

Other researchers[10] have found that deposition of ECM proteins, such as collagens, fibronectin, tenascin, laminin and other adhesion complex glycoproteins, or hyaluronate may contribute to the development and disappearance of postoperative corneal haze. Changes in dermatan sulphate (fetal proteoglycan) vs. Keratan sulphate ratio have been shown to have a similar effect.[36]

Plasminogen-Plasmin System and Tryptase

Different proteolytic mechanisms (such as plasminogen-plasmin system, matrix metalloproteinases, mast cell proteinases, leukocyte-mediated mechanisms, or complement activa-

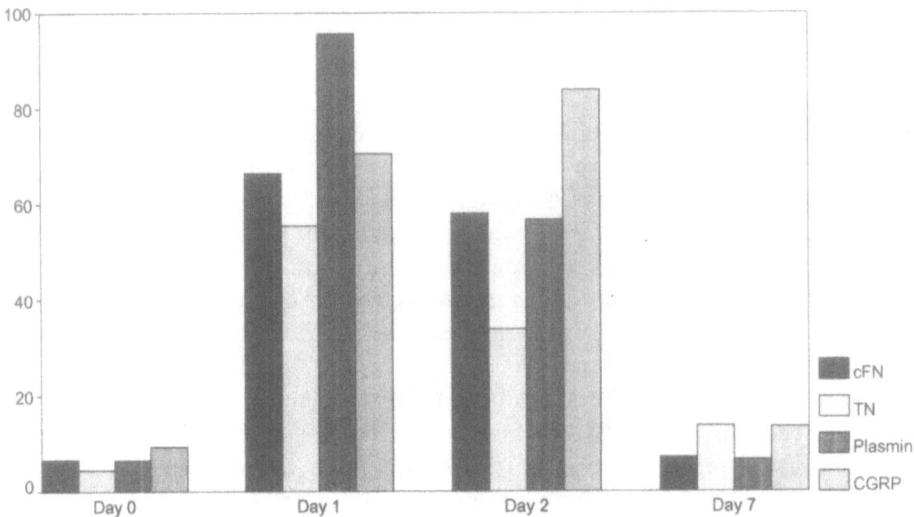

Figure 1. Mean pre- and postoperative flows in the collection capillary (μl/min).

tion) are though to be important for regulation of wound healing. During initial healing, complex proteolytic enzyme cascades are activated for advancement of epithelial cells on the stromal surface. The cells of the leading edge are supposed to use plasminogen-plasmin system for this directional proteolysis.[37–40] Hepatocyte-derived plasminogen is activated by plasminogen activators urokinase (uPA), tissue activator (tPA), or protease nexin to proteolytically active plasmin. Plasminogen activators are regulated by plasminogen activator inhibitors PAI-1

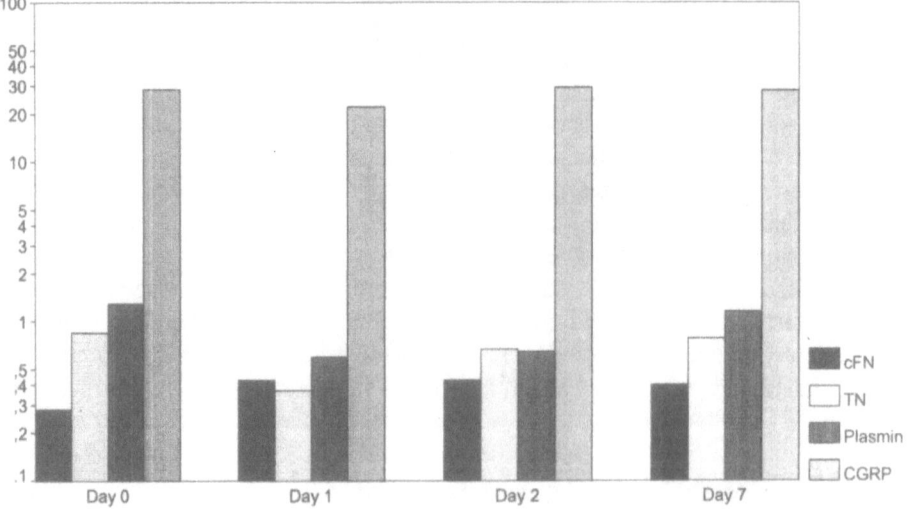

Figure 2. Mean pre- and postoperative concentrations (μg/ml) of cellular fibronectin (cFN), tenascin (TN) and calcitonin gene-related peptide (CGRP), and activities (IU/l) of plasmin.

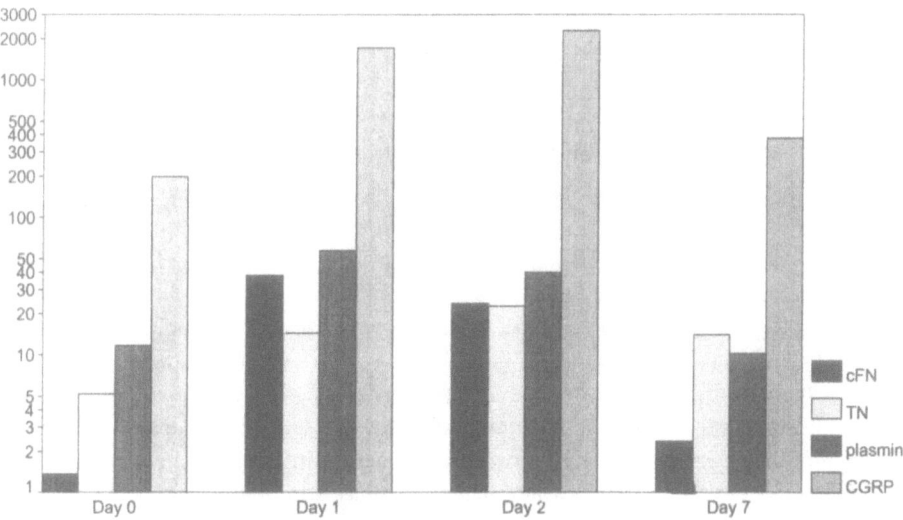

Figure 3. Mean pre- and postoperative releases (ng/min or μIU/l for plasmin) of cellular fibronectin (cFN), tenascin (TN), plasmin and calcitonin gene-related peptide (CGRP).

or PAI-2. Plasmin activity is inhibited by serum proteins such as α_2-antiplasmin, α_2-macroglobulin, albumin or α_1- antitrypsin. All these components are present in tear fluid.[41–46] All principle corneal cell types synthesize α_2-macroglobulin, which is a multifunctional inhibitor against serine-, metallo-, aspartic and thiol proteinases.[47] Epithelial cells also produce α_1-antitrypsin, an inhibitor of serine proteinases and leukocyte elastase.[48] Imbalance between activators of plasminogen and inhibitors of active plasmin is supposed to lead to exaggerated tissue proteolysis and inhibition of wound healing, which can probably be prevented by a serine proteinase inhibitor aprotinin.[38,49] Plasminogen activator inhibitors are upregulated by cytokines, such as TGF-β and TNF.[50, 51]

PRK induces increased release of plasmin in tear fluid (Figure 3).[42] It is elevated only as long as the epithelial defect has not healed (2–3 days). In spite of enhanced synthesis, plasmin activity per volume of tears decreases during the first postoperative days after PRK because of reflex tearing (Figures 1 and 2). This probably prevents excessive proteolysis at the surface of the wound.

Tryptase, another serine proteinase, is one of the major protein components stored in mast cell granules. Increased levels of immunoreactive tryptase have been measured in tears during active ocular allergy, following conjunctival provocation with allergen or compound 48/80, or after mechanical irritation, such as rubbing of eyes.[52] Initial results indicate that tryptase activity, measured by a fluorometric assay, is significantly decreased after PRK, while tryptase release remains practically the same during the postoperative days. This seems natural while there are no mast cells in central cornea. Conjunctival mast cells do not appear to be stimulated by laser photoablation.

Growth Factors and Cytokines

Cytokines are polypeptides involved in signal transmission between cells. The expanding list of cytokines includes growth factors, interleukins, tumor necrosis factor-α, and interferons. Cytokines may transmit signals to neighboring cells (paracrine stimulation) or within the cell itself (autocrine regulation), even without secretion (intracrine effect), or exert an effect via body fluids to other target tissues (endocrine effects).

Corneal epithelial and stromal cells synthesize a number of growth factors or their receptors. Li and Tseng subdivided the expression of 12 cytokines and their receptors in four patterns.[53] Type I included cytokines expressed exclusively by epithelial cells (transforming growth factor-α (TGF-α), interleukin-1β (IL-1β), platelet-derived growth factor-B (PDGF-B), while their receptors were predominantly (epidermal growth factor receptor (EGFR), IL-1R) or exclusively (PDGFR-β) expressed by fibroblasts. Type II included growth factors that were expressed equally by both epithelial cells and fibroblasts (insulin-like growth factor-I (IGF-I), TGF-β1, -β2, basic fibroblast growth factor (bFGF) and their receptors). Type III included keratocyte growth factor (KGF) and hepatocyte growth factor (HGF) which were expressed exclusively by fibroblasts, while their respective receptors were predominantly expressed by epithelial cells. These three groups thus contained growth factors that were potentially involved in paracrine interactions between epithelial and stromal cells. Type IV cytokines macrophage colony stimulating factor (M-CSF) and interleukin-8 (IL-8)) were expressed by fibroblasts and/or epithelial cells but their receptors were expressed by inflammatory cells. In this study transcript expression of TNF-α was not detected by epithelial cells or fibroblasts.

Several cytokines are present in tear fluid.[54–58] However, little is known about the changes in growth factor levels after corneal wounding. The roles of EGF and TGF-α have been reviewed elsewhere.[59–61] Studies have shown that the release of TGF-β1, VEGF, TNF-α and HGF in human tear fluid increases significantly following excimer laser-induced corneal wound.[56–58] Their release is returned to the preoperative level by seventh postoperative day when the epithelial defect has also healed. The concentrations of TGF-β1 and TNF-α remain on the constant level, while those of HGF and VEGF decrease during the first two postoperative days. The VEGF concentration returns to the preoperative level by the seventh postoperative day, but the HGF level is still lower on DAY 7 than preoperatively. The mean pre- and postoperative flows in the collection capillary, cytokine concentrations, and releases are shown in Figures 4–6.

Possible sources of tear fluid growth factors are the lacrimal gland(s), corneal epithelial and stromal cells, conjunctival or inflammatory cells, or conjunctival vessels. Corneal wounding has been shown to stimulate at least EGF and TNF-α mRNA expression in the lacrimal gland.[62,63] It is assumed that production of other growth factors in the lacrimal gland is enhanced by corneal wounding in a similar fashion. At least EGF, TGF-α, FGF, TGF-β1, and HGF are expressed in the lacrimal gland.[61,64–66] Growth factors also exert signal transduction between cells in different corneal layers as shown by Li and Tseng.[53] HGF, for example, is a paracrine mediator secreted by fibroblast cells to modulate the functions of epithelial cells. Corneal epithelial wounding appears to stimulate the production of HGF in keratocytes.[66] TGF-β1 and TGF-βRII are expressed by both epithelial cells and stromal fibroblasts,[53,67] while TGF-β1 protein has also been detected in both epithelium and stromal matrix.[68] TGF-β is a multifunctional cytokine synthesized in a latent prepromonomer, the C-terminal fragments of which can be cleaved off to form the active TGF-β dimer. TGF-β can be activated by proteolytic enzymes such as plasmin.[69] Corneal wounding also stimulates epithelial and stromal TNF-α mRNA expression.[70] TNF-α is a proinflammatory cytokine, produced by activated macrophages and monocytes, lymphocytes, neutrophils, endothelial cells, smooth muscle cells, and cultured wound fibroblasts.[71,72] TNF-α is an example of those tear fluid cytokines that can potentially also be derived from conjunctival or inflammatory cells.[73]

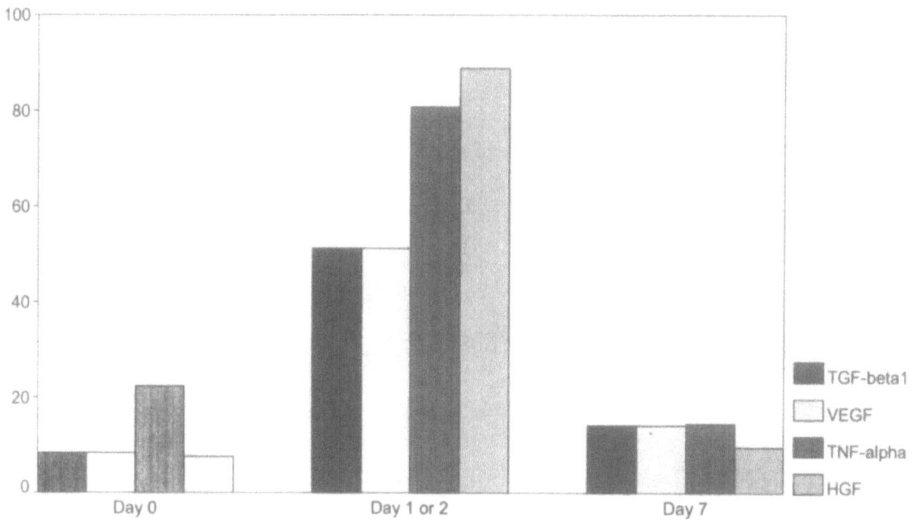

Figure 4. Mean pre- and postoperative flows in the collection capillary (μl/min).

What is the function of these tear fluid growth factors during the early postoperative period after PRK? HGF exerts its effects on the corneal epithelial cells by increasing their proliferation and motility, but inhibiting their differentiation.[74] TGF-β1, on the other hand, inhibits the proliferation of corneal epithelium.[75] However, HGF possibly prevents this inhibitory effect and releases the corneal epithelial cells from TGF-β1-induced growth arrest.[76] In corneal stroma TGF-β stimulates myofibroblast transformation

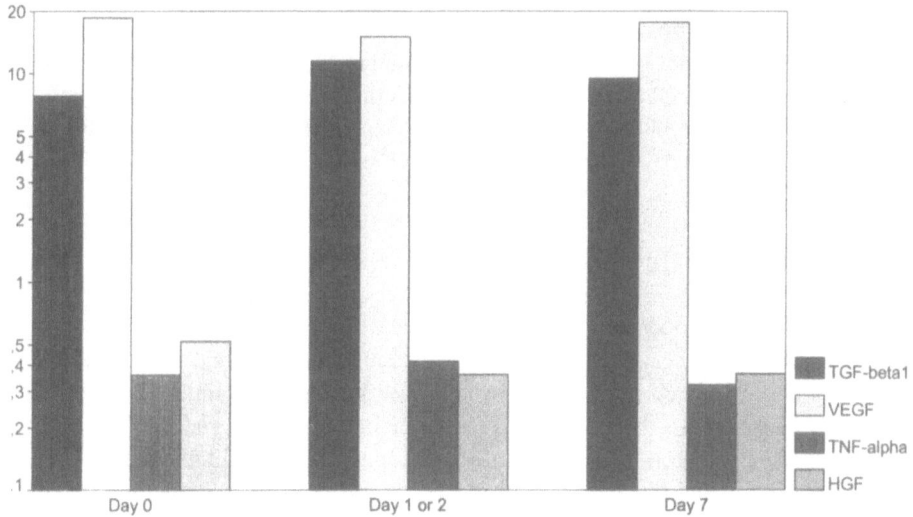

Figure 5. Mean pre- and postoperative concentrations (ng/ml) of transforming growth factor-β (TGF-β), vasoendothelial growth factor (VEGF), tumor necrosis factor-α (TNF-α) and hepatocyte growth factor (HGF).

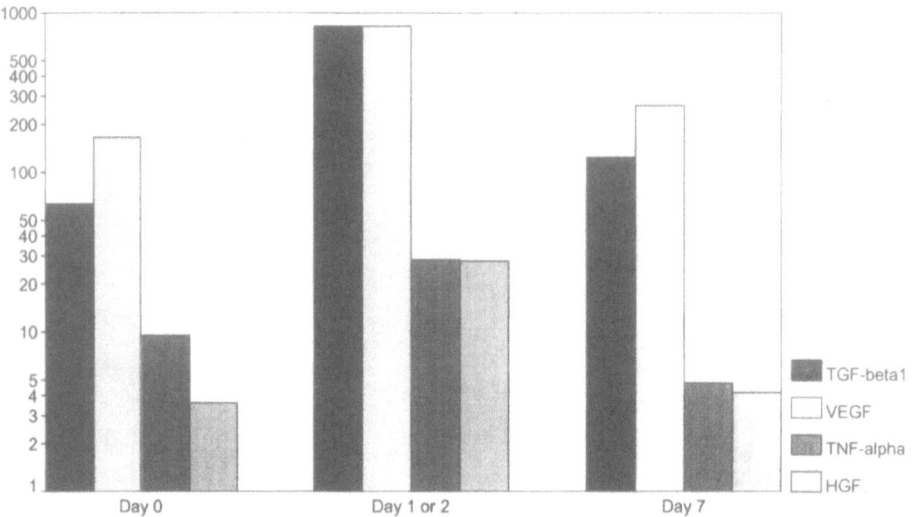

Figure 6. Mean pre- and postoperative releases (pg/min) of transforming growth factor-β (TGF-β), vasoendothelial growth factor (VEGF), tumor necrosis factor-α (TNF-α) and hepatocyte growth factor (HGF).

of keratocytes and production of ECM proteins, such as fibronectin, which mediates spreading of the epithelial cells during the initial stages of wound healing.[77,78] TGF-β also downregulates IL-1α-induced matrix metalloproteinase expression by corneal keratocytes.[79] Vasoendothelial growth factor (VEGF) is a likely candidate for a retinal angiogenic factor,[80] but its role in the corneal healing is unknown. In the skin it enhances vasopermeability and induces angiogenesis. The presence of VEGF in normal tears as well as the presence of VEGF and its receptor FLT-1 in cultured keratocytes suggests a regulatory role in the stroma.[56,81] TNF-α has been shown to stimulate fibronectin-induced migration of corneal epithelial cells and fibroblast proliferation.[25,82] It inhibits extracellular matrix protein production and stimulates collagenase or prostaglandin E_2 secretion,[83,84] both known to be enhanced after PRK. Both TGF-β and TNF-α are potential candidates involved in formation of postoperative haze: TGF-β appears to stimulate corneal scar formation,[85] whereas low amounts of TNF-α has been connected to hypertrophic scarring of skin.[86]

Corneal Nerves and Calcitonin Gene-Related Peptide (CGRP)

There is a growing body of evidence that corneal sensory innervation and neuropeptides released from these nerves have important roles in wound healing. It has been shown that sensorily denervated corneas heal slowly.[87,88] Both trigeminal and sympathetic ganglion neurons can increase the mitotic rate of epithelial cells *in vitro*.[89] CGRP, together with EGF, has been shown to increase corneal epithelial wound healing *in vitro*.[90] Wound healing is also accelerated by nerve growth factor and suppressed by depletion of sensory neuropeptides by capsaicin.[91,92] Furthermore, the sensory nerves and muscarine-type cholinergic receptors located in corneal epithelial cells and regulated by corneal sensory nerves have been supposed to have a direct influence on the production of epithelial adhesion structures and healing.[93–95] Direct innervation of epithelial cells and keratocytes has recently been proposed.[96] Nerve fibers invaginating these cells might thus modulate the release of cytokines from these cells into the anterior stroma or epithelium.

Excimer laser PRK sharply ablates the stromal nerve.[8] Nerve ending destruction probably produces the intense postoperative pain and release of neurotransmitters in the tear fluid.[8,97] Release of CGRP in tears is enhanced after PRK but once the corneal surface is reepithelialized, it is returned to the preoperative level (Figure 3).[8] However, it is possible that the release continues under the healed epithelium, although the tear fluid analysis does not appear to reveal much about the intracorneal situation once the epithelium has grown over the ablated area. Despite the marked hypersecretion of tears, the concentration of CGRP does not decrease after PRK, indicating a concomitant increase in CGRP release by corneal sensory nerves and/or lacrimal glands (Figures 1 and 2).

Following photoablation, neural recovery takes place. Epithelial innervation is regenerated in about three months, but the subepithelial nerve plexus and the stromal nerves, the majority of which are located in the anterior third of the stroma, regenerate very slowly.[8] They show coarse and oily patterns, send numerous thin regenerative leashes which are found as late as one year after PRK, and may never achieve normal morphology. During the first two months reflex tearing is also decreased. Corneal sensitivity has been reported to fluctuate even 6 months after PRK.[98]

The neural damage, postoperative pain, release of CGRP and prostaglandin E_2[99] following PRK may indicate activation of metabolic pathways leading to formation of nitric oxide and/or free radicals. However, this has not yet been confirmed. Topical nonsteroidals (NSAIDs) have been shown to reduce postoperative pain after PRK without affecting much wound healing.[100] Their frequent long-term administration has, however, been reported to cause corneal complications.

CONCLUSION

At present understanding of wound healing mechanisms is far from complete. The latest results based on the pre- and postoperative tear fluid analysis of PRK patients show that corneal wounding induces increased release of several growth modulating factors potentially involved in the healing response. It seems possible that corticosteroids or NSAIDs—the current therapies for prevention of haze—can be replaced by more specific drugs, such as growth factors, their inhibitors or receptor blockers, once we know the cytokines or other mediators responsible for the scar formation, or learn to inhibit the epithelial messengers that stimulate stromal scar formation. The studies on LASIK wounds demonstrating absence of stromal cell stimulation seem promising in this respect.[7]

ACKNOWLEDGMENTS

Sources of Support: The Mary and Georg Ehrnrooth Foundation; The Friends of the Blind, Finland; The Eye and Tissue Bank Foundation, Finland; and the Eye Foundation of Finland.

REFERENCES

1. S.L. Trokel, Srinivasan, R., and Braren B., Excimer laser surgery of the cornea. *Am. J. Ophthalmol.* 96:710 (1983).

2. T Niizuma, Ito, S., Hayashi, M.,et al., Cooling the cornea to prevent side effects of photorefractive keratectomy. *J. Refract. Corneal Surg.* 10(Suppl):262 (1994).

3. T. Tervo, Mustonen, R., and Tarkkanen., A., Management of dry eye may reduce haze after excimer laser photorefractive keratectomy (letter). *Refract. Corneal Surg.* 9:306 (1993).

4. S. J. Tuft, Gartry, DS, Rawe I.M., and Meek, K.M., Photorefractive keratectomy: implications of corneal wound healing. *Br. J. Ophthalmol.* 77:243 (1993).

5. T. Latvala, Tervo, K., and Tervo, T., Reassembly of the $\alpha_6\beta_4$ integrin and laminin in the rabbit corneal basement membrane after excimer laser surgery. A twelve-month follow-up. *CLAO J.* 21:125 (1995).

6. T. Latvala, Tervo, K., and Tervo, T., Expression of cellular fibronectin and tenascin in the rabbit cornea after excimer laser PRK: a twelve months results. *Br. J. Ophthalmol.* 79:65 (1995).

7. T. Latvala, Barraquer-Coll C, Tervo K, and Tervo T. Corneal wound healing and nerve morphology after excimer laser *in situ* keratomileusis (LASIK) in human eyes. *J. Refr. Surg.* In press (1996).

8. K. Tervo, Latvala, T., and Tervo, T., Recovery of corneal innervation following photorefractive keratoablation. *Arch. Ophthalmol.* 112:1466 (1994).

9. K. Tervo, Perez-Santonja, J.J., Alio Sanz, J.L., et al., Nerve morphology after LASIK in rabbit corneas. (Abstract) *Invest. Ophthalmol. Vis. Sci.* 37(Suppl.):64 (1996).

10. I. K. Gibson, Inatomi, T., Extracellular matrix and growth factors in corneal wound healing. *Curr. Opin. Ophthalmol* 6:3 (1995).

11. M. Ohji, SundarRaj, N., Hassel, J.R., and Thoft, R.A., Basement membrane synthesis by human corneal epithelial cells *in vitro*. *Invest. Ophthalmol. Vis. Sci.* 35:479 (1994).

12. J.R. Hassell, Schrecengost, P.K., Rada, J., et al., Biosynthesis of stromal matrix proteoglycans and basement membrane components by human corneal fibroblasts. *Invest. Ophthalmol. Vis. Sci.* 33:547 (1992).

13. R. Wise, Wilson, S.E., He, Y-G., and Weng, J., Interleukin-1 alpha induces apoptosis in human corneal stromal fibroblast cells. (Abstract). *Invest. Ophtalmol. Vis. Sci.* 35 (Suppl):1980 (1994).

14. M. Campos, Hertzog, L., Garbus, J.J., and McDonnell, P.J., Corneal sensitivity after photorefractive keratectomy. *Am. J. Ophthalmol.* 114:51 (1992).

15. K.Y. Chan, Järveläinen, M., Chang, J.H., and Edenfield, M.J., A cryodamage model for studying corneal nerve regeneration. *Invest. Ophthalmol. Vis. Sci.* 31:2008 (1990).

16. T. Linna, and Tervo, T. Results of real-time confocal microscopy of human corneal wound healing after excimer laser photorefractive keratectomy. Submitted (1996).

17. G-B van Setten, Koch, J.W., Tervo, K., et al., Expression of tenascin and fibronectin in the rabbit cornea after excimer laser surgery. *Graefe's Arch. Clin. Exp. Ophthalmol.* 230:178 (1992).

18. T.D. Fitzsimmons, Fagerholm, P., Härfstrand, A., and Schenholm, M., Hyaluronic acid in the rabbit cornea after excimer laser superficial keratectomy. *Invest. Ophthalmol. Vis. Sci.* 33:3011 (1992).

19. E. Ruoslahti, Fibronectin and its receptors. *Annu. Rev. Biochem.* 57:375 (1988).

20. T. Vartio, Laitinen, L., Närvänen O, et al., Differential expression of the ED sequence-containing form of cellular fibronectin in embryonic and adult human tissues. *J. Cell. Sci.* 88:419 (1987).

21. J.W. Tamkun, and Hynes, R.O., Plasma fibronectin is synthesized and secreted by hepatocytes. *J. Biol. Chem.* 258:4641 (1983).

22. J.D. Cameron, Hagen, S.T., Waterfield, R.R., and Furcht, L.T., Effects of matrix proteins on rabbit corneal epithelial cell adhesion and migration. *Curr. Eye Res.* 7:293 (1988).

23. K. Watanabe, Nakagawa, S., and Nishida, T., Stimulatory effects of fibronectin and EGF on the migration of corneal epithelial cells. *Invest. Ophthalmol. Vis. Sci.* 28:205 (1987).

24. T. Nishida, Nakamura, M., Murakami, J., et al., Epidermal growth factor stimulates corneal epithelial cell attachment to fibronectin through a fibronectin receptor system. *Invest. Ophthalmol. Vis. Sci.* 33:2464 (1992).

25. X Wang, Kamiyama, K., Iguchi, I., et al., Enhancement of fibronectin-induced migration of corneal epithelial cells by cytokines. *Invest. Ophthalmol. Vis. Sci.* 35: 4001 (1994).

26. M. Chiquet, and Fambrough, D.M., Chick myotendinous antigen. II. A novel extracellular glycoprotein complex consisting of large disulfide-linked subunits. *J. Cell. Biol.* 98:1937 (1984).

27. F.S. Jones, Burgoon, M.P., Hoffman, S., et al., A cDNA clone for cytotactin contains sequences similar to epidermal growth factor-like repeats and segments of fibronectin and fibrinogen. *Proc. Natl. Acad. Sci. USA* 85:2168 (1988).

28. H.P. Erickson, and Bourdon, M.A., Tenascin: an extracellular matrix protein prominent in specialized embryonic tissues and tumors. *Annu. Rev. Cell. Biol.* 5:71 (1989).

29. A. Kaplony, Zimmermann, D.R., Fischer, R.W., et al., 220,000 isoform expression correlates with corneal cell migration. Development 1991;112:605 (1991).

30. P. End, Panayotou, G., Entwistle, A., et al., A modulator of cell growth. *Eur. J. Biochem.* 209:1041 (1992).

31. T. Linna, and Tervo, T., Unpublished observation.

32. T. Virtanen, Ylätupa, S., Mertaniemi, P., et al., Tear fluid cellular fibronectin levels after photorefractive keratectomy. *J. Refr. Surg.* 11:106 (1995).
33. M. Vesaluoma, Ylätupa, S., Mertaniemi, P., et al., Increased release of tenascin in tear fluid after photorefractive keratectomy. *Graefe's Arch. Clin. Exp. Ophthalmol.* 233:479 (1995).
34. M. Fukuda, Fullard, R.J., Willcox, M.D.P., et al., Fibronectin in the tear film. *Invest. Ophthalmol. Vis. Sci.* 37:459 (1996).
35. M. Fukuda, Miyamoto, Y., Miyara, Y., et al., Hyaluronic acid concentration in human tear fluids. (Abstract) *Invest. Ophthalmol. Vis. Sci.* 37(Suppl):848 (1996).
36. T. Tervo, Mertaniemi, P., and Vesaluoma, M., Inflamacion en cirugia refractiva. In: *Inflamaciones Oculares,* J.L. Alio y Sanz, Carreras Egana, B., and Ruiz Moreno, J.M., eds.,. Edika Med., Barcelona (1995).
37. M.B. Berman, Kenyon, K., Hayashi, K., and L'Hernault, N., The pathogenesis of epithelial defects and stromal ulceration. In *The Cornea: Transactions of the World Congress on the Cornea III,* H.D. Cavanagh, ed., Raven Press, New York (1988).
38. T. Tervo, and van Setten, G-B., Aprotinin for inhibition of plasmin on the ocular surface: principles and clinical observations. In: *Healing Processes of the Cornea.*R.W. Beuerman, Crosson, C.E., and Kaufman, H.E., eds., Portfolio Publishing Company of Texas, The Woodlands (1989).
39. A. Vaheri, Bizik, J., Salonen, E.M., et al., Regulation of the pericellular activation of plasminogen and its role in tissue-destructive processes. *Acta. Ophthalmol.* 1992 (Suppl):34 (1992).
40. J. Pöllänen, Stephens, R.W., and Vaheri, A., Directed plasminogen activation at the surface of normal and malignant cells. *Adv. Cancer Res.* 57:273 (1991).
41. T. Tervo, van Setten, G-B, Päällysaho, T., et al., Wound healing of the ocular surface. *Ann. Med.* 24:19 (1992).
42. T. Tervo, Virtanen, T., Honkanen, N., et al., Tear fluid plasmin activity after excimer laser photorefractive keratectomy. *Invest. Ophthalmol. Vis. Sci.* 35:3045 (1994).
43. J.U. Prause, Serum albumin, serum antiproteases and polymorphonuclear leucocyte neutral collagenolytic protease in the tear fluid of normal healthy persons. *Acta. Ophthalmol. Copenh.* 61:261 (1983).
44. J.U. Prause, Cellular and biochemical mechanisms involved in the degradation and healing of the cornea. The polymorphonuclear leukocyte and tear fluid serum antiproteases in human melting central corneal ulcers. *Acta. Ophthalmol.* 168(Suppl) :1 (1984).
45. G-B. van Setten, Salonen, E.M., Vaheri, A., et al., Plasmin and plasminogen activator activities in tear fluid during corneal wound healing after anterior keratectomy. *Curr. Eye Res.* 8:1293 (1989).
46. D.J. Stevens, Marshall, J.M., Benjamin, L., et al., Plasminogen activator in human tears. *Eye* 6:653 (1992).
47. W. Borth, Alpha 2-macroglobulin, a multifunctional binding protein with targeting characteristics. *Faseb.. J.* 6:3345 (1992).
48. S.S. Twining, Fukuchi, T., Yue, B.Y., et al., Corneal synthesis of alpha 1-proteinase inhibitor (alpha 1-antitrypsin). *Invest. Ophthalmol. Vis. Sci.* 35:458 (1994).
49. T. Tervo, van Setten, G.B., Tervo, K., and Tarkkanen, A.. Experience with plasmin inhibitors. *Acta. Ophthalmol. Suppl.* 1992:47 (1994).
50. M. Laiho, Saksela, O., Andreasen, P.A,, and Keski-Oja, J., Enhanced production and extracellular deposition of the endothelial-type plasminogen activator inhibitor in cultured human lung fibroblasts by transforming growth factor-beta. *J. Cell. Biol.* 103:2403 (1986).
51. S.F. Hackett, and Campochiaro, P.A., Modulation of plasminogen activator inhibitor-1 and urokinase in retinal pigmented epithelial cells. *Invest. Ophthalmol. Vis. Sci.* 34:2055 (1993).
52. S.I. Butrus, Ochsner, K.I., Abelson, M.B., and Schwartz, L.B., The level of tryptase in human tears. An indicator of activation of conjunctival mast cells. *Ophthalmology* 97:1678 (1990).
53. D-Q. Li, and Tseng, S.C.G., Three patterns of cytokine expression potentially involved in epithelial-fibroblast interactions of human ocular surface. *J. Cell. Phys.*163:61 (1995).
54. G-B. van Setten, Viinikka, L., Tervo, T., et al., Epidermal growth factor is a constant component of normal human tear fluid. *Graefe's Arch. Clin. Exp. Ophthalmol.* 227:184 (1989).
55. G-B. van Setten, and Schultz, G., Transforming growth factor is a constant component of human tear fluid. *Graefe's Arch. Clin. Exp. Ophthalmol.* 232:523 (1994).
56. M. Vesaluoma, Teppo, A-M., Grönhagen-Riska, C., and Tervo, T., Release of TGFβ and VEGF in tear fluid following photorefractive keratectomy. (Abstract) *Invest. Ophthalmol. Vis. Sci.* 37(Suppl):847 (1996).
57. M. Vesaluoma, Teppo, A-M., Grönhagen-Riska, C., and Tervo, T., Increased release of tumor necrosis factor-α in human tear fluid after excimer laser-induced corneal wound. *Br. J. Ophthalmol.* 81:1 (1997).
58. Q. Liang, Tervo, T., Vesaluoma, M., et al., Tear hepatocyte growth factor (HGF) production increases markedly after excimer laser photorefractive keratoplasty (PRK). (Abstract) *Invest. Ophthalmol. Vis. Sci.* 37(Suppl): 847 (1996).
59. G. Schultz, Khaw, P.T., Oxford, K., et al., Growth factors and ocular wound healing. *Eye* 8:184 (1994).

60. G.S. Schultz, Rotatori, D.S., and Clark, W., EGF and TGFα in wound healing and repair. *J. Cell. Biochem.* 45:364 (1991).

61. G-B. van Setten, Macauley, S., Huphreys-Beher, M., et al., Detection of transforming growth factor-α mRNA and protein in rat lacrimal glands and characterization of transforming growth factor-α in human tears. *Invest. Ophthalmol. Vis. Sci.* 37:166 (1995).

62. H.W. Thompson, and Beuerman, R.W., Regulation of growth factor production correlates in lacrimal gland with wound responses from the eye. (Abstract) *J. Cell. Biochem.* 16B(Suppl):187 (1992).

63. H.W. Thompson, Beuerman, R.W., Cook, J., et al., Transcription of message for tumor necrosis factor-alpha by lacrimal gland is regulated by corneal wounding. *Adv. Exp. Med. Biol.* 350:211 (1994).

64. G-B. van Setten, Tervo, K., Virtanen, I., et al., Immunohistochemical demonstration of epidermal growth factor in the lacrimal and submandibular glands of rats. *Acta Ophthalmol. (Copenh.)* 68:477 (1990).

65. Z. Ji, Yoshino, K., Monroy, D., and Pflugfelder, S.C., Transforming growth factor β (TGFβ) expression in the human lacrimal gland. (Abstract) *Invest. Ophthalmol. Vis. Sci.* 35(Suppl):1792 (1994).

66. Q. Li, Weng, J., Bennett, G.L.,et al., Hepatocyte growth factor (HGF) and HGF receptor protein in lacrimal glands, tears, and cornea. *Invest. Ophthalmol. Vis. Sci.* 37:727 (1996).

67. S.E. Wilson, He, Y-G., and Lloyd, S.A., EGF, EGF receptor, basic FGF, TGFbeta-1, and IL-1 alpha mRNA in human corneal epithelial cells and stromal fibroblasts. *Invest. Ophthalmol. Vis. Sci.* 33:1756 (1992).

68. S.E. Wilson, Schultz, G.S., Chegini, N., et al., Epidermal growth factor, transforming growth factor-alpha, transforming growth factor-beta, acidic fibroblast growth factor, basic fibroblast growth factor and interleukin-1 proteins in the cornea. *Exp. Eye. Res.* 59:63 (1994).

69. R.M. Lyons, Keski-Oja, J., and Moses, H.L., Proteolytic activation of latent transforming growth factor-beta from fibroblast-conditioned medium. *J. Cell. Biol.* 106:1659 (1988).

70. W. Ayliffe, Espaillat, A., Foster, C.S., and Lee, S.J., Polymerase chain reaction analysis of TNF-α gene expression in rat corneal wound healing. (Abstract) *Invest. Ophthalmol. Vis. Sci.* 34(Suppl.):1376 (1993).

71. J. Vilcek, and Lee, T.H., Tumor necrosis factor. New insights into the molecular mechanisms of its multiple actions. *J. Biol. Chem.* 266:7313 (1991).

72. T.J. Fahey, III., Turbeville. T., and McIntyre, K., Differential TNF secretion by wound fibroblasts compared to normal fibroblasts in response to LPS. *J. Surg. Res.* 58:759 (1995).

73. W. Bernauer, Wright, P., Dart, J.K., et al., Cytokines in the conjunctiva of acute and chronic mucous membrane pemphigoid: an immunohistochemical study. *Graefe's Arch. Clin. Exp. Ophthalmol.* 231:563 (1993).

74. S.E. Wilson, He, Y.G., Weng, J., et al., Effect of epidermal growth factor, hepatocyte growth factor, and keratinocyte growth factor on proliferation, motility and differentiation of human corneal epithelial cells. *Exp. Eye Res.* 59:665 (1994).

75. F.E. Kruse, and Tseng, S.C.G., Transformierender Wachstumsfaktor beta 1 und 2 hemmen die Proliferation von Limbus- und Hornhautepithel. *Ophthalmologe* 91:617 (1994).

76. J. Taipale, and Keski-Oja, J., Hepatocyte growth factor releases epithelial and endothelial cells from growth arrest induced by transforming growth factor β1. *J. Biol. Chem.* 271:4342 (1996).

77. J.V. Jester, Barry, P.A., Cavanagh, H.D., and Petroll, W.M., Role of TGF-β1 in myofibroblast transformation and corneal wound healing. (Abstract). *Ocular Cell & Molecular Biology Symposium II, San Diego, California* (1995).

78. M. Ohji, SundarRaj, N., and Thoft, R.A., Transforming growth factor-β stimulates collagen and fibronectin synthesis by human corneal stromal fibroblasts. *Curr. Eye Res.* 12:703 (1993).

79. M.T. Girard, Matsubara, M., and Fini, M.E., Transforming growth factor-beta and interleukin-1 modulate metalloproteinase expression by corneal stromal cells. *Invest. Ophthalmol. Vis. Sci.* 32:2441 (1991).

80. P.A. D'Amore, Mechanisms of retinal and choroidal neovascularization. *Invest. Ophthal. Vis. Sci.* 35:3974 (1994).

81. J. Bednarz, Weich, H.A., Rodokanaki-von Schrenck, A., and Engelmann, K., Expression of genes encoding growth factors and growth factor receptors in differentiated and dedifferentiated human corneal endothelial cells. *Cornea* 14:372 (1995).

82. B.J. Sugarman, Aggarwal, B.B., Hass, P.E., et al., Recombinant tumor necrosis factor-α: effects on proliferation of normal and transformed cells in vitro. *Science* 230:943 (1985).

83. A. Mauviel, Daireaux, M., Redini, P., et al., Tumor necrosis factor inhibits collagen and fibronectin synthesis in human dermal fibroblasts. *FEBS Lett.* 236:47 (1988).

84. J.M. Dayer, Beutler, B., and Cerami, A., Cachectin/tumor necrosis factor stimulates collagenase and prostaglandin E_2 production by human synovial cells and dermal fibroblasts. *J. Exp. Med.* 162:2153 (1985).

85. J.V. Jester, Petroll, W.M., Barry, P.A., et al., Inhibition of corneal fibrosis by topical application of blocking antibodies to TGF-β in the rabbit LK model. (Abstract). *Invest. Ophthalmol. Vis. Sci.* 36(Suppl.):867 (1995).

86. C. Castagnoli, Stella, M., Berthod, C., et al., TNF production and hypertrophic scarring. *Cell. Immunol.* 147:51 (1993).
87. L. Paton, The trigeminal and its ocular lesions. *Br. J. Ophthalmol.* 10:305 (1926).
88. R.W. Beuerman, and Schimmelpfennig, B., Sensory denervation of the rabbit cornea affects epithelial properties. *Exp. Neurol.* 69:196 (1980).
89. J. Garcia-Hircshfeld, Lopez-Briones, L.G., and Belmonte, C., Neurotrophic influences on corneal epithelial cells. *Exp. Eye Res.* 59:597 (1994).
90. A.A. Miculec, Monroe, F.A., and Tanelian, D.L., EGF and CGRP increase in vitro corneal epithelial wound healing. (Abstract) *Invest. Ophthalmol. Vis. Sci.* 34(Suppl):3323 (1993).
91. A.K. Li, Koroly, M.J., Schattenkerk, M.E., et al., Nerve growth factor: acceleration of the rate of wound healing in mice. *Proc. Natl. Acad. Sci. U S A* 77:4379 (1980).
92. J. Gallar, Pozo, M.A., Rebollo, I., and Belmonte, C., Effects of capsaicin on corneal wound healing. *Invest. Ophthalmol. Vis. Sci.* 31:1968 (1990).
93. K.S. Baker, Anderson, S.C., Romanowski, E.G., et al.,. Trigeminal ganglion neurons affect corneal epithelial phenotype. Influence on type VII collagen expression *in vitro. Invest. Ophthalmol. Vis. Sci.* 34:137 (1993).
94. K. Araki, Ohashi, Y., Kinoshita, S., et al., Epithelial wound healing in the denervated cornea. *Curr. Eye. Res.* 13:203 (1994).
95. G.J. Lind, and Cavanagh, H.D., Nuclear muscarinic acetylcholine receptors in corneal cells from rabbit. *Invest. Ophthalmol. Vis. Sci.* 34:2943 (1993).
96. L.J. Mller, Pels, L., and Vrensen, G.F.J.M., Ultrastructural organization of human corneal nerves. *Invest. Ophthalmol. Vis. Sci.* 37:476 (1996).
97. P. Mertaniemi, Ylätupa, S., Partanen, P., and Tervo, T., Increased release of immunoreactive calcitonin gene-related peptide (CGRP) in tears after excimer laser keratectomy. *Exp. Eye Res.* 60:659 (1995).
98. T. Ishikawa, Park, S.B., Cox, C., et al., Corneal sensation following excimer laser photorefractive keratectomy in humans. *J. Refr. Corneal. Surg.* 10:417 (1994).
99. A.F. Phillips, Szerenyi, K., Campos, M., et al., Arachidonic acid metabolites after excimer laser corneal surgery. *Arch. Ophthalmol.* 111:1273 (1993).
100. D.H. Richard, Assouline, M., Renard, G., et al., Prospective randomized trial of topical soluble 0.1 % indomethacin for the control of pain following excimer photoablation of the cornea. (Abstract). *Invest. Ophthalmol. Vis. Sci.* 35(Suppl):1672 (1994).

34

ESSENTIAL ROLE OF A PROTEIN KINASE C (PKC) SIGNAL TRANSDUCTION SYSTEM IN CORNEAL EPITHELIAL MIGRATION

Keiko Ofuji, Masatsugu Nakamura, Takashi Nagano, and Teruo Nishida

Department of Ophthalmology
Yamaguchi University School of Medicine
Yamaguchi, Japan

ABSTRACT

The migration of corneal epithelial cells is an important step in corneal wound healing under various pathologic conditions. Several extracellular factors are known to modulate corneal epithelial migration. However, to understand the healing process, it is important to know how the cells respond to these factors. This study investigated the possible role of three intracellular signal transduction systems: protein kinase C (PKC), cAMP-dependent protein kinase (PKA), and cGMP-dependent kinase (PKG). The length of the path of corneal epithelial migration was measured on rabbit corneal blocks incubated with PKC inhibitors (H-7, calphostin C) or an activator of PKC (phorbol 12-myristate 13-acetate). We also used HA-1004, an inhibitor of PKA and PKG, and cAMP or cGMP analogues that would mimic the effect of PKA and PKG activation. PKC inhibitors reduced epithelial migration in a dose-dependent fashion, and the PKC activator stimulated it. On the contrary, neither the PKA or PKG inhibitor, nor the cAMP and cGMP analogues, had any effect. The increased migration induced by PKC activator and the decrease induced by PKC inhibitor suggest that, under these conditions, a signal transduction system via the PKC pathway plays an important role in corneal epithelial migration.

INTRODUCTION

The migration of corneal epithelial cells is an important first step in corneal epithelial wound healing under various pathologic conditions. Several factors have been reported to modulate corneal epithelial migration. Extracellular matrix proteins, such as fibronectin and hyaluronan, provide a suitable extracellular environment for epithelial cell attachment and initiation of migration. The addition of fibronectin or hyaluronan stimulates corneal epithelial migration *in vitro*[1-4] and *in vivo*.[5-7] Epidermal growth factor (EGF) and interleukin 6 (IL-6) have been reported to activate the expression of integrin, i.e., fibronectin receptors, in corneal epithelial cells,[8] and to stimulate epithelial migration *in vitro* and *in vivo*.[2,9-11]

To better understand the mechanisms of corneal epithelial wound healing, it is important to identify the intracellular signal transduction system(s) that are activated by extracellular factors to express the biological functions in the cells. Several signal transduction systems in corneal epithelial cells are known: Cyclic AMP (cAMP) and cyclic GMP (cGMP) serve as second messenger for cAMP-dependent protein kinase C (PKA) or cGMP-dependent protein kinase (PKG) systems. Protein kinase C (PKC) is another important signal transduction system in many cells[12-14] and in corneal epithelial cells.[15]

This study attempted to identify which second signal transduction system might play an essential role during corneal epithelial migration. An organ culture system of rabbit corneas was used to investigate the effects of activators or inhibitors of PKA, PKG, and PKC on corfneal epithelial migration.

MATERIALS AND METHODS

Materials

Male Japanese albino rabbits weighing 2 to 3 kg were obtained from Seiwa, Kitakyushu City, Fukuoka, Japan. The animals were treated in conformation with the ARVO Statement for the Use of Animals in Ophthalmic and Vision Research. Phorbol 12-myristate 13-acetate (PMA), 8-bromo cyclic AMP (8br-cAMP), 8-bromo cyclic GMP (8br-cGMP), calphostin C were purchased from Sigma Chemical Co. (St. Louis, MO). H-7 and HA-1004 were obtained from Seikagaku Corporation (Tokyo, Japan). TC-199 culture medium was obtained from the Research Foundation for Microbial Diseases of Osaka University (Suita, Osaka, Japan). Multiwell tissue culture dishes (24 wells, #3524) were from Costar Corporation, Cambridge, MA.

Measurement of Epithelial Migration in Organ Culture of the Cornea

Rabbit corneas were cultured and the length of the path of epithelial migration was measured as described previously.[1] Briefly, rabbits were killed with an intravenous overdose of pentobarbital sodium (Nembutal sodium solution; Abbott Laboratories; North Chicago, IL). Eyes were enucleated, and a sclerocorneal section was excised. After being washed several times with sterile phosphate-buffered saline (PBS), the corneas were cut into 2 x 4 mm blocks with a razor blade. The corneal blocks were placed in plastic 24-well tissue culture dishes with 1 ml of serum-free TC-199 culture medium with or without the reagents at the concentrations indicate (see Results). The corneal blocks were cultured at 37°C, usually for 24 hours, and then fixed overnight with a mixture of 100% ethanol and glacial acetic acid (95:5 vol/vol) at 4°C. They were dehydrated and embedded in paraffin. Three 4-μm sections, 200 μm apart, were cut from each block. After deparaffinization, the specimens were stained with hematoxylin-eosin and observed under a light microscope. Photographs were taken with black and white film. The length of the path of epithelial migration was measured on the photograph. Results were expressed in micrometers as means ± SEM of six measurements.

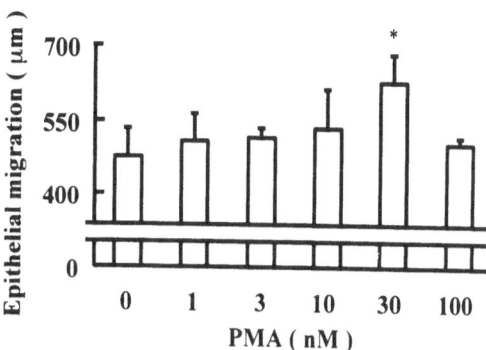

Figure 1. Effects of a PKC activator (phorbol 12-myriastate 13-acetate, PMA) on corneal epithelial migration. The corneal blocks were cultured for 24 hours in the absence or presence of various concentrations of PMA. The length of the path of epithelial migration was measured as described in Materials and Methods section. Each point represents mean ± SEM of six determinations. *:p<0.05 by Dunnett multiple comparisons test with the control.

Statistical Analysis

Statistical analysis was carried out by Dunnett multiple comparison test. In some cases, Student's t test was applied.

RESULTS

First examined was the effect of a PKC activator on corneal epithelial migration. Figure 1 shows the effect of the addition of a phorbol ester, PMA, at 1, 3, 10, 30, or 100 nM for 24 hours. PMA stimulated epithelial migration in a dose-dependent fashion. At 30 nM, PMA significantly ($p < 0.05$) stimulated epithelial migration by 32%, compared to cultures without PMA. However, 100 nM of PMA, epithelial migration was decreased nearly to control levels. The difference between cultures at 30 nM and at 100 nM was statistically significant ($p < 0.05$, by Student's t test).

Next, the study examined the time course of epithelial migration in the absence or presence of PMA (30 nM). The length of the path of epithelial migration was measured on corneal blocks cultured for 0.5, 1, 4, 12, 18, or 24 hours. No epithelial migration was observed until hour 18, regardless of whether PMA was present or not. In control cultures without PMA, the length of the path of epithelial migration increased significantly between hour 18 and hour 24. In the presence of PMA, the lag phase was the same as in control cultures; however, the rate of increase in the length of the path was significantly higher (Figure 2). These results demonstrated that corneal epithelial migration was facilitated by activation of PKC through the addition of PMA.

The effect of the period of exposure to PMA was then investigated. After 0.5, 1, 4, 12, or 18 hours of cultivation in the presence of PMA (30 nM) the culture media were changed, and cultivation continued without PMA for the remainder of the 24-hour period. Exposure to PMA for the first hour of cultivation resulted in a significant increase in the length of the path of epithelial migration, compared with controls. No difference in epithelial migration was observed among those cultured with PMA for the first 1, 4, 12, 18, or entire 24 hours (Figure 3).

When cAMP analogue (8-Br cAMP, 0.1 or 1mM), adenyl cyclase activator (forskolin, 10 mM) or cGMP analogue (8-Br cGMP, 0.1 or 1μM) was added to the culture medium to increase the intracellular concentrations of cAMP or cGMP, no significant difference in the length of the path of the epithelial migration was observed after 24 hours' culture (Table 1). These results demonstrated that only an activator of PKC (PMA) stimu-

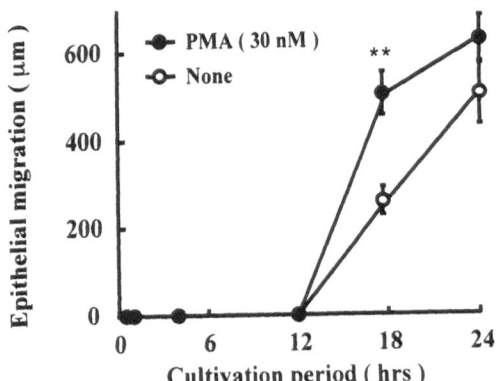

Figure 2. The chronological changes in the length of the path of the epithelial migration in the absence or presence of PMA (30 nM). The corneal blocks were cultured for indicated period of time with or without PMA, and the length of the path of epithelial migration was measured. Each point represents mean ± SEM of six determinations. *:p<0.05, **p<0.01 by Dunnett Multiple comparison test with the control.

lated epithelial migration, and that at least 1 hour exposure to PMA was required to initiate the activation of epithelial migration.

Inhibitors of PKC, PKA, and PKG affected corneal epithelial migration as expected. HA-1004, which is a potent inhibitor of PKA and PKG, but a weak inhibitor of PKC, had no significant effect on epithelial migration up to the highest concentration examined (30 μM). This suggests that PKA and PKG play no significant role in corneal epithelial migration (Figure 4). H-7, an inhibitor of PKC, significantly decreased the length of the path of epithelial migration in a dose-dependent fashion. When H-7 was added at a concentration of 10 μM or 30 μM, the length of the path of the epithelial migration was 59% and 18%, respectively, of migration in cultures without H-7 (Figure 4). Calphostin C, a more specific inhibitor of PKC than is H-7, also decreased the length of the path of epithelial migration in a dose-dependant fashion. At concentrations of 10 μM or above, the difference from control cultures was statistically significant (p < 0.05, Figure 5).

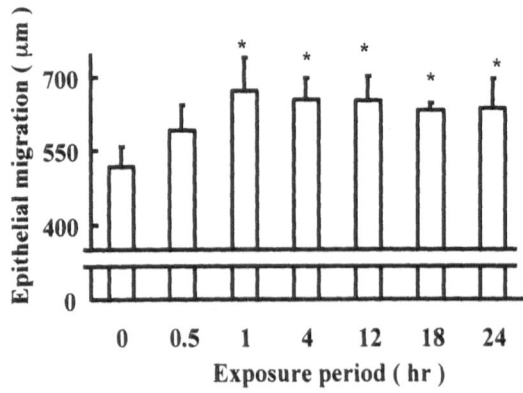

Figure 3. Effects of exposure period to PMA (30 nM). The corneal blocks were cultured for 24 hours and the length of the path of epithelial migration was measured. PMA was initially present in the culture migration was measured. PMA was initially present in the culture medium for the indicated period; then the medium was changed to one without PMA, and cultivation continued. Controls were cultured for 24 hours without PMA, and another group was cultured with 30 nM of PMA for 24 hours. Each point represents mean ± SEM of 6 determinations. *:p<0.05, by Dunnett multiple comparison test with controls incubated in the absence of PMA.

Table 1. Effects of cAMP or cGMP analogues on

Addition	Length of path of epithelial migration (μm)
8Br-cAMP (0.1 mM)	523.2 ± 27.5
8Br-cAMP (1 mM)	530.4 ± 29.2
forskolin (10 μM)	513.2 ± 40.2
8Br-cGMP (0.1 mM)	524.2 ± 36.2
8Br-cGMP (1 mM)	550.9 ± 39.6
None	499.1 ± 35.3

The corneal blocks were cultured for 24 hours in TC199 containing 8Br-cAMP (0.1, 1 mM) forskolin (10μM), or 8Br-cGMP (01,1 mM). Control was only cultured in unsupplemented TC199. The length of the path of epithelial migration was measured as described in Materials and Methods section. Each data represents mean ±SEM of 6 determinations.

DISCUSSION

These findings demonstrated that the activation of PKC is an essential part of the intracellular signal transduction system for corneal epithelial migration, and that the cAMP or cGMP system itself is not responsible for epithelial migration. The presence of PKC activator significantly increased corneal epithelial migration, and PKC inhibitors significantly decreased it in this organ culture system using rabbit corneas. The addition of cAMP or cGMP analogues did not affect corneal epithelial migration.

The present results are in good agreement with those reported by Hirakata et al.,[16] who reported that PKC activity was an important factor in regulating corneal epithelial wound healing. They cultured mechanically debrided epithelium of rat corneas in the presence of PKC inhibitors, such as staurosporine, sphinganine or H-7, or in the presence of the PKC activators, PMA or 1-oleoyl-2-acetyl-sn-glycerol (OAG). Akhtar and colleagues found that phorbol esters, such as PMA, stimulated PKC activity in the bovine corneal epithelial cells.[13,14] They reported that PKC inhibitors significantly reduced the rate of epithelial wound closure; PKC activators, however, had no significant effect. These investigators suggested that PKC in the corneal epithelial cells had been fully activated by corneal wounding, so that additional PKC activators produced no significant stimulation of wound closure. The results in the current organ culture model are not inconsistent with

Figure 4. Effects of H-7 and HA-1004 on the corneal epithelial migration. Corneal blocks were cultured in the absence or presence of various concentrations of H-7 or HA-1004 for 24 hours, and the length of the path of the corneal epithelial migration was measured. Each point represents mean ± SEM of 6 determinations. *:p<0.05, **:p<0.01 by Dunnett multiple comparison test with the control.

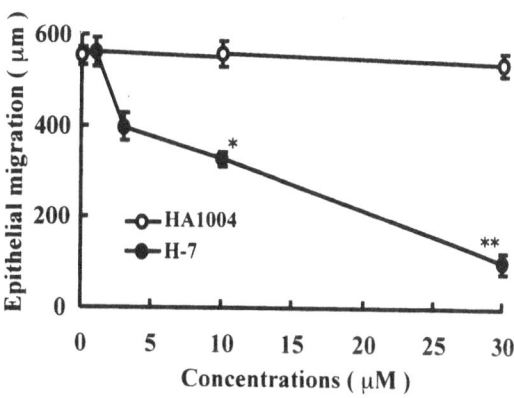

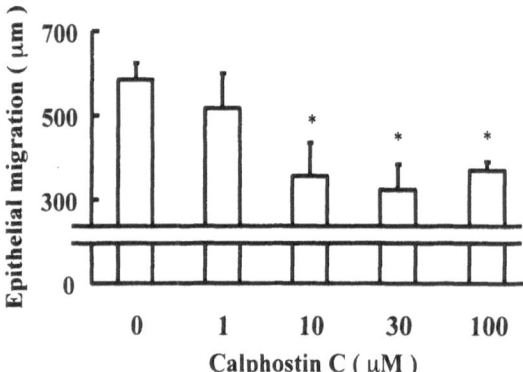

Figure 5. Effects of calphostin C on corneal epithelial migration. Corneal blocks were cultured in the absence or presence of various concentrations of calphostin C for 24 hours, and the length of the path of the corneal epithelial migration was measured. Each point represents mean ± SEM of 6 determinations. *:$p < 0.05$, by Dunnett multiple comparison test with the control.

this suggestion. As these figures demonstrate, the length of the path of epithelial migration in unsupplemented control cultures was around 500 to 550 μm after 24 hours' cultivation. The inhibition of this epithelial migration by the presence of PKC inhibitor (Figures 4 and 5) suggests that cellular PKC might have been well activated during the preparation of the corneal blocks. Therefore, further activation by PMA did not affect the corneal epithelial migration greatly. As shown in Figures 1–3, the increase was significant, but small.

As shown in Figures 1 and 3, PKC activation required a minimal period of exposure to PMA (1 hour), as well as a certain level of PMA concentration (30 nM in these experiments). Corneal epithelial migration was decreased at the higher concentration of 100 nM, which was the concentration used by Hirakata et al.[16] There was a lag phase of at least 12 hours before the epithelial migration was actually initiated. PKC activator did not affect the lag phase, but it significantly increased the epithelial migration measured at 18 and 24 hours (Figure 2).

Lin and Bazan have reported the presence of various subtypes of PKC activity in the corneal epithelium.[12] The total PKC activity was unchanged after rabbit corneal epithelium was denuded, but α-PKC activity increased in the migrating epithelial cells. It seems to be important to consider the differential activation of PKC subtypes.

H-7 is a potent inhibitor of PKC, but it also inhibits PKA and PKG.[17] Calphostin C has been reported to be a more specific inhibitor of PKC than is H-7.[18] Both H-7 and calphostin C inhibited corneal epithelial migration (Figures 4 and 5), leading to the conclusion that PKC plays an essential role in corneal epithelial migration. HA-1004, which is a potent inhibitor of PKA and PKG, is structurally similar to H-7, so it has often been used as a control for H-7. However, Hirakata et al. reported that HA-1004 had no effect on corneal epithelial wound healing *in vitro*.[16] It was also found that HA-1004 did not affect corneal epithelial migration (Figure 4). The addition of cAMP or cGMP analogues also failed to affect. Thus, under the conditions described, PKA and PKG systems do not appear to be responsible for corneal epithelial migration. These results on the roles of PKA and PKG are in good agreement with those reported by others.

Jumblatt and Neufeld have reported that cholera toxin, a specific activator of adenylate cyclase, stimulated corneal epithelial wound healing *in vivo* when epithelial abrasion was made by heptanol debridement, but did not affect healing when the epithelial wound was made mechanically with a blade.[19] The latter result is compatible with the current results using an organ culture model *in vitro*. However, another study showed that cholera toxin or forskolin, which elevated intracellular levels of cAMP, inhibited the rate of wound closure, but increased the cell adhesion in rabbit corneal epithelial tissue culture.[20] O'Brien et al. have reported that timoptic, which decreases intracellular adenyl cyclase activity, had no effect on corneal reepithelialization when the epithelium was scraped with blade *in vivo.*[21]

The paradoxical ability of cholera toxin to stimulate wound closure *in vivo* may be caused by the difference between the experimental models. Epithelial wounds *in vivo* are closed initially by epithelial cells migrating from the periphery, rather than by proliferation in the wound site. This study used full-thickness corneas cut into small blocks, so that the epithelium migrated over the cut stroma at the sides of the blocks, where the native basement membrane was absent. The presence or absence of epithelial basement membrane might influence the results.

REFERENCES

1. T. Nishida, Nakagawa, S., Awata, T., et al., Fibronectin promotes epithelial migration of cultured rabbit cornea *in situ. J. Cell Biol.* 97:1653 (1983).
2. T. Nishida, Nakamura, M., Mishima, H., and Otori, T., Differential modes of action of fibronectin and epidermal growth factor on rabbit corneal epithelial migration. *J. Cell. Physiol.* 145:549 (1990).
3. T. Nishida, Nakamura, M., Mishima, H., and Otori, T., Hyaluronan stimulates corneal epithelial migration. *Exp. Eye Res.* 53:753 (1991).
4. M. Nakamura, Mishima, H., Nishida, T., and Otori, T., Binding of hyaluronan to plasma fibronectin increases the attachment of corneal epithelial cells to a fibronectin matrix. *J. Cell. Physiol.* 159:415 (1994).
5. T. Nishida, Nakagawa S., Nishibayashi, C., et al., Fibronectin enhancement of corneal epithelial wound healing of rabbits *in vivo. Arch. Ophthalmol.* 102:455 (1984).
6. M. Nakamura, Hikida, M., and Nakano, T., Concentration and molecular weight dependency of rabbit corneal epithelial wound healing on hyaluronan. *Curr. Eye Res.* 11:981 (1992).
7. M. Nakamura, Nishida, T., Hikida, M., and Otori, T., Combined effects of hyaluronan and fibronectin on corneal epithelial wound closure of rabbit *in vivo. Curr. Eye Res.* 13:385 (1994).
8. T. Nishida, Nakamura, M., Murakami, J., et al., Epidermal growth factor stimulates corneal epithelial cell attachment to fibronectin through a fibronectin receptor system. *Invest. Ophthalmol. Vis. Sci.* 33:2464 (1992).
9. P.C. Ho, Davis, W.H., Elliott, J.H., and Cohen, S., Kinetics of corneal epithelial regeneration and epidermal growth factor. *Invest. Ophthalmol. Vis. Sci.* 13:804 (1974).
10. T. Nishida, Nakamura M., Mishima, H., and Otori, T., Interleukin 6 promotes epithelial migration by a fibronectin-dependent mechanism. *J. Cell. Physiol.* 153:1 (1992).
11. T. Nishida, Nakamura, M., Mishima, H., et al., Interleukin 6 facilitates corneal epithelial wound closure *in vivo. Arch. Ophthalmol.* 110:1292 (1992).
12. N. Lin, and Bazan, H.E.P., Protein kinase C subspecies in rabbit corneal epithelium: increased activity of alpha subspecies during wound healing. *Curr. Eye Res.* 11:899 (1992).
13. R.A. Akhtar, and Wilmoth, T.L., Phorbol esters inhibit ionomycin-induced hydrolysis of phosphoinositides and phosphatidylcholine in bovine corneal epithelial cells. *Curr. Eye Res.* 11:135 (1992).
14. R.A. Akhtar, and Choi, M.W., Stimulation of phospholipase D by phorbol esters and ionomycin in bovine corneal epithelial cells. *Curr. Eye Res.* 11:553 (1992).
15. H.E. Bazan, Dobard, P., and Reddy, S.T., Calcium- and phospholipid-dependent protein kinase C and phosphatidylinositol kinase: two major phosphorylation systems in the cornea. *Curr. Eye Res.* 6:667 (1987).
16. A. Hirataka, Gupta, A.G., and Proia, A.D., Effect of protein kinase C inhibitors and activators on corneal re-epithelialization in the rat. *Invest. Ophthalmol. Vis. Sci.* 34:216 (1993).
17. H. Hidaka, Inagaki, M., Kawamoto, S., and Sasaki, Y., Isoquinolinesulfonamides, Novel and potent inhibitors of cyclic nucleotide dependent protein kinase and protein kinase C. Biochemistry 23:5036 (1984).
18. E. Kobayashi, Nakano, H., Morimoto, M., and Tamaoki, T., Calphostin C (UCN-1028C), a novel microbial compound, is a highly potent and specific inhibitor of protein kinase C. *Biochem. Biophys. Res. Commun.* 159:548 (1989).
19. M.M. Jumblatt, and Neufeld, A.H., Characterization of cyclic AMP-mediated wound closure of the rabbit corneal epithelium. *Curr. Eye Res.* 1:189 (1981).
20. M.M. Jumblatt, and Neufeld, A.H., A tissue culture assay of corneal epithelial wound closure. *Invest. Ophthalmol. Vis. Sci.* 27:8 (1986).
21. W.J. O'Brien, DeCarlo, J.D., Stern, M., and Hyndiuk, R.A., Effects of timoptic on corneal reepithelialization. *Arch. Ophthalmol.* 100:1331 (1982).

35

STROMAL-EPITHELIAL INTERACTIONS IN THE CORNEA

Steven E. Wilson

Eye Institute and Department of Cell Biology
The Cleveland Clinic Foundation
Cleveland, Ohio

ABSTRACT

Communication between corneal epithelial cells and keratocytes is likely to contribute to normal maintenance, wound healing, corneal tissue organization, and the pathophysiology of corneal disease. Interactions between these cells are mediated via cytokines, growth factors, and their receptors. Other mechanisms of communication may also occur.

Hepatocyte growth factor (HGF) and keratinocyte growth factor (KGF) are classical paracrine mediators produced by the keratocytes that regulate the proliferation, motility, and differentiation of corneal epithelial cells via the HGF receptor and KGF receptor (stromal to epithelial interactions). HGF is also produced by the lacrimal gland and is a component in the tear film. After corneal wounding, however, HGF protein and HGF and KGF mRNA production is stimulated in keratocyte cells. Upregulation of HGF and KGF production in the keratocyte cells is likely mediated by the release of IL-1 from the injured epithelial cells. Thus, IL-1 serves as a molecular transducer that signals keratocytes that the epithelium has been injured and stimulates the stromal cells to increase production of HGF and KGF to modulate corneal epithelial wound healing.

Epithelial to stromal interactions are also important in the cornea. It has recently been demonstrated that the disappearance of anterior keratocytes following corneal epithelial injury is mediated via programmed cell death (apoptosis) characterized by chromatin condensation, nucleosomal fragmentation, the formation of apoptotic bodies, and DNA fragmentation. Our data suggest that IL-1, and possibly soluble Fas ligand, released from corneal epithelial cells by injury, trigger apoptosis in the keratocytes via IL-1 receptor and Fas, respectively, expressed by the stromal cells.

It is hypothesized this system is physiologically activated by infection of corneal epithelial cells by viral pathogens such as herpes simplex virus and that death of the anterior keratocytes functions to limit the extension of virus. Injury to the epithelium during refractive surgical procedures such as photorefractive keratectomy (PRK) could be perceived by the cornea as a massive viral infection of the epithelium that results in apoptosis

Advances in Corneal Research, edited by Lass
Plenum Press, New York, 1997

of the anterior keratocytes. Keratocyte apoptosis may be the initiating event in the subsequent wound healing response and a promising site for interventions to control wound healing following refractive surgery. These observations provide a physiologic explanation for the difference that has been noted in wound healing response between surface ablation procedures (i.e., PRK) where the central corneal epithelium is injured and procedures such as LASIK in which the central corneal epithelium is maintained. This epithelial-stromal interactive system also provides a working hypothesis for the pathogenesis of ectatic diseases such as keratoconus where various abnormalities that might shift the balance between keratocyte proliferation and apoptosis could lead to a slow loss of the total number of keratocytes and, therefore, to stromal thinning.

Clinicians and scientists have long speculated regarding the importance of communications occurring between corneal epithelial and stromal cells (stromal-epithelial interactions) and the significance of these interactions in maintenance of normal corneal structure and function, pathophysiology of corneal disease, and corneal wound healing.[1] Over the past few years specific growth factor/cytokine-receptor systems have been detected in corneal cells *in vivo* and *in vitro* and some of their functions identified. This paper will review what is currently known about these corneal modulators of stromal-epithelial interactions and some of the processes they regulate.

Hepatocyte Growth Factor (HGF), Keratinocyte Growth Factor (KGF), and Their Receptors: Stromal-Epithelial Interactions in the Cornea

HGF and KGF have been characterized as classical mediators of stromal-epithelial interactions that function in many tissues. HGF and KGF are heparin-binding paracrine mediators secreted by fibroblast cells to regulate the functions of epithelial cells.[2-9] For example, HGF and KGF modulate proliferation and other functions in skin keratinocytes.[3,9] HGF has been shown to be identical to scatter factor, a fibroblast-derived factor that disperses cohesive colonies of epithelial cells.[10] HGF, KGF, and their receptor messenger RNAs (mRNA) have been detected *in vitro* and *ex vivo* in corneal cells.[12] HGF and KGF mRNA are expressed in corneal stromal fibroblast and endothelial, but not epithelial, cells. HGF receptor and KGF receptor mRNAs are expressed in all three major cell types in the cornea.[12] In addition, alternatively spliced mRNAs coding for a soluble form of the KGF receptor consisting only of the extracellular domain of the receptor and a HGF receptor that is truncated within the intracellular domain appear to be expressed in corneal epithelial cells.[6,12] The functions of the alternative receptors thought to be coded from these mRNAs are currently under investigation (Liang Q, Weng J, Wilson SE, unpublished data, 1996). Presumably, they are expressed by the corneal epithelial cells to modulate the responses of the cells to the corresponding growth factors (KGF and HGF) or possibly, in the case of the alternative HGF receptor mRNA, to activate different signal transduction pathways in response to the growth factor.[6]

Monoclonal antibodies that are useful for immunohistologic localization are available for HOF and HGF receptor.[13] HGF receptor protein is expressed in all three major cell types of the human cornea, but at highest levels in epithelium (Fig. 1A). HGF protein is detectable in keratocytes (Fig. 1 B) and endothelial, but not epithelial, cells. HGF production by keratocyte cells is markedly upregulated in response to mechanical corneal epithelial wounding (Fig. 1C).[13] Interestingly, HGF can be detected in association with the ocular surface in the unwounded cornea.[13] HGF is detectable in tears and is produced by the lacrimal gland.[13] Therefore, it is likely that the HGF associated with the surface epithelial cells in the unwounded cornea is derived from the lacrimal gland, although other sources such as conjuncti-

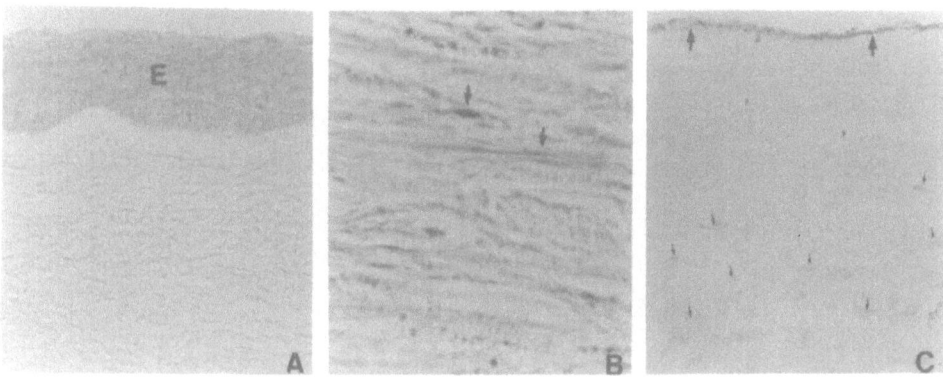

Figure 1. Immunohistochemical staining for HGF and HGF receptor protein expression in the cornea. A. HGF receptor is expressed in human corneal epithelial cells (E). 400X B. HGF is only detectable at low levels in keratocyte cells (arrows) in unwounded human cornea at high magnification. X1000. C. Forty-eight hours after corneal epithelial wounding HGF production is upregulated in mid to posterior stromal keratocytes (small arrows) in rabbit cornea. Note that keratocyte HGF is undetectable in the anterior corneal stroma consistent with apoptosis of the anterior keratocytes in response to epithelial wounding.[17] The entire thickness corneal epithelium stains for HGF (large arrows). Epithelial cell-associated HGF is bound to glysoaminoglycans (HGF is a heparin-binding growth factor) and HGF receptor on the epithelial cell surface. Keratocytes and tears are sources of epithelial cell-bound HGF. (Figures reprinted by permission. Previously published in Wilson, et al., *Investigative Ophthalmology and Visual Sciences* 37:727–39, 1996.

val blood vessels could also contribute tear HGF. HGF staining is detected throughout the epithelial layer in the cornea after a mechanical surface injury such as scrapping (Fig, 1C). Since the epithelial cells do not produce HGF, it is likely that the HGF associated with healing corneal epithelial cells is derived from the lacrimal gland and keratocytes.[13]

Antibodies that are useful for KGF and KGF receptor immunohistology are not yet available. Therefore, confirmation of KGF and KGF receptor protein expression in the cornea has not been obtained.

What functions are regulated by HGF and KGF in the cornea? *In vivo* studies have demonstrated that HGF stimulates proliferation and motility of corneal epithelial cells (Fig. 2).[14] In addition, HGF inhibits differentiation of corneal epithelial cells.[14] KGF was also shown to stimulate proliferation of corneal epithelial cells. Neither HGF nor KGF has an effect on proliferation of stromal fibroblast cells.[14] Thus, it is unclear what functions are served by the HGF receptors and KGF receptors expressed by keratocyte cells. These receptors could possibly mediate feedback loops regulating expression of HGF and KGF by the keratocyte cells, but this has not been confirmed. Corneal endothelial cells proliferate in response to both HGF and KGF Studies have not been performed testing the effect of HGF or KGF on normal or wounded corneas *in vivo*.

Epithelial-Stromal Interactions in the Cornea: The IL-1 and Fas Systems

Just as HGF and KGF mediate stromal-epithelial interactions, it is likely that there are epithelial to stromal interactions in the cornea regulated by cytokines or growth factors produced by epithelial cells. Observations suggesting that such interactions occur were made some time ago. Nakayasu[15] and Crosson[16] first demonstrated that the underlying keratocyte cells disappear over a period of several hours when corneal epithelial cells are wounded by mechanical scraping (Fig. 3A and 3B). Recently, it has been demonstrated

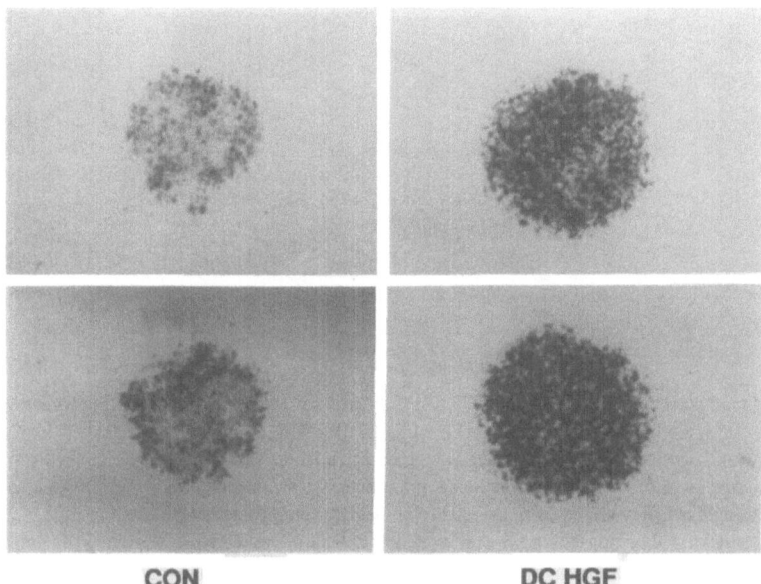

Figure 2. Corneal epithelial response to HGF. First passage human corneal epithelial cells were plated in the center of cloning cylinders in six-well plates. After 24 hours the cloning cylinders were removed and cells were exposed to vehicle (CON) or 5 mg/ml double-chain processed HGF (DC HGF) in serum-free defined medium. The HGF-treated colonies expanded compared with the vehicle-treated colonies. Expansion of the colonies has been shown to occur through HGF-modulated increases in proliferation and motility.[14]

Figure 3. Apoptosis of the underlying keratocytes in response to mechanical epithelial scrapping. A. Unwounded rabbit cornea stained with propidium iodide. X200 Note anterior keratocytes. B. Rabbit cornea four hours after mechanical epithelial scrapping stained with propidium iodide. The corneal stroma reproducibly becomes thinner and keratocytes more spindle shaped. Anterior stromal surface indicated by open arrows. Note the diminished number of keratocytes in the anterior corneal stroma. Posterior keratocytes and one that is still detectable anteriorly is indicated by arrows. X200. **C-F.** Transmission electron micrographs of keratocytes in wounded and unwounded mouse corneas. (C) In the unwounded mouse cornea, normal anterior keratocytes (arrow) underlie intact corneal epithelium (E). Magnification 4000X. (D). Superficial stromal keratocytes at one hour after epithelial scrapping reveal advanced programmed cell death. Dense chromatin condensations (arrows) that have undergone fragmentation are the only detectable remnants of the keratocyte cell. Magnification 4000X. (E) Normal keratocyte at approximately one third depth from the anterior corneal surface in an unwounded mouse cornea. Note normal chromatin pattern within the nucleus (N) and a mitochondrion (arrow). Magnification 25,000 X. (F) keratocyte at approximately 1/3 corneal depth from the anterior stromal surface at one hour after epithelial scrapping. Note dense chromatin condensation (C) within the nucleus compared with the normal keratocyte. Very little cytoplasm is present outside the nucleus. Cellular blebbing (large arrow) is occurring at the cell surface. Numerous membrane bound structures (apoptotic bodies, small arrows) are visible within the cell space and within the adjacent collagen lamellae. Magnification 25,000 X. (G) Apoptosis [anoikis], as detected by TUNEL staining for fragmented DNA, was detectable in superficial epithelial cells (arrows) in unwounded cornea. Apoptosis, however, was not detected in the underlying stroma. Horizontal bars indicate location of anterior stromal surface. 400X (H) DNA fragmentation consistent with apoptosis was detected by TUN EL assay in superficial keratocytes (arrow) four hours after an epithelial scrape wound. Staining of endothelial cells was also noted after corneal epithelial scraping in a few cells in some specimens (not shown). Original magnification 400X Figures reprinted by permission. Previously published in Wilson, et al., *Experimental Eye Research*, 62,325–338,1996.

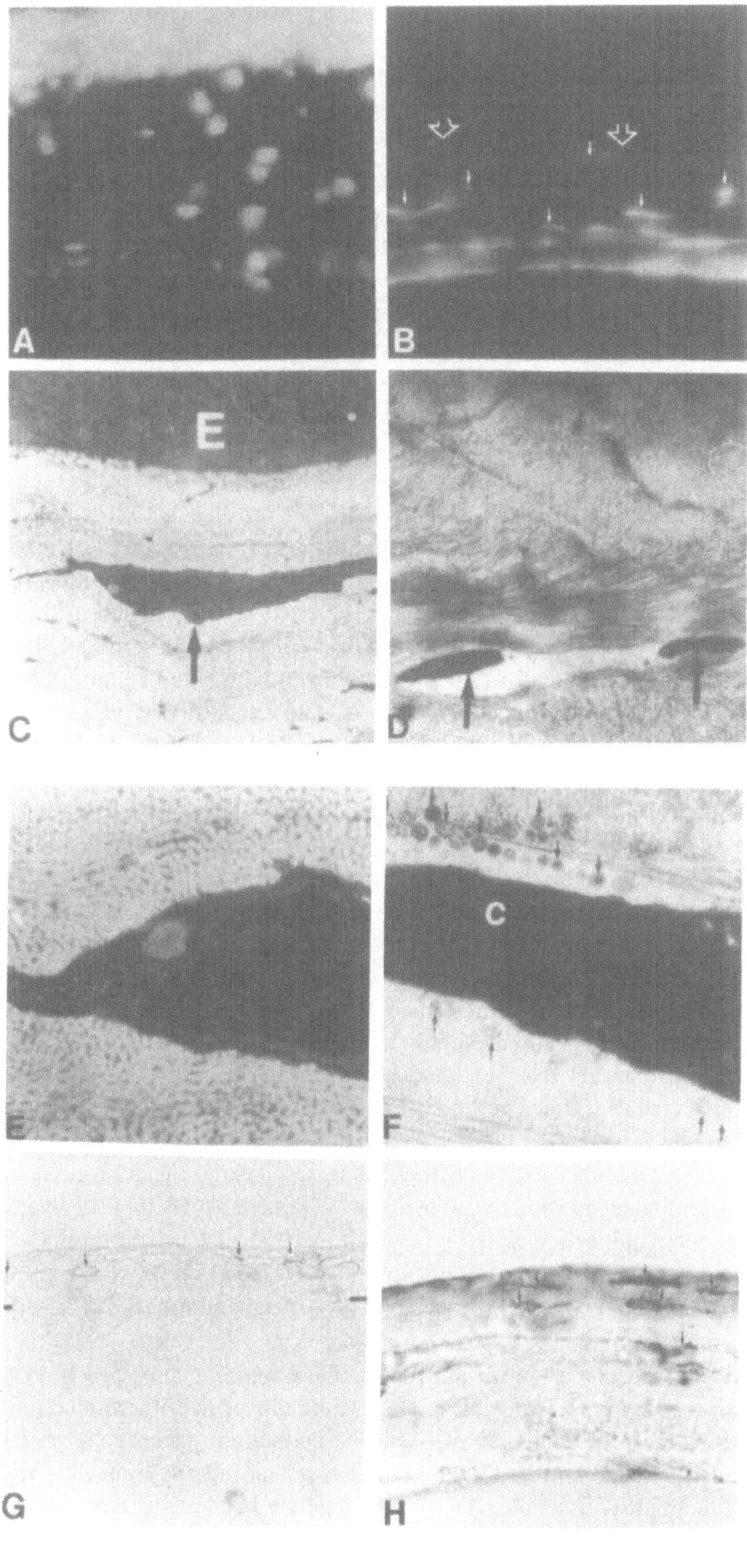

(Fig. 3 C, D, E, F) that this disappearance is mediated by programmed cell death (apoptosis) of the keratocyte cells characterized by cell shrinkage, chromatin condensation and fragmentation, and cellular blebbing with the formation of membrane bound structures which appear to contain intracellular organelles (apoptotic bodies).[17] In addition, DNA fragmentation suggestive of apoptosis was detected in the anterior keratocytes by TUNEL assay (Fig. 3G and 3H). Maximal anterior keratocyte apoptosis is noted approximately 4 hours after epithelial injury in mice and rabbits. The anterior corneal stroma is repopulated by activated keratocytes within three days after corneal epithelial injury.

In what were initially thought to be unrelated experiments, the effect of interleukin-1 (IL-1) alpha on stromal fibroblast cell proliferation *in vitro* was tested. The research team was motivated to undertake these experiments because the pattern of expression of IL-1 alpha and IL-1 type I receptor in primary cultures of corneal cells and corneal tissue sections suggested IL-1 as a potential mediator of epithelial to stromal interactions. Corneal epithelial and endothelial cells constitutively express IL-1 alpha mRNA[18] and protein.[19] Stromal fibroblast cells express type I IL-1 receptor, but not IL-1 alpha.[20] These initial *in vitro* and *ex vivo* studies of IL-1 alpha expression motivated our investigations on the effects of IL-1 alpha on stromal fibroblasts. Subsequent studies,[21] however, have suggested that under certain conditions stromal fibroblast cells are competent to produce IL-1 alpha. In the *in vitro* experiments designed to monitor proliferative response to the cytokines, we observed that IL-1 alpha and IL-1 beta in medium with 0.5% serum stimulated death in stromal fibroblast cells beginning after approximately 6–8 days of exposure.[17] This cell death was associated with fragmentation of DNA suggesting that cell death was mediated by apoptosis. The effect of IL-1 alpha was inhibited by IL-1 receptor antagonist. IL-1 alpha did not stimulate death of corneal epithelial or endothelial cells *in vitro*.

When mouse IL-1 alpha was microinjected into the central corneal stroma of BALB/c mice an interesting response was noted.[17] On staining with hematoxylin and eosin there was redistribution of keratocytes with a marked decrease in density in the center of the cornea at the site of injection and increased density just beneath the epithelium (Fig. 4A). This redistribution was not observed in vehicle injected corneas (Fig. 4B). The TUNEL assay demonstrated that keratocytes within the central stroma adjacent to injection site of IL-1 alpha, but not vehicle, had DNA fragmentation consistent with apoptosis.[17] The keratocytes beneath the epithelium formed nearly a straight line with an acellular layer of stroma between the keratocytes and the epithelial basement membrane (Fig 4A).[17] It appeared as if the depot of IL-1 alpha could have had a negative chemotactic effect on the keratocytes that did not undergo apoptosis. Possibly, whether the keratocyte cell undergoes apoptosis or negative chemotaxis in response to the IL-1 alpha is dependent on the localized concentration of the cytokine. The keratocytes that survived appeared to have assumed an equilibrium position between the IL-1 alpha depot in the mid stroma and the overlying epithelium. One interpretation of this observation was that modulators produced by the epithelial cells (i.e., IL-1 alpha, IL-1 beta, and perhaps other modulators) repelled the keratocytes from the opposite direction.

In this study, researchers were unable to inhibit anterior stromal keratocyte apoptosis in response to corneal epithelial scrape wounds by prior microinjection of large quantities of IL-1 receptor antagonist beneath the epithelium. One of the principles that has been revealed by gene knockout animal models is that there is frequently redundancy of important functions at the molecular level. Thus, we began to explore the possibility that there could be other systems that mediated keratocyte apoptosis in response to epithelial injury.

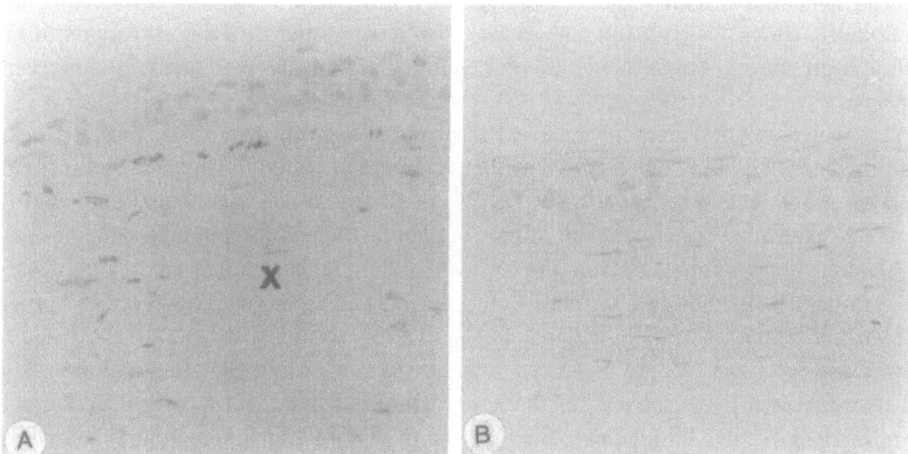

Figure 4. Effect of mouse IL-1 alpha injection into the corneal stroma of BALB/c mice. (A) Microinjection of mouse IL-1 alpha into the central cornea of a BALB/c mouse resulted in localized stromal edema, apparent redistribution of corneal fibroblasts, and decrease in the number of central corneal fibroblasts compared with injection of vehicle alone (B) at four hours after injection. Needles were passed into the cornea at the limbus and were advanced to the central cornea through the stroma under direct microscopic observation prior to injection. The approximate site of injection is noted by X. Note that in the cornea injected with IL-1 alpha, many of the corneal fibroblasts have formed a line in the anterior cornea parallel to the basal epithelium. There is a lucent area, however, between the corneal fibroblasts and the epithelial cells. Even the few fibroblasts that appear to have moved anterior to this location remain separated from the epithelium (hematoxylin and eosin). TUNEL assay on the same sections demonstrated that keratocytes at the site of IL-i alpha injection underwent apoptosis (not shown).[17] Figures reprinted by permission. Previously published in Wilson, et al., Experimental Eye Research, 62, 325–338, 1996.

Specific cell types can be stimulated to undergo apoptosis in response to a variety of signals. Stimuli commonly differ between different cells. For example, T lymphocytes undergo apoptosis in response to glucocorticoids, radiation, and binding of Fas ligand to the Fas receptor.[18] Regardless of the cell-specific upstream pathway, most programmed cell death appears to be mediated by a final common pathway that includes an interleukin-1 beta converting enzyme (ICE)-like protease, bad, bax, bcl-2 and other modulators. Some of the components within the final common pathway have yet to be identified. Virtually every cell examined to date has constitutively expressed the components of the final common pathway.[19] The Fas ligand and Fas (the receptor for the Fas ligand) have been best characterized in the immune system.[20,21] Both the receptor (Fas) and Fas ligand are synthesized as membrane-bound proteins and interactions occur by juxtacrine (direct cell to cell contact) between adjacent cells. Recently, however, it has been demonstrated that Fas ligand is also expressed as a soluble protein produced by alternative mRNA splicing and, therefore, paracrine interactions are possible.[18,22] Expression and function of Fas and Fas ligand in the cornea has recently been explored on the basis of new reports of expression of this system in non-immune tissues such as liver and skin.[23–25] It has been demonstrated that Fas and Fas ligand mRNA are expressed in primary cultures of corneal epithelial, stromal fibroblast, and endothelial cells.[26] Using immunohistochemistry we have also detected Fas receptor protein expression in all three major cell types of the cornea in fresh frozen human corneal sections.[26] Fas ligand protein, however, was only detected in corneal epithelial and endothelial cells. Interestingly, the pattern of expression of the Fas and Fas ligand proteins in fresh frozen human tissue mirrors that of IL-1 type I receptor and IL-1 alpha/IL-1 beta. Griffith and coworkers[27] also recently reported the expression of Fas ligand and protein in corneal epithelial and endothelial cells, as well as many other cells of the eye.

To evaluate competency of the Fas/Fas ligand system in the cornea, the effect of a monoclonal antibody to Fas that activates the receptor was tested.[26] This anti-Fas antibody stimulates apoptosis of corneal stromal fibroblast, epithelial and endothelial cells withIN 24 hours of exposure. The expression of Fas, but not Fas ligand protein in keratocytes suggest that signaling would occur from the corneal epithelium or endothelium to keratocytes, but not in the opposite direction. Since both Fas and Fas ligand are expressed in corneal epithelial and endothelial cells and the Fas-activating antibody stimulates apoptosis of each of these cell types, we are presented with a puzzle regarding signaling within each of these tissues. Does paracrine or juxtacrine signaling occur between corneal endothelial cells or epithelial cells? If so what is the function of this intralayer signaling and how is it controlled? Further study will be required to unravel the physiology of the Fas/Fas ligand system in the cornea, but many interesting details regarding corneal function are likely to be revealed by these investigations.

Possible IL-1 and Fas System Functions in the Cornea

IL-1 alpha and IL-1 beta lack signal sequences for transport from cells by traditional pathways and, therefore, the cytokines are released primarily through cell damage or cell death.[28] There is also evidence that IL-1 can be released in limited amounts through exocytosis.[29]

What naturally occurring injuries are likely to be encountered by the corneal epithelium during the life of an organism that would lead to the release of IL-1 and other mediators of response to injury? Certainly, corneal infection by viral organisms would be a common hazard with the potential to seriously threaten the survival of the organism. We have hypothesized that apoptosis of underlying keratocytes in response to epithelial injury functions as a defense mechanism to limit the extension of viral infections by pathogens such as herpes simplex virus that have the capacity to infect corneal epithelial and keratocyte cells.[13] Recent experiments have demonstrated that primary corneal infection with herpes simplex in rabbits stimulates apoptosis of keratocytes underlying areas of epithelial injury (Wilson SE, Hill J, Beuerman R, unpublished data). Interestingly, the smallpox and cowpox viruses direct the expression of proteins that would interfere with IL-1 alpha and IL-1 beta signaling.[30,31] It is intriguing that the latter viruses tend to produce characteristic scaring attributable to deeper extension of the infection in the skin and cornea and the herpes simplex virus, which is not known to code factors that would interfere with IL-1 signaling, tends to produce infections limited to the epithelium. Clinical observations fit nicely with this hypothesis, since primary and recurrent herpes simplex infections of the cornea are frequently limited to the epithelium.[32,33]

The presence of a system that detects injury to the epithelium and stimulates programmed cell death of the underlying keratocytes is of obvious importance to refractive surgery. In excimer laser photorefractive keratectomy (PRK) the corneal epithelium is frequently removed by mechanical debridement. Transepithelial ablation can also be utilized. It seems reasonable to suggest that the cornea may perceive this epithelial injury as massive viral infection. We hypothesize that the resulting apoptosis of the underlying epithelial cells is an initiating event in the subsequent wound healing process. Keratocytes repopulate the anterior cornea over the first few days following PRK, but these cells tend to be "activated" and present at higher density.[34,35] Activation of the keratocytes is thought to correlate with production of increased collagen and other matrix components that contribute to stromal haze and regression.[34,35] Research efforts to regulate apoptosis of the underlying keratocytes could lead to better control of the wound healing response that occurs following PRK and possibly increase the efficacy and safety of the procedure.

Laser-assisted *in situ* keratomeleusis (LASIK) is a lamellar refractive surgical procedure in which a hinged flap of corneal stroma and attached epithelium is raised with an automated microkeratome. Laser ablation is performed within the stromal bed before depositing the flap back into position. If appropriate steps are taken to protect the flap, only the peripheral corneal epithelium is injured during this procedure. Thus, based on our recent observations, we would expect the wound healing response to be decreased in the central cornea if the epithelium is preserved intact. Preliminary studies in rabbits suggest that this is the case (Helena M, Pedroza L, Wilson SE, unpublished data). However, keratocyte apoptosis is noted along the lamellar interface in the central stromal in some cases Similarly, early clinical studies suggest that there is decreased scarring and increased stability and predictability associated with LASIK compared with surface ablation.[36,37] Alterations in the epithelial-stromal response due to reduced injury to the central corneal epithelium could be an important determinant of the distinctive clinical response noted with LASIK compared to surface ablation procedures like PRK.

What other corneal functions could the epithelial-stromal communication system regulate? One of the most intriguing questions regarding normal corneal physiology, and in fact the physiology of virtually all organs of higher organisms, is what systems are in place to maintain tissue organization. In other words, what maintains the epithelium, stroma, and endothelium in their respective anatomical positions and what prevents the keratocytes, for example, from invade the epithelium or the endothelium? It seems reasonable to suggest that there are active systems in place to regulate the tissue organization of the organ. The hypothesis here is that the IL-1 and Fas systems participate in this process. IL-1 alpha and IL-1 beta, having no signal sequence for transport from the cell, are primarily released when the cell is injured. Studies have demonstrated, however, that IL-1 can be released in limited amounts through exocytosis.[29] It is hypothesized that small amounts of IL-1 alpha and beta are released from corneal epithelial and endothelial cells by exocytosis (or in the case of the epithelium through normal turnover of the epithelial cells during maturation) in the absence of injury and that these cytokines participate to maintain keratocytes within the stroma through a combination of negative chemotaxis and apoptosis. Thus, it is speculated that keratocytes are repelled by IL-1 alpha, IL-1 beta, and perhaps other factors such as soluble Fas ligand released by the epithelium and endothelium and that keratocyte cells that approach too closely to the limiting cellular layers are induced to undergo apoptosis. Even though animal knockouts for Fas, Fas ligand, and IL-1 receptor have not revealed evidence of corneal structural abnormalities, redundancy in the molecular control of essential functions commonly results in normalcy in the face of the interruption of an individual regulatory system. It will likely be necessary to generate double or even triple knockouts for such abnormalities to become manifest. Pathophysiologic observations suggestive of such interactions are commonly noted on histologic examination of recipient corneal buttons in cases of pseudophakic bullous keratopathy, corneal endothelial allograft rejection, Fuchs' dystrophy, or other diseases that destroy the corneal endothelium. Retrocorneal fibrous proliferation is frequently noted on the posterior surface of the cornea. Other investigators have suggested that the fibroblastic cells in these membranes are derived from transformed endothelial cells.[38] It seems just as likely that these cells could, in some cases, be derived from keratocytes that transverse to the posterior surface of the cornea in the absence of the inhibitory influences from the endothelium. Similarly, subepithelial pannus associated with ectopic localization of keratocytes directly beneath the epithelium is frequently noted in advanced cases of bullous keratopathy or Fuchs' dystrophy.[17,39,40] There may be complete loss of Bowman's acellular layer in some cases. It is speculated that the epithelium becomes dysfunctional as corneal edema progresses and that epithelial cell production of inhibitory cytokines such as IL-1 is diminished. Alternatively, the localization of these factors may become disordered with factors passing into the tear film rather than into the anterior corneal stroma. Further investigation is needed to characterize this hypothetical corneal tissue organizational system and to conclusively establish whether the IL-1 and Fas cytokine/receptor systems contribute to these processes. Preliminary observations elucidating the expression and functions of these systems suggest that they may indeed have key roles.

Finally, the observations reported here regarding potential functions of the IL-1 system in the cornea and prior observations of Fabre et al.[41] and Bereau et al.[42] suggest a possible role for this system in the pathogenesis of keratoconus and provide a different perspective from which to view candidate defects underlying the disease. While exploring the association between keratoconus, ectopic disease, and IL-1, these investigators noted that stromal fibroblasts from eyes with keratoconus have four-fold greater numbers of IL-1 receptors than stromal fibroblasts from normal eyes.[41,42] It is likely that there is a delicate balance between keratocyte proliferation and apoptosis within the cornea if the total numbers of cells populating the stroma is to remain nearly constant over the adult life span. A similar balance between these processes has been noted in other tissues.[43–45] The observations of Fabre,[41] Bereau,[42] and coworkers suggest that the keratocytes of keratoconus patients could have increased sensitivity to IL-1 alpha and IL-1 beta. It is hypothesized that the balance between apoptosis and proliferation in the corneal stroma could be perturbed in response to stimuli promoting the release of IL-1 from the epithelium or endothelium. This in turn could result net loss of stromal mass. If this hypothesis is correct, then the loss would likely be very slow in order to correspond with the clinical progression of the disease that is usually measured in decades. Such a slow loss of keratocytes

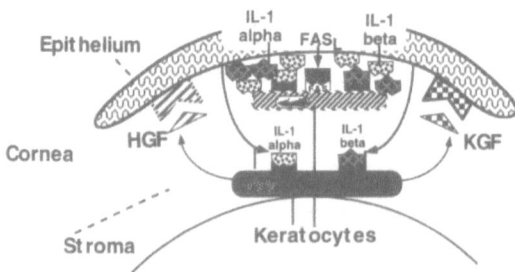

Figure 5. Schematic diagram of stromal-epithelial interactions in the cornea involving IL-1 alpha, IL-beta, Fas ligand, HGF, KGF, and the corresponding receptors after corneal epithelial wounding. Epithelial injuy results in release of IL-1 alpha and IL-1 beta from the epithelial cells and into the corneal stroma. Fas ligand may also be released as a soluble mediator by the corneal epithelium. Anterior keratocytes (diagonal lines with condensed chromatin) undergo programmed cell death that may be mediated by exposure to apoptosis-inducing epithelial-derived modulators (IL-1 and Fas ligand).[17,26] Posterior stromal keratocytes survive. Exposure to lower levels of IL-1 alpha or IL-1 beta stimulates increased production of HGF and KGF by the keratocytes. As paracrine mediators of stromal-epithelial interaction, HGF and KGF in turn facilitate epithelial healing through modulation of corneal epithelial proliferation, motility, and differentiation.[12,14]

would likely be undetectable by histopathologic analysis of diseased corneas at particular points in time. An attractive feature of this hypothesis is that it provides a unifying hypothesis for the association between keratoconus and factors such as eye rubbing, atopic disease, and rigid contact lens wear that have also been associated with keratoconus.[46–48] Each of these factors is associated with mechanical corneal epithelial cell injury or increased cell turnover, which could augment the release of mediators such as IL-1. If a shift in the equilibrium between proliferation and apoptosis of keratocytes has a role in the pathogenesis of keratoconus, then the prediction could also be made that genetic defects resulting in increased release of IL-1 from the epithelium, increased sensitivity of keratocytes to IL-1, or activation of any of the downstream effectors of keratocyte apoptosis could underlie the development of keratoconus. This is our working hypothesis regarding the pathogenesis of keratoconus. A great deal or work will be required to refute or validate this hypothesis, but a wealth of information regarding the normal physiology of the cornea is also likely to be generated from such studies.

ACKNOWLEDGMENTS

Supported by US Public Health Service grant EY10056 from the National Institutes of Health, Bethesda, Maryland and The Cleveland Clinic Foundation.

REFERENCES

1. I. Gipson, Epithelial response to injury. In *Corneal Biophysics Workshop: Proceedings Corneal Biomechanics and Wound Healing*, L.A. McNicol, and Strahlman, E., National Eye Institute, National Institutes of Health (1989).
2. T. Nakamura, Nishizawa, T., Hagiya, M., et al., Molecular cloning and expression of hepatocyte growth factor. *Nature* 342:440 (1989).
3. K. Matsumoto, Hashimoto, K., Yoshikawa, K., and Nakamura, T., Marked stimulation of growth and motility of human keratinocytes by hepatocyte growth factor. *Exp. Cell. Res.* 196:114 (1991).
4. J.S. Rubin, Chan, AM-L., Bottaro, D.P., et al. A broad-spectrum human lung fibroblast -derived mitogen is a variant of hepatocyte growth factor. *Proc. Natl. Acad. Sci.* 88:415 (1991).
5. R. Montesano, Matsumoto, K., Nakamura, T., and Orci, L., Identification of a fibroblast-derived epithelial morphogen as hepatocyte growth factor. *Cell* 67:901 (1991).
6. S.E. Wilson, Weng, J., Chwang, E., et al., Hepatocyte growth factor (HGF), keratinocyte growth factor (KGF), and their receptors in human breast cells and tissues: alternative HGF and KGF receptors. *Molecular and Cellular Biology Res.* 40:337 (1994).
7. K. Matsumoto, Hashimoto, K., Yoshikawa, K., and Nakamura, T., Marked stimulation of human keratinocytes by hepatocyte growth factor. *Exp. Cell. Res.* 196:114 (1991).
8. J.S. Rubin, Chan, AM-L., Bottaro, D.R., et al., A broad-spectrum human lung mitogen is a variant of hepatocyte growth factor. *Proc. Natl. Acad. Sci.* 88:415 (1991).
9. C. Marchese, Rubin, J., Ron, D., et al., Human keratinocyte growth factor activity on proliferation and differentiation of human keratinocytes: dDifferentiation response distinguishes KGF from EGF family. *J. Cell. Physiol.* 144:326 (1990).
10. P.W. Finch, Rubin, J.S., Miki, T., et al., Human KGF is FOF-related with properties of a paracrine effector or epithelial cell growth. *Science* 245:752 (1989).
11. K.M. Weidner, Arakaki, N., Hartmann, G., et al., Evidence for the identity of human scatter factor and human hepatocyte growth factor. *Proc. Natl. Acad. Sci.* 88:7001 (1991).
12. S.E. Wilson, Walker, J.W., Chwang, E.L., and He, Y-G., Hepatocyte growth factor (HGF), keratinocyte growth factor (KGF), their receptors, FGF receptor-2, and the cells of the cornea. *Invest. Ophthalmol. Vis. Sci.* 34:2544 (1993).
13. Q. Li, Weng, J., Bennett, G.L., et al., Hepatocyte growth factor (HGF) and HGF receptor protein in lacrimal gland, tears, and cornea. *Invest. Ophthalmol. Vis. Sci.*,37:727 (1996).

14. S.E. Wilson, He, Y-G., Weng, J., et al., Effect of epidermal growth factor, hepatocyte growth factor, and keratinocyte growth factor, on proliferation, motility, and differentiation of human corneal epithelial cells. *Exp. Eye Res.*;59:665 (1994).

14. K. Nakayasu, Stromal changes following removal of epithelium in rat cornea. *Jpn. J. Ophthalmol.* 32:113 (1988).

15. C.E. Crosson, Cellular changes following epithelial abrasion. In *Healing Processes in the Cornea*, R.W. Beuerman, Crosson, C.E., and Kaufman, H.E., eds., Gulf Publishing Co., Houston, TX (1989).

16. S.E. Wilson, He, Y-G., Weng, J., et al., Epithelial injury induces keratocyte apoptosis: Hypothesized role for the interleukin-1 system in the modulation of corneal tissue organization. *Exp. Eye Res.* 62:325 (1996).

18. S. Nagata, and Golstein, P., The Fas death factor. *Science* 267:1449 (1995).

19. J.J. Cohen, Apoptosis: physiologic cell death. *J. Lab Clin. Med.* 124:761 (1994).

20. T. Brunner, Mogil, R.J., LaFace, D., et al., Cell-autonomous Fas (CD95) Fas-ligand interaction mediates activation-induced apoptosis in T-cell hybridomas. *Nature* 373:441 (1995).

21. T.S. Griffith, Brunner, T., Fletcher, S.M., et al., Fas ligand-induced apoptosis as a mechanism of immune privilege. *Science* 270:1189 (1995).

22. M. Tanaka, Suda, T., Takahashi, T., and Nagata, S., Expression of the functional soluble form of human Fas ligand in activated lymphocytes. *EMBO J.* 14:1129 (1995).

23. R. Ni, Tomita, Y., Matsuda, K., et al., Fas-mediated apoptosis in primary cultured mouse hepatocytes. *Exp. Cell. Res.* 215:332 (1994).

24. M. Oishi, Maeda, K., and Sugiyama, S., Distribution of apoptosis-mediating Fas antigen in human skin and effects of anti-Fas monoclonal antibody on human epidermal keratinocyte and squamous cell carcinoma cell lines. *Arch. Dermatol. Res.* 286:396 (1994).

25. K. Sayama, Yonehara, S., Watanabe, Y., and Miki, Y., Expression of Fas antigen on keratinocytes *in vivo* and induction of apoptosis in cultured keratinocytes. J. Invest. Dermatol. 103:330 (1994).

26. S.E. Wilson, Li, Q., Weng, J., et al., The Fas/far ligand system and other modulators the cornea, *Investigative Ophthalmology and Visual Sciences*, in press.

27. T.S. Griffith, Brunner, T., Fletcher, S.M., et al., Fas ligand-induced mechanism of immune privilege. *Science* 270:1189 (1995).

28. C.A. Dinarello, The interleukin-1 family: 10 years of discovery. *FASEBJ* 8:1314 (1994).

29. A. Rubartelli, Cozzolino, F., Talio, M., and Sitia, R., A novel secretory pathway for interleukin-1 beta, a protein lacking a signal sequence. *EMBO J.* 9:1503 (1990).

30. R.F. Massung, Esposito, J.J., Liu, L., et al., Potential virulence determinants in terminal regions of variola smallpox virus genome. *Nature* 366:748 (1993).

31. C.A. Ray, Black, R.A., Kronheim, S.R., et al., Viral inhibition of inflamation: Cowpox virus encodes an inhibitor of the interleukin-1 beta converting enzyme. *Cell* 69:597 (1992).

32. K.R. Wilhelmus, Diagnosis and management of herpes simplex stromal keratitis. *Cornea* 6:286 (1987).

33. R.D. Stulting, Kindle, J.C., and Nahmias, A.J., Patterns of herpes simplex keratitis in inbred mice. *Invest. Ophthalmol. Vis. Sci.* 26:1360 (1985).

34. K.D. Hanna, Pouliquen, Y.M., Waring, G.O., 3rd., et al., Corneal wound healing in monkeys after repeated excimer laser photorefractive keratectomy. *Arch. Ophthalmol..* 110:1286 (1992).

35. R.A. Del Pero, Gigstad, J.E., Roberts, A.D., et al., A refractive and histopathologic study of excimer laser keratectomy in primates. *Am. J. Ophthalmol.* 109:419 (1990).

36. S. Vale, McDermott, M.L., and Taylour, F., Visual and refractive results of combined PRK and ALK in moderate to high myopia. *Invest. Ophthalmol. Vis. Sci.* 36:S579 (1995).

37. J.M. Khoury, Azar, D.T., Jain, S., and Tuli, S.W., Modified automated keratomiliusis: Sphero-refractive resection under a hinged flap. *Invest. Ophthalmol. Vis. Sci.* 36:S866 (1995).

38. E.P. Kay, Rabbit corneal endothelial cells modulated by polymorphonuclear leukocytes are fibroblasts. Comparison with keratocytes. *Invest. Ophthalmol. Vis. Sci.* 27:891 (1986).

39. G.O. Waring, Rodrigues, M.M., and Laibson, P.R., Corneal dystrophies. II. Endothelial dystrophies. *Surv. Ophthalmol.* 23:147 (1978).

40. S.E. Wilson, Bourne, W.M., Fuchs' dystrophy. *Cornea* 7:2 (1988).

41. E.J. Fabre, Bereau, J., Pouliquen, Y., and Lorans, G. Binding sites for human interleukin 1 alpha, gamma interferon and tumor necrosis factor on cultured fibroblasts of normal cornea and keratoconus. *Curr. Eye. Res.* 10:585 (1991).

42. J. Bereau, Fabrec E.D., Hecquet, C., et al., Modification of prostiglandin E2 and collagen synthesis in keratoconus fibroblasts associated with an increase of interleukin 1 alpha receptor number. *CR Acad. Sci. III.* 316:425 (1993).

43. K.A. Knox, Johnson, G.D., and Gordon, J., A study of protein kinase C isozyme distribution in relation to Bcl-2 expression during apoptosis of epithelial cells *in vivo. Exp. Cell. Res.* 207:68 (1993).

44. E. Gould, and McEwen, B.S., Neuronal birth and death. *Curr. Opin. Neurobiol.* 3:676 (1993).

45. I.D. Bowen,. Apoptosis or programmed cell death? *Cell. Biol. Intl.* 17:365 (1993).

46. J.T. Coyle, Keratoconus and eye rubbing. *Am. J. Ophthalmol.* 97:527 (1989).

47. Koreman, N.M., A clinical study of contact-lens-related keratoconus. *Am. J. Ophthalmol.* 101:390 (1986).

48. M.S. Macsai, Varley, G.A., and Krachmer, J.H., Development of keratoconus after contact lens wear. Patient characteristics. *Arch. Ophthalmol.* 108:534 (1990).

36

REGULATORY MECHANISM OF PROCOLLAGENASE SYNTHESIS BY KERATOCYTES

Hiroshi Mishima, Kosuke Abe, and Toshifumi Otori

Department of Ophthalmology
Kinki University School of Medicine
Osaka, Japan

ABSTRACT

Keratocytes play an important role in collagen metabolism in the corneal stroma. It has been reported that various cellular functions of keratocytes are regulated by extracellular matrices and cytokines. To understand the regulatory mechanism of collagenase synthesis by keratocytes, this study investigated the effects of extracellular collagen and cytokines on procollagenase synthesis by keratocytes. To perform this evaluation, subcultured human keratocytes were embedded in a type I collagen matrix. The cells were cultured for 24 hours with unsupplemented MEM. Various cytokines (IL-1β, EGF, TGF-β, PDGF) were added to the medium. The amount of procollagenase in the medium was estimated by ELISA using a monoclonal antibody against human procollagenase. Results reveal that when keratocytes were cultured in a collagen matrix, the amount of procollagenase in the medium depended on either the incubation period or the number of cells. Furthermore, the amount of enzyme increased in proportion to the concentration of extracellular collagen. The amount of enzyme in the medium also increased by the addition of heat-denatured collagen. The addition of either IL-1β, EGF, or PDGF stimulated procollagenase synthesis by the cells. On the other hand, enzyme synthesis was inhibited by the addition of TGF-β. The present results seem to indicate that procollagenase synthesis by keratocytes is regulated by extracellular collagen and various kinds of cytokines.

INTRODUCTION

Collagen is the major constituent of the corneal stroma. The normal integrity of stromal collagen fibrils is important to maintaining corneal transparency. Keratocytes are thought to contribute to collagen metabolism (i.e., collagen synthesis and degradation) in the stroma, while matrix metalloproteases (MMPs), including collagenase, are thought to

Advances in Corneal Research, edited by Lass
Plenum Press, New York, 1997

play a central role in the breakdown of the extracellular matrices of the corneal stroma. Keratocytes have been reported to produce various types of MMPs, such as MMP-1, MMP-2, MMP-3, or MMP-9.[1-4] In corneal wound healing, keratocytes were reported to synthesize both collagenase and collagen for tissue remodeling.[1,2] Collagenase was also detected in the ulcerating cornea.[5] The production of MMPs in keratocytes has been extensively investigated. However, the mechanism by which the production of MMPs in keratocytes is regulated has not been fully understood.

In vivo, cells are embedded in an extracellular matrix and recognize its constitutive macromolecules through specific membrane components such as integrins, anchorins, proteoglycans, and so forth. Multiple roles have been ascribed to these cell-matrix interactions that are involved in processes such as embryogenesis, cell adhesion, migration, differentiation, and tumor invasion.[6-8] Keratocytes *in vivo* are also surrounded by extracellular matrix proteins. However, the cellular functions of keratocytes have been investigated using cells cultured on a plastic plate. Previously, keratocytes were cultured in a type I collagen matrix, which revealed that extracellular collagen influenced various functions of keratocytes such as modifications of cell shape and mitotic activity.[9] Keratocytes in a collagen matrix connected to each other with gap junctions, which are observed between the cells *in vivo*.[10] These findings clearly indicate that keratocytes in a collagen matrix could be a model of cellular behavior *in vivo*.

The fact that growth factors and cytokines play important roles in the regulation of various cellular functions has been clarified recently. Among these agents, interleukin 1 (IL-1), epidermal growth factor (EGF), transforming growth factor β (TGF-β), and platelet-derived growth factor (PDGF) were reported to regulate the collagen metabolism of fibroblasts.[11-18] However, these experiments were performed using cells cultured on plastic plates and their cellular response to these cytokines in a collagen matrix remains unclear.

In the present study, keratocytes were cultured in a collagen matrix and the activity of the procollagenase synthesis estimated in order to understand the effect of extracellular collagen on procollagenase synthesis by keratocytes. In addition, the effects of IL-1, EGF, TGF-β, or PDGF on procollagenase synthesis by keratocytes cultured in a collagen matrix were investigated.

MATERIALS AND METHODS

Materials

Human keratocytes were the kind gift from Dr. Scheffer C.G. Tseng (Bascom Palmer Eye Institute; Miami, FL, USA). Eagle's minimum essential medium MEM was purchased from the Research Foundation for Microbial Diseases of Osaka University (Suita, Osaka, Japan). A porcine type I collagen solution (3 mg/ml in HCl, pH 3.0) was obtained from Nitta Gelatin Co. (Yao, Osaka, Japan). Human epidermal growth factor (EGF) and transforming growth factor β (TGF-β) were purchased from Earth Pharmaceutical Co. (Akoh, Hyogo, Japan); platelet-derived growth factor-BB (PDGF) was from Signa (St. Louis, MO, USA); cycloheximide was from Nakarai Tesque (Kyoto, Japan); human recombinant IL-1β was the kind gift of Otsuka Pharmaceutical Co. (Osaka, Japan); antihuman procollagenase monoclonal antibodies (4H11, 5d1G10) and procollagenase purified from human fibrosarcoma cells (HT1080) were the kind gifts of Kanebo Co. (Osaka, Japan).

Cell Culture in a Collagen Gel

Human keratocytes were cultured and passed in MEM containing 10% fetal calf serum (FCS) as described previously.[9] In all experiments, keratocytes were cultured within six passages. Cultivation of keratocytes in a collagen matrix was performed as previously described[9] with some modifications. A type I collagen solution was mixed with a 10-fold concentration of MEM and neutralized with 0.2N NaOH. Suspensions of keratocytes were added and the collagen solution was plated in a 24-multiwell plate (300 μl/well) and incubated at 37°C for 1 hour to form a gel. Three hundred microliters of MEM was placed over the gel, and the cells were cultivated for another 24 hours. Then the culture medium was collected and centrifuged to eliminate cell debris. The number of cells, the length of cultivation time, or the collagen concentration was varied in certain experiments. In later experiments in this series, EGF(100 ng/ml), IL-1β, TGF-β, or PDGF (each at 10 ng/ml) was added.

Procollagenase Synthesis by Keratocytes

The procollagenase synthesis by keratocytes was estimated by measuring the amount of the enzyme in the culture medium by ELISA. The monoclonal antibody that recognized the active site of procollagenase (4H11, 100 μl/well) was immobilized on micro plate wells by incubating overnight at 4°C. After washing three times with 0.05% tween 20 in PBS, the plates were incubated with the conditioned medium (100 μl/well) for 1 hour at room temperature. Then the plates were washed and incubated with biotin-conjugated monoclonal antibody (5D1G10, 100 μl/well) which recognized N-amino terminus of procollagenase. After washing, the plates were further incubated with 1 mg/ml of horseradish peroxidase-conjugated streptavidin in sodium bicarbonate (0.05M, pH 8.3) for 1 hour at room temperature. Then, the plates were incubated with 0.4 mg/ml of o-phenylenediamine dichloride and 0.1% H_2O_2 in citrate phosphate buffer (0.15M, pH 5.0) for 15 minutes. The enzyme reaction was terminated by the addition of 100 ml of 2N sulfuric acid and the amount of procollagenase was assayed by a colorimetric method using a microplate reader (NP-500; Kurabo; Tokyo, Japan) at 490 nm. Purified procollagenase from human fibrosarcoma cells (HT1080) was used as a standard.

Statistics

Data were shown as mean ± SEM of triplicate measurements. Statistical significance was determined by Student's t test.

RESULTS

Various numbers of keratocytes (1×10^3 to 3×10^4 cells) were placed on a plastic plate or embedded in a collagen matrix. After 24 hours of cultivation, the procollagenase concentration in the medium was measured (Fig. 1). The enzyme concentration increased in proportion to the number of cells cultured both on a plastic plate and in a collagen matrix. However, the enzyme concentration in the medium of keratocytes cultured in a collagen matrix was higher than that of the cells cultured on a plastic plate. When cycloheximide was added to the medium at the concentration of 10 μg/ml, procollagenase was not detected in the medium under any of the cultivating conditions. The effect of cul-

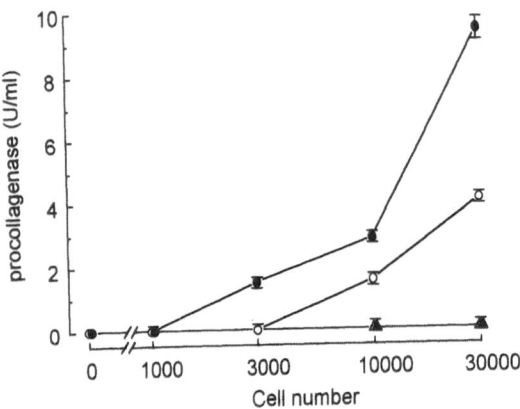

Figure 1. The procollagenase synthesis by keratocytes. Various numbers of cells were cultured on a plastic plate (open circle) or in a collagen matrix (closed circle) for 24 hours. Procollagenase concentration in the medium was measured by ELISA. Cycloheximide (10 μg/ml) was added to the medium (open triangle: on a plasltic plate; closed triangle: on a collagen gel).

tivation periods on the procollagenase synthesis by keratocytes was investigated. The cells (1 x 10^4 cells) were cultured on a plastic plate or in a collagen matrix for indicated periods (Fig. 2). After 9 hours of cultivation both on a plastic plate and in a collagen matrix, the procollagenase concentration in the medium increased in proportion to the cultivation periods. Furthermore, at 16, 24, and 48 hours of cultivation, the enzyme concentration of the cells cultured in a collagen matrix was higher than that on a plastic plate. These findings indicated that keratocytes cultured both on a plastic plate and in a collagen gel synthesized procollagenase. It was also suggested that the cells in a collagen matrix synthesized much more enzyme than those on a plastic plate. Then the dose effect of extracellular collagen on procollagenase synthesis by keratocytes was investigated. The cells were cultured in various concentrations of collagen matrices for 24 hours and the enzyme concentration in the medium was measured (Fig. 3). Zero mg/ml of collagen indicated the amounts of procollagenase from the cells cultured on a plastic plate. The amount of procollagenase in the medium increased in proportion to the concentration of collagen. At the concentration of 2.2 mg/ml of collagen, the amount of the enzyme in the medium was about 3 times grater than that of the control (0 mg/ml of collagen). These findings indicated that extracellular collagen stimulated procollagenase synthesis by keratocytes.

Next the study investigated whether or not denatured collagen also stimulated the procollagenase synthesis as well as native collagen. For this, native collagen was denatured by heating at 60°C for 15 minutes and the solution was neutralized and diluted with the MEM. Keratocytes were cultured on plastic plates and various concentrations of dena-

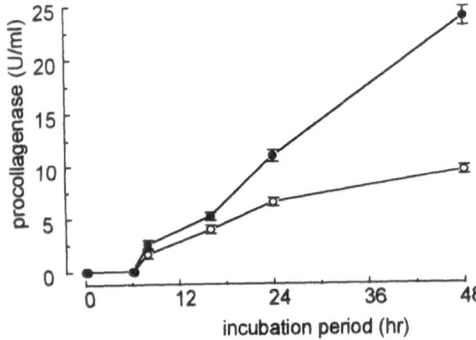

Figure 2. The effect of incubation on procollagenase synthesis by keratocytes. Keratocytes (1 x 10^4 cells) were cultured on a plastic plate (open circle) or in a collagen matrix (closed circle) for up to 48 hours. At 6, 9, 12, 24, and 48 hours of cultivation, the medium was collected and the enzyme concentration was measured.

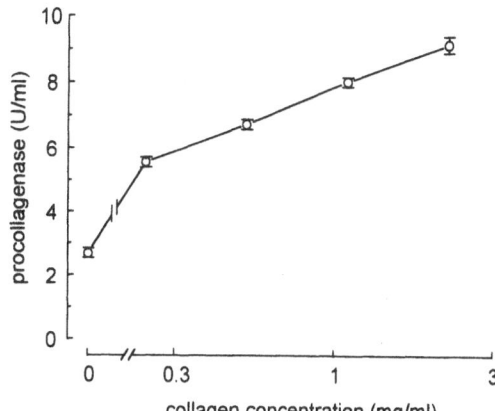

Figure 3. Effect of collagen on procollagenase synthesis by keratocytes. Keratocytes (1×10^4 cells) were embedded in various concentrations of collagen matrices and were cultured for 24 hours. The enzyme concentration was measured.

tured collagen were added to the medium. After 24 hours of cultivation, the enzyme concentration in the medium was increased by the addition of denatured collagen in a dose-dependent manner (Fig. 4).

Also investigated were the effects of IL-1β, EGF, PDGF, or TGF-β on procollagenase synthesis by keratocytes cultured in a collagen marix (Fig. 5). Either of EGF (100 ng/ml), IL-1β (10 ng/ml), PDGF (10 ng/ml), or TGF-β (10 ng/ml was added to the medium and cultivation was carried out for 24 hours. The addition of either IL-1β, PDGF, or EGF increased the enzyme concentration in the medium as much as 1.5-fold over the control. These increases were statistically significant ($p < 0.01$). On the other hand, the additional of TGF-β significantly decreased the enzyme concentration by 25% ($p < 0.01$).

DISCUSSION

In the present study, it was found that extracellular collagen stimulated procollagenase synthesis by keratocytes. Denatured collagen also stimulated the enzyme synthesis by the cells. Furthermore, the procollagenase synthesis by keratocytes in a collagen gel was modulated by various types of growth factors and cytokines. These findings seem to suggest that procollagenase synthesis by keratocytes *in vivo* might be regulated by both extracellular collagen and cytokines.

Matrix metalloproteases (MMPs) are the family of enzymes that mainly contribute to the degradation of the extracellular matrix. The production of MMPs by keratocytes has

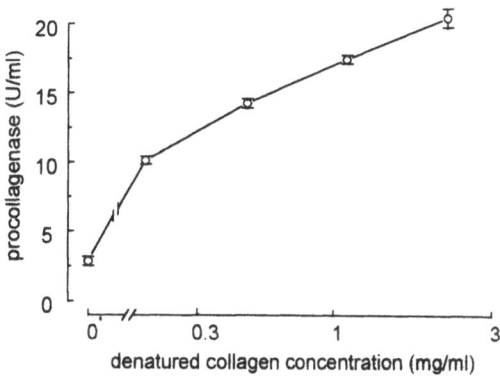

Figure 4. The effect of denatured collagen on procollagenase synthesis by keratocytes. Keratocytes (1×10^4 cells) were cultured on a plastic plate and various concentrations of denatured collagen were added. After 24 hours of cultivation, the procollagenase concentration int he medium was measured.

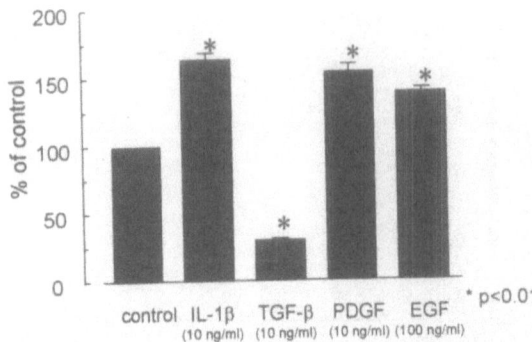

Figure 5. Effects of cytokines on procollagenase synthesis by keratocytes. Keratocytes (1×10^4 cells) were cultured in a Collagen matrix. Either of EGF (100 ng/ml), IL-1β (10 ng/ml), PDGF (10 ng/ml), or TGF-β (10 ng/ml) was added to the medium and cultivation was carried out for 24 hours.

been extensively investigated both *in vitro* and *in vivo*. It has been reported that keratocytes produce collagenase (MMP-1) geratinase (MMP-2, MMP-9) stromelysin (MMP-3). The present results confirmed the results described in the previous reports.[2-4] However, in the previous *in vitro* studies, keratocytes were cultured on plastic plates. The present study compares the enzyme synthesis by cells cultured in a collagen matrix with that by cells on a plastic plate and found that procollagenase synthesis by keratocytes was stimulated by cultivating them in a collagen matrix. It has recently been proposed that the extracellular matrix contributes to the regulation of various cellular functions, such as attachment, migration, mitosis, or protein synthesis. It has previously been reported that extracellular collagen changed the shape of keratocytes and inhibited their mitotic activity.[9] In the present study, extracellular collagen stimulated the procollagenase synthesis by keratocytes. Furthermore, the addition of denatured collagen also stimulated the enzyme synthesis by cells. Stimulatory effects of collagen on the collagenase synthesis by other types of cells has also been reported.[19-22] Biswas et al.[15] also reported that both native and denatured forms of collagen stimulated enzyme production. The mechanism of the stimulatory effect of collagen on collagenase synthesis by cells has not been fully understood. Integrins, a group of extracellular matrix receptors, are thought to play an important role in the interaction between the extracellular matrix and the cells.[23] Werb et al.[24] found that collagenase expression depended on the capacity to cross-link and cluster α5β1 receptors on the cell surface of synovial fibroblasts. Larjava et al.[25] reported that antibodies against β1 and 1α integrin subunits were found to stimulated expression of the 92 kDa type IV collagenase in keratinocytes. Schiro et al.[26] reported that integrin α2β1 was involved in the interaction between collagen and the cell and it mediated the contraction of collagen matrices. These findings may suggest that extracellular collagen stimulate procollagenase synthesis by keratocytes via cell surface integrins.

In contrast to the idea that cell-matrix interactions modulate the collagenase production by the cells, enzyme expression may be regulated by cytokines and growth factors. The present results showed that either EGF, IL-1, or PDGF stimulated procollagenase synthesis by keratocytes and TGF-b inhibited the enzyme synthesis. Upregulation of collagenase gene expression by fibroblasts was reported to be mediated by various inflammatory agents, including IL-1, TNF-α, and PDGF.[13,14,16-18,23] In human fibroblasts, EGF also induces expression of collagenase.[12] TGF-β was reported to downregulate collagenase gene expression in human synovial cells.[15] These findings suggested that the response of keratocytes in a collagen matrix to these cytokines might be similar to those of fibroblasts on plastic plates.

ACKNOWLEDGMENTS

We thank Dr. Scheffer C.G. Tseng (Bascom Palmer Eye Institute; Miami, FL, U.S.A.) for the gift of human keratocytes; Dr. Yukihisa Wada (Kanebo Co.; Osaka, Japan) for anti-human procollagenase antibodies and procollagenase; and Otsuka Pharmaceutical Co (Osaka, Japan) for human recombinant IL-1β. This work was supported in part by a grant-in-aid from the Department of Education, culture and Science of Japan and by a grant from the Osaka Eye Bank; Osaka, Japan.

REFERENCES

1. J. Sakai, Hung, J., Zhu G., et al., Collagen metabolism during healing of lacerated rabbit cornea. *Exp. Eye Res.* 52:237 (1991).
2. M.T. Girard, Matsubara M, Kublin, C., et al., Stromal fibroblasts synthesize collagenase and stromelysin during long-term tissue remodeling. *J. Cell Sci.* 104:1001 91993).
3. M.B. Berman, Regulation of corneal fibroblast MMP-1 collagenase secretion by plasmin. *Cornea* 12:420 (1993).
4. M.E. Fini, Yue, B.Y.J.T., and Suger, J., Collagenolytic-gelatinolytic metalloproteinases in normal and keratoconus cornea. *Curr. Eye Res.* 11:849 (1992).
5. M. Berman, Leary, R., and Gage, J., Latent collagenase in the ulcerating rabbit cornea. *Exp. Eye Res.* 25:435 (1977).
6. E.D. Hay, Extracellular matrix, cell skeletons, and embryonic development. *Am. J. Med Genet.* 34;14 (1989).
7. N.J. Bissell, and Barcellos-Hoff, M.H., The influence of extracellular matrix on gene expression: is structure the massage? *J. Cell Sci.* S8:327 (1987).
8. L.A. Liotta, Tumor invasion and metastasis - role of extracellular matrix. *Cancer Res.* 46:1 (1986).
9. T. Nishida, Ueda, A., Fukuda, M., et al., Interaction of extracellular collagen and corneal fibroblasts: morphologic and biological changes or rabbit corneal cells cultured in a collagen matrix. *In Vitro Cell Dev. Biol.* 24:1009 (1988).
10. A. Ueda, Nishida, T., Otori, T., and Fujita, H., Electron microscopic studies on the presence of gap junction between corneal fibroblasts in rabbits. *Cell Tissue Res.* 249:473 (1987).
11. C.C. Chua, Geiman, D.E., Keller, G.H., and Ladda, R.L., Induction of collagenase secretion in human fibroblast cultures by growth promoting factors. *J. Biol. Chem.* 26:5213 (1985).
12. A.C. Colige, Lambert, C.A., Nusgens, B.V., and Lapieré, C.M., Effect of cell-cell and cell-matrix interactions on the response of fibroblasts to epidermal growth factor in vitro; expression of collagen type I, collagenase, stromelysin, and tissue inhibitor of metalloproteinases. *Biochem. J.* 285:215 (1992).
13. A. Circolo, Welgus, H.G., Pierce, G.F., et al., Differential regulation of the expression of proteases/anteproteinases in fibroblasts. Effects of interleukin 1 and platelet-derived growth factor. *J. Biol. Chem* 266:12283–8.
14. E.M. Tan, Qin, H., Kennedy, S.H., et al., Platelet derived growth factors-AA and -BB regulate collagen and collagenase gene expression differentially in human fibroblasts. *Biochem. J.* 310:585, 1995.
15. D.R. Edwards, Murphy, G., Reynolds, J.J., et al., Transforming growth factor modulates the expression of collagenase and metalloproteinase inhibitor. *EMBO J.* 6:1899 (1987).
16. J.M. Dayer, de Rochemontiex, B., Burrus, B., et al., Human recombinant interleukin 1 stimulates collagenase and prostaglandin E2 production by human synovial cells. *J. Clin Invest.* 77:658 (1986).
17. M. Gowen, Wood, D.D., Ihrie, E.J., et al., Stimulation by human interleukin 1 of cartilage breakdown and production of collagenase and proteoglycanase by human chondrocytes but not human osteoblasts in vitro. *Biochem. Biophys. Acta* 797;186 (1984).
18. J.A. West-Mays, Strissel, K.J., Sadow, P.M., and Fini, M.E., Competence for collagenase gene expression by tissue fibroblasts requires activation of an interleukin 1 alpha autocrine loop. *Proc. Natl. Acad. Sci. USA* 92:6768 (1995).
19. C. Biswas, and Dayer, J.M., Stimulation of collagenase production by collagen in mammalian cell cultures. *Cell* 18:1035 (1979).
20. C. Mauch, Adelmann-Grill, B., Hatamochi, A., and Krieg T., Collagenase gene expression in fibroblasts is regulated by a three-dimensional contact with collagen. *FEBS Lett.* 250:301 (1989).

21. U. Saarialho-Kere, Kovacs, S., Pentland, A.P., et al., Cell-matrix interactions modulate interstitial collagenase expression by human keratinocytes actively involved in wound healing. *J. Clin. Invest.* 92:2858 (1993).
22. C.A. Lambert, Soudant, E.P., Nusgens, B.F., and Lapiére, C.M. Pretranslational regulation of extracellular matrix macromolecules and collagenase expression in fibroblasts by mechanical forces. *Lab. Invest.* 66:444 (1992).
23. R.O. Hynes, Integrins: versatility, modulation, and signaling in cell adhesion. *Cell* 69:11 (1992).
24. Z. Werb, Tremble, P.M., Benrendsten, E., et al., Signal transduction through the fibronectin receptor induces collagenase and stromelysin gene expression. *J. Cell Biol.* 109:877 (1989).
25. H. Larjava, Lyons, J.G., Salo, T., et al., Anti-integrin antibodies induce type IV collagenase expression in keratinocytes. *J. Cell Physiol.* 157:190 (1993).
26. J.A. Schiro, Chan, B.M., Roswit, W.T., et al., Integrin $\alpha 2\beta 1$ (VLA-2) mediates recognization and contraction of collagen matrices by human cells. *Cell* 67:403 (1991).
27. M.E. Fini, Strissel, K.J., Girard, M.T., et al., Interleukin 1α mediates collagenase synthesis simulated by phorbol 12-myristate 13-acetate. *J. Biol. Chem.* 265:11291 (1994).

37

MOLECULAR MECHANISMS CONTROLLING THE GENE EXPRESSION PROGRAM FOR CORNEAL REPAIR

M. Elizabeth Fini, Jeffery R. Cook, William B. Rinehart, Peter M. Sadow,
Katherine J. Strissel, and Judith A. West-Mays

Developmental Biology Laboratory
Vision Research Laboratories
New England Medical Center
Tufts University School of Medicine
Boston, Massachusetts

ABSTRACT

The wound healing response following surgical injury to the cornea can be quite variable and difficult to predict. The goal of this paper is to elucidate basic mechanisms which control activation of the corneal stromal cell to the repair phenotype and its subsequent competence to mediate repair tissue remodeling. These studies focused on expression of the matrix metalloproteinase, collagenase. The experiments performed in this study lead to the proposal of a new paradigm for understanding the modulation of repair gene expression by the wound environment, that is, regulation through autocrine cytokine intermediates. This model suggests a novel point at which drug intervention can be used to alter the repair process.

MOLECULAR MECHANISMS

Cornea Is Resistant to Repair

The recent increase in the use of surgical procedures to correct vision has resulted in renewed interest in investigation into basic mechanisms of wound healing in the corneal stroma. This has occurred because it has become increasingly clear that the nature of the wound healing response following surgical injury to the cornea can be quite variable and difficult to predict. Repair in any organ is a fibrotic response to injury, and results in deposition of an unspecialized repair tissue which acts much like a spot weld.[1] The ability of an animal to deposit repair tissue rapidly can preserve its life. However, deposition of repair tissue is quite different from regeneration, and does not restore the functions of the damaged tissue. This is especially apparent in corneal stroma, a tissue with a highly organized structure essential to the passage of light.[2-4] Probably as a means of preserving this structure, the corneal stroma is an extremely static tissue which undergoes normal self-renewal at a rate that is much slower than that of other organs.[5] Even after some types of injury, such as that resulting from radial keratotomy, stromal fibroblasts typically remain quiescent (at least in the human) and the stromal incision becomes filled with epithelium originating from the wound edge.[6,7] Unfortunately, this form of healing is mechanically weak and leaves the repaired area vulnerable to further injury. On the other hand, when stromal cells are activated to proliferate, as often occurs after laser surgery in humans[6,7] or penetrating keratectomy in rabbits,[8] they deposit a disorganized repair tissue which interferes with vision. This repair tissue is remodeled progressively over time, a process that imparts increased strength. Interestingly, in some experimental animal models, such as the young rabbit, remodeling also leads to an improvement in clarity (B), and thus might be considered a form of functional regeneration. Clinical observation suggests that such remodeling can occur in humans as well, although controlled experiments are generally lacking.

What determines the variable nature of the wound healing and remodeling response in cornea, and how can it be controlled? It would seem that answers to these questions could make possible a more successful outcome following corneal corrective surgeries. In the following, we review some findings from our own lab and others which have given us insight into this problem.

Initiation of the Gene Expression Program for Corneal Repair

As in other organs, injury to cornea initiates an overlapping sequence of cellular processes that enables rapid repair of the injured structure.[9] A very early event is the attraction of inflammatory cells into the damaged area, a process that begins within hours after injury. Inflammatory cells, including macrophages and neutrophils, release proteolytic enzymes reactive against extracellular matrix molecules, and macrophages can also phagocytose tissue debris. These functions, when kept under control help to debride the damaged tissue in an acute wound. Excessive inflammation, however, can create chronic wound-healing situations.[10-12] In organs with an epithelial component, such as cornea[13] or skin,[9] epithelial resurfacing of the damaged area also begins very rapidly after injury. In cornea, this occurs first by epibolic spreading of cells from the stratified corneal epithelium located adjacent to the injured area onto the wound bed. These cells form a one or two cell layer over the injured surface. Central corneal wounds in rats and rabbits are completely resurfaced within 24–48 hours after injury through this process. Proliferation of epithelial cells occurs later, leading to a return of normal stratification to the repair epithelium. The corneal repair epithelium deposits a new basement membrane beneath itself, probably in collaboration with cells located in the stroma.[14-18] Laminin-5 is deposited beneath the cells as they migrate and laminin- I and type VII collagen are deposited shortly thereafter.[19] However, the assembly and remodeling of the basement membrane necessary for strong adhesion between epithelium and stroma takes much longer.[18,20] Synthesis of enzymes with the capacity to degrade components of the basement membrane, as well as the stromal matrix, is also induced in the repair epithelium. These include plasminogen activators[21] and matrix metalloproteinases (MMPs),[19,22-25] in healing corneal epithelium of rabbits, rats, and humans, gelatinase B (MMP-9) is the prominent MMP. This enzyme is reactive against basement membrane collagens and its expression occurs in the migrating epithelial tip. In the healing epidermis of skin.[26]

MMP-I is also synthesized at this location, but this enzyme has not been detected in the epithelium of rabbit corneal wounds.[24] Collagenase has, however, been detected in the epithelium of human corneas with repair defects, although not at the migrating tip.[19] Finally, collagenase mRNA has been detected in organ-cultured rabbit corneas treated with Platelet Activating Factor.[27] It has been suggested that the induced epithelial enzymes can participate in debridement, epithelial cell migration, and remodeling of the newly-deposited epithelial basement membrane. However, their exact role in repair is not known since current data are only correlative.

While the epithelium is resurfacing the wound bed, the process of repair in the stroma is also beginning with activation of stromal cells (keratocytes) at the wound edge. In a rat model, the region of activation was described as occupying a narrow border a few hundred microns wide on either side of the damaged area.[28] Initiation of the activation process is detectable at 6 hours after injury as an increase in the number and size of nucleoli per cell, and an increase in cell size. Within 24 hours, 75–80% of the corneal stromal cells originally present at the wound edge are activated. These cells acquire a more fibroblastic shape, migrate into the area of damage, and proliferate; after a few weeks there are many more cells per unit area in repair tissue than in the normal stroma. Similar observations have been made in studies on the rabbit model.[8,29–31] Most recently, Jester and coworkers described the reorganization of the actin cytoskeleton that contributes to the fibroblastic shape.[32] As stromal cells became activated, it was found that cortical actin bundles were lost and stress fibers appeared. The molecular organization of these stress fibers was like that found in subcultured cells. A similar cytoskeletal organization is seen in the fibroblasts of skin repair tissue.[33]

Activation of the stromal cell to the repair fibroblast phenotype involves an upregulation in protein synthesis as evidenced by incorporation of radioactively-labeled macromolecular precursors.[34] Recent studies have revealed that repair fibroblasts synthesize several new proteins that contribute to the fibroblastic phenotype (Table 1). One of these, documented in the cat model by Jester and co-workers, is the α5 integrin subunit.[35] Induced expression of α5 integrin in repair fibroblasts makes possible heterodimerization with the β1 subunit, which is synthesized by both uninjured and injured stromal cells. These observations agree with findings of Masur and colleagues in studies on the integrins made by freshly-isolated and subcultured stromal fibroblasts of rabbit.[36] The α5β1 integrin heterodimer acts as the cell surface receptor for fibronectin. Acquisition of this receptor may, therefore, be key to the reorganization of the actin cytoskeleton that occurs with stromal cell activation, by allowing the formation of focal adhesions to fibronectin. Its

Table 1. New proteins synthesized by repair fibroblasts

Integrin α5
    makes possible formation of the α5β1 heterodimer in cell culture, this enables
        cells to attach to and spread on fibronection
    hypothesized to contribute to wound contraction

Smooth muscle actin
    found in smooth muscle cells such as those in uterus
    hypothesized to give repair fibroblasts contractile properties

The matrix metalloproteinases, collagenase, and stromelysin
    cleave native collagen I (collagenase) and other ECM molecules (stromelysin)
    hypothesized to mediate long term remodelling of repair tissue

---

role in the wound may be to contribute to the capacity of the fibroblast to migrate and to organize the fibronectin fibrils. Another new protein that is expressed in the repair fibroblast is smooth muscle actin.[37] In skin wounds, it has been suggested that this protein imparts contractile properties to the cell, and the timing and location of its synthesis in cornea correlates with wound contraction.[35]

Much of the synthetic activity of the repair fibroblast is involved with the production of extracellular matrix (ECM);[38] this helps fill in tissue ablated by injury and joins the wound edges. The ECM synthesized by repair fibroblasts has a rather different composition from that synthesized sized by stromal cells of the normal, uninjured stroma. The lamellae of normal stroma are composed of type l and type V collagen; these two molecules associate into heterotypic fibrils of uniquely narrow diameter, and this is thought to be important for corneal transparency.[4] In young rabbits, about 11% of the total collagen in uninjured corneal stroma is type V. This increases to about l6% in repair tissue.[39] Of the proteoglycans that form the ground substance of the normal corneal stroma, the two primary types are the cornea-specific molecule, lumican (keratan sulfate proteoglycan), and a molecule that is also found in sclera arid skin, decorin (dermatan sulfate proteoglycan). Maintenance of the appropriate ratio (3:2) between lumican and decorin is thought to be important for determining the precise degree of corneal hydration needed for tissue transparency.[40,41] In stromal repair tissue, decorin is a much more prominent component of the ECNIM than lumican.[42] Fibronectin is only a minor component of the normal corneal stroma, though it is a major component of the repair tissue.[32] Following injury, fibronectin is deposited from the tear film[16] but much is also synthesized by the repair fibroblast.[32] Similarly, tenascin is found in the repair tissue, but not in normal stroma.[43] It is likely that these changes in the ECM proteins synthesized and deposited by the stromal fibroblasts, which synthesize the repair tissue, contribute to its opacity.

In addition to depositing ECM, repair fibroblasts also turn on new synthesis of enzymes that can degrade ECM. Prominent among these are the MMPs. Collagenase (MMP-l) and stromelysin (MMP-3) are not synthesized by stromal cells in the uninjured cornea, but their synthesis is upregulated in the repair fibroblast.[25] Synthesis of the only MMP found in the uninjured cornea, gelatinase A (MMP-2), is also upregulated[22] during repair. Collagenase is reactive specifically against the native type I collagen triple helix, and stromelysin can degrade a broad range of matrix components, including proteoglycans.[25] Gelatinase A also has a broad reactivity, but is especially active against denatured collagen molecules. These proteinases may participate in debridement of damaged extracellular matrix components. However, their more important function is probably to help mediate the remodeling of newly-deposited repair tissue which occurs by progressive degradation and resynthesis.[44] In young rabbits, this remodeling results in a clearing of the repair tissue to transparency and thus a functional regeneration.[8] This suggests a very important function for MMPs in the stromal repair tissue; however, as for the epithelial MMPs, the evidence that they participate in this function remains correlative.

In organs such as skin, factors released by blood platelets or macrophages are thought to provide important activating cytokines such as PDGF.[1] However, cornea lacks a blood supply or resident phagocytic cells, which may be a major reason for the resistance of the cornea to repair, but then what does initiate this process in cases where it occurs? Evidence suggests that an epithelial mesenchymal interaction controls fibroblast activation. Thus, the repair fibroblasts that migrate into the injured area from the wound edge accumulate beneath the wound epithelium,[45] making it appear as though they were attracted by this tissue. New extracellular matrix of the repair tissue is first laid down by these cells; progressive healing toward the back of the cornea follows. Experiments in rats have shown that if epithelium is removed daily after corneal injury, stromal cells at the wound edge do not undergo morphological activation.[28] Furthermore, ^{35}S-Sulfate labeling of the stromal cells at the wound edge does not occur in the absence of the epithelium,[34] demonstrating a lack of synthetic activity. Stromal cell activation will occur, however, if the epithelium is allowed to grow back.[28] These findings have suggested that the repair epithelium which resurfaces the wound bed produces substances that control fibroblast activation, thus initiating the program for repair gene expression.

What is the molecular nature of the substances controlling fibroblast activation? To identify activating substances, this study focuses on collagenase. Expression of collagenase seemed like an excellent marker for stromal cell activation, since the gene is completely silent in the uninjured tissue, but is expressed in repair fibroblasts within 24 hours of injury. In work performed a number of years ago, Johnson-Wint, Gross, and colleagues used a corneal cell co-culture model to search for substances produced by epithelial cells that affect the capacity of stromal cells to produce collagenase, as measured by an enzymatic assay.[46–48] They demonstrated that substances, which could either stimulate or inhibit the elaboration of latent collagenolytic activity by stromal cells freshly isolated from the cornea, were released simultaneously by epithelial cells.[46–49] Follow-up on this study by measuring collagenase synthesis directly[50] revealed that stromal cells freshly isolated into culture do not synthesize collagenase, but that culture medium conditioned by corneal epithelial cells contained factors that could not only stimulate collagenase synthesis, but could also inhibit collagenase synthesis stimulated by treating stromal cells with the inflammatory cytokine, interleukin-1 (IL-1).

Collagenase expression in cultured fibroblasts derived from a variety of sources is known to be stimulated by a broad range of different cytokines.[51] Corneal epithelial cells produce mRNA or protein for a number of these. In an attempt to identify the key collagenase-regulating cytokines produced by epithelial cells, conditioned medium was treated with agents that would interfere with the activity of specific candidate cytokines. The effects of these treatments were then assayed by examining the capacity of the medium to control collagenase synthesis. Using this approach, the major stimulator was identified as an IL-1 isoform, IL-1α,[52] and the major inhibitor of IL-1-stimulated collagenase synthesis as the TGF-β isoform, TGF-β_2.[53]

IL-1α[54] and TGF-β[55] are well-characterized cytokines known to influence many other cell functions besides the stimulation of collagenase gene activation. Their actions often appear to be opposite; IL-1 has been generally associated with inflammatory and degradative functions, while TGF-β stimulates activities such as deposition of extracellular matrix. Thus, it seems possible that these two cytokines could control the diverse activities connected with stromal cell activation. This hypothesis remains to be tested *in vivo*. Nevertheless, anything that controls the balance of activity between IL-1α and TGF-β should have far reaching effects on corneal repair. Both IL-1α and TGF-β genes are expressed by the corneal epithelium *in situ*, in the intact, uninjured state. What factors would regulate the balance of IL-1α and TGF-β produced by the corneal epithelium under wound healing conditions? To address this question, this study returned to the early work of Johnson-Wint, Gross and colleagues. They showed that expression of net stimulatory activity for collagenase synthesis bears an interesting relationship to the density at which epithelial cells are plated in culture.[46] Co-culture of freshly-isolated corneal stromal cells with low numbers of corneal epithelial cells was more stimulatory than co-culture with high numbers. To determine the molecular basis for this observation, IL-1α release by epithelial cells plated at increasing density was measured.[52] It was found that the total amount of IL-1α released by corneal epithelial cells in culture, on a per cell basis, was considerably higher at low cell densities than at high cell densities. This effect on IL-1α release did not appear to be primarily a result of an overall increase in the amount of IL-1α synthesized, since cell density had a much smaller effect on the amount of IL-1α that was cell-associated. In contrast, the release of inhibitory activity for IL-1-stimulated collagenase synthesis was not affected by cell density. These results indicate that changes in the degree of cell to cell contact can control the release of IL-1α and that this is responsible for shifting the balance of stimulatory and inhibitory cytokines toward net stimulatory activity for collagenase synthesis.

The selective effect of cell density on expression of IL-1α seems important because the reduced contact between cells of a low density culture could mimic the situation at the edge of a healing wound epithelium. Thus, the molecular mechanisms controlling cell contact modulation of IL-1α release will be important to elucidate. One hypothesis is that caderine, the molecules that mediate adhesion between epithelial cells, might be involved in transmitting the signal. Since total collagenase inhibitory activity (controlled by TGF-β) was not affected by cell density, cell contact must be selective for release of only certain cytokines. However, it is important to consider potential regulatory mechanisms for TGF-β activity that might be controlled by other factors besides cell density. Unlike IL-1α, TGF-β is released from cells as a latent cytokine which must be converted to an activated form in the extracellular space. The primary cell culture model revealed that much of the TGF-β released into the culture medium was in the active form.[53] Would this be true in the cornea, as well, or would activation of TGF-β be as important a regulatory step as release? Such interesting questions remain to be answered.

Modulation of Repair Gene Expression

New gene expression by repair fibroblasts is not simply an on or off phenomena, but instead proceeds according to precise temporal and spatial patterns which differ for each gene. For example, expression of α-smooth muscle actin precisely parallels the temporal invasion of the wound area by stromal fibroblasts, but expression continues in each cell for only a few weeks correlating with the process of wound contraction.[37] In contrast, the amount of gelatinase A proenzyme within the repair tissue, which forms following penetrating injury to the rabbit cornea, increases over the first week after wounding in parallel with fibroblast invasion.[22] It then remains constantly elevated at three-fold above normal levels over an eight week time course. Eventually, expression gradually declines, though it is still elevated at nine months after injury, correlating with the process of repair tissue remodeling. These results suggest that different repair genes are subject to independent regulatory factors. Interestingly, in both the examples cited, the changes are remarkably localized within the wound boundaries,[22] suggesting that modulation of the gene expression program for repair is controlled by some aspect of the wound environment rather than simply by a defeasible factor from the epithelium

What aspects of the wound environment might control repair gene expression? To approach this question, attention was again focused on factors which might regulate the collagenase gene. Early passage subcultured fibroblasts derived from a variety of tissues have been used to study mechanisms regulating collagenase expression.[51,56] In these cells, synthesis of MMPs can be stimulated by a large variety of different agents and conditions that would likely be found in damaged tissues (Table 2). Major groups of stimulators that have already been considered are the inflammatory cytokines and growth factors such as IL-1 , TGF or PDGF. Another potentially relevant group of stimulators includes conditions or agents which seem to have in common the capacity to cause reorganization of the actin

Table 2. Some stimulators of collagenase synthesis

Inflammatory cytokines and growth factors
  TNF-alpha
  IL-1
  PDGF
  EGF

Agents that affect cell shape and actin polymerization
  cytochalasin B
  trypsin
  contraction of collagen gel

Some agents which ligate cell surface integrins
  antibody to α5β1 (fibronection receptor)
  fibronectin fragments (not intact fibronectin)
  antibody to α4β1 (tenascin receptor)
  tenascin

Tumor-promoting phorbol esters
  phorbol myristate acetate

cytoskeleton. These include treatment with proteinases, phagocytosis of latex beads, or treatment with cytochalasin B (CB), which causes depolymerization of filamentous actin. Shape change is also produced when fibroblasts cultured in a collagen gel are allowed to contract the gel by freeing its edges from the culture dish. *In vivo*, this situation might be reproduced by release of the tension exerted by fibroblasts on their matrix during wound contraction, or as they reorganize their matrix during the period of repair tissue remodeling. Another member of this group of stimulators is the tumor promoter, phorbol myristate acetate (PMA). PMA activates protein kinase C (a signal transduction molecule common to pathways used by a number of stimulators) due to its similarity to the second messenger, diacylglycerol. This results in direct stimulation of the transcriptional promoter of the collagenase gene by activation of the transcription factor, AP-1 , however, a change in cell shape is a secondary effect of PMA treatment, and this could activate collagenase expression through a separate pathway.

How could shape change stimulate collagenase expression? An important finding relevant to this question is that collagenase expression is not directly induced in response to agents such as PMA or CB, but is preceded by a lag time of 6–20 hrs.[50, 57] In addition, the major increase in the level of collagenase mRNA is blocked by co-treatment of cells with inhibitors of protein synthesis. These findings demonstrate the requirement for synthesis of an intermediate protein for induction of collagenase synthesis. In considering the possibilities as to the nature of this protein, it was noted that many of the conditions and agents that stimulate collagenase expression by fibroblasts also have in common the capacity to stimulate expression of various cytokines.[58] In fact, several publications have described autocrine substances made by fibroblasts that could stimulate collagenase expression when added exogenously to cultures.[47,59,60] Therefore, the hypothesis that a cytokine acts as the intermediate in the stimulation of collagenase expression that occurs in response to shape change was proposed.

To test this hypothesis, corneal fibroblasts were treated with agents that could specifically neutralize candidate cytokines, at the same time that we treated them with CB, trypsin, or PMA.[61] It was found that treatment with IL-1 receptor antagonist (IL-1ra) completely abrogated CB or trypsin-stimulated collagenase expression, and reduced PMA-stimulated collagenase expression by about 90%. IL-1ra is a naturally occurring substance which competes with IL-1 for binding to its receptor, but does not send a signal into the cell. Therefore, the capacity of IL-1α. to neutralize the action of CB, trypsin, or PMA to stimulate collagenase expression suggested that a form of IL-1 was the necessary intermediate cytokine that we sought to identify. There are two forms of IL: IL-l and IL-lα. However, it was found that corneal fibroblasts synthesize only IL-1α. Treatment with CB, trypsin, or PMA-induced cells to make IL-1α. Neutralizing antibody to IL-lar blocked this induction indicating that it was IL-lα that was responsible for inducing the cells to make collagenase. In addition to its ability to stimulate collagenase expression, IL-lα also was found to regulate itself. Therefore, a function of shape change is activation of the IL-lα autocrine loop. Regulation through the autocrine loop was not specific for corneal cells, but was the regulatory mechanism used by a variety of fibroblasts in culture including cells from lung, tendon, and synovium.[62]

Implications of the IL- lα Autocrine Loop for Therapeutic Intervention

Current understanding of collagenase gene regulation through the IL- lα autocrine loop is diagrammed in Figure 1. The concept of regulation through the IL-lα autocrine intermediate, constitutes a new paradigm for understanding collagenase gene expression. It was realized some years ago that regulation of collagenase expression in response to stimulators occurs primarily by indirect mechanisms. However, this fact has been given little attention in the excitement over new findings on the role of transcription factors in collagenase gene activation, which function independent of new protein synthesis.[63] The data show that different signals may start on their individual pathways into the cell, but

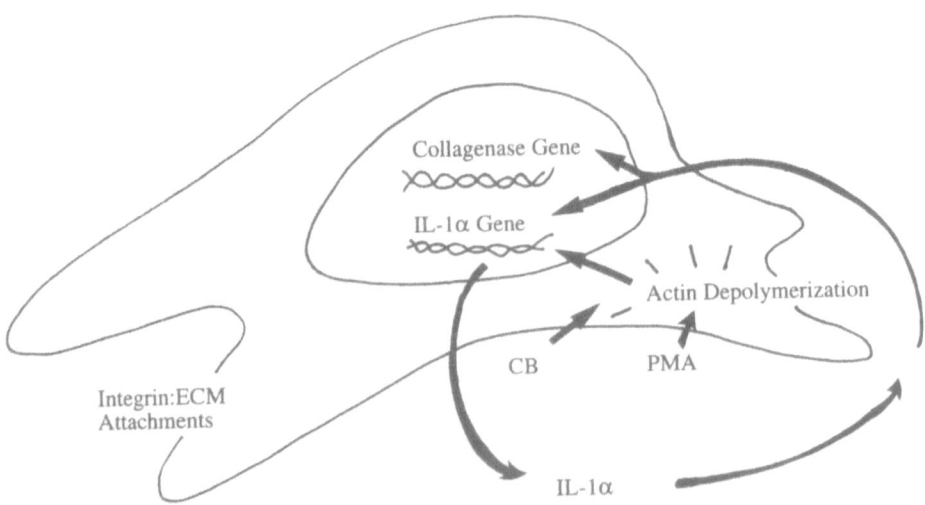

Figure 1. Model for autocrine feedback loop controlling collagenase expression. Agents or conditions that cause the depolymerization of actin stress fibers (which impinge on the cell membrane at the site of integrin:ECM attachment alter cell shape, conferring a rounded appearance. We have found that these agents also cause release of IL-1α. Release of IL-1α activates the IL-1α gene, setting up a positive feedback loop. Maintenance of the IL-1α autocrine loop is required collagenase expression in response to shape change agents.

then are shunted back outside to re-initiate signaling via a common pathway starting from the IL- l receptor. This inside out mechanism would make the initial signal available to other cells in addition to the one stimulated. The coordination of cell activities required for their function together as a tissue would thus be facilitated.

Reorganization of actin constitutes only one of the many possible stimulators and conditions that are known to control collagenase expression in fibroblast cultures, and some of these are particularly relevant to wound healing. As discussed above, a variety of cytokines and growth factors present in the wound environment which could potentially stimulate collagenase. Do these use the IL-1α intermediate, or do they take a different pathway to signal to the collagenase gene? Another particularly interesting stimulator with respect to wound healing is ligation of integrin receptors. Plating of cells on proteolytic fragments of fibronectin, or intact tenascin, stimulate collagenase expression through their respective cell surface integrin receptors.[64,65] Neither of these ECM molecules are found in the uninjured cornea, however, as discussed above, both appear in the repair tissue. Could IL-1α act as an intermediate in the case of this type of stimulation? Researchers currently are working on these problems.

Results point to the importance of IL-1α as an intermediate in controlling the re-modeling phenotype, indicating that elucidation of the IL-1α signaling pathway will provide key knowledge for any rational effort at drug discovery aimed at controlling the remodeling process. Some progress has been made in recent years, however, much has still to be learned.[66]

The IL-1α Autocrine Feedback Loop Is Activated in Repair Fibroblasts

Cells in culture can do nothing more than they can do in the tissue *in situ*, nevertheless, the significance of cell behaviors in culture is not always obvious. The difficulty lies in our ability to pinpoint the *in vivo* situation being reproduced. For this reason, even though it was believed that the cell culture model was offering us a glimpse into the mechanisms of regulation of collagenase expression in the tissue, it was known that this had to be confirmed with an *in vivo* study. Is the IL-α autocrine feedback loop really an important mechanism controlling collagenase expression in repair tissue?

An important finding with respect to this question was again first reported by Johnson-Wint, Gross, and colleagues.[46] They showed that CB could not stimulate the elaboration of latent collagenolytic activity by stromal cells freshly-isolated from the cornea, even though it could do so in early passage subcultures. However, CB could stimulate freshly-isolated cultures in the presence of a biologically active cytokine. Interestingly, conditioned medium from passaged corneal cell cultures could substitute for the purified cytokine. These results lead to the proposal that subculturing of cells stimulates the synthesis of a biologically active cytokine which could act as a cofactor for CB. In fact, when collagenase synthesis was assayed directly, it was found that CB was not essential for stimulation; primary cultures treated only with IL-1 synthesize levels of collagenase similar to passaged cultures.[50] Nevertheless, in view of conclusions from our work about the role of IL-1α in mediating collagenase synthesis in passaged cultures,[62] researchers were still led to a similar (although more specific) hypothesis as the Gross group; that the inability of primary cells to respond properly to CB is due to their incompetence to synthesize the IL-1α intermediate.

The proposed hypothesis turned out to be essentially correct. As predicted, it was found that primary cultures cannot synthesize IL-1α in response to CB. Not only do shape change stimulators fail to induce IL- lα but, neither does exogenously-added IL-1 in primary cultures. Together, these results indicate that primary cultures are deficient in their capacity to activate or to sustain the IL-1α feedback loop. Since the primary cells cannot make collagenase in response to CB, then this response must be entirely dependent on the IL-1α intermediate. Interestingly, it appears that the low level of collagenase gene stimulation by PMA in primary cells is not regulated by the small amount of IL-1α that is produced; this stimulation could not be blocked with IL-1α antagonists. These studies reveal that both IL-1α dependent and independent pathways control collagenase expression, but that the indirect IL-1α pathway is the major mechanism.[61]

Could the nature of fibroblast activation involve acquisition of competence to express IL-1α? To test this hypothesis, we used a wound model of penetrating keratectomy in the rabbit as described by Cintron and colleagues.[8] In this procedure, a trephine is used to remove a 2 mm portion of cornea, much as would be done prior to grafting in humans. However, in this case the space is not grafted but is allowed to fill with a fibrin plug derived from precursors in the aqueous humor. Plug polymerization occurs very rapidly and the anterior chamber reforms within about 15 minutes. Epithelium from the edges of the wound migrates over the plug and completely closes within 24–48 hours. Fibroblasts begin to migrate into the plug within 24 hours, and within two weeks, the clot has been largely replaced by stromal repair tissue. At this two week time point, the cells in the tissue are essentially all fibroblasts, as the minor inflammation which follows injury has subsided by this time. A similar trephine used to create the wound can also be used to punch out the repair tissue that has formed; the wound boundaries are clearly demarcated since the repair tissue is opaque. In this way collection of a pure population of repair fibroblasts is possible.

Using the penetrating keratectomy model, freshly-isolated stromal cells from uninjured cornea and from injured cornea are compared for expression of collagenase. It was reasoned that, if repair fibroblasts had acquired competence for IL-1α, expression, they would be making lots of collagenase since they had been exposed to proteases during their isolation which should stimulate synthesis and release of IL-1α. Sure enough, it was found that repair fibroblasts from injured cornea produced large amounts of collagenase constitutively, in contrast to those from the uninjured cornea which were completely negative for collagenase expression.[25] Repair fibroblasts also made IL-1α expression of which could be blocked by addition of IL-α.[67] Importantly, expression of collagenase could also be blocked with neutralizing agents to IL-1α. From these data, it was concluded that fibroblast activation in the repair tissue is much like fibroblast activation in cell culture and involves acquisition of competence to make IL-1α.

Autocrine IL-1α Initiates a Morphogenetic Cytokine Cascade

Figure 2 presents the current model for collagenase gene regulation in the corneal wound. Based on results of experiments described above, it was proposed that naive stromal cells from freshly injured tissue are dependent on paracrine interaction with the epithelium for the IL-1α needed to stimulate expression of the repair gene, collagenase. Some time after injury occurs however, stromal cells undergo a change in which they acquire competence for IL-1α synthesis. Once this happens, they are independent of the epithelium. Competence for IL-1α expression may be very important for modulation of collagenase synthesis during the long-term process of repair tissue remodeling, which follows completion of epithelial repair. However, collagenase is only one of the many genes that must be regulated during repair. Might autocrine IL-Iα expression have a more general importance in regulating the repair phenotype?

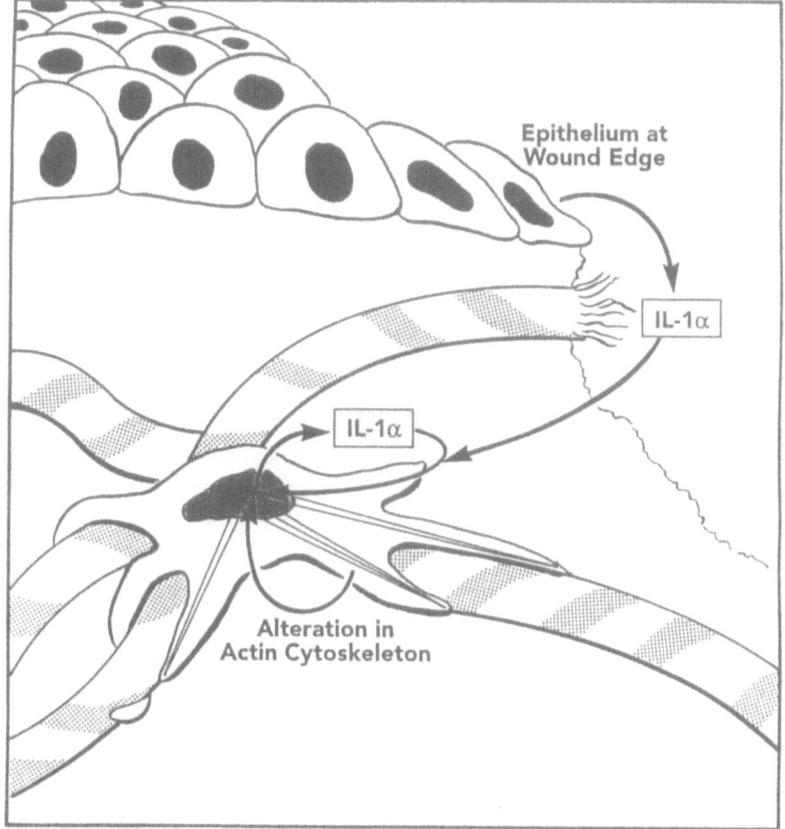

Figure 2. Model for the role of IL-1α in controlling expression of collagenase in the corneal wound. Loss of epithelial cell:cell contacts at the edge of a corneal wound stimulates release of IL-1α which can then stimulate the stromal fibroblast to synthesize collagenase. Later during the repair process, however, the stromal cell acquires competence to make its own IL-1α, thus rendering it independent of the epithelium for collagenase expression. The state of competence allows the stromal fibroblast to activate the IL-1α autocrine loop in response to conditions that alter cell shape.

In thinking about the possibility of a more general role for IL-1α, the fact that this cytokine might act to control gene expression in two different ways was considered. The most obvious is direct control on expression of other effector genes, such as collagenase. However, it is well known that cytokines also control expression of other cytokines. This suggested that IL-1α might act as part of an autocrine cytokine network. Could it be located at a central or apical node on this network? Northern blot analysis of cultures of early passage stromal fibroblasts stimulated with PMA or CB showed us that these cells did indeed express other cytokine genes that are known to be inducible by exogenous IL-1α treatment, including PDGF, IL-6, SAA3, and IL-8 (KJ Strissel, JA West-Mays, and ME Fini, unpublished). The latter two cytokines were considered further. SAA3 is itself a stimulator of collagenase synthesis in fibroblasts.[59] IL-8 is chemotactic for inflammatory cells and stimulates fibroblast migration.[68] Inhibition of IL-1α activity by treatment with IL-1ra or IL-1α antibody inhibited stimulated expression of SAA3[69] or IL-8[67] by PMA or CB, indicating that autocrine IL-1α at least partially controls expression of these cytokines in early passage corneal stromal cells. Is this regulatory network used in the repair tissue? Like early passage fibroblasts, repair fibroblasts freshly-isolated from the tissue were found to express both SAA3 and IL-8. IL-8 expression can be inhibited by treatment with IL-1ra, demonstrating that the capacity for IL-8 expression is at least partially dependent on the relative competence of corneal stromal fibroblasts to make autocrine IL-1α. IL-1ra, therefore, can act as the initiator of a morpho-genetic cascade with the capacity to control more than just collagenase expression in the repair fibroblast. Its position at the apex of a cytokine cascade means that IL-1ra might serve as a useful target for pharmacological treatments to control repair inhibition of IL-1α expression.

Understanding of IL-1α Expression

Understanding that collagenase gene expression is regulated through the IL-1α autocrine loop suggests that this could be a new point at which collagenase gene expression could be manipulated pharmacologically. There are three well-known inhibitors of collagenase expression in early passage fibroblasts: dexamethasone, TGF-β, and retinoic acid. It has been widely believed that each of these inhibitory substances blocks collagenase synthesis through a direct inhibition of intracellular signaling. However, in view of the results discussed above, we began to question the validity of this idea. In a recent study,[70] it was asked whether the more important inhibitory pathway might be an indirect one, acting on the collagenase gene through inhibition of IL-1α expression. Co-treatment of early passage stromal fibroblasts with TGF-β or dexamethasone, at the same time as CB or PMA, was found to inhibit the stimulation of IL-1α expression. Retinoic acid, in contrast, did not have this effect. Nevertheless, all three agents did effectively inhibit collagenase expression stimulated by exogenously-added IL-1, indicating their capacity to interfere with the action of the autocrine intermediate. All three agents were also effective in suppressing the small increase in collagenase expression stimulated by PMA in freshly-isolated stromal cell cultures that is independent of the IL-1α intermediate. Taken together, these findings imply that it should be possible to block collagenase expression without inhibiting expression of other genes upregulated during wound healing. Further studies along these lines should aid in the development of rational methods to control aspects of corneal repair.

Acquisition of Competence for IL-1α Expression in the Repair Fibroblast

The preceding sections have discussed the finding that cells acquire the competence while in culture to make IL-1α and that this is essential to their ability to express at least some of the genes responsible for the repair phenotype, including collagenase. To examine the circumstances of competence acquisition more carefully, freshly-isolated stromal cells were plated into culture and assayed for their competence for CB-inducible collagenase expression over time. Collagenase expression was followed at the level of the individual cell by using the technique of immunostaining. It was found that acquisition of CB-inducibility does not even require that cells be subcultured, but develops progressively over the course of the first week in primary culture. This gradual acquisition of competence is not reflected at the single cell level as a gradual increase in CB-inducibility. Instead, competence is acquired autonomously by each cell with the total number of competent cells increasing progressively over time (MT Girard and ME Fini, unpublished observations). These findings suggest that competence involves the gradual attainment of a limiting threshold in each cell for some new activity required for production of IL-1α.

Since the lack of IL-1α protein synthesis in primary cells is paralleled by a lack of IL-lα mRNA, the ways in which the steady state level of IL- lα mRNA might be controlled in the cell came under consideration. IL-1α belongs to a group of cytokine genes that share an (A+U)-rich sequence in the 3' untranslated regions of their mRNAs.[71] In macrophages, these sequences have been shown to mediate rapid mRNA turnover, effectively preventing mRNA accumulation despite active gene transcription. PMA was shown to increase the half-life of IL-1 mRNA, and this was responsible for its ability to increase the accumulation of IL- 1 message in the cell.[71] Treatment of macrophages with the inhibitor of protein synthesis, cycloheximide, also stimulated accumulation of the cytokine mRNAs with (A+U)-rich sequence, presumably by preventing the resynthesis of rapidly-degraded proteins required for the specific mRNA turn-over mechanism to operate. It was found that cycloheximide also stimulated accumulation of IL-1α mRNA in early passage corneal fibroblast cultures. Fibroblasts containing undetectable levels of IL-1α, when untreated, were found to contain large amounts of IL- lα mRNA after treatment with cycloheximide for l hour, and even more mRNA was present after treatment for two hours. Cells that already contained IL-1α mRNA when untreated were found to contain considerably more IL-1α mRNA after cycloheximide treatment for one hour.[62] The results of this experiment suggest that the IL-1α gene is actively transcribed in cultures of early passage corneal fibroblasts, and that the steady-state level of IL-1α mRNA is determined by changes in the mRNA half-life in response to stimulators such as CB or PMA. Interestingly, it was found that cycloheximide could not induce IL-1α mRNA in stromal cells freshly-isolated from the cornea. This suggests that incompetence for induction of IL1-α expression in response to CB or PMA is due to the fact that the IL-1α gene in not being transcribed.

The experiments described above led to the hypothesis that the new activity needed for stromal cell competence may be a factor required for IL-1α gene transcription. Therefore, the IL-1α gene transcriptional promoter has become our current experimental focus. Surprisingly, although the human IL-1α gene was characterized some years ago,[72] essentially nothing about the mechanisms regulating its transcription has been reported in the literature. All that is known is that the DNA upstream of the transcription start site contains potential binding sites for transcription factors NF-kappaB and AP- 1, as well as a region similar to the adenovirus major late promoter, which is thought to bind USF proteins. We are now investigating the role of these transcription factors in the fibroblast transition.

Another question that still must be answered is what condition of the wound initiates the stromal cell transition to competence for IL-1α expression? The initiator of the cell culture transition may be quite different from the initiator *in situ*. Could the initiator in the later case be one of the cytokines released by the repair epithelium? This question recalls the finding that, while exogenous IL-1α will turn on collagenase expression in freshly-isolated stromal cells, it will not turn on IL-α expression. However, perhaps prolonged exposure to IL-1α may enable a cell to reach the hypothesized threshold for competence. This is a hypothesis which could potentially be tested in vivo using methods to interfere with IL-1α activity in the wound.

SUMMARY AND PERSPECTIVE

We have investigated the mechanisms whereby cell-cell and cell-matrix interactions can modulate expression of genes that define the repair phenotype, using collagenase as our gene of focus. We have found that the mechanism by which these types of interactions control collagenase expression is through their capacity to control release of an intermediate cytokine, IL-1α. Released IL-lα can also activates a cytokine network which not only further stimulates collagenase expression but also affects other cell behaviors associated with the repair phenotype. This new paradigm for the control of repair gene expression suggests a novel point at which drug intervention can be used to modulate the repair process. It will be important to determine whether other cytokines are utilized as intermediates in this way, and which repair genes they control. Furthermore, an understanding of mechanisms regulating expression and release of these intermediate cytokines will be essential to our understanding of the transition to the repair phenotype, and its modulation over time.

REFERENCES

1. T.F. Deuel, Kawahara, R.S., Mustoe, T.A., and Pierce, G.F., Growth factors and wound healing: platelet-derived growth factor as a model cytokine. *Annu. Rev. Med.* 42:567(1991).
2. G.B. Benedek, Theory of transarency of the eye. *Appl. Optics* 10:459 (1971).
3. J.M. Fitch, Birk, D.E., Mentzer, A., et al., Corneal collagen fibrils: dissection with specific collagenases and monoclonal antibodies. *Invest. Ophthalmol. Vis. Sci.* 29:1125 (1988).
4. D.E. Birk, Fitch, J.M., Babiarz, J.P., et al., Collagen fibrillogenesis *in vitro*: interaction of type I and V collagen regulates fibril diameter. *J. Cell Sci.* 95:649 (1990).
5. P.F. Davison, and Galbavy, E.J., Connective tissue remodeling in corneal and scleral wounds. *Invest. Ophthalmol. Vis. Sci.* 27:1478 (1986).
6. T. Grosvenor, How predictable are the results of excimer laser photorefractive keratectomy? A review. *Optometry and Vision Science* 72:698 (1995).
7. P.S. Binder, Radial keratotomy and excimer laser photorefractive keratectomy for the correction of myopia. *J. Refr. Corn. Surg.* 10:443 91994).
8. C. Cintron and Kublin, C.L., Regeneration of corneal tissue. *Dev. Biol.* 61:346 (1977).
9. R.A.F. Clark, Overview and general consideration of wound repair. In *The Molecular and Cellular Biology of Wound Repair,* R.A.F. Clark, and Henson, P.M., eds., Plenum, New York (1988).
10. M.B. Berman, Collagenase and corneal ulceration. In *Collagenase in Normal and Pathological Connective Tissues,* D.E. Wooley, and Evanson, J.M., eds., John Wiley, Chichester (1980).
11. C.S. Foster, Zelt, R.P., Mai-Phan, T., and Kenyon, K.R., Immunosuppression and selective inflammatory cell depletion: studies on a guinea pig model of corneal ulceration after alkali burning. *Arch. Ophthalmol.* 100:1820 (1982).
12. V. Falanga, Chronic wounds: pathophysiologic and experimental considerations. *J. Invest. Dermatol.* 100;721 91993).
13. M.A. Lemp, Cornea and sclera. *Arch. Ophthalmol.* 94:473 (1976).
14. M.A. Kurpakus, Stock, E.L., and Jones, J.C.R., Analysis of wound healing in an *in vitro* model: early appearance of laminin and a 125 kD polypeptide during adhesion complex formation. *J. Cell. Science* 96:651 (1990).
15. M.A. Kurpakus, Quaranta, V., and Jones, J.C.R., Surface relocation of α6β4 integrins and assembly of hemidesmosomes in an in vitro model of wound healing. *J. Cell. Biol.* 115:1737 A91991).
16. L.S. Fujikawa, Foster, C.S., Gipson, I.K., and Colvin, R.B., Basement membrane components in healing rabbit corneal epithelial wounds: immunofluorescence and ultrastructural studies. *J. Cell. Biol.* 98:128 (1984).
17. I.K. Gipson, Spurr-Michaud, S.S., and Tisdale, A.S. Hemidesmosomes and anchoring fibril collagen appear synchronously during development and wound healing. *Dev. Biol.* 126:253 (1988).
18. I.K. Gipson, Spurr-Michaud, S.Sj., and Keough, M., Reassembly of anchoring structures of the corneal epithelium during wound repair in the rabbit. *Invest. Ophthalmol. Vis. Sci.* 30:425 (1988).
19. M.E. Fini, Parks, W.C., Rinehart, W.B., et al., Role of matrix metalloproteinases in failure to re-epithelialize following corneal injury. *Am. J. Path.* 149:1287 (1996).
20. A.A. Khodadoust, Silverstein, A.m., Kenyon, K.R., and Dowling, J.E., Adhesion of regenerating corneal epithelium: The role of basement membrane. *Am. J. Ophthalmol* 65:339 (1968).
21. M. Berman, Kenyon, K., Hayashi, K., L'Hernault, N., The pathogenesis of epithelial defects in stromal ulceration. In *The Cornea: Transactions of the World Congress on the Cornea III,* H.D. Cavanaugh, Ed., Raven Press, Ltd., New York (1988).

22. M. Matsubara, Girard, K.T., Kublin, C.L., et al. Differential roles for two gelatinolytic enzymes of the matrix metalloproteinase family in the remodelling cornea. *Develop. Biol.* 147:425 (1991).

23. M. Matsubara, Ziesks, J., and Fini, M.E., Mechanism of basement membrane dissolution preceding corneal ulceration. *Invest. Ophthalmol. Vis. Sci.* 32:92 (1991).

24. M.E. Fini, Girard, M.T., and Matsubara, M., Collagenolyltic/gelatinolytic enzymes in corneal wound healing. *Acta Ophthalmologica* 70(Suppl. 202):26 (1992).

25. M.T. Girard, Matsubara, M., Kublin C., et al., Stromal fibroblasts synthesize collagenase and stromelysin during long-term remodeling of repair tissue. *J. Cell. Sci.* 104:1001 (1993).

26. U.K. Saarialho-Kere, Chang, E.S., Welgus, H.G., and Parks, W.C., Distinct localization of collagenase and tissue inhibitor of mtalloproteinases expression in wound healing associated with ulcerative pyogenic granuloma. *J. Clin. Invest.* 90:1952 (1993).

27. H.E.P. Bazan, Yao, Y., and Bazan, N.G., Platelet-activating factor induces collagenase expression in corneal epithelial cells. *Proc. Natl. Acad. Sci.* 90:8678 (1993).

28. V. Weimar, Healing processes in the cornea. In *The Transparancy of the Cornea*, S. Duke-Elder, and E.S., Perkins, eds., Blackwell Scientific Publications, Oxford (1960).

29. G.K. Smelser, and Ozanic, V., New concepts in anatomy and histology of the cornea. In *the Cornea*, J.H. King, and McTigue, J.W., eds., Butterworths, Washington (1965).

30. H. Matsuda, and Smelser, G.K., Electron microscopy of corneal wound healing. *Exp. Eye Res.* 33:427 (1973).

31. J.V. Jester, Rodrigues, M.M., and Herman, I.M., Characterizaion of avascular corneal wound healing fibroblasts: new insights into the myofibroblast. *Am. J. Pathol.* 127:140 (1987).

32. R.M.R. Garana, Petrolll, M., Chen, W.-T., et al., Radial keratotomy: II. Role of the myofibroblast in corneal wound contraction. *Invest. Ophthalmol. Vis Sci* 33:3271 91992).

33. M.P. Welch, Odland, G.F., and Clark, R.A.F., Temporal relationships of f-actin bundle information, collagen, and fibronectin matrix assembly, and fibrinectin expression in wound contraction. *J. Cell. Biol.* 110;133 91990).

34. G.K. Smelser, Role of the epithelium in incorporation of sulfate in the corneal connective tissue. In *The Transparency of the Cornea*, S. Duke Elder and Perkins, E.S., eds., Blackwell Scientific Publications, Oxford (1960).

35. J.V. Jester, Barry P.A., Lind, G.J., et al., Corneal keratocytes: *in situ* and *in vitro* organization of cytoskeletal contractile proteins. *Invest. Ophthalmol. Vis. Sci.* 35:730 91994).

36. S.K. Masur, Cheung, J.K.H., and Antohi, S., Identification of integrins in cultured corneal fibrblasts and in isolated keratocytes. *Invst.* Ophthalmol. Vis. Sci. 34:2690 (1993).

37. J.V. Jester, Petroll, W.M., Barry, P.A., and Cavanagh, H.D., Expression of α-smooth muscle (α-SM) actin during corneal stromal wound healing. *Invest. Ophthalmol. Vis. Sci.* 36:709 (1995).

38. R. Ross, Everett, N.B., and Tyler, R., Wound healing and collagen formation. *J. Cell. Biology* 44:645 (1970).

39. C. Cintron, Hong, B-S., and Kublin, C.L., Quantitative analysis of collagen from normal developing corneas and corneal scars. *Current Eye Res.* 1:1 (1981).

40. B.O. Hedbys, The role of polysaccharides in corneal swelling. *Exp. Eye. Res.* 1:81 (1961).

41. F.A. Bettelheim, and Plessy B., The hydration of proteolglycans of bovine cornea. *Biochim. Biophys. Acta* 381:203 (1975).

42. J.R., Hassell, Cintron, C., Kublin, C., and Newsome, D.A. Proteoglycan changes during restoration of transparency in corneal scars. *Arch. Biochem. Biophys.* 222:362 (1983).

43. T. Latvala, Tervo, K., Mustonen, R., and Tervo, T., Expression of cellular fibronectin and tenascin in the rabbit cornea after excimer laser photorefractive keratectomy: a twelve months tudy. *Brit. J. Ophthalmol.* 79:65 (1995).

44. R.J. Cionni, Katakami, C., Labrich, J.B., and Kao, W-Y., Collagen metabolism following corneal lacerations in rabbits. *Curr. Eye Res.* 5:549 91986).

45. J.H. Dunnington, Tissues responses in ocular wounds. *Am. J. Ophthalmol* 43:667 (1957).

46. B. Johnson-Muller, and Gross, J., Regulation of corneal collagenase production: epithelial-stromal cell interactions. *Proc. Natl. Acad. Sci. USA* 75:4417 (1978).

47. B. Johnson-Wint, Regulation of stromal cell collagenase production in adult rabbit cornea: in vitro stimulation and inhibition by epithelial cell products. *Proc. Natl. Acad. Sci. USA* 77:5331 (1980).

48. B. Johnson-Wint. Autocrine regulation fcollagenase production by passaged corneal stromal cells in vitro. *Invest. Ophthalmol. Vis. Sci.* 28(Suppl):230 (1987).

49. I. Kuter, Johnson-Wint, B., Beupre, N., and Gross, J., Collagenase secretion accompanying changes in cell shape occurs only in the presence of a biologically active cytokine. *J. Cell. Sci.* 92:423 (1989).

50. M.E. Fini, and Girard, M.T., The pattern of metalloproteinase expression by corneal fibroblasts is altered with passage in cell culture. *J. Cell Sci.* 97:373 (1990).

51. C.M. Alexander, and Werb, Z., Extracellular matrix degradation. In *Cell Biology of Extracellular Matrix*, E.D. Hay, ed., Plenum Press, New York (1991).

52. K.J. Strissel, Rinehart, W.B., Giarard, M.T., and Fini, M.E., Regulation of paracrine cytokine balance controlling collagenase synthesis by corneal cells. *Invest. Ophthalmol. Vis. Sci.* In press. (1997).

53. K.J. Strissel, Rinehart, W.B., and Fini, M.E., A corneal epithelial inhibitor of stromal cell collagenase synthesis identified as TGF-β2. *Invest. Ophthalmol. Vis. Sci.* 36:151 (1995).

54. C.A. Dinarello, and Savage, N., Interleukin-1 and its receptor. *Crit. Rev. Immunol.* 9:1 (1989).

55. M.B. Sporn, and Roberst, A.B., Peptide growth factors and their receptors. In *Handbook of Experimental Pharmacology, Vols. 1 and 2*, Springer-Verlag, Berlin (1990).

56. C.E. Brinckerhoff, Fini, M.E., Ruby, P.L., et al., Coordinate regulation of metalloproteinase gene expression in synovial cells. In *Development and Diseases of Cartilage and Bone Matrix, Vol. 4*, A. Sen, and Thornhill, T., eds., Alan R. Liss, New York (1987).

57. J. Aggeler, Frisch, S.M., and Werb Z., Collagenase is a major gene product of induced rabbit synovial fibroblasts. *J. Cell Biol.* 98:1662 (1984).

58. C. Nathan, and Sporn, M., Cytokines in context (review). *J. Cell. Biol.* 113:25 (1991).

59. C.E. Brinckerhoff, Mitchell, T.I., Karmilowicz, M.J., et al., Autocrine induction of collagenase by serum amyloid. *Science* 243:655 (1989).

60. P. Angel, Rahmsdorf, J., Poting, A., et al., 12–0-tetradicanolyphorbol-13-acetate (TPA)-induced gene sequences in human primary diploid fibroblasts and their expression in SV40-transformed fibroblasts. *J. Cell Biochem.* 29:351 (1985).

61. J.A. West-Mays, Strissel, K.J., Sadow, P.lM., and Fini, M.E., competence for collagenase gene expression by tissue fibroblasts requires activation of an IL-1 alpha autocrine loop. *Proc. Natl. Acad. Sci. USA* 92:6768 (1995).

62. M.E. Fini, Strissel, K.J., Girard, M.T., et al., Interleukin-1α mediates collagenase synthesis stimulated by phorbol myristate acetate. *J. Biol. Chem.* 269:11291 (1994).

63. P. Ange, and Karin, M., The role of June, Fos and the AP-1 complex in cell-proliferation and transformation. *Biochim. Biophys. Acta* 1072:129 (1991).

64. Z. Werb, Tremble, P.M., Behrendtsen, O., et al., Signal transduction through the fibronectin receptor induces collagenase and stromelysin gene expression. *J. Cell. Biol.* 109:877 (1989).

65. P. Tremble, Chiquet-Dhrismann, R., and Werb, Z., The extracellular matrix ligands fibronectin and tenascin collaborate in regulating collagenase gene expression in fibroblasts. *Mol. Cell. Biol.* 5:439 (1994).

66. K. Kuno, and Matsushim, K., The IL-1 receptor signalling pathway. *J. Leukocyte Biol.* 56:542 (1994).

67. J.A. West-Mays, Sadow, P.M., Tobin, T.W., et al., An endogenous IL-1α feedback loop regulates collagenase and IL-8 gene expression in stromal fibroblasts during corneal repair. In press. *Invest. Ophthalmol. Vis. Sci.* (1997).

68. J.R. Dunlevy, and Couchman, J.R., Interleukin-8 induces motile behavior and loss of focal adhesions in primary fibroblasts. *J. Cell Sci.* 108:311 (1995).

69. K.J. Strissel, Girard, M.T., West-Mays, J.A., et al., Role of serum amyloid A as an intermediate in the IL-1 and PMA-stimulated signalling pathways regulating expression of rabbit fibroblast collagenase. *Exp. Cell Res.* Submitted.

70. J.A. West-Mays, Sadow, P.M., Mullady, D.K., and Fini, M.E., Inhibitors of collagenase synthesis operate through IL-1 alpha dependent and independent pathways. *J. Biol. Chem.* Submitted.

71. G. Shaw, and Kamen, R., A conserved Au sequence from the 3 untranslated region of GM-CSF mRNA mediates selection of mRNA degradation *Cell* 46:659 (1986).

72. Y. Furutani, Natake, M., Yamayoshi, M., et al., Cloning and chaacterization of the cDNAs for human and rabbit interleukin-1 precursor. *Nucleic Acids Res.* 13:5869 (1986).

SECTION V: MOLECULAR BIOLOGY, CELLULAR BIOLOGY, AND GENETICS

Abstracts of Other Conference Presentations and Posters

MODULATION OF CORNEAL VASCULARIZATION BY CONJUNCTIVALIZATION

Andrew J.W. Huang, Cheng-Hui Li, and Eleut Hernandez

Basconi Palmer Eye Institute, University of Miami, Miami FL

When extensive ocular surface trauma destroys the cornea and limbus, limbal deficiency can develop and lead to corneal vascularization and conjunctivalization of the cornea. We hypothesized that conjunctival epithelial ingrowth may modulate the process of corneal vascularization during corneal wound healing. By immunohistochemistry and RT-PCR, we noted abundant basic fibroblast growth factor (bFGF) and vascular endothelial growth factor (VEGF) in the normal rabbit conjunctiva and vascular cornea with proliferating conjunctival epithelium, but not in the normal cornea. These findings suggest ocular surface epithelium may exert a paracrine modulation on the corneal vascularization. We further investigated the modulating mechanisms of conjunctival differentiation during corneal wound healing and corneal vascularization induced by conjunctivalization. Using a battery of antibodies to transforming growth factor-betas (TGF-beta) and their related proteins, we noted that TGF-beta 1 and its latency-associated protein (LAP) as well as TGF-beta 2 were expressed in the basal layers of ocular surface epithelium and conjunctival goblet cells in rabbits. In contrast, type II receptor of TGF-beta was noted in the superficial ocular surface epithelium and deep stroma. By ELISA, we noted that bFGF was expressed abundantly in the conditioned media of explant cultures of normal conjunctiva and vascular cornea, but only minim ally in the normal cornea and limbus. The contrast, TGF-beta 2 was preferentially expressed by the normal cornea and limbus. The expression of bFGF and TGF-beta 2 showed an inverse relationship between avascular and vascular tissues. In addition, TGF-beta 2 of normal conjunctiva and vascular cornea had higher biological activities and were more resistant to neutralization by an anti-TGF-beta 2 neutralizing antibody. The bcl-2 oncogene has been known to inhibit programmed cell death (apoptosis) without affecting cellular proliferation. In normal human ocular surface epithelia, we noted that bcl-2 expression was limited to the basal epithelia of limbus and conjunctiva and not found in the cornea. Expression of bcl-2 correlated well with the proliferative capacity of epithelial explant cultures. These findings suggest that ocular surface epithelial differentiation is orchestrated via a cytokine network, which in turn may modulate the expression of angiogenic cytokines in corneal vascularization induced by conjunctivalization.

LIPOSOME-MEDIATED ENTRY OF THE SV40 LARGE T-ANTIGEN INTO CORNEAL ENDOTHELIAL CELLS LOCALIZES TO THE NUCLEUS AND INDUCES DNA SYNTHESIS

Timothy P. Fleming,[1,3] Choun-Ki Joo,[1,4] Jay S. Pepose,[1,2] and Joseph Williams[1]

[1]Departments of Ophthalmology and Visual Sciences, [2]Department of Pathology, [3]Department of Genetics, Washington University School of Medicine, St. Louis, MO 63110 [4]Department of Ophthalmology, Catholic University Medical College, Seoul, Korea

Primate corneal endothelial cells (CEC) do not regenerate *in vivo,* therefore cell loss must be compensated by corneal endothelial cell enlargement and migration. Prom clinical perspective, CEC loss or dysfunction can reach the point where the endogenous cells can no longer adequately deturgesce the cornea, requiring penetrating keratoplasty to restore visual function.

The goal of our study is to explore an alternative strategy to promote the growth of endogenous CEC. Our method has been to utilize a "protein therapy" approach where we introduce a potent intracellular mitogen, the SV40 large T antigen, to promote growth of the quiescent CEC. The principle of this strategy was substantiated by us and other labs which demonstrated that the expression of the SV40 large T antigen could promote growth in cultures of human CEC.

Using liposome-mediated transfer of beta-galactosidase, We have shown that proteins can be delivered to cornea cells both *in vitro* and in an *ex vivo* environment. By using purified SV40 large T-antigen in culture, we have shown that the liposome delivered T-antigen can localize to the nucleus and promote cell division. By utilizing this method *ex vivo* in murine, rabbit, and feline models, we will demonstrate n the feasibility of this technique in promoting cell growth of cells normally considered non-proliferating, or senescent. This technique has broad applications to other models of wound healing and growth promotion of degenerative cells.

NUCLEOTIDE-BASED THERAPY STRATEGIES FOR REGULATING CORNEAL WOUND HEALING

Gregory Schultz and Roy Tarnuzzer

Institute for Wound Research, University of Florida, Gainesville, FL

Stromal scarring is a natural consequence of comes l injury. With the development of excimer laser keratectomy and radial keratotomy, the ability to limit scarring has become crucial for optimal clinical outcome. Data indicates that transforming growth factor beta (TGF-b) plays a major rote in stimulating corneal scar formation. Conventional approaches for limiting scarring in ocular wounds; are based on the use of agents that reduce inflammation and synthesis of extracellular matrix proteins such as anti-inflammatory steroids or anti-metabolites including 5-fluorouracil or mitomycin-C. The lack of selectively and side effects of these drugs are drawbacks for their use in the cornea. Oligonucleotide-based strategies offer new concepts for the inhibition of corneal scarring. Selective inhibition of gene expression by oligonucleotide are based on three basic strategies: antisense RNA, ribozymes, and external guide sequence-ribonuclease P. Antisense oligonucleotide typically are short (usually 17 to 25 nucleotdes) synthetic sequences of RNA or DNA that are complementary to a specific mRNA or DNA sequence. Several mechanisms have been proposed to account for antisense oligonucleotide-mediated inhibition of gene expression. These include inhibition of transcription, RNA processing or translation. A major limitation of conventional antisense therapy is that a single antisense molecule affects only one mRNA transcript within a cell. Therefore, if a gene product is highly expressed, antisense oligonucleotide may not significantly alter overall expression of the gene product. Ribozymes are specialized antisense molecules that also contain a core structure that possesses enzyme-like RNase activity. Ribozymes can be custom-designed as "gene-specific endonucleases" to base-pair with a specific cellular mRNA then the catalytic core structure cleaves the mRNA, releases the fragments of mRNA freeing the ribozyme to bind and cleave additional mRNA molecules in a true catalytic manner In vitro experiments have shown that ribozymes will selectively reduce levels of mRNA molecules and their proteins in cells. The external guide sequence-RNase P system (EGS-RNase P) takes advantage of the ubiquitous presence in cells of RNase P, an enzyme that cleaves tRNA precursors to generate the 5' termini of mature tRNA molecules. EGS with regions complementary to targeted mRNAs are recognized by RNase P and cleaved. We have constructed a synthetic ribozyme complementary to the type II TGF-b receptor and shown that it will cleave target mRNA in vitro. Oligonucleotide-based therapies to regulate corneal scarring hold much promise but requires additional development

TUMOR SUPPRESSOR GENE FUNCTION IN THE CORNEA

Sandy T. Feldman,[1,2] Alexis Diwa,[1] Leyla Celikkoi,[1] and Carl Edman[2]

[1]Departments of Ophthalmology and [2]Cancer Center, University of California, San Diego School of Medicine, La Jolla, CA

The purpose is to discuss the role of tumor suppressor genes in the regulation of cellular proliferation and differentiation of corneal cells.

The analysis of cell cycle markers and their inhibitors was also assessed by RT-PCR of each cell layer isolated from donor human corneas. The phosphorylation state of Rb protein was determined by immunostaining human corneas with antibodies directed against the underphosphorylated form of Rb protein.

Rb protein is not phosphorylated in the corneal endothelium. Expression of the cyclin dependent kinase inhibitor p21 was detected in adult human corneal endothelial cells but not young (donor age 10 months and 3 years). Keratocytes also failed to show constitutive expression of p21.

The Rb protein and p21 may function to prevent cellular proliferation of corneal endothelium. Yet terminal differentiation of corneal endothelium occurs prior to occurrence of p21 expression. The *in vivo* inhibition of keratocyte growth occurs by a p21 independent mechanism.

SYNERGISTIC EFFECT OF SUBSTANCE P WITH EPIDERMAL GROWTH FACTOR ON CORNEAL EPITHELIAL MIGRATION

M. Nakamura,[1] T. Nishida,[1] K Ofuji,[1] T.W. Reid,[2] C.J. Murphy,[3] and M.J. Mannis[4]

[1]Department of Ophthalmology, Yamaguchi University School of Medicine, Yamaguchi, Japan, [2]Department of Ophthalmology, Texas Tech University, Lubbock, TX, [3]Department of Surgical Science, School of Vet. Medicine, University of Wisconsin-Madison, WI [4]Department of Ophthalmology, University of California Davis, Sacramento, CA

Purpose: In order to investigate the role of neural regulation on the corneal epithelium, we examined the effect of substance P (SP) on corneal epithelial migration using an organ culture system of rabbit corneas. We investigated the synergistic effects of SP with 1) growth factors; epidermal growth factor (EGF), basic fibroblast growth factor (bFGF), transforming growth factor-ß (TGF-ß) and insulin-like growth factor-1 (IGF-1), 2) extracellular matrix proteins; fibronectin, vitronectin, laminin and collagen type IV, and 3) cytokines; interleukin- 1α (IL- 1α), IL- 1β and interleukin-6 (IL-6).

Methods: Rabbit corneal blocks were cultured in the absence or presence of various reagents for 24 hours. At the end of this time the corneal blocks were fixed, dehydrated, embedded in paraffin and stained by H-E, and the length of the path of epithelial migration was measured.

Results: The addition of SP alone did not affect epithelial migration up to a concentration of 50 µg/ml. EGF, fibronectin, vitronectin, collagen type IV, and IL-6 stimulated epithelial migration, but bFGF, TGF-ß, IGF-1, laminin, IL-1α, and IL-1α did not. The stimulatory effect of EGF on the epithelial migration was further enhanced by the presence of SP. The synergistic effect of SP and EGF on corneal epithelial migration was abolished by the addition of a SP antagonist or enkephalinase. Other neurotransmitters (vasoactive intestinal peptide, calcitonin gene related peptide, acetylcholine chloride, norepinephrine, serotonin) or tachykinins (neurokinin A, neurokinin B, kassinin, eledoisin, physalaemin) were also examined, but only SP exhibited a synergistic effect with EGF on corneal epithelial migration.

Conclusion: These results demonstrate that SP synergistically interacts with the EGF stimulation of corneal epithelial migration *in vitro* in a specific manner, suggesting a possible role of SP as a modulator of epithelial wound healing.

EFFECT OF MITOMYCIN C ON VIABILITY AND PROLIFERATION OF CULTURED HUMAN PTERYGIA FIBROBLASTS

R.E. Smith II, S.G. Waller, P.S. Dixon, P.M. Kloess, and C.A. Manning

Department of Ophthalmology, Wilford Hall Medical Center, San Antonio, TX

Purpose: The purpose of this study is to determine the minimum concentration and exposure time for the intraoperative use of mitomycin C used to prevent recurrent pterygia after primary excision. **Methods:** Human pterygia fibroblasts and conjunctival epithelium were exposed to mitomycin C *in vitro* at concentrations and durations of exposure used clinically. Cell proliferation was determined by quantification of tritiated thymidine up-take and cell viability was assessed using a standard Alamar Blue assay system. **Results:** Mitomycin C was not cytocidal to pterygia fibroblasts or normal conjunctival epithelial cells at any of the three concentrations (0.1 mg/ml, 0.2 mg/ml, 0.4 mg ml) during any of the exposure times of 1, 3, and 5 minutes. All exposures to mitomycin C were antiprolif-erative. Pterygia fibroblast proliferative inhibition ranged from 46.0% with 0.1 mg/ml MMC exposure to 63.5% with 0. 4 mg/ml MMC exposure at 1 minute exposure. Normal conjunctival epithelial cell proliferation inhibition ranged from 47.0% with 0.1 mg/ml MMC exposure at three minutes to 58.8% with 0.4 mg/ml MMC exposure at one m-inute—slightly less than the pterygium inhibition. Percent inhibition did not increase sig-nificantly with longer exposure times. MMC 0.2 mg/ml at one minute exposure and MMC 0.1 mg/ml at three minute exposure both result in 50% proliferation inhibition at the low-est concentration and exposure level **Conclusions:** Mitomycin C probably does not reduce recurrence rate of pterygium by its cytotoxic effect on pterygia fibroblasts, rather the ef-fect may be due to the inhibition of proliferation of both the fibroblasts as well as the con-junctival epithelial cells and possibly the limbal epithelial basal stem cells.

bFGF, TGF-β1 AND TENASCIN IN WOUND HEALING OF HUMAN CORNEA

Henry Maseruka,[1] Richard E. Bonshek,[2] Andrew B. Tullo,[2] and A.B.A. Ridgway[2]

[1]Department of Pathological Sciences, University of Manchester, UK, [2]Department of Ophthalmology, Manchester Royal Eye Hospital, UK

Purpose: Tenascin (TN), a glycoprotein known to influence cellular activities in de-velopment and wound healing, has been shown to be expressed transiently in wound heal-ing of human skin and of animal corneas. In preliminary studies we have shown that a similar situation exists for the human cornea. *In vitro* studies have shown that TN is in-duced, *inter alia*, by TGF-b1 and bFGF. This study was therefore undertaken to determine if such a relationship exists *in vivo* in the human cornea. **Method:** Corneas from globes with penetrating/perforating corneal injury and corneal trephines in which there had been previous surgery were selected to encompass a range of time between injury arid removal. Globes enucleated for choroidal melanoma provided normal corneas. Antibodies to I) bFGF; ii) TGF-β1 and iii) human TN were applied to 6 μm microtome sections and bind-ing revealed by a standard avidin-biotin peroxidase complex (ABC) technique. **Results:** In general, bFGF and TGF-ß1 staining patterns were similar, in that, where positive, they tended to co-localise in basal and suprabasal epithelium, epithelial basement membrane and, faintly, in the endothelium. Positivity was seen in cases where there was loss of Bow-man's membrane, especially overlying areas of anterior stromal scarring, and in a case where there was epithelial downgrowth following relaxing corneal incisions. However, in recently injured corneas, faint basal epithelial staining for TGF-ß1, but not bFGF, was found in areas adjacent to points of perforation/penetration; There was no definite rela-tionship between either cytokine and TN, In recently injured corneas and in healed mature scarring, TN immunoreactivity was absent, except in areas where there was dehiscence of epithelium or malapposed stroma. In these areas bFGF and TGF-ß1 were negative. Con-clusion: No definite relationship was found between the expression of TN and that of bFGF and TGF-ß1. This probably indicates the importance of other regulating factors, eg.,

IL-1α, IL-4, IL-6, etc., or may reflect differences between the situations *in vitro* and *in vivo*

ROLE OF SIGNAL TRANSDUCTION SYSTEM IN COLLAGEN DEGRADATION BY KERATOCYTES

T. Nagano, J.L. Hao, and T. Nishida

Department of Ophthalmology, Yamaguchi University, Japan

Purpose: To understand the regulatory mechanism of corneal ulceration, we investigated the role of intracellular signal transduction systems in collagen degradation by rabbit keratocytes cultured in collagen gels three dimensionally. For this purpose, we examined the effects of activators and/or inhibitors of protein kinase C (PKC) or protein kinase A (PKA) on the collagen degradation by keratocytes.

Methods: Rabbit keratocytes (1×10^5 cells/well) were cultured in type I collagen gel three dimensionally with culture medium MEM containing plasminogen (60 µg/ml) for 24 hours. Activators and/or inhibitors of PKC or PKA, such as phorbol 12-myristate 13-acetate (PKA), forskolin, 8Br-cAMP, H-7, were added to the culture medium at various concentrations. After the cultivation, the culture medium was ultrafiltrated to remove native collagen fibrils. Then the ultrafiltrates were acid hydrolyzed and the amount of hydroxyproline was measured spectrophotometrically. Collagen degrading activity was expressed as µg hydroxyproline/well.

Result: Collagen degradation by keratocytes was increased by the addition of PKA in a dose dependent manner, and reached the plateau at the concentration of 0.1 µM. When structurally similar PKA analog (4α-PMA) was added to the culture medium as a negative control, no change in collagen degradation was observed. The addition of PKC inhibitor (H-7) decreased the collagen degradation. The addition of the PKA activators, forskolin and 8Br-cAMP, had no effect on the collagen degradation.

Conclusion: These results demonstrated that PKC plays a significant role in collagen degradation by keratocytes, but PKA system might not participate in collagen degradation.

TRANSECTION OF CORNEAL ENDOTHELIAL CELLS WITH BCL-2 GENE

C.-K. Joo[1], Y.-J. Oh[2], K.-S. Cho[1], M.-J. Jeon[1], and J.-H. Kim[1]

[1]Department of Ophthalmology Catholic University Medical College, [2]Department of Biology YonSei University

Corneal endothelial (CEN) cells play an important role in preserving the transparency of the cornea. However, corneal endothelium is contact with the aqueous humor in which oxidant species are continuously being generated by UV light and inflammatory cells and is, therefore, susceptible to oxidative damage. In order to determine what role, if any, protooncogene Bcl-2 might play in CEN cells during serum deprived cell death and phototoxic damage such like Uvirradiation, we employed bovine CEN cells and murine CEN cells established by transformation with SV large T antigen (supercells). Two types of CEN cells were tranfected with either the eukayotic expression vector containing human Bcl-2 cDNA (a gift from Dr. Korsmeyer) or a control vector. These expression vectors were previously constructed by replacing the splenic focus forming virus (SFFV) promoter in SFFVBcl-2n1 and SFFVNco with a 760 bp Sau3A1 fragment containing the human cytomegalovirus major immediate early enhancer/promoter. Neomycin-resistant colonies were selected and subsequently expanded in DMEM supplemented with 10% heat inactivated fetal bovine serum and 250 ug/ml G418. Positive stable CEN cells expressing Bcl-2 (CEN/Bcl-2) were initially determined by using reverse transcription-polymerase chain reaction and further characterized by immunofluorescent staining and western blot analysis by using monoclonal antibody 6C8 (a gift from Dr. Korsmeyer). Among 14 CEN/Bcl-2 stable cell lines, two clones expressed high level of 26 Kda full-length protein within their cytoplasm. As expected, control cells (CEN/Neo) did not express human Bcl-2. Using these resulting stable cell lines (CEN/Bcl-2 #5, #12) and cells expressing the control vector (CEN/Neo) the effects of Bcl-2 gene on the prevention of CEN cell death under the condition of serum deprivation or free radical stress would be also presented. (Supported by grants from Korean Medical Association).

VIRUS - MEDIATED GENE TRANSFER TO THE CORNEAL ENDOTHELIUM

Frank Larkin[1], Sandra Rayner[2], and Andrew George[2]

[1]Department of Pathology, Institute of Ophthalmology and [2]Department of Immunology Royal Postgraduate Medical School, London, United Kingdom

Purpose: To examine the feasibility of gene transfer to animal and human cornea by adenovirus vectors. **Methods:** Specimens of human, rabbit and rat cornea were incubated for 3h in solutions of recombinant replication-deficient type 5 adenovirus containing a marker gene encoding *E.coli* ß-galactosidase (ß-gal). Control specimens were incubated in virus-free medium. Following *ex vivo* storage in culture medium at 37°C, gene expression was examined by histology and an assay of ß-gal production. Genetically modified rabbit corneas were used as donor allografts for *in vivo* assessment in 14 recipients. **Results:** Marker gene expression was restricted to the endothelium (75–100% of cells positive at 3 days). Following storage, ß-gal assay indicated CMV-driven expression to be maximal at 3–7 days, falling to undetectable levels at 28 days. Genetically modified donor rabbit corneas attained normal clarity on day 1 following transplantation and showed deturgescence at a similar tempo to mock-infected donor corneas. **Conclusions:** At least short-term virus-mediated transfer of novel genes is feasible, in an 'eye bank' setting. No adverse effect of the viral vector or gene transfer procedure was evident in rabbits following transplantation. This system is now being investigated for transfer of therapeutic genes to corneal endothelium. (Supported by Special Trustees of Moorfields Eye Hospital and the Iris Fund for Prevention of Blindness.)

GENE EXPRESSION IN THE RAT DURING CORNEAL GRAFT REJECTION

G. Rocha,[1] J.C. Sánchez-Thorin,[1] Y. Yamamoto,[2] B. Bowyer,[1] Lamar Chandler,[1] S. Pross,[2] S.X. Stevens,[1] H. Friedman,[2] J. Deschênes,[3] and J.J. Rowsey[1]

[1]Departments of Ophthalmology and [2]Microbiology and Immunology, University of South Florida, Tampa, FL, [3]Department of Ophthalmology, McGill University, Montréal, Canada

Background: The changes that occur in the gene expression of cytokines and other immune-related factors during corneal graft rejection are not completely understood. **Purpose.** To standardize the parameters of mRNA analysis in the rat cornea and iris/ciliary body (I/CB) during corneal graft rejection. **Methods:** Lewis rats were grafted with Brown Norway corneal buttons. At the peak of rejection, the eyes were dissected into cornea and I/CB, homogenized and frozen at -70° C. A single-step acid-guanidinium thiocyanate-phenol-chloroform RNA extraction method was used. Both qualitative (using agarose gel electrophoresis) and quantitative (using HPLC) RT-PCR were used to assess the total RNA from cornea and I/C B, and to measure the expression index of early activation markers (IL-1 alpha, IL-1 ß, TGF-alpha), macrophage activity (inducible nitric oxide syntheses), Th-1 (IL-2, IL-12, IF-gamma) and Th-2 (IL-4, IL-10) cell activation, as well as genes associated with ocular immune privilege (TGF-ß, FAS.). **Results:** The average total RNA concentration obtained was 8.6 ug/cornea and 3.52 ug/ I/CB. Optimal conditions for cytokine RT-PCR were: denaturation (94°C for 5 min), annealing (60°C for 5 min) and extension (72°C) for 30–35 cycles. The results were reported as the expression index of each individual mRNA as compared to the housekeeping gene ß-microglobulin. **Conclusions.** A single rat eye provides enough total RNA for corneal and I/CB mRNA analysis by RT-PCR. This reproducible technique may prove to be a valuable tool in the study of cytokine time-kinetics and therapeutic measures during corneal graft rejection. *Supported in part by an unrestricted grant from Research to Prevent Blindness and Colciencias (Colombia).*

TISSUE INHIBITORS OF METALLOPROTEINASES-1 AND -2 ENHANCE THE SPREADING OF CORNEAL EPITHELIUM

Shizuya Saika,Yuka Okada, Natsuko Hashizume, Osamu Yamanaka, Yoshitaka Ohnishi, and Akira Ooshima

Departments of Ophthalmology and Pathology, Wakayama Medical Oollege, 7-Banco 27, Wakayama, Japan

Purpose: Tissue inhibitors of metallproteinases (TIMP) -l and -2 are secreted in injured corneal stroma, modulating the reconstruction of connective tissue by inhibiting matrix-degrading enzymes. It has been reported that TIMPs have a growth-promotive effects on various types of cultured cells. Here, we examined the effects of TIMPs, epidermal growth factor (EGF), and keratinocyte growth factor (KGF) on the spreading of squamous epithelium of organ-cultured rabbit cornea. **Methods:** Spreading of corneal epithelium was evaluated by the method of Nishida, et al. (J Cell Biol 97: 1653–1657, 1983) with a minor modification. Rabbit small corneal blocks were incubated in TC-199 culture medium in the presence or absence of various concentrations of TIMP-1 (0–1000 ng/ ml), TIMP-2 (0–2000 ng/ ml), EGF (0–100 ng/ ml) or KGF (0–500 ng/ ml) for 24 h. Corneal blocks were fixed with formalin. Cryosections of the blocks were stained with HE, and observed under light microscopy. The pass of the spreading epithelium on the stromal cut surface was measured. **Results:** Corneal epithelium spread on the stromal cut surface of each corneal block. Each agent, TIMP-1, TIMP-2, or EGF enhanced the spreading of corneal epithelium at the concentrations of 100, 50, or 10 ng/ ml with maximum effects, respectively. Percentages of the epithelial spreading at the concentrations of maximum effects were 171, 141, or 130%, respectively. KGF had no significant promotive effect on such epithelial spreading. **Conclusions:** Exogenous TIMPs promoted the spreading of organ-cultured rabbit cornea in situ, suggesting endogenous TIMPs may influence the healing of corneal epithelium *in vivo*, and also that topical administration of exogenous TIMPs may have a beneficial therapeutic effects on corneal epithelial damages.

THE RECONSTRUCTION OF HUMAN CORNEAL EPITHELIAL AND STROMAL LAYERS *IN VITRO*

Mayumi Kajikawa, Masahiro Okamoto, Keizo Takahashi, Shigeki Okamoto, Yuichi Ohashi, and Yoichi Minami

Department of Ophthalmology, Ehime University School of Medicine, Ehime; Department of Ophthalmology, Saga Medical School, Saga, Japan

Purpose: An *in vitro* reconstituted corneal model offers a simplified system to evaluate cell to cell relationship between corneal epithelial cells and keratocytes. Therefore, we attempted to establish this model using three dimensional collagen gel matrix culture.
Methods: Corneal epithelial cells and keratocytes were harvested by trypsinization from donated human eyes and primary-cultured in SHEM medium. Then, cultured keratocytes were embedded in type I bovine collagen gel at the cell density of 5 x 10~ cells /ml and laid onto a nitrocellulose membrane of a plastic dish (Millicell-CM, Millipore). On the next day, epithelial cells were seeded on the collagen gel and cultured until they reached a subconfluency before exposure to an air-liquid interface. After 10 to 14 day application of an air-liquid interface, the reconstructed corneal layers were fixed with 10% formaline-neutral buffer solution, embedded in paraffm, and stained by hematoxylin-eosin for histological observations.
Results: The epithelial layer became stratified and consisted of 4 to 6 cell layers on the collagen gel. The epithelial cells at the top layer were found more flattened than those at the bottom layer. Keratocytes in the collagen gel formed a network in parallel to the corneal surface, resembling human corneal stroma.
Conclusion: Human corneal epithelial and stromal layers were successfully reconstructed *in vitro* and could be maintained for at least 4 weeks. Our model is a useful tool for the investigation of fundamental cell biology of the human cornea.

THE EFFECT OF GELSOLIN OVER-EXPRESSION IN SV40-TRANSFORMED RABBIT CORNEAL KERATOCYTES

Penny K. Mar,[1] I. Huang,[1] P. Roy,[1] H. Yin,[2] H.D. Cavanagh,[1] and J.V. Jester[1]

Departments of [1]Ophthalmology and Physiology[2]; University of Texas Southwestern Medical Center; Dallas, Texas

Purpose: Previous studies have shown that during corneal wound healing, normal keratocytes transform to myofibroblasts, as characterized by the expression of a-smooth muscle actin (a-SM actin). The association with myofibroblast transformation, a putative contractile apparatus composed of microfilament bundles (stress fibers) and focal contacts forms. Gelsolin activity severs actin filaments and thus may disrupt the integrity of this contractile apparatus, interfering with myofibroblast transformation. The goal of the current studies was to assess the effects of gelsolin overexpression on a myofibroblast-like keratocyte cell line. **Methods:** TRK43 is an SV40-transformed rabbit keratocyte cell line which phenotypically resembles TGFß-induced normal keratocytes, in that these cells constitutively express a-smooth muscle actin and contract collagen lattices under serum-free conditions. TRK43 cells were transfected by electroporation with pREP4-GS, a gelsolin overexpressing construct. Transfectants were selected by hygromycin resistance. The protein levels of gelsolin and a-SM actin in selected transfectants, which varied morphologically from epithelioid-like to fibroblast-like, were assessed by Western blots. F-actin distribution in these cells was determined by staining with FITC-phalloidin. Candidates of interest were then immunochemically stained for a-SM actin and tested for collagen lattice-contracting ability. **Results:** One transfectant of particular interest, GSTF9, demonstrated an epithelioid-like morphology, in addition to a striking lack of stress fibers, as shown by immunochemical staining for F-actin and a-SM actin. The level of gelsolin expression in these cells appeared to be 3–4 fold that of TRK43, the parental cell line, while the level of a-SM actin protein was undetectable, as demonstrated by Western blot. In addition, GSTF9 displayed less collagen lattice contraction. After 24 hours, the GSTF9 cells contracted the lattice by 33% as opposed to 58% for TRK43 cells (n=3), demonstrating about a 50% inhibition of lattice contraction. **Conclusions:** These results suggest that full-length actin filaments are required for *in vitro* wound contraction, as cells with elevated gelsolin levels demonstrated a decrease in collagen lattice contraction. This effect was accompanied by a lack of detectable a-SM actin protein, which suggests that the disruption of the contractile apparatus by gelsolin overexpression may serve to down-regulate a-SM actin expression and myofibroblast transformation. (Supported by NEI EY07348 (JV3), Senior scientist awards (JVJ, HDC) and an unrestricted grant from Research to Prevent Blindness, Inc.)

RGD PEPTIDES INHIBIT TGFß1-INDUCED A-SMOOTH MUSCLE (A-SM) ACTIN EXPRESSION, CELL PROLIFERATION AND TYROSINE PHOSPHORYLATION OF FOCAL ADHESION PROTEINS IN RABBIT KERATOCYTES

J. Huang, P.A. Barry-Lane, H.D. Cavanagh, W.M. Petroll, and V. Jester

University of Texas Southwestern Medical Center at Dallas, Dallas, Texas

Purpose: In previous studies we have shown that TGFß[1] induces the expression of a-SM actin, fibronectin and α5ß1 integrin, characteristic of myofibroblast transformation.

Using RGD peptides, we studied the effects of inhibitors of cell-matrix interaction on the $TGF\beta_1$-induced transformation of normal rabbit keratocytes (NRK). **Methods:** We cultured NRK with serum-free media, and then treated primary cultures with 1 ng/ml $TGF\beta_1$ with and without RGD peptides. Measurements were then made of a-SM actin expression, cell proliferation and tyrosine phosphorylation of adhesion proteins using immunocytochemistry and Western Blotting. **Results:** We report that GRGDdSP (50 μM to 100 μM), which specifically blocks cell attachment to fibronectin, inhibits TGFß1-induced a-SM actin expression while GPenGRGDSPCA (1 μM to 1 mM), which specifically blocks binding to vitronectin, has no effect. GRGDdSP also blocked TGFß1-induced cell proliferation but had no effect on TGFß1-induced fibronectin synthesis. NRK treated with $TGF\beta_1$ and RGD showed decreased focal adhesion assembly and stress fiber formation. This was associated with the disappearance of the tyrosine phosphorylated proteins as recognized by Western blotting with monoclonal anti-phosphotyrosine, 4G10. Major proteins that are tyrosine phosphorylated following $TGF\beta_1$ treatment included $p_{125}FAK$, a 130 kD protein consistent with p130 and a novel 160 kD protein. Min or proteins included a 67 kD and a 220 kD tyrosine phosphorylated proteins which have molecular weights consistent with paxllin and tensin, respectively. The exact identity of these proteins is currently being investigated. **Conclusions:** Overall thee data indicate that the induction of myofibroblast transformation and perhaps cell proliferation following TGFß1 treatment is a two step process involving: (1) enhanced expression of extracellular matrix and matrix receptors, and (2) the 'outside to inside' signaling by αSß 1-fibronectin mediated by tyrosine phoshorylation or activation of 'stretch' receptors. Studies evaluating these possibilities are ongoing. Supported by NEI EY07348 (WJ) and Senior Scientist Awards (WJ, HDC) and an unrestricted grant from Research to Prevent Blindness, Inc.

PHOTO-ONCOGENE EXPRESSION DURING CORNEAL

Yuka Okada, Shizuya Saika, Yoshitaka Ohnishi, and Emiko Senba

Departments of Ophthalmology and Anatomy, Wakayama Medical College, 7-Banco 27, Wakayama, 640, Japan

Purpose: While transformation of epithelial cells to a motile form is the first step in wound healing of the corneal epithelium, the migratory mechanism in these cells is not fully understood. We examined the expression of proto-oncogene mRNAs in the rat cornea during epithelial and stromal wound healing after simple epithelial ablation, penetrating injury or alkali burn. **Methods:** Eighty-eight male Wistar rats were divided into three groups of treatment; (1) ablation of central corneal epithelium, the basement membrane remaining intact, (2) penetrating injury at the central cornea and (3) alkali burn in the central cornea produced by 1N NaOH. The affected eyes were then enucleated after various intervals of healing. Frozen sections were processed for in situ hybridization with c-fos, c-jun, fos B, jun B and jun D mRNAs or were stained with anti-c-Fos and anti-c-Jun antibodies. **Results:** The signals for c-fos, c-jun and fos B reached a peak 30 to 60 min after ablation, but were no longer evident at 120 min. Jun BrnRNA was detected in the epithelium around the defect 60 min after the ablation, later than the other proto-oncogenes, and reached its peak after 90 min. The message for jun D, was detected in normal epithelium, and was not affected by wounding. C-Fos and c-Jun imuunoreactivities were detected in the epithelium around the epithelial defect from 60 to 120 min after these treatments. The distribution of these proto-oncogene products were varied in these three types of injury. The immunoreactivities for these peptides were also detected in the keratocytes after epithelial ablation in the denuded stroma. In the alkali burned corneas, the imnunoreactivities were detected in the keratocytes in the whole corneal stroma, while almost no keratocytes around the penetrating injury showed such immunoreaction. **Conclusion:** These findings indicate that transcriptional activation of epithelial cells and keratocytes are indicated in the early phase after epithelial ablation before the cells start to migrate, and that these proto-oncogene products may play important roles in wound healing in cornea.

Session VI

Contact Lenses

38

THE EFFECT OF CONTACT LENSES ON THE CONJUNCTIVA

Peter C. Donshik

Division of Ophthalmology
University of Connecticut Health Center
Farmington, Connecticut

ABSTRACT

The purpose of this paper is to review the effects contact lenses have on the conjunctiva. A review of the literature of the effects of contact lenses on conjunctival sensitivity, epithelial cells, bacterial flora, and inflammation reveals that contact lenses have no effect on bulbar conjunctival sensitivity, but appear to cause a decrease in the sensitivity of the tarsal conjunctiva and the lower lid margin. However, contact lens wear does cause an increase in mucous production and an increase in mucous-containing vesicles in the epithelial cells, as well as an increase in goblet cells. They may also cause squamous metaplasia with enlarged flattened epithelial cells, without evidence of keratinization, as well as snake-like changes in the conjunctival epithelium. Contact lenses do not have a significant effect on the conjunctival flora, but may affect the eye's ability to eliminate microorganisms that are introduced. In addition, contact lens care solutions can cause a toxic or allergic reaction causing conjunctival erythema and chemosis with involvement of the cornea. Chlorhexidine and thimerosal appear to be two solutions with the highest incidence of allergic response. Also, either a poor contact lens fit or the use of thimerosal can cause a syndrome that mimics superior bulbar conjunctivitis of Theodore. The contact lens, especially when coated, can cause giant papillary conjunctivitis. Results of this review indicate that in the majority of patients, contact lens wear has little effect on the conjunctiva. However, a contact lens is a foreign body and can cause changes that can affect the conjunctiva

INTRODUCTION

All contact lenses can have a potential effect on a variety of aspects of the conjunctiva. This paper looks at how contact lenses affect conjunctival sensitivity, epithelial cells, bacterial flora, and conjunctival inflammation.

Advances in Corneal Research, edited by Lass
Plenum Press, New York, 1997

Conjunctival Sensitivity

In the normal eye, limbal conjunctival sensitivity appears to be greatest at the temporal margin and is reduced with age. Lawrenson and Ruskall evaluated limbal touch sensitivity and found that contact lenses do not appear to affect the sensitivity of the limbal conjunctiva.[1] In 1994, McGowan and associates studied the palpebral conjunctiva and lid margin.[2] They looked specifically at the sensitivity of the occlusal surface of the lid (the area mid-way between the eyelashes and the tarsal conjunctival opening), the marginal angle palpebral conjunctiva, and the mid-tarsal conjunctiva. Their findings revealed that the most sensitive area appears to be the marginal angle of the lid. They also showed that the lower lid had a higher sensitivity than the upper lid at the marginal angle and at the occlusal surface, but the mid-tarsal conjunctiva appeared to be equally sensitive in both lids.[2] In addition, contact lens wear causes a reduction in the sensitivity of the lower lid margin[3] — the decrease in sensitivity appears to be greatest during the first two weeks of wearing contact lenses.[4]

Conjunctival Epithelial Cells

Contact lenses have been shown to have an effect on conjunctival epithelial cells. Greiner and co-workers[5] reported that the rubbing of the contact lens on the upper tarsal conjunctiva causes an increase in mucous production with an increase in the mucous-containing vesicles in the epithelial cells. Using impression cytology, Connor and co-workers[6] found a two-fold increase in goblet cells in subjects wearing polymacon contact lenses with a water content of 38% (FDA Group I). This process took approximately five months before a statistically significant increase in the goblet cells was observed. By six months, however, a two-fold increase was noted. The increase in the goblet cells probably accounts for the increased mucous that is often observed in contact lens wearers. While conjunctival mucous has a beneficial effect in coating the contact lenses in order to make them more comfortable, the mucous may also have an adverse effect by causing conjunctival inflammation. It is important to note that, while Connor and co-workers reported an increase in goblet cells, none of the patients discontinued contact lens wear or reported complications with their contact lenses. Thus, the increase in goblet cell response in that study cannot be interpreted as an adverse phenomenon. More likely, it was an adaptive response of the conjunctival goblet cells to wearing contact lenses. In 1992, Knop and Reale[7] revealed that soft contact lenses in asymptomatic contact lens wearers can cause cellular changes. Specifically, they reported the presence of squamous metaplasia with distinctively enlarged flattened cells without evidence of keratinization. These researchers also reported snake-like changes of the epithelium, which they felt were due to the chronic mechanical irritation by the contact lens.

Bacterial Flora

Studies on the effect of contact lenses on the conjunctival bacterial flora, for the most part, have shown that contact lenses do not seem to have a significant effect. Winkler and Dixon[8] showed that the short-term daily wear of polymethyl methacrylate (PMMA) contact lenses did not alter the bacterial flora. On the other hand, Kepetansky[9] and co-workers reported an increase in the quantity of bacteria after six months of rigid contact lens wear. The wearing of a therapeutic contact lens also does not appear to alter the normal conjunctival flora.[10,11,12] Recent studies have supported the concept that contact lens wear has a minimal effect on the conjunctival flora. Fleiszig and Efron[13] reported that the conjunctival flora is similar in daily wear contact lens wearers and non-contact lens wearers. However, positive cultures were actually obtained more frequently from members of the control group who were former lens wearers compared to both current contact lens wearers and those who had never worn lenses. This suggests that prolonged contact lens wear may produce an increase in bacterial flora that is present only after cessation of lens wear. There was no difference in the prevalence of potential pathogenic flora between lens wearers and non-lens wearers. There were, however, more positive cultures for potential pathogens among former contact lens wearers. Over 70% of the storage cases of contact lens wearers were contaminated and potential pathogens were isolated from 6% of these cases. However, there did not appear to be any correlation between the organisms found in lens storage cases and the organisms found on the lens or the conjunctival flora. This would also suggest that the eyes of lens wearers were able to eliminate foreign organisms that may be introduced during lens insertion. However, if this mechanism is compromised then infection could occur. These studies suggest that contact lens wear can cause changes in the conjunctival flora that may suppress factors that can inactivate or clear foreign bodies or organisms from the eye. It does not appear that the contact lens specifically changes the conjunctival flora, or that this change in any way leads to an infection or the development of an infection. However, bacterial isolates were found more often in contact lens wearers. Larkin and Leeming[14] cultured the lid margin, bulbar conjunctiva, and tear film of contact lens wearers and non-wearers. They found that contact lens wearers had higher bacterial counts at all locations, although the isolates from the bulbar conjunctiva were not statistically significant, while those from the lid margin and tear film were statistically significant. Rigid gas permeable contact lenses, when worn on an extended wear basis, appeared to have an effect on the microbial flora of the conjunctiva. Fleiszig and Efron[15] cultured the conjunctiva of patients before and after they wore extended wear rigid gas permeable lenses. The subjects wore their contact lenses for six nights of extended wear and then cleaned and disinfected their lense. Cultures were taken before onset of lens wear and repeated after two months of extended contact lens wear. While approximately 5% of normal, healthy eyes harbor potential pathogenic bacteria,[16] 26% of their subjects had organisms that could be considered potentially pathogenic after two months of extended contact lens wear. However, none of the patients had a corneal infection. In addition, after two months of contact lens wear, the number of eyes that cultured negative increased, and the number of eyes harboring only normal conjunctival organisms decreased. This further supported their hypothesis that contact lens wear might have an effect that reduces the normal flora and/or reduces the efficiency with which the eye can normally remove microorganisms from the conjunctival sac.

Conjunctival Inflammation

Contact lenses, or the solutions associated with their care, can create conjunctival inflammation, causing either an allergic or a toxic reaction. It has been estimated that 10% to 40% of contact lens wearers have experienced an adverse reaction using one or more of the common care regimens.[17] The incidence could even be higher if patients mix and match different solutions from different care regimens. The common culprits causing conjunctivitis are benzalkonium chloride, chlorhexidine, thimerosal and, of course, hydrogen peroxide if it is not neutralized. The usual symptoms consist of conjunctival erythema and chemosis. Often, the cornea is involved, with epithelial erosions, microcysts, opacities, and pseudodendrites.

Superior limbic keratoconjunctivitis, secondary to contact lens wear, is a condition that mimics the idiopathic form described by Dr. Theodore.[18,19] It can occur from either a poor fitting lens, or thimerosal sensitivity.[20,21] Patients complain of contact lens intolerance, foreign body sensation, lens coating, and ocular redness, especially involving the superior bulbar conjunctiva. Examination reveals erythema of the superior tarsal conjunctiva, with a fine papillary reaction. The superior bulbar conjunctiva is often injected, and the vessels are prominent. This area of the conjunctiva can stain with either fluorescein or Rose bengal. The superior limbus may be edematous, and the superior cornea can be involved with punctate keratopathy, filaments, or vascular ingrowth. Once diagnosis has been made, the treatment is to discontinue lens wear until the eye is free of inflammation. Often, a short course of topical steroids is helpful; contact lenses can then be refitted. For these patients, frequent lens replacement or disposable contact lenses are often beneficial. A care system utilizing non-preserved chemical disinfection is recommended. Rigid gas permeable contact lenses can be an alternative if symptoms recur with soft contact lenses.

Giant papillary conjunctivitis (GPC) was first reported by Dr. Spring[22] in 1974. The syndrome is defined by a typical complex of symptoms associated with inflammation and anatomical changes on the upper tarsal conjunctiva. These symptoms can begin weeks or years after initiation of lens wear. The syndrome affects contact lens wearers of any age, without preference for either sex. It is usually bilateral, but unilateral cases have been reported.[23] Patients typically complain of increased lens awareness, excessive lens movement, and mucous production in association with ocular irritation, redness, burning, and itching. They often complain of mucous at the inner canthus on awakening in the morning, and their contact lenses are frequently coated. Examination of the upper tarsal conjunctiva reveals inflammation and the presence of large papules. In the early stages, the symptoms of GPC may precede the signs. The upper tarsal conjunctiva may only display hyperemia. As the disease progresses, there is a loss of the normal vascular arcade, and the fine vessels radiating perpendicular to the tarsal margin become more difficult to visualize. A papillary reaction also occurs. Since only 0.6% of the normal population of individuals who have not worn contact lenses have a papillary reaction of 0.3 mm or larger on their upper tarsal conjunctiva,[24] a papillary reaction of 0.3 mm or larger is consistent with a diagnosis of GPC. Biopsies from the upper tarsal conjunctiva shows the presence of basophils, eosinophils, mast cell, and plasma cells.[25] Tears from patients with active GPC show elevated levels of immunoglobulins, specifically IgE, IgG, and, in the more severe cases, IgM. These tear immunoglobulins are locally produced by the external eye and are not elevated in asymptomatic contact lens wearers. They are related to the severity of the symptoms. After contact lenses have been removed and the ocular inflammation has abated, the tear immunoglobulins will return to normal levels.[26] In addition, levels of complement factor, including C3, Factor B and C3 anaphylatoxin (C3a) are also elevated in the tears of GPC patients.[27] Tear lactoferrin levels are increased, while tear lysozyme levels appear to remain normal.[28] In addition, chemotactic factors have been detected in the tears of contact lens wearers with active GPC. Specifically, neutrophilic chemotactic factor (NCF) is present at 1.5 times the levels found in tears of normal individuals; in asymptomatic contact lens wearers, NCF levels are only three times higher than in normal tears.[29] If NCF derived from rabbit conjunctival cells is injected into the uninjured tarsal conjunctiva of rabbits, morphological changes are observed that are similar to those seen in GPC. Histological analysis of the conjunctiva from these rabbits shows infiltration of neutrophils, eosinophils, and plasma cells.[30]

In patients with GPC, coated contact lenses are consistently present. As the syndrome progresses, the coating becomes more of a problem with patients finding it increasingly difficult to keep their lenses clean. There does not appear to be any morphological or biochemical difference between the coating found on the lenses from patients with GPC and those from patients who are asymptomatic.[31-34] However, when coated contact lenses from patients who have GPC are placed on the eyes of Rhesus monkeys, the monkeys will develop injection, thickening and a papillary reaction of the upper tarsal conjunctiva resembling GPC. In addition, elevated levels of IgE and IgG can be found in their tears. If a biopsy is taken from the tarsal plate, a cellular infiltrate consisting of eosinophils and plasma cells that is similar to the infiltrate observed in biopsies from the tarsal conjunctiva of patients with GPC is observed.[35] New contact lenses, or lenses worn by patients without GPC, do not elicit these changes.

At present, the cause of GPC is unknown. The question of whether GPC is purely an immunological disease or whether mechanical trauma or irritation contributes to it has been a subject of frequent debate. A possible hypothesis of the pathophysiology of contact lens-associated GPC is as follows: the contact lens becomes coated and an immunological reaction occurs causing the production of tear immunoglobulins (IgE, IgG, and, in severe cases, IgM). In addition, the complement system is activated by the formation of C3 anaphylatoxin. C3 anaphylatoxin, in addition to IgE and some classes of IgG, can interact with mast cells and basophils to cause the release of vasoactive amines. In addition, a coated contact lens can cause conjunctival trauma and the consequent release of NCF, which then attracts the eosinophils, mast cells, and basophils, as well as lymphocytes and plasma cells that are found on the histological examination of biopsies from GPC patients. These cells interact with IgG, IgE, and C3a, resulting in the release of vasoactive amines which are responsible for initiating the complex of symptoms. These symptoms result in further coating of the contact lens and thus perpetuate this cycle of events. Lactoferrin, a potent inhibitor of C3a, has been found to be decreased in the tears of patients with GPC. The management of GPC can be directed at decreasing the coating on the contact lens, which will decrease the antigen load, and trauma to the conjunctival surface, or it can be directed at modulation of the immune reaction.

The management of giant papillary conjunctivitis was studied in 200 symptomatic patients. Various management options were evaluated. They consisted of the following: decreasing contact lens wearing time, replacing the contact lens with a lens of identical type, instituting a new cleaning regimen, discontinuing the contact lenses for a period of time before refitting the patient with a new and different contact lens of the same material, or changing the lens polymer. If the wearing time was decreased or the contact lens was replaced with a similar type of lens without first discontinuing lens wear, patients had a rapid return of symptoms. However, if the contact lens was discontinued for a period of time (3 to 4 weeks) and then the patient was refitted with either a soft lens of a different polymer, a rigid gas permeable contact lens, or a disposable frequent replacement lens, then, overall, 94% were able to continue wearing contact lenses for a significant period of time. If one looked at specific management strategies, one found that changing the polymer from a HEMA material to a glyceryl methylmethacrylate (GMMA) material resulted in 80.6% of the patients successfully wearing their lenses. If a rigid gas permeable contact lens was utilized, 82.1 % were able to continue wearing their lenses. If a frequent replacement or a disposable lens was utilized, then 90.9% of the patients were able to continue wearing their lenses. On the other hand, if the same contact lens was refitted, only 68.8% were able to continue wearing their lenses, and if a soft lens of similar HEMA material was utilized, only 71.4% were able to continue wearing their lenses. Thus, changing the contact lens polymer, or using a frequent replacement/disposable contact lens had the greatest success.[36]

Topical corticosteroids, topical non-steroidal anti-inflammatory agents, and topical mast cell stabilizers are strategies available to modulate the immune response. The use of topical steroids has not been widely advocated because the potential complications of steroids far outweighs the potential benefit of keeping an individual in contact lenses. Mast cell stabilizers have been reported to be quite helpful in maintaining patients with giant papillary conjunctivitis.[37,38] Thus, using multiple options, such as changing the lens polymer to a glyceryl methylmethacrylate, utilizing a rigid gas permeable lens, or utilizing a soft lens on a frequent replacement/disposable basis, results in a success rate of over 90%. In individuals who still have a return of symptoms after changing the lens polymer, the use of a topical mast cell stabilizer or a non-steroidal anti-inflammatory drug as an adjunctive therapy to clean contact lenses can help these patients continue in contact lens wear.

Thus, the evidence presented would suggest that all contact lenses can affect the conjunctiva in a variety of ways.

REFERENCES

1. L.G. Lawrenson, and Ruskell, C.L., Investigation of limbal touch sensitivity using a Cochet-Bonnet aesthesiometer. *Br. J. Ophthalmol.* 77:339 (1993).
2. D.P. McGowan, Lawrenson, J.G., and Ruskell, G.L., Touch sensitivity of the eyelid margin and palpebral conjunctiva. *Acta Ophthalmology* 72:57 (1994).
3. J.M. Dickson, Ocular changes due to contact lenses. *Am. J. Ophthalmol.* 58:424 (1964).
4. G.E. Lowther, and Hilt, R.M., Sensitivity threshold of the lower lid margin in the course of adaptation to contact lenses. *Am. J. Ophthalmol.* 45:587 (1968).
5. J.V. Greiner, and Allansmith, M.R., Effect of contact lens wear on the conjunctival mucous system. *Ophthalmol.* 88:821 (1981).
6. C.G. Connor, Campbell, J.B., Steel, C.A., and Burke, J.H., The effect of daily wear contact lenses on goblet cell density. *J. Am. Optometric. Assoc.* 65:792 (1994(.
7. P.E. Knop, and Brewitt, H., Conjunctival cytology in asymptomatic wearers of soft contact lenses. *Graefes Arch. Clin. Exper. Ophthalmol.* 230:340 (1992)
8. O.H. Winkler, and Dixon, J.M., Bacteria of the eye. *Arch. Ophthalmol.* 72:817 (1964).
9. F.M. Kepetansky, Suie, T., Gracy, A.D., and Bitonte, J.L., Bacteriologic studies of patients who wear contact lenses. *Am. J. Ophthalmol.* 57:255 (1964).
10. P.S. Binder, and Worthen, D.M., A continuous wear hydrophilic lens. Prophylactic topical antibiotics. *Arch. Ophthalmol.* 94:2109 (1976).
11. G. Hovding, Conjunctival and contact lens bacterial flora during continuous "bandage lens" wear. *Acta Ophthalmol.* 60:439 (1982).
12. M. Rydberg, Bacteriology in continuous wear of soft contact lenses. *Contact Intraocul. Lens Med. J.* 1:150 (1975).
13. S.M.J. Fleiszig, and Efron, N., Microbial flora in eyes of current and former contact lens wearers. *J. Clin. Microbiol.* 30:1156 (1992)
14. D.F. Larkin, and Leeming, J.P., Quantitative alterations of the commensal eye bacteria in contact lens wear. *Eye* 5:70 (1991).
15. S.M.J. Fleiszig, and Efron, N., Conjunctival flora in extended wear of rigid gas permeable contact lenses. *Optometry Vis. Sci.* 69:354 91992).
16. G. Smolin, Okumoto, M., and Nozik, R.A., Microbial flora in extended wear soft contact lens wearers. *Am. J. Ophthalmol.* 88:543 (1979).
17. B.D. Coward, Neumann, R., and Callender M: Solutions intolerance among users of four chemical soft tens care regimens. *Am. J. Optom. Physiol. Opt.* 61 :523–527 (1984).
18. F.H. Theodore, Superior limbic keratoconjunctivitis. *Eye, Ear, Nose and Throat Month* 42:25 (1964).
19. F.H. Theodore, and Ferry, A.P., Superior limbic keratoconjunctivitis - Clinical and pathological correlations. *Arch. Ophthalmol.* 84:481(1970).
20. S. Stenson, Superior limbic keratoconjunctivitis associated with soft contact lens wear. *Arch. Ophthalmol.* 101:402 (1983).

21. D.D. Sendele, Kenyon, K.R., and Mobilia, E.R., Superior limbic keratoconjunctivitis in contact lens wearers. *Ophthalmology* 90:616 (1983).
22. T.F. Spring, Reaction to hydrophilic lenses. *Med. J. Aust.* 1:499 (1974).
23. P.C. Palmisano, Ehlers, W.H., and Donshik, P.C., Causative factors in unilateral giant papillary conjunctivitis. *CLAO J.* 19:103 (1993).
24. D.R. Korb, Allansmith, M.R., Greiner, J.V., et at., The prevalence of conjunctival changes in wearers of hard contact lenses. *Am. J. Ophthalmol.* 90:336 (1980).
25. M.R. Allansmith, Korb, D.R, and Greiner, J.V., Giant papillary conjunctivitis induced by hard or soft contact lens wear: quantitative histology. Ophthalmology 85:766 (1978).
26. P.C. Donshik, and Ballow, M., Tear immunoglobulins in giant papillary conjunctivitis induced by contact lenses. *Am. J. Ophthalmol.* 96:460 (1983).
27. M. Ballow, Donshik, P.C., and Mendelson, L., Complement proteins in C3 anaphylatoxin in the tears of patients with conjunctivitis. *J. Allergy Clin. Immunol.* 76:473 (1985).
28. P. Rapacz, Tedesco, J., Donshik, P.C., et al., Tear lysozyme and lactoferrin levels in giant papillary conjunctivitis and vernal conjunctivitis. *CLAD J.* 14:207 (1988).
29. S.A. Elgebaly, Donshik, P.C., Rahhal, F., et al., Neutrophilic chemotactic factors in the tears of giant papillary conjunctivitis patients. *Invest. Ophthalmol. Vis. Sci.* 32:208 (1991).
30. W.H. Ehlers, Donshik, P.C., Gillies, C, et al., The induction of an inflammatory reaction by chemotactic factors derived from conjunctival cells. *Invest. Ophthalmol. Vis. Sci.* 31:241 (1990).
31. P.J. Caroline, Robbin, J.B., Greiner, J.V., et al., Microscopic and elemental analysis of deposits on extended wear soft contact lenses. *CLAO J.* 11:311–316 (1985).
32. O.G. Gudmundsson, Woodward, D.F., Fowler, S.A., et al., Identification of proteins in contact lens surface deposits by immunofluorescence microscopy. *Arch. Ophthalmol.* 103:196 (1985).
33. J.T. Barre, Dugan, P.R., Reindeer, W., et al., Protein and element analysis of contact lenses of patients with superior limbic keratoconjunctivitis and GPC. *Optom. Vis. Sci.* 66:133 (1989).
34. S.A. Fowler, Greiner, J.V., and Allansmith, M.R., Soft contact lenses from patients with giant papillary conjunctivitis. *Am. J. Ophthalmol.* 88:1056 (1979).
35. M. Bellow, Donshik, P.C., Rapacz, P., et al., Immunological response in Cynomolgus monkeys to lenses from patients with contact lens-induced giant papillary conjunctivitis. *CLAO J.* 15:64 (1989).
36. P.C. Donshik., Giant papillary conjunctivitis. *Trans. Am. Ophthalmol. Soc. Xcll* (1994).
37. D.M. Meisler, Berzins, U.J., Krachmer, J.H., et al., The treatment of giant papillary conjunctivitis. *Arch. Ophthalmol.* 100:1609 (1982).
38. C.J. Kruger, Ehlers, W.H., Luistro, A.F., et al., The treatment of giant papillary conjunctivitis with Cromolyn sodium. *CLAO J.* 1 8:46 (1992).

SECTION VI: CONTACT LENSES

Abstracts of Other Conference Presentations and Posters

CHANGING PATTERNS OF WEARING SCHEDULES IN SOFT CONTACT LENS WEARERS

R. Linsy Farris

Department of Ophthalmology of the College of Physicians and Surgeons of Columbia University, Harlem Hospital Medical Center, and the Edward S. Harkness Eye Institute, Presbyterian Hospital, New York, NY

Soft contact lens wearers are greatly influenced by the media and recommendations of their contact lens fitter in deciding how to wear their contact lenses. Soft contact lens manufacturing improvements and competition in the marketplace have resulted in low-cost, high-quality lenses which may be worn and replaced as it suits the patient.

Patient histories reveal a varied pattern of daily, every two to three days, weekly, monthly or less frequent. replacement, with varying patterns of cleaning, rinsing and storage. Variations are also evident in the use of daily or extended wear with the determining factors being the skill of insertion and removal technique and the contact lens fitter's preferences.

The tolerance of the individual eye and patient is a predominant factor in the success of soft contact lens wear and remains the final determinant of the wearing schedule.

CONTACT LENS WEAR MODALITIES AND REPLACEMENT SCHEDULES: DEFINITIONS AND RECOMMENDATIONS

Donald J. Doughman[1] and John S. Massare[2]

[1]University of Minnesota, [2]CLAO

There is confusion regarding the definitions of soft contact lens wear modalities and lens replacement schedules. There are three wear modalities as follows: 1) Daily Wear - Lenses worn *only* during waking hours with *no overnight wear*. 2) Extended Wear - Lenses are worn continually, i.e., 24 hours daily for a specified number of days, (usually no more than seven days, i.e., six nights of overnight wear). 3) Flexible Wear -Patient has the choice to wear the lenses on a daily wear or extended wear basis, e.g., daily wear during the week with extended wear over the weekend. There are three replacement schedules as follows: 1) Conventional or Traditional Replacement - No specific scheduled replacement. 2) Frequent Replacement - Lenses replaced after a specific time period, e.g., every month. 3) Disposable Replacement - Lenses replaced after one use. Confusion occurs when patients (and sometimes practitioners) refer to "Disposable Wear Lenses," when what they really mean is "Disposable Replacement Lenses." Disposable Replacement Lenses may be *worn* on a daily or an extended wear basis. There are advantages and disadvantages to each wear modality and replacement regimen, along with cost and convenience factors. These issues, as well as specific recommendations for their use, will be discussed.

CORNEAL TOPOGRAPHY: ITS VALUE IN FITTING AND FOLLOWING CONTACT LENS PATIENTS

Scott McRae

Oregon Health Sciences Center, Portland, Oregon

Corneal topography has played a dramatic role in our understanding of fitting both hard and soft contact lenses. Current corneal topography assessments are undergoing considerable evolution in both hardware and software algorithms used to display and calculate corneal curvature. The corneal topography systems evolving are playing a critical role in our understanding of modern contact lens fittings. New developments with corneal topography will also be discussed.

CORNEAL EPITHELIAL ALTERATIONS IN CONTACT LENS WEAR – FREE RADICAL AND PROGRAMMED CELL DEATH HYPOTHESIS

Kazuo Tsubota

Non-oxygen permeable contact lenses may produce corneal epithelial problems. However, many patients develop injection and epithelial breakdown 6–8 hours after removal of the lens. What mechanism makes the delay? We have hypothesized that the oxygen re-perfusion may be the major cause of cell damage through free-radical formation.

Various statistics showed that the extended wear soft contact lens is the major risk factor for ulcerative keratitis. What are the basic mechanism for the increased risk? As observed by specular microscope, our previous study showed that the corneal epithelium enlarges only in extended wear-soft contact lenses. We have hypothesized that the enlargement of the epithelium is caused by the delayed desquamation due to the inhibition of programmed cell death of corneal epithelium.

I will discuss the results of our two new hypothesis of corneal epithelium responding to contact lens wear.

CORNEAL STROMAL AND ENDOTHELIAL RESPONSES TO CONTACT LENSES

B. A. Holden

Cornea and Contact Lens Research Unit and Cooperative Research Centre for Eye Research and Technology, School of Optometry, University of New South Wales, Sydney, NSW, 2052, Australia

Research[1,2] has clearly shown that the short term endothelial response to contact lenses (blebs) is associated with the effect of lowering pH on cell volume regulation. The polymegethous changes with chronic hypoxic contact lens wear have not yet been satisfactory explained. Stromal responses such as edema (striae and folds) and even chronic thinning are clearly Inversely related to the oxygen transmissiblity of contact lenses worn. The most persistent and difficult response to understand is that of "inflammatory" cell recruitment to the sub-epithelial anterior stroma as a result of contact lens induced Insult to the epithelium. The key future questions are how much of the corneal response to contact lenses will be eliminated by highly oxygen permeable materials and what do we need to do to eliminate contact lens induced inflammation.

CORNEAL INFECTION IN CONTACT LENS WEARERS: CENTRAL, PERIPHERAL, INFECTIOUS, STERILE

Roger Buckley

Corneal infection is by far the most serious of all of the complications of contact lens wear. As the numbers of the contact lens wearers rises (a three-fold increase in lenses dispensed was recorded between 1982 and 1988 in the United Kingdom) so the numbers of cases of contact lens-associated keratitis increases (a literature search indicates a greater than four-fold increase in the number of reported cases between 1986 and 1989). The presence of a contact lens on the eye renders the cornea susceptible to infection by organisms that do not normally cause keratitis in lens non-wearers; these include *Pseudomonas aeruginosa* and *Acanthamoeba* species. The roles of organism adherence and biofilm production have been investigated, as has the part played by the lens case as a reservoir of infection. In addition to 'classical' infection, the entity of sterile keratitis is recognised as an important complication of contact lens wear. This paper reviews the current position of all of these vitally important clinical problems.

CHANGING PATTERNS OF CONTACT LENS WEARERS IN JAPAN

Kiyoshi Watanabe, Hikaru Hamano, and Yasuo Tano

Department of Ophthalmology, Osaka University Medical School, Osaka, Japan

To our knowledge, Japan is the only country in which hard lens wear is more common than soft lens wear. In general, Japanese ophthalmologists believe hard contact lenses to be safer than soft contact lenses. Although high-water-content soft contact lenses with improved Dk values have been produced, it was necessary to make them thicker to improve durability, thus reducing the oxygen supply to the cornea. Furthermore, these lenses were subject to lens deposits, which caused a decline in visual performance. Disposable soft contact lenses made from high-water-content materials with consistently high performance that were developed in the U.S. have recently been introduced into the Japanese market. We reviewed the charts of 23,068 patients in order to investigate the incidence of corneal complications in Japan. Compared with hard contact leases, these newer disposable soft contact lenses provide a greater degree of comfort, are safer, and do not cause conjunctival injection associated with 3 and 9 o'clock staining.

SILSOFT LENSES FOR PAEDIATRIC APHAKIA

Murali Krishnamachary and Lakshmi Ramachandran

L.V. Prasad Eye Institute, Hyderabad, India

Purpose: To evaluate the role of silicone elastomer contact lenses in managing paediatric aphakia.

Methods: In a retrospective study done between Jan, 1992 and March, 1995, 37 children (54 eyes) fitted with silsoft (elastofilcon A, Bausch & Lomb) lenses were evaluated. We analysed the lens parameters, mode of *wear,* complications, frequency of lens replacement, and visual results.

Results: Mean age was *3.15* years (range, 3 months to 9 years). Seventeen patients had bilateral aphakia. Majority (64.8 %) of the patients were fitted within six weeks of surgery. Mean follow-up was 12.1 months. Small (11.3 mm) and steep (7.5 and 7.7 mm) lenses were used for fitting majority of the patients (87.5 %). Twenty five patients were on extended wear (3 days to 4 weeks). Better than 20/100 vision was obtained in seven patients with unilateral and three patients (six eyes) with bilateral aphakia. Central and steady fixation was noted in six patients with unilateral and eight patients (16 eyes) with bilateral aphakia. Three patients developed corneal ulcers, of which two were infectious, and one had a stuck-on lens. Lenses had to be replaced for lens loss (35 lenses) and excess deposits (75 lenses).

Conclusion: Silsoft lenses play an important role in management of paediatric aphakia. Frequent lens replacements and corneal complications are the limiting factors.

SELECTED RADIUS BANDAGE SOFT CONTACT LENSES FOLLOWING PHOTOREFRACTIVE KERATECTOMY

Florence Malet, Beatrice Cochener, and Joseph Colin

The prevention of postoperative pain is an important factor following photorefractive keratectomy (PRK). Our routine treatment is currently the combination of a soft contact lens with diclofenac eye drops. However, in some cases, a "tight lens syndrome" may occur.

We have conducted a prospective study to compare the post-PRK pain and tolerance of the contact lens after fitting, in two groups of patients:

- either a standard radius (8.80 mm) soft hydrophilic contact lens (Acuvue[R] - Vistakon), diameter : 14 mm.
- or a SHCL (Acuvue[R]) selected according to the pre-operative keratometric values: R : 8.4, 8.8 or 9.1 mm with diameters of 14.0 or 14.4 mm.

In both groups, the power of the lens was + or - 0.5 diopters. The bandage lenses were worn during three days and then removed.

Clinical evaluation was made at day 2 to analyze: 1 - the contact lens fitting (lens mobility); 2 - the ocular response (limbal injection, chemosis...); 3 - the postoperative pain.

Results : Selected radius bandage SHCL gave better results than standard radius SHCL when comparing the three evaluated criteria. No case of corneal infection occurred.

THE a, ß, γ CELL HYPOTHESIS FOR RENEWAL OF IRE CORNEAL EPITHELIAL SURFACE

Rougwei Ren, Mathew W. Petroll, James V. Jester, and H. Dwight Cavanagh

Department of Ophthalmology, University of Texas Southwestern Medical Center at Dallas, TX

Purpose. Three populations of corneal surface epithelial cells have previously been identified with scanning electron microscopy and specular microscopy. We tested the hypothesis that these three cell types represent the age distribution of cells on the corneal surface, using *in vivo* confocal microscopy (TSCM) and corneal irrigation cytology. **Methods.** An *in vivo* tandem scanning confocal microscope with 24X objective was used to examine 10 eyes of 10 patients and 12 eyes of 6 rabbits. Images were recorded on video tapes and digitized. Single image frames were selected and analyzed with a silicon graphic workstation. Prior to TSCM examination desquamated corneal cells from the surface were harvested using a specially modified corneal irrigation chamber (CIC). Cells were stained by acridine orange and cell sizes were analyzed using video microscopy. **Results.** The corneal epithelial surface is composed of α (dark), β (medium), and γ (bright) cells. The shedding of cells was observed exclusively from γ cell populations. The γ cell size was measured because these cells have identifiable and minimum overlapped cell border. The mean cell size was $1502\pm237(\mu m^2)$ for rabbit and 903 ± 154 (μm^2) for human. The mean cell size of desquamated corneal epithelial cells was 1436 ± 286 (pm^2) for rabbit and $875\pm$ 117 (μm^2) for human. The fact that desquamated cells and the γ cells had similar sizes support the idea that the γ cell population represents the most aged cells which are in the final process of shedding from the epithelial surface. The percentage of α, b, γ area was also measured in each image. The mean areas occupied by α, β, γ cells were 8.7%, 29.0%, 62.3% for rabbit, and 14.3%, 31.5%, 54.2% for hun'an, respectively. **Conclusions.** Corneal epithelial surface cells can be classified as α cells, β cells, γ cells; cell brightness appears to correlate with increased cell age (maturation). There is a dynamic shedding of γ cells, exposing α and β cells, and transformation of α cells to β, and β cells to γ cells. Measurements of γ cell sizes and relative α,β,γ areas by *in vivo* TSCM may provide quantitative assessment of the turnover of the corneal epithelial surface related to contact lens wear, ocular toxicity, and surface epithelial abnormalities and disease processes. (Supported by NEI EY10738 (HDC), Bausch & Lomb Inc., The Pearle Vision Foundation, Senior scientist awards (JVJ, HDC) and an unrestricted grant from Research to Prevent Blindness, Inc.)

THE EFFECT OF HYDROGELS WORN ON EXTENDED WEAR BASIS ON CORNEAL EPITHELIAL CELL EXFOLIATION AND POLYMORPHONUCLEAR LEUCOCYTE INDUCTION IN PRECORNEAL TEAR FILM

Lakshmi Ramachandran,[1] Deborah F. Sweeney,[2] Gullapalli N.Rao,[1] and Brien A. Holden[2]

[1]Bausch & Lomb Contact Lens Centre, L.V.Prasad Eye Institute, Hyderabad, India,
[2]Cornea and Contact Lens Research Unit, Sydney, Australia

Purpose: To study the effect of two types of disposable hydrogel lenses used on extended wear basis on the corneal epithelial cell (EC) exfoliation rate and poymorphonuclear leucocytes(PMN) induction into the tear film on a group of experienced lens wearers. **Methods:** Six patients wearing unilateral Acuvue (Etafilcon, 58% H_2O content, Group IV) vs SeeQuence 2 (Polymacon, 38% H_2O content, Group I) disposable hydrogel lenses on a six night extended wear basis for a mean period of 15 months were enrolled. Four normal non-contact lens wearers were enrolled as controls. At the end of 6 nights of extended wear schedule the contact lenses were removed immediately on awakening and placed in 5ml phosphate buffered saline and vortexed. The cornea was then irrigated using the non-contact corneal irrigation chamber for 10 seconds and the solution collected. The samples obtained, both from the contact lens and cornea, were passed through a polycarbonate membrane filter ($5\mu m$). The membranes were then stained using Diff-Quik (Giemsa) and enumerated for cells under a light microscope. Non- contact corneal irrigation was performed following *8* hours eye closure in controls in a similar manner. **Results:** Mean number of EC and PMN following 8 hours of eye closure in normals was 336 and 688 respectively. There was a significant increase in EC exfoliation (GrIV/GrI: 1135/1213) and PMN induction (GrIV/GrI: 1113/1915) with lens wear ($p < 0.5$). The difference was not significant in the EC exfoliation and PMN induction between the two types of lenses. **Conclusions:** The state of altered epithelial turn over (increased EC) and subclinical inflammation (increased PMN) may predispose eyes wearing extended wear disposable hydrogel contact lenses to inflammatory and infectious diseases of the cornea.

COMFORT IN DAILY VERSUS TWO-WEEKLY REPLACED CONTACT LENSES

Chris O. Imafidon,[1] Bernice K. Glover,[2] Joe E. Imafidon,[3] Cyprian Asota,[4] Khan Briggs,[3] and Emmanuel Mukoro

[1]Cambridge, UK; [2]New Jersey; [3]Ile-Ife, Nigeria; [4]Optom, Cambridge, UK

A double-masked study was conducted to compare comfort and initial adaptation of a medium water content lens replaced every wearing day (Twelve hourly) with the same type of lens replaced bi-weekly in patients who had no previous contact lens experience. 50 subjects wore a single-use lens on one eye while the fellow eye wore one lens for one week (this was removed and disinfected daily). This was followed by a cross-over study of the fellow eye wearing a single-use and vice versa.

There was no significant difference in the subjective comfort of lenses replaced daily compared to those lenses replaced fortnightly. The average time for the achievement of maximum comfort was 12.5 +A 3.00 in either eye. The length of adaptation time did not differ significantly in both eyes.

The rate of biofilm formation and other natural lubrication agents on lens surface seem to have been adequate to achieve initial comfort in single-use lenses within the first fifteen minutes post-insertion in over 90% of cases.

ADHERENCE OF *PSEUDOMONAS AERUGINOSA* TO SHED RABBIT CORNEAL EPITHELIAL CELLS AFTER OVERNIGHT WEAR OF CONTACT LENSES

James V. Jester, Hongwei Ren, Mathew W. Petroll, and H. Dwight Cavanagh

Department of Ophthalmology, University of Texas Southwestern Medical Center at Dallas, Dallas, Texas

Purpose: Previous studies (Imayasu et al. Ophthalmology, 1994) have shown that contact lens oxygen transmissibility correlates with binding of *P. aeruginosa* (ATCC 27853) to the rabbit cornea after overnight lens wear. Studies of human lens wear stratified by oxygen transmissibility will be required to validate these animal results. In humans bacterial binding to shed cells obtained through corneal irrigation cytology may provide an indirect measure of in vitro binding. The purpose of this study was to establish relationships between binding to shed cells and to the corneal surface in an animal model. **Methods.** Lenses used were rigid lens A (Dk/L=10); rigid lens B (97); soft lens A (9), soft lens B (20). soft lens C (39) with six rabbits in each group. After overnight lens wear, the corneal surface was irrigated with a specially modified corneal irrigation chamber (CIC) to harvest surface cells before exposure to bacterial suspensions (1×10^7 CFU/ml) for 30 minutes. The number of bacteria adherent to the cornea were assessed by CFU determination. Cells collected from the corneal surface (9 ml) were incubated with I ml bacterial suspension containing 108 (CFU/ml) for 30 minutes. The number of bacteria adherent to shed cells was assessed by staining with acridine orange and direct counting by epifluorescence microscopy. **Results.** The differences in the number of bacteria adhering to shed epithelial cells between treated and control eye were 2.90± 1.20, and 0.23 ± 0.41 for rigid A and B, and 5.97+1 54 367+232 1.74 ± 1.54 (bac./cell) for soft lens A,B, and C. Overnight contact lens were induced a significant increase in bacterial binding to shed corneal epithelial cells for rigid A and soft A,B,C. There were significant differences between rigid A and rigid B, soft A and soft C, soft B and soft C ($p<0.05$, ANOVA). The binding of bacteria to shed cells was significantly correlated with the binding of bacteria to the cornea confirming previous results (R=0.908, $p<0.05$). Conclusions. These results show that P. aeruginosa adherence to shed corneal epithelial cells is enhanced after overnight lens wear and that bacterial binding to shed corneal epithelial cells is a valid method for studying contact lens induced corneal infections in humans. Supported by NEI EY10738

(FIDC), Bausch & Lomb Inc., The Pearle Vision Foundation, Senior scientist awards (W3, HDC) and an unrestricted grant from Research to Prevent Blindness, Inc.

RECOVERY OF CORNEAL ENDOTHELIAL MORPHOLOGY AFTER DISCONTINUATION OF PMMA OR HEMA CONTACT LENS WEAR

M.Th.P. Odenthal, I.M. Gan, J. de Brabander, J. Oosting, A. Kijlstra, and W.H. Beekhuis

The Rotterdam Eye Hospital, Rotterdam and Department of Ophthalmology Academic Medical Center, Amsterdam; The Netherlands

Purpose: In the end of the eighties wearers of low gas-permeable contact lenses were advised to stop wearing these lenses because of the negative effects on the morphology of the corneal endothelium. Purpose of this study is to analyse the endothelial changes after discontinuation of low gas permeable contact lens wear. **Methods**: At the time of discontinuation and at least five years after, non-contact specular photographs of the corneal endothelium were made in 20 patients, 2 male and 18 female. Before discontinuation of low gas permeable contact lens wear, 15 persons were wearing PMMA contact lenses for at least 10 years (average duration 20.9 years, range 17–27 yrs), and the remaining 5 persons HEMA lenses for at least 5 years (average duration 10.0 yrs, range 6–12). By computer-analysis of 400 times enlarged endothelial photographs, parameters for polymegathism and pleomorphism were calculated. Per eye, 3 pictures before and 3 pictures after discontinuation of low gas permeable contact lens wear were analysed. Results: 19 patients were refitted with high gas permeable contact lenses. In this group, 15 patients were refitted with RGP contact lenses and 4 patients with high water content soft lenses. One patient switched to spectacle wear. Significant recovery of the corneal endothelial morphology after discontinuation of PMMA or HEMA contact lens wear was found (p <0.05). Improvement was most marked in patients with severe polymegathism. Mean cell density was unchanged. **Conclusion:** Endothelial polymegathism and pleomorphism due to PMMA or HEMA contact lens wear are partly reversible.

This study was sponsored by Stichting H.O.F., Rotterdamse Vereniging Blindenbelangen, Hoornvliesstichting Nederland, Bausch & Lomb and Essilor, and was performed during the Van Loenen Martinet Cornea Fellowship, The Rotterdam Eye Hospital.

Session VII

Microbial Keratitis–Viral

39

THE BIOLOGY AND PATHOLOGY OF VARICELLA ZOSTER VIRUS IN THE GANGLION

Thomas J. Liesegang

Department of Ophthalmology
Mayo Clinic Jacksonville
Jacksonville, Florida 32224

ABSTRACT

The varicella zoster virus (VZV) is present almost uniformly in select human ganglion tissue following hematogenous or nerve seeding. The morphology and physiochemical properties of this labile alpha herpes virus are known. Herpes simplex virus (HSV) and VZV share a common ancestry with much homology; anticipation of the VZV gene function is based on extensive knowledge of HSV. The intracellular activity of the virion has been detailed with the anticipated effect of antiviral drugs. VZV reactivates infrequently because of multiple characteristic differences with HSV. Latency in non-neuronal cells explains the extensive ganglionic damage with VZV reactivation. The hallmark of VZV recurrence is a decline in cell-mediated immunity; this cell-mediated immunity can be boosted by VZV vaccine or natural exposure to exogenous or endogenous VZV. Unfortunately, studies of VZV are hampered by the labile cell free viral yield as well as by the absence of a complete animal model. The pathophysiology of postherpetic neuralgia may have mechanisms other than acute neuralgia, with subgroup mechanisms involving local nociceptors, peripheral nerve fibrosis, collateral axonal sprouting, disordered spinal cord input, central nervous system hyperexcitability, persistence of VZV in mononuclear cells, and the role of the deficient cell-mediated immunity.

INTRODUCTION

Varicella zoster virus (VZV) is exceedingly labile and difficult to obtain in a cell-free form. In addition, a complete animal model similar to human VZV has not yet been developed. Because of these factors, less is known about VZV than is known about herpes simplex virus (HSV). However, newer research techniques and extrapolation to knowledge of HSV have permitted a more complete understanding of VZV primary infection as varicella, latency, and recurrence as zoster. This report summarizes the fragments of understanding of the virology, genome, and pathophysiology of the infection, latency, and recurrence, as well as some comments about the animal model of the disease and the pathogenesis of postherpetic neuralgia.

VIROLOGY

The varicella zoster virus is an exclusively human virus with 95% of the US population infected as evidenced by circulating virus specific antibody[1] or probing of the trigeminal ganglion with polymerase chain reaction. The virus is highly contagious with over 80% of household contacts acquiring the virus.[2] A notable exception is in natives of the subtropics and tropics, where varicella is much less prevalent.[3] The significance of a late age of onset of varicella on the subsequent course of zoster is unknown.[4] Although highly infectious, the spread of varicella apparently requires intimate rather than casual contact. Transmission is largely through inhalation of infectious aerosols, but direct contact with active varicella-zoster lesions also leads to infection. Herpes zoster is infectious to varicella susceptibles, though analysis of household contacts suggests that the risk is only about a third of varicella.[5] As suggested years ago, restriction of zoster to a few dermatomes during naturally-occurring disease reflects infection of the partially immunized host.

There are over 80 herpes viruses that infect a wide range of vertebrate hosts.[6] Most are restricted to a single host in nature with man as the exception since humans are infected by at least seven herpes viruses of various classifications: HSV I, HSV II, and VZV are alpha viruses; cytomegalovirus (CMV) is a beta virus; Epstein-Barr virus (EBV) is a gamma virus and herpes virus 6 and 7 have recently been isolated and are closely related to CMV. VZV is a member of the alpha herpes virus group based on shared characteristics of cytopathology *in vitro*, host range, replicative cycles with mucocutaneous eruptions, physiochemical structure and genomic organization, sensory neurotropism and latency, and ability to translocate bidirectionally via nerve between the sites of latency in sensory ganglia and infection at the epithelial surface.

VZV exhibits typical herpes morphology consisting of an electron dense toroidal core of double stranded DNA genome surrounded by a protein capsid. The nucleocapsid is approximately 100 nm in diameter and consists of 162 hexagonal capsomeres with a central hollow organized in an icosahedron with 5:3:2 symmetry. The virus contains an amorphous envelope obtained by budding through the inner membrane of the cell nucleus. Radially oriented glycoprotein spikes project about 8 nm on its outer surface. The viral tegument is the electron-dense translucent area located between the capsid and the envelope. The entire intact viral particle measures 180–200 nm in diameter.

The propagation of VZV in tissue culture is limited to human and primate cells. Because the virus is highly cell-associated, low titers are obtained and the virus is usually propagated only when infected cells are used as the inoculum. Most clinical and research laboratories use human embryo lung fibroblasts for both primary and quantitative replication. Other cell lines are used to propagate VZV for special purposes such as attenuation or to induce adaption. The particle-infectivity ratio of 10^7 for VZV infected cells[7] is quite high compared to that reported for HSV at 10^1.[8] There may be important structural differences in the envelopes of VZV that cause it to be so labile or, alternatively, that cause virion assembly to be such an inefficient process. The advantages of cell-free VZV is its stability during storage and its ability to produce a quantitatively controlled infection in tissue culture.[9] Sonic disruption of cells can yield cell-free VZV, but this appears to be an inefficient inoculum.[10] Fortunately, virally- induced transformation of tissue culture cells is rare, although it has been described.[11]

Because VZV is exceedingly labile, only limited study of VZV was possible until recombinant DNA technology allowed cloning and expression of viral genes. Uncoating of the virion occurs following virion attachment to the plasma membrane and penetration into the cytoplasm of the cell, and the nucleocapsid is transported through the cytoplasm to the nuclear membrane. Then the viral genome is carried into the nucleus of the cell where it becomes circularized and the major phase of DNA synthesis occurs by a rolling circle mechanism to produce head-to-head concatemers of cleaved unit-length molecules. The earliest visible viral particles appear in the infected-cell nucleus and are characterized by a dense central core surrounded by a single membrane. VZV replication is dependent on a cascade of gene expression that is triggered by a number of transregulatory genes. These genes induce the expression of a subsequent set of genes which encode the enzymes necessary for viral DNA replication. These, in turn, set the stage for the subsequent production, trimming, and assembly of the structural proteins into infectious virions. Envelopment is initiated by budding through the inner lamella of the nuclear membrane and further viral glycoprotein assembly and processing occurs in the cytoplasm in association with rough endoplasmic reticulum, Golgi complex, and lysosomal vacuoles. The second virion coat is acquired during passage through the nuclear membrane and not at the cell surface, though the envelopment may also occur in intracytoplasmic vacuoles.[12] The virions travel through the cytoplasm, fuse with the plasma membrane, and are released by exocytosis.[13] Viral particles, both in the cytoplasm and in the extracellular fluid, have two membranes and resemble particles in vesicle fluid. The complete virus replication cycle takes about 30 hours, with DNA synthesis beginning at 10 hours post infection and peaking at 18 hours.[14] Despite the relatively rapid replication cycle of VZV in cell culture, large amounts of infectious virus are difficult to obtain since little infectious virus is released from VZV-infected cells *in vitro*. Most extracellular VZV virions have a pleomorphic morphology with only about 10% having complete cores.[15]

The glycoproteins of VZV have been examined in the greatest detail because these envelope proteins are essential to understanding the VZV-specific immunity and the production of improved vaccines.[16] The VZV glycoproteins are synthesized late in the virus replication cycle. There are six to eight mature viral glycoproteins, which are divided into three major groups based on their reactivity with monoclonal antibodies. All the glycoproteins have homologs in HSV-I.[17] The most abundant and immunogenic group has been labeled gpI, which is analogous to and weakly homologous to HSV I gE.[18] The VZV gpII glycoprotein is important in the initial adsorption phase of cell infection and is required for viral growth, perhaps via viral entry and cell fusion; it is analogous with HSV IgB. The VZV gpIII glycoprotein is important in the cell to cell spread of the virus. The gpIV is somewhat analogous to products of HSV I Us 7 gene. The VZV gpV gene has some homology with HSV IgC. In cells producing herpes viruses, the viral glycoproteins are usually present in the plasma membrane as well as internal cell membranes and can be associated with a variety of new cell surface activities.[19]

GENOME

The genome of VZV is composed of four segments of double stranded DNA: long unique, short unique, long repeat, and short repeat. The unique segments are flanked at both ends by inverted long repeats and short repeats, respectively. The VZV greatly prefers that the unique long segment be maintained in one orientation and therefore produces two predominate genome isomers. About 5% of the time the long unique region inverts with respect to the short unique region for no evident reason.[10,20] Both HSV I and VZV have four genome isomers in the virion, albeit in different proportions.[6] The genome is linear when packaged by the virus but circularizes upon entering the cell where it undergoes a rolling circle replication to complete the cycle.

The restriction enzyme profiles derived for a large number of VZV isolates from widely varying geographic locations have revealed strain patterns which have been qualitatively and quantitatively very similar although not identical.[10,21,22] The DNA structure remains relatively stable upon multiple viral passages,[22] and antigenic variation of VZV isolates has not been demonstrated, as it has been for HSV. VZV isolates from an individual with varicella and subsequent zoster have been shown by restriction endonuclease mapping to be identical.[23] The same individual can be infected with different strains of VZV at the same time, although most hosts demonstrate only a single VZV strain.[24,25] Biologic and biophysical markers that can be used to distinguish the wild type and Oka vaccine strains of VZV.[26]

The complete sequence of VZV DNA is known. The 125,000 base pairs of the VZV makes it the smallest of the human herpes viruses,[27] about 17% smaller than HSV. VZV is not a unique size, but may vary between 124,000 and 126,000 base pairs.[6] The base composition is 46% guanine + cytosine indicating a major evolutionary divergence from the other neurotrophic viruses; HSV I and II have 67 and 69% guanine + cytosine, respectively.

Both VZV and HSV are descendants of a common ancestor from 37 to 70 million years ago.[28,29] The homology between the short unique VZV and HSV segments and their adjacent repeats is extensive.[27] There are apparent inversions of different regions of the genome. A "core" set of genes is derived from the common ancestor and other genes or sequences have been adapted. Seven genes are essential for HSV I DNA replication and each of these genes has a homolog in VZV, implying that the biochemical processes of DNA replication are similar.[30] VZV has five genes that have no HSV counterparts and HSV has several genes that have no counterpart in VZV.[6] Genes with no counterpart are an obvious place to look for the phenotypic differences between the viruses, although the enzymatic properties of similar proteins can differ.[6]

The VZV genome contains approximately 70 genes distributed fairly equally between the two DNA strands.[27] Since three genes are found at the repeat elements (internal repeat and terminal repeat), two copies of each exist: hence, 67 unique VZV genes (and proteins) are predicted. Knowledge about specific gene functions has been accomplished primarily by comparison with homologous sequences of the HSV.[6] Another strategy has been the preparation of synthetic peptides to produce antibodies to putative VZV proteins. Blocking antibodies to VZV thymidine kinase have been detected in the sera of patients with herpes zoster.[31] The functional roles of VZV specific proteins have not been characterized in detail. VZV is known to induce a virus-specific thymidine kinase similar to other herpes viruses and the presence of this enzyme has been used as a marker for biochemical transformation. These kinases act to phosphorylate nucleosides and the nucleoside analogs are preferentially phosphorylated and may become active inhibitors of viral DNA polymerase.

Most anti-VZV drugs are activated by the viral thymidine kinase and inhibit the viral DNA polymerase. Acyclovir is phosphorylated by the viral-encoded thymidine kinase to acyclovir monophosphate and then to the triphosphate by cellular enzymes. ACV triphosphate either inhibits the DNA polymerase directly or is incorporated into viral DNA, resulting in chain termination. Drugs dependent on viral thymidine kinase phosphorylation and targeted at viral polymerase include acyclovir, valacyclovir, penciclovir, famciclovir, sorivudine, and bromyvinyldeoxyuridine (BVDU). Drugs that are not dependent on viral thymidine kinase phosphorylation and targeted at viral polymerase include vidarabine, foscarnet, and hydroxyphosphonylmethoxypropyl (HPMP). Other agents may act on thymidylate synthase or ribonucleotide reductase.

PATHOPHYSIOLOGY

The respiratory symptoms in varicella suggest that the oropharynx is the likely portal of entry of the virus, although virus usually cannot be cultured from respiratory secretions.[32] By polymerase chain reaction (PCR), however, VZV has been found in the nasopharynx of 90% during the early clinical onset.[33,34] Viral replication occurs at the primary inoculation site followed by transportation via the blood and lymphatics (primary viremia) to all organs, including the ganglia during acute varicella. Viremia has been demonstrated in varicella patients for 1 to 11 days prior to the rash, being carried predominantly in the lymphocytes.[35,36] The virus is taken up by cells of the reticuloendothelial system (liver, spleen and lymphatics), where it undergoes multiple cycles of replication during the remainder of the incubation period. Viral replication is limited somewhat by nonspecific and a developing specific immune response. In most individuals the defenses are soon overwhelmed and a more extensive secondary viremia develops.[37] This secondary viremia is accompanied by cutaneous and mucosal lesions, as well as by prodromal symptoms. The ganglia may also become infected at this time.[38] Focal concentrations of cutaneous lesions may be related to local injury, including trauma and ultraviolet light.[39] Complications of varicella are more common in neonates and the immunosuppressed because of a deficient cell-mediated immune response; the increased severity of varicella in the normal adult, however, remains a mystery.

The cutaneous lesions of varicella begin with infection of the capillary endothelial cells, with subsequent spread to the epithelial cells of the epidermis. Intracellular and extracellular edema develop, producing the vesicle between the stratum corneum and the basal layers of the epidermis. Infected cells develop intranuclear inclusions and multinuclear giant cells which are fused epithelial cells mediated by viral glycoproteins. Multinucleated giant cells may contain as many as 30 nuclei, each with an inclusion body. Chromatin granules marginate against the nuclear membrane as an extrachromosomal structure. Early in the course, the nuclei may contain homogenous basophilic material, but more often they are found with a rounded eosinophilic body surrounded by a wide clear zone. Perivascular infiltration of round cells occurs in the dermis. As leakage from vessels occurs, the vesicles are filled with polymorphonuclear cells, macrophages, and fibrin as it becomes cloudy. Lesions can proceed from papule to crust in 8–12 hours. Uncomplicated varicella heals without scarring except in patients with a severe dermal response or propensity to develop keloids, or in patients who develop secondary bacterial skin infections. Varicella lesions elsewhere are similar depending on the tissue involved. The ganglia can also be simultaneously infected by transport of the virus from the skin to the contiguous sensory nerves and then axonal transport to the ganglia. During the acute varicella infection, both neuronal and non-neuronal cells harbor infection. In one study, 0.6% of neuronal and 0.3% of non-neuronal cells contained replicating VZV, but in only one instance were the two infected cell types adjacent.[38]

VZV DNA is detected in blood mononuclear cells even in uncomplicated cases for several weeks after the rash[40] and may be a significant cause of morbidity and mortality in the immunocompromised.[41] VZV has been detected in macrophages, B cells, and T cells but does not appear to replicate within human mononuclear cells.[40] The relative roles of these mononuclear transport mechanisms in the pathogenesis of primary infection, in reactivation, and in the complications of zoster requires further research.

The cardinal pathologic feature of herpes zoster is ganglionic inflammation and hemorrhagic necrosis, often associated with neuritis, localized leptomeningitis, unilateral segmental myelitis, and degeneration of related motor and sensory roots. VZV has been cultured from the ganglia only in rare isolated cases of acute zoster.[42] Electron microscopy and immunofluorescence have demonstrated VZV particles and antigen in acute disease in CNS tissues, the trigeminal ganglion and its nerve axons, in Schwann cells, and in the arterial walls of ocular and CNS tissue.[43] Adjacent ganglia often show similar changes, and adjacent segments of the spinal cord or brainstem are involved with direct viral invasion. The sensory nerves show degeneration and demyelination both peripherally and centrally. Demyelination is seen in areas of mononuclear cell infiltration and microglial proliferation. Electron microscopy and fluorescent antibody confirm the presence of virus and viral antigen in neuronal and satellite cells and within the corresponding sensory nerves prior to the development of cutaneous lesions. The demonstration of afferent ganglionic fibers to intra- and extracranial blood vessels provides an explanation for the interaxonal spread of virus and the resultant granulomatous arteritis which may be a viral or viral induced immunopathologic event. [44] Granulomatous arteritis can develop during both primary infection and during VZV reactivation. VZV specific DNA has been found in circulating mononuclear cells during zoster[45] and by PCR in mononuclear cells even in the absence of recent zoster.[46]

The skin lesions of zoster develop because of retrograde transport of VZV from the ganglia to the skin. The VZV has the ability to cause dermal ischemia and necrosis and a tendency to cause skin scars and other manifestations of infarctive necrosis of tissues. The skin lesions are identical to that of varicella. Herpes zoster occurs with the greatest frequency in those dermatomes in which the rash of varicella is most dense, presumably related to a large inoculum and a corresponding increase in infected neurons at the time of initial seeding. Even if the immune response is able to abort the cutaneous lesions of zoster, there may still be a necrosis and inflammatory response at the ganglion (zoster sine herpete). If the amnestic response is delayed or deficient, then both more severe local disease and cutaneous dissemination is seen.

LATENCY

Operationally, during latency, virions are not seen by electron microscopy, but virus may be extricated by explantation of latently infected cells or cocultivation of latently infected cells with some indicator cells. While HSV can be isolated from trigeminal ganglionic explants of normal adults at autopsy,[47] VZV cannot be rescued from explants of ganglia.[48] Studies of VZV latency have required the use of nucleic acid hybridization to detect genomic VZV DNA and virus-specific transcripts.[49–54] Polymerase chain reaction technology has provided detection of VZV in 87% of trigeminal ganglia and 53% of thoracic ganglia. *In situ* hybridization has successfully detected VZV RNA and DNA in neurons of latently infected trigeminal[55] and thoracic ganglia.[56] Latency is, therefore, more readily established within trigeminal ganglia than in thoracic dorsal root ganglia. Latent

VZV DNA is less abundant than HSV DNA as determined by PCR and not all ganglia from a single host are positive.

Five regions (or more correctly, five regions of viral transcripts) of the genome may be active during VZV latency, suggesting that the entire genome probably persists within latently infected ganglia.[52] The genome resides in these ganglia in very low copy number. Several of the VZV transcripts detected in latently infected ganglia are from the genes manifested early in an active infection. The incidence of clinical reactivation (as learned from HSV latency) seems to be inversely related to the abundance of one or more of the initial early (?repressor) proteins. Another study suggests that only a single VZV-specific transcriptional region is active in adult trigeminal and thoracic ganglia during latency.[57] This single transcript would be analogous to HSV latency although in a different region of the genome. Using *in situ* hybridization techniques, no VZV transcription patterns were detected in the trigeminal ganglia of infants ranging in age from 3 weeks to 7 months of age but were detected in the ganglia of 15 of 20 normal adults ranging in age from 9 to 74 years.[38] Both VZV-specific RNA and DNA have been detected in ostensibly normal human sensory ganglia.[58] Latency with multiple viral strains occurs with HSV infection[59] and studies suggest it can also occur with VZV infection.[25, 60] The cellular factors that influence the switch of viral gene expression from latency to lytic infection is unclear but likely involves an interaction that allows the expression of pivotal viral mediators of reactivation.

The primary target cell for VZV latency is debated. The cells infected by VZV or HSV in the ganglia during the primary infection may differ from those involved during latency. During varicella, evidence of VZV replication is detected in a large number of both neuronal and non-neuronal cells of the human trigeminal ganglion.[38] During reactivation both satellite and neuronal cells (0.6%) expressed VZV RNA from several regions of the genome,[38] whereas during latency between .01% and .3% of only non-neuronal cells exhibited VZV transcripts.[51] A single report described VZV transcripts only in non-neuronal cells (satellite cells, endothelial cells and fibroblast-like cells) and not in neurons during latency.[38,61] This satellite cell may be the Schwann cell that invests each neuron in the ganglion with their cytoplasmic processes. Integration into the host DNA is crucial if the virus resides in a replicating cell such as the satellite cells. A further study in an in vitro model of VZV latency found that VZV could only be reactivated from combined neuronal and non-neuronal cells but not from either alone.[62] Tissue culture studies[63] and early animal studies, on the other hand, suggest that VZV may be latent exclusively in the neurons.[64] The clinical and histopathologic picture of VZV reactivation is consistent with the role of both these cells in reactivation with cell to cell spread allowing ample opportunity to infect many neurons and encompass the entire dermatome.[65]

RECURRENCE

VZV reactivates clinically much less often than HSV and lacks asymptomatic shedding. VZV does not consistently reactivate in response to provocative stimuli, suggesting a mechanism dissimilar to that of HSV. The non-neuronal site of latency may explain the less frequent reactivation of VZV compared to HSV because it is less subject to the neural triggers that provoke HSV reactivation.[38] With several genes actively expressed during latency, VZV may exploit multiple, and perhaps more potent regulatory strategies to sustain its latent state. Although varicella is latent in many ganglia, it manifests as zoster in a segmental and unilateral fashion. This is peculiar since it is not stimulated by irritation of the neuron, but rather is initiated by an immunosuppressed state that should effect all ganglia equally. Whereas HSV typically reactivates within 1–4 weeks of immunosuppression, VZV typically reactivates at 2–4 weeks of immunosuppression again suggesting that the regulatory apparatus involved in VZV latency is apparently more potent than that for HSV. The infrequency of VZV reactivation may then have several explanations.[49] VZV does not replicate well within sensory neurons; VZV is latent in non-neuronal cells; there is no gene equivalent to LATs gene; there are several regions transcriptionally active during latency; the regulatory apparatus involved in VZV latency is more potent than it is for HSV.

Zoster arises at any age, with the likelihood increasing proportional to the age of the individual and inversely with the individual's immune competence. The most important and strongest antibodies to VZV are directed against the three major glycoproteins and the main nucleocapsid protein. These specific antibodies do not correlate with protection from reinfection, severity of clinical varicella, or the development of zoster.[66] Specific cell-mediated immunity appears after the exanthem and does correlate with the clinical severity and the ability to limit the VZV infection.[67] In addition, VZV specific cell-mediated immunity also provides protection against reinfection and zoster. In young adults, serum anti-VZV antibody is a good surrogate for cell-mediated immunity, but in the elderly, the presence of antibody does not indicate cell-mediated immunity to VZV. The importance of cell-mediated immunity in the containment of VZV latency is confirmed by the many clinical circumstances of reactivation. There is evidence of a transient hyporesponsiveness of cell-mediated immunity during the acute phase of herpes zoster[68,69] that is rapidly restored.[70]

With age there is a progressive decline in the capacity of the immune system to react with foreign antigens associated with an increased reactivity with autoantigens.[71] Herpes zoster appears to be a marker of the gradual decay in immune defenses, especially VZV specific T lymphocytes.[72–75] VZV-specific CMI responses are diminished in about a third of subjects over age 60[74] as measured by skin-test reactivity and VZV-induced lymphocyte blastogenesis, whereas humoral antibodies generally persist but are without significance.[76] Lymphocytes from people 65 years old are less responsive in culture to the varicella zoster antigen than are lymphocytes from young people, strengthening the association among thymic involution, T-cell dysfunction, and the exacerbation of herpes zoster in the elderly. The reduced rate of exposure of elderly individuals to acute VZV infections may be one factor accounting for the decline in T cell recognition of this virus. As a corollary, stimulating T-cell immunity to VZV by the VZV vaccine may reduce the likelihood of reactivation. However, at present here is no direct evidence that the immune system can alter the virus host cell interaction to shift the balance between latency and reactivation. Alpha and gamma interferon are detected after primary VZV infection and may also play a role in the control of VZV replication but their role in recurrence remains unknown.[77]

During reactivation VZV undergoes an initial phase of replication within the affected sensory ganglion, producing active ganglionitis. Zoster involves an explosive and destructive spread of virus across the sensory ganglia, including numerous satellite cells, and this is very different from the pathology of HSV infection and explains the neurological complications and the pain. Extensive monocytic and lymphocytic infiltration, focal hemorrhage, and nerve cell destruction occur. Transitory circulating monocytes and lymphocytes traffic through the ganglia, become infected by VZV, and lead to the associated viremia and dissemination. VZV-specific DNA may persist in peripheral monocytes for years.[78] Hematogenous spread of virus accounts for the appearance of a few vesicles remote from the affected dermatome in 17–35% of patients.[79] Immunocompromised patients have a risk of dissemination of up to 40%,[80] with 10% of these high-risk patients developing visceral involvement, particularly of the lungs, liver, and the brain. The pain intensifies as the VZV spreads down the sensory nerve, producing radiculoneuritis. The virus is released around the sensory nerve endings where a second phase of replication results in the histopathologic skin changes identical to those of primary varicella.

Subclinical reactivations of VZV occur in both immunocompromised and immunocompetent patients.[81–83] Both endogenous reactivations as well as exogenous reexposure by either association with a patient with varicella or with zoster[84–86] or by the VZV vaccine are important mechanisms in maintaining enhanced T-cells ready to respond to endogenous VZV reactivations.[73] This potential for a boost in T cell response to VZV persists in the elderly.[87] The small dose of infectious virus released with zoster is immediately contained by circulating antibody or cell-mediated immunity. Zoster sine herpete, neurologic VZV-produced disease or systemic VZV-produced disease without rash are all recognized clinical entities accompanied by VZV-specific antibody,[88] boost in T cell response, and by peripheral blood mononuclear cells with incomplete VZV DNA.[40]

There have been a few reports of epidemics of zoster, which suggests that zoster can be exogenously acquired.[89] None of the outbreaks were documented by VZV strain typing and probably represent manifestations of a fairly common disease since 10–20% of people will develop at least one attack in their lifetime.[90] There is still no convincing evidence that a person can develop zoster as a result of close contact with patients having varicella or zoster.

ANIMAL MODELS

VZV is highly species specific and naturally infects only humans and the gorillas. Obtaining high titers of VZV *in vitro* has proven elusive because the VZV is so highly cell associated. Therefore, a complete animal model for VZV disease has yet to be developed. In addition, most attempts to produce varicella in animals has led to production of antibody but little clinical sign of infection or pathologic changes. Seroconversion has been demonstrated in the rat, rabbit, and guinea pig. Animal-to-animal spread, viremia, and exanthem have been demonstrated in the guinea pig, although this model system has been critically inoculum-titer dependent.

The guinea pig model with VZV inoculated onto the cornea produced superficial corneal disease in all inoculated animals which resolved within 9 days; 60% of the animals developed pneumonitis which evolved over 4–15 days. VZV was recovered by cocultivation from conjunctival cultures and from trigeminal ganglia, superior cervical ganglia, midbrain, and cerebellum up to 20 days following inoculation.[91] A rabbit model has also been successful in producing infection of the cornea and the trigeminal ganglia. Persistence has been more difficult to establish although may be possible in the rat.[92]

The simian (Old World monkey) varicella virus produces varicella-like disease but does not infect humans. VZV resembles closely this simian varicella virus, including a limited DNA homology distributed throughout the genome.[93] Simian varicella virus uniformly causes a severe disease with a high fatality rate in their natural hosts, but reactivation as zoster has not been demonstrated. Latent simian DNA can be detected by PCR from multiple levels of the neuroaxis, paralleling the findings with VZV in humans.[94] Reactivation of simian varicella appears as a whole body rash suggesting recurrence from multiple ganglia, or, more likely, that hematogenous spread of virus is important in the pathogenesis. The simian virus can become latent in multiple ganglia without the development of clinical varicella, paralleling the known phenomenon of subclinical varicella infection in humans.[54] This may have implications for humans in that the live attenuated VZV vaccine offered in the U.S. results in VZV latency with the same (and probably additional) potential to reactivate as the naturally occurring VZV.

POSTHERPETIC NEURALGIA

The description of latent VZV transcripts present in the non-neuronal cells is consistent with the neuralgia associated with zoster. Replication first in the surrounding satellite cells can facilitate spread to adjacent susceptible neuronal and non-neuronal cells and eventually large portions of the ganglion can be destroyed.[30,38] Multiple sensory neurons can become reactivated and convey the virus to all quadrants of the cutaneous dermatome.

Nociceptors account for the pain and dysthesia that precedes the cutaneous rash (pre-eruptive). The massive inflammatory response in the cutaneous tissue is a cause of much of the actual tissue damage during acute zoster. Tissue damage-excited nociceptors are primary afferent neurons that respond to insult and become sensitized in the presence of inflammation.[95] Sensitized nociceptors spontaneously discharge (they are usually silent), have a lowered activation threshold (allodynia), and have an exaggerated response to the stimuli that exceeds the pain threshold (hyperalgesia). The inflammatory response excites and sensitizes the nociceptives that innervate the nervi nervorum, the sheath surrounding the nerve and ganglion contributing to the poorly localized, deep, aching pain.[96]

There is damage within the ganglion from direct neurolytic injury to neurons and axons and from indirect injury due to the inflammatory reaction accompanied by intraneural or intraganglionic hemorrhage. Frequent, brief, high frequency discharges occur in the neuron's membrane. The allodynia and the hyperalgesia are enhanced by a central hyperexcitability from activity transmitted by unmyelinated C-fiber nociceptors to the spinal cord.[97] The hyperexcitability spreads, probably via interneurons, to include cells that were not directly activated by the nociceptor input that initially incited the change. Rubbing the affected area expands the area of pain. In herpes zoster (HZ), there is preferential loss of large inhibitory fibers, resulting in diminished segmental inhibition with increased nociceptive transmission into the dorsal horn. Small fibers are excitory, transmit pain, and contain substance P, a tachykinin amenable to therapy. There may be an additional contribution from the immune response because of local or distal effects of cytokine production.[71]

The mechanisms of pain in postherpetic neuralgia (PHN) may or may not be related to the acute neuralgia. There may be subgroups of patients with distinct pathophysiologic mechanisms.[98,99] The nociceptor sensitivity and central hyperexcitability of acute neuralgia usually resolve gradually.[95] There may be persistent sensitization of C-fiber nociceptors,[100] although this mechanism has not been established in PHN. Release of substance P from C-fiber nociceptors leads to vasodilation and, in at least some patients with PHN, the skin is vasodilated and warm, suggesting this mechanism. There may be acquisition of abnormal sensitization to sympathetic nerve activity or to plasma catecholamines. The transdermal application of aspirin and lidocaine can significantly reduce pain in some patients by quieting abnormal nociceptor activity.[101]

Fibrosis occurs in the peripheral nerve but does not appear to be inflammatory. There is also fibrosis of the dorsal root ganglion and the dorsal horn of the spinal cord is disordered without atrophy. There is a continued increase in the small nerve fibers and a reduction in large fibers, allowing increased transmission through the unopposed smaller nerve fibers.[102,103] This disordered fiber input into a diseased dorsal root ganglion and dorsal horn may be more contributory than the inflammatory fibrotic scarring disease of the peripheral nerve axons.[96,102,103]

Extensive fibrosis within the nerve leads to intraneural neuromas with fascicles of regenerating axons. These axonal sprouts display several types of pathologic activity including abnormal sensitivity to mechanical stimuli, to cold, and to changes in the microenvironment.[95] Discharges in neighboring axons can activate these axon sprouts. Collateral innervation into the herpetic denervation area by the adjacent nerves is known to be associated with abnormal pain sensations from abnormal collateral nociceptors and/or to an abnormality in the somatosensory processing regions of the central nervous system. The death of neurons also results in the degeneration of their intraspinal terminal arbors, depriving spinal neurons of some of their synapses. These deafferented spinal neurons are known to develop spontaneous and stimulus-evoked epileptiform discharges in similar situations.[95]

The central nervous system plays a key role in PHN since section of herpetic nerves does not relieve the pain. In many patients, stimulus-evoked pains occur in large areas of skin surrounding the territory of the infected nerve, suggesting abnormal sensory processing in the CNS.[98, 104] There is an abnormal persistence of nociceptor-evoked central hyperexcitability (N-methyl-d-asparate type synapses) with a heightened severity of response to mild stimuli.[105]

VZV-specific proteins have been found in the mononuclear cells of zoster patients with PHN months or years after the rash, suggesting the persistence, reactivation, and expression of VZV.[106] The period of mononuclear persistence coincides with the period of the acute pain and may be related both to the amount of acute pain,[78] and to the lack of reduction in PHN.[107]

The relationship of PHN to the declining VZV-specific immune response in the elderly seems intuitive but remains unclear. The severity of cutaneous zoster and the immune state may not predict the risk or the magnitude of PHN.[108] Other studies have noted that PHN is most common in the elderly, the immunocompromised, and those with more severe pain or rash at the time of onset of the illness.[109]

The therapeutic implications of this research are several. It is not surprising that antiviral therapy cannot consistently reduce the prevalence or severity of PHN. Killing the virus in the early ganglionic phases of disease or the persistent virus in mononuclear cells has rationale in theory and more recent studies with early very high dose antiviral are beginning to suggest a clinical effect on PHN.[110] Aggressive pain control at the onset of HZO, especially in those elderly patients prone to PHN, may reduce the magnitude of the initiation phase of nociceptor-evoked central hyperexcitability and lessen the probability that some subsequent factor will be able to maintain abnormal central processing. A two-pronged strategy aimed at both the central and peripheral pain mechanisms should be considered. Topical application of a local anesthetic plus a tricyclic antidepressant are one such combination effective against peripheral pain. Amitryptine blocks reuptake of norepinephrine and serotonin. N-methyl-d-aspartate receptor antagonists like dextromethorphan are partially effective in suppressing nociceptor-evoked central hyperexcitability.

REFERENCES

1. S.E. Straus, Ostrove, J.M., Inchauspe, G., et al., NIH conference. Varicella-zoster virus infections. Biology, natural history, treatment, and prevention. *Ann. Intern. Med.* 108:221 (1988).
2. R. Mench, Nassim, C., Niku, S., et al., Seroepidemiology of varicella. *J. Infect. Dis.* 153:153 (1986).

3. J.N. Longfield, Winn, R.E., Gibson, R.L., et al. Varicella outbreaks in Army recruits from Puerto Rico. Varicella susceptibility in a population from the tropics. *Arch. Intern. Med.* 150:970 (1990).

4. T.H. Weller, Varicella and herpes zoster: a perspective and overview. *J. Infect. Dis.* 166:S1 (1992).

5. J.E. Gordon, Chickenpox: an epidemiologic review. *Am. J. Med. Sci.* 244:362 (1962).

6. A.J. Davison, Varicella-zoster virus. The Fourteenth Fleming lecture. *J. Gen. Virol.* 72:475 (1991).

7. C. Grose, Friedrichs, W.E., and Smith, G.C., Purification and molecular anatomy of the varicella-zoster virion. *Biken. J.* 26:1 (1983).

8. D.H. Watson, Russel, W.C., and Wildy, P., Electron microscopic particle counts on herpes virus using the phosphotungstate negative staining technique. *Virology* 19:250 (1963).

9. L. Gelb, Varicella zoster virus. In *Virology*, B. Fields, editor. Raven Press, New York (1990).

10. N.J. Schmidt, and Lennette, E.H., Improved yields of cell-free varicella-zoster virus. *Infect. Immun.* 14:709 (1976).

11. K. Yamanishi, Matsunaga, Y., Ogino, T., and Lopetegui, P. Biochemical transformation of mouse cells by varicella-zoster virus. *J. Gen. Virol.* 56:421 (1981).

12. F. Jones, and Grose, C., Role of cytoplasmic vacuoles in varicella-zoster virus glycoprotein trafficking and virion envelopment. *J. Virol.* 62:2701 (1988).

13. C. Grose, and Ng , T.I., Intracellular synthesis of varicella-zoster virus. *J. Infect. Dis.* 166:S7 (1992).

14. A. Vafai, Wroblewska, Z, Wellish, M., et al., Analysis of three late varicella-zoster virus proteins, a 125,000-molecular-weight protein and gp1 and gp3. *J. Virol.* 52:953 (1984).

15. M.L. Cook, and Stevens, J.G., Labile coat: reason for noninfectious cell-free varicella-zoster virus in culture. *J. Virol.* 2:1458 (1968).

16. C. Grose, Glycoproteins encoded by varicella-zoster virus: biosynthesis, phosphorylation, and intracellular trafficking. *Annu. Rev. Microbiol.* 44:59 (1990).

17. P.G. Spear, Membrane proteins specified by herpes simplex viruses. I. Identification of four glycoprotein precursors and their products in type 1-infected cells. *J. Virol.* 17:991 (1976).

18. P.M. Keller, Davison, A.J., Lowe, R.S., et al., Identification and structure of the gene encoding gpII, a major glycoprotein of varicella-zoster virus. *Virology* 152:181 (1986).

19. R. Manservigi, and Cassai, E., The glycoproteins of the human herpesviruses. *Comp. Immunol. Microbiol. Infect. Dis.* 14:81 (1991).

20. Y. Hayakawa, and Hyman, R.W., Isomerization of the UL region of varicella-zoster virus DNA. *Virus Res.* 8:25 (1987).

21. S.E. Straus, Hay, J., Smith, H., and Owens, J., Genome differences among varicella-zoster virus isolates. *J. Gen. Virol.* 64:1031 (1983).

22. S. Yamamoto, Kabuta, H., and Shingu, M., Restriction endonuclease analysis of varicella-zoster virus DNAs. *Kurume Med. J.* 38:45 (1991).

23. S.E, Straus, Reinhold, W., Smith, H.A., et al., Endonuclease analysis of viral DNA from varicella and subsequent zoster infections in the same patient. *N. Engl. J. Med.* 311:1362 (1984).

24. B. Pichini, Ecker, J.R., Grose, C., and Hyman, R.W., DNA mapping of paired varicella-zoster virus isolates from patients with shingles. *Lancet* 2:1223 (1983).

25. R. Hondo, Yogo, Y., Kurata, T., and Aoyama, Y., Genome variation among varicella-zoster virus isolates derived from different individuals and from the same individuals. *Arch. Virol.* 93:1 (1987).

26. Y. Hayakawa, Torigoe, S., Shiraki, K., et al., Biologic and biophysical markers of a live varicella vaccine strain (Oka): identification of clinical isolates from vaccine recipients. *J. Infect. Dis.* 149:956 (1984).

27. A.J. Davison, and Scott, J.E., The complete DNA sequence of varicella-zoster virus. *J. Gen. Virol.* 67:1759 (1986).

28. G.A. Gentry, Lowe, M., Alford, G., and Nevins, R., Sequence analyses of herpesviral enzymes suggest an ancient origin for human sexual behavior. *Proc. Natl. Acad. Sci. (USA)* 85:2658 (1988).

29. A.J. Davison, and McGeoch, D.J., Evolutionary comparisons of the S segments in the genomes of herpes simplex virus type 1 and varicella-zoster virus. *J. Gen. Virol.* 67:597 (1986).

30. J.M. Ostrove, Molecular biology of varicella zoster virus. *Adv. Virus Res.* 38:45 (1990).

31. C.F. Kallander, Gronowitz, J.S., and Torfason, E.G., Human serum antibodies to varicella-zoster virus thymidine kinase. *Infect. Immun.* 36:30 (1982).

32. T. Ozaki, Matsui, Y., Asano, Y., et al., Study of virus isolation from pharyngeal swabs in children with varicella. *Am. J. Dis. Child.* 143:1448 (1989).

33. T. Ozaki, Miwata, H., Matsui, Y., et al., Varicella zoster virus DNA in throat swabs [see comments]. *Arch. Dis. Child.* 66: 333 (1991).

34. S. Kido, Ozaki, T., Asada, H., et al., Detection of varicella-zoster virus (VZV) DNA in clinical samples from patients with VZV by the polymerase chain reaction [see comments]. *J. Clin. Microbiol.* 29:76 (1991).

35. Y. Asano, Itakura, N., Hiroishi, Y., et al., Viremia is present in incubation period in nonimmunocompromised children with varicella. *J. Pediatr.* 106:69 (1985).

36. T. Ozaki, Ichikawa, T., Matsui, Y., et al., Lymphocyte-associated viremia in varicella. *J. Med. Virol.* 19:249 (1986).

37. S. Feldman, and Epp, E., Detection of viremia during incubation of varicella. *J. Pediatr.* 94:746 (1979).

38. K.D. Croen, Ostrove, J.M., Dragovic, L.J., and Straus, S.E., Patterns of gene expression and sites of latency in human nerve ganglia are different for varicella-zoster and herpes simplex viruses. *Proc. Natl. Acad. Sci. (USA)* 85:9773 (1988).

39. B. Gilchrest, and Baden, H.P., Photodistribution of viral exanthems. *Pediatrics* 54:136 (1974).

40. D.H. Gilden, Hayward, A.R., Krupp, J., et al., Varicella-zoster virus infection of human mononuclear cells. *Virus Res.* 7:117 (1987).

41. M.G. Myers, Viremia caused by varicella-zoster virus: association with malignant progressive varicella. *J. Infect. Dis.* 140:229 (1979).

42. H. Shibuta, Ishikawa, T., Hondo, R., et al., Varicella virus isolation from spinal ganglion. *Arch. Gesamte Virusforsch* 45:382 (1974).

43. K. Nagashima, Nakazawa, M., and Endo, H., Pathology of the human spinal ganglia in varicella-zoster virus infection. *Acta Neuropathol. (Berl)* 33:105 (1975).

44. M.R. Mayberg, Zervas, N.T., and Moskowitz, M.A., Trigeminal projections to supratentorial pial and dural blood vessels in cats demonstrated by horseradish peroxidase histochemistry. *J. Comp. Neurol.* 223:46 (1984).

45. D.H. Gilden, Devlin, M., Wellish, M., et al., Persistence of varicella-zoster virus DNA in blood mononuclear cells of patients with varicella or zoster. *Virus Genes* 2:299 (1989).

46. M.E. Devlin, Gilden, D.H., Mahalingam, R., et al., Peripheral blood mononuclear cells of the elderly contain varicella-zoster virus DNA. *J. Infect. Dis.* 165:619 (1992).

47. K.G. Warren, Devlin, M., Gilden, D.H., et al., Herpes simplex virus latency in patients with multiple sclerosis, lymphoma and normal humans. In, *Oncogenesis and Herpesviruses III, Part 2: Cell-Virus Interactions, Host Response to Herpesvirus Infection and Associated Tumors, Role of Co-Factors.* Vol. 24, G. De-The, Henle, W., Rapp, R., eds., International Agency for Research in Cancer, Lyon (1978).

48. S.A. Plotkin, Stein, S., Snyder, M., and Immesoete, P., Attempts to recover varicella virus from ganglia. *Ann. Neurol.* 2:249 (1977).

49. K.D. Croen, and Straus, S.E., Varicella-zoster virus latency. *Annu. Rev. Microbiol.* 45:265 (1991).

50. D.H. Gilden, Vafai, A., Shtram, Y., et al., Varicella-zoster virus DNA in human sensory ganglia. *Nature* 306:478 (1983).

51. R.W. Hyman, Ecker, J.R., and Tenser, R.B., Varicella-zoster virus RNA in human trigeminal ganglia. *Lancet* 2:814 (1983).

52. R. Mahalingam, Wellish, M., Wolf, W., et al., Latent varicella-zoster viral DNA in human trigeminal and thoracic ganglia. *N. Engl. J. Med.* 323:627 (1990).

53. R. Mahalingam, Wellish, M.C., Dueland, A.N., et al., Localization of herpes simplex virus and varicella zoster virus DNA in human ganglia. *Ann. Neurol.* 31:444 (1992).

54. A. Mafai, Murray, R.S., Wellish, M., et al., Expression of varicella-zoster virus and herpes simplex virus in normal human trigeminal ganglia. *Proc. Natl. Acad. Sci. (USA)* 85:2362 (1988).

55. R.B. Tenser, and Hyman, R.W., Latent herpesvirus infections of neurons in guinea pigs and humans. *Yale J. Biol. Med.* 60:159 (1987).

56. D.H. Gilden, Rozenman, Y., Murray, R., et al., Detection of varicella-zoster virus nucleic acid in neurons of normal human thoracic ganglia. *Ann. Neurol.* 22:377 (1987).

57. R. Cohrs, Mahalingam, R., Dueland, A.N., et al., Restricted transcription of varicella-zoster virus in latently infected human trigeminal and thoracic ganglia. *J. Infect. Dis.* 166:S24 (1992).

58. K.D. Croen, Ostrove, J.M., Reinhold, W.C., et al., Different sites of latency of herpes simplex virus and varicella-zoster virus in human trigeminal ganglia as defined by in-situ hybridization. *Proceedings of the 12th International Herpesvirus Workshop* (1987).

59. M.E. Lewis, Leung, W.C., Jeffrey, V.M., and Warren, K.G., Detection of multiple strains of latent herpes simplex virus type 1 within individual human hosts. *J. Virol.* 52:300 (1984).

60. L.D. Gelb, Dohner, D.E., Gershon, A.A., et al.,. Molecular epidemiology of live, attenuated varicella virus vaccine in children with leukemia and in normal adults. *J. Infect. Dis.* 155:633 (1987).

61. S.E. Straus, Clinical and biological differences between recurrent herpes simplex virus and varicella-zoster virus infections [clinical conference]. *J.A.M.A.* 262:3455 (1989).

62. E. Somekh, Tedder, D.G., Vafai, A., et al., Latency of varicella-zoster virus in vitro in cells derived from human fetal dorsal root ganglia (abstract 779). *Program and abstracts of the 31st Interscience Conference on Antimicrobial Agents and Chemotherapy (Chicago).* American Society of Microbiology, Washington, D.C. (1991).

63. B. Wigdahl, Rong, B.L., and Kinney-Thomas, E., Varicella-zoster virus infection of human sensory neurons. *Virology* 152:384 (1986).

64. M.P. Merville-Louis, Sadzot-Delvaux, C., Delree, P., et al., Varicella-zoster virus infection of adult rat sensory neurons *in vitro. J. Virol.* 63:3155 (1989).

65. J.L. Meier, and Straus, S.E., Comparative biology of latent varicella-zoster virus and herpes simplex virus infections. *J. Infect. Dis.* 166:S13 (1992).

66. P.A. Brunell, Novelli, V.M., Keller, P.M., and Ellis, R.W., Antibodies to the three major glycoproteins of varicella-zoster virus: search for the relevant host immune response. *J. Infect. Dis.* 156:430 (1987).

67. M. Larkin, Heckels, J.E., and Ogilvie, M.M., Antibody response to varicella-zoster virus surface glycoproteins in chickenpox and shingles. *J. Gen. Virol.* 66:1785 (1985).

68. O. Baadsgaard, Lindskov, R., and Geisler, C., Reduction of the number of immunocompetent cells in the acute stage of herpes zoster. *Arch. Dermatol. Res.* 279:374 (1987).

69. A.R. Hayward, and Herberger, M., Lymphocyte responses to varicella zoster virus in the elderly. *J. Clin. Immunol.* 7:174 (1987).

70. G.W. Jordan, and Merigan, T.C., Cell-mediated immunity to varicella-zoster virus: *in vitro* lymphocyte responses. *J. Infect. Dis.* 130:495 (1974).

71. M.E. Weksler, Immune senescence. *Ann. Neurol.* 35:S35 (1994).

72. A.E. Miller, Selective decline in cellular immune response to varicella-zoster in the elderly. *Neurology* 30:582 (1980).

73. A.M. Arvin, Cell-mediated immunity to varicella-zoster virus. *J. Infect. Dis.* 166:S35 (1992).

74. B.L. Burke, Steele, R.W., Beard, O.W., et al., Immune responses to varicella-zoster in the aged. *Arch. Intern. Med.* 142:291 (1982).

75. R. Berger, Florent, G., and Just, M., Decrease of the lymphoproliferative response to varicella-zoster virus antigen in the aged. *Infect. Immun.* 32:24 (1981).

76. A.A. Gershon, and Steinberg, S.P., Antibody responses to varicella-zoster virus and the role of antibody in host defense. *Am. J. Med. Sci.* 282:12 (1981).

77. A.M. Arvin, Kushner, J.H., Feldman, S., et al., Human leukocyte interferon for the treatment of varicella in children with cancer. *N. Engl. J. Med.* 306:761 (1982).

78. D.H. Gilden, Mahalingam, R., Dueland, A.N., and Cohrs, R., Herpes zoster: pathogenesis and latency. *Prog. Med. Virol.* 39:19 (1982).

79. G. Oberg, and Svedmyr, A., Varicelliform eruptions in herpes zoster--some clinical and serological observations. *Scand. J. Infect. Dis.* 1:47 (1969).

80. R.J. Whitley, Varicella-zoster virus infections. In, *Antiviral agents and viral diseases of man.* G.J. Galasso, Whitley, R.J., and Merigan, T.C., eds., Raven Press, New York (1990).

81. D.H. Gilden, Dueland, A.N., Devlin, M.E., et al., Varicella-zoster virus reactivation without rash. *J. Infect. Dis.* 166:S30 (1992).

82. A. Wilson, Sharp, M., Koropchak, C.M., et al., Subclinical varicella-zoster virus viremia, herpes zoster, and T lymphocyte immunity to varicella-zoster viral antigens after bone marrow transplantation. *J. Infect. Dis.* 165:119 (1992).

83. P. Ljungman, Lonnqvist, B., Gahrton, G., et al., Clinical and subclinical reactivations of varicella-zoster virus in immunocompromised patients. *J. Infect. Dis.* 153:840 (1986).

84. A.M. Arvin, Koropchak, C.M., and Wittek, A.E., Immunologic evidence of reinfection with varicella-zoster virus. *J. Infect. Dis.* 148:200 (1983).

85. A.A. Gershon, Steinberg, S.P., and Gelb, L., Clinical reinfection with varicella-zoster virus. *J. Infect. Dis.* 149:137 (1984).

86. K.A. Weigle, and Grose, C., Molecular dissection of the humoral immune response to individual varicella-zoster viral proteins during chickenpox, quiescence, reinfection, and reactivation. *J. Infect. Dis.* 149:741 (1984).

87. A. Hayward, Levin, M., Wolf, W., et al., Varicella-zoster virus-specific immunity after herpes zoster. *J. Infect. Dis.* 163:873 (1991).

88. J.P. Luby, Ramirez-Ronda, C., Rinner, S., et al., A longitudinal study of varicella-zoster virus infections in renal transplant recipients. *J. Infect. Dis.* 135:659 (1977).

89. S. Schimpff, Serpick, A., Stoler, B., et al., Varicella-zoster infection in patients with cancer. *Ann. Intern. Med.* 76:241 (1972).

90. M.W. Ragozzino, Melton, L,J., Kurland, L.T., et al., Risk of cancer after herpes zoster: a population-based study. *N. Engl. J. Med.* 307:393 (1982).

91. D. Pavan-Langston, and Dunkel, E.C., Ocular varicella-zoster virus infection in the guinea pig. A new *in vivo* model. *Arch. Ophthalmol.* 107:1068 (1989).

92. M.G. Myers, and Connelly, B.L., Animal models of varicella. *J. Infect. Dis.* 166:S48 (1992).

93. W.L. Gray, and Oakes, J.E., Simian varicella virus DNA shares homology with human varicella-zoster virus DNA. *Virology* 136:241 (1984).
94. R. Mahalingam, Smith, D., Wellish, M., et al., Simian varicella virus DNA in dorsal root ganglia. *Proc. Natl. Acad. Sci. (USA)* 88:2750 (1991).
95. G.J. Bennett, Hypotheses on the pathogenesis of herpes zoster-associated pain. *Ann. Neurol.* 35:S38 (1994).
96. A.K. Asbury, and Fields, H.L., Pain due to peripheral nerve damage: an hypothesis. *Neurology* 34:1587 (1984).
97. C.J. Woolf, Recent advances in the pathophysiology of acute pain [comment]. *Br. J. Anaesth.* 63:139 (1989).
98. M.C. Rowbotham, and Fields, H.L., Post-herpetic neuralgia: the relation of pain complaint, sensory disturbance, and skin temperature. *Pain* 39:129 (1989).
99. B.S. Galer, and Portenoy, R.K., Acute herpetic and postherpetic neuralgia: clinical features and management. *Mt. Sinai. J. Med.* 58:257 (1991).
100. M.A. Cline, Ochoa, J., and Torebjork, H.E., Chronic hyperalgesia and skin warming caused by sensitized C nociceptors. *Brain* 112:621 (1989).
101. M.C. Rowbotham, Topical agents for post-herpetic neuralgia. In: *Herpes zoster and postherpetic neuralgia,* Watson, C.P.N., ed., Elsevier, Amsterdam (1993).
102. R.K. Portenoy, Duma, C., and Foley, K.M., Acute herpetic and postherpetic neuralgia: clinical review and current management. *Ann. Neurol.* 20:651 (1986).
103. P.N. Watson, and Evans, R.J., Postherpetic neuralgia. A review. *Arch. Neurol.* 43:836 (1986).
104. C.P.N. Watson, and Deck, J.H., The neuropathology of herpes zoster with particular reference to postherpetic neuralgia and its pathogenesis. In: *Herpes zoster and postherpetic neuralgia. Pain research and clinical management. Vol. 8.* C.P.N. Watson, ed., Elsevier, Amsterdam (1993).
105. R.H. Gracely, Lynch, S.A., and Bennett, G.J., Painful neuropathy: altered central processing maintained dynamically by peripheral input [published erratum appears in *Pain* 1993 Feb; 52(2):251–3] [see comments]. *Pain* 51:175 (1992).
106. A. Vafai, Wellish, M., and Gilden, D.H., Expression of varicella-zoster virus in blood mononuclear cells of patients with postherpetic neuralgia. *Proc. Natl. Acad. Sci. (USA)* 85:2767 (1988).
107. D.H. Gilden., Herpes zoster with postherpetic neuralgia--persisting pain and frustration [editorial; comment]. *N. Engl. J. Med.* 330:932 (1994).
108. H.H. Balfour, Jr., Varicella zoster virus infections in immunocompromised hosts. A review of the natural history and management. *Am. J. Med.* 85:68 (1988).
109. S.P. Harding, Lipton, J.R., and Wells, J.C., Natural history of herpes zoster ophthalmicus: predictors of postherpetic neuralgia and ocular involvement. *Br. J. Ophthalmol.* 71:353 (1987).
110. Anonymous. Guidelines for the management of shingles. report of a working group of the British Society for the Study of Infection (BSSI). *J. Infect. Dis.* 30:193 (1995).

SECTION VII: MICROBIAL KERATITIS—VIRAL

Abstracts of Other Conference Presentations and Posters

HERPES SIMPLEX VIRUS LATENCY AND RECURRENCE

D.L. Easty,[1] C. Shimeld,[1] J. Whiteland,[1] S. M. Nicholls,[1] and T. J. Hill[2]

[1]Department of Ophthalmology, Bristol Eye Hospital, UK and [2]Department of Pathology and Microbiology, University of Bristol, UK

Purpose: To study HSV-1 reactivation and recurrent disease in mice. **Methods:** We have made quantitative observations *in situ* on the immunological events in the cornea during the development of recurrent corneal disease induced by UV irradiation of latently infected mice. Eyes with such disease were examined by immunohistochemistry using monoclonal antibodies to identity mouse immune cells and a polyclonal antibody to detect virus antigen. **Results:** On day 4, virus antigens were seen in the corneal epithelium of all mice, and in some animals antigens were also present in the iris and/or the conjunctival epithelium. The number of foci of infection ranged from 1–5. At this time, granulocytes were the predominant infiltrating cells; they were present throughout the corneas with large numbers associated with epithelial lesions. By day 7, in some corneas, ulcers had healed and associated stromal disease was limited to slight focal oedema and/or cellular infiltration(mild disease). In others, ulcers remained and stromal disease was severe with opacification and vessel ingress. On day 7, in corneas with mild disease there was a significant infiltrate of T cells and granulocytes were rare. In contrast, T cells were sparse in corneas with severe disease and large number of granulocytes were still present. These differences persisted until at least day 10. **Conclusions:** We have shown considerable variation in the amount of antigen in eyes with recurrent disease which may influence the magnitude of the immune response. The early presence of granulocytes, suggests that these cells play a role in initial clearance of virus. In this method, the severity of immunopathology is associated with the continued presence of large numbers of granulocytes rather than T cells. In addition we have shown that the surgical trauma of corneal grafting appears to be the most potent stimulus of recurrent disease after transplantation. Virus occasionally recurs in the recipient epithelium, but does not penetrate the basement membrane to the stroma. The graft-host junction appears to be a 'weak spot' where antigen readily reaches the stroma, perhaps, from nerve endings severed in the operation. Infiltrating cells then act as a conduit to the endothelium, which may become infected and prejudice the graft.

CLINICAL PRESENTATION OF OCULAR HERPES SIMPLEX INFECTION

Andrew Tullo

The cardinal features of ocular herpes simplex were well described long before the discovery of the causative agent in the 1920's. Despite many years of shared clinical experience it could be argued that we have made limited progress in managing clinical manifestations despite a vastly improved knowledge of herpes simplex virus (HSV). We still rely heavily on clinical signs for diagnosis. We do not know if the epidemiology of herpes simplex keratitis (HSK) is changing significantly. We recognise several influential host factors including the fact that HSK is more common in men than women, but do not know why. We understand the ability of HSV to establish latent infection in sensory neurones and possibly the cornea, but have as yet been unable to use this knowledge in prevention of disease. We acknowledge the importance of the immune system in pathogenesis but do not yet know how to best manipulate it. Topical steroids have been, and still are used inappropriately, and antiviral agents have their limitations. We are now faced with new information from molecular biological techniques which demonstrate viral DNA where we do and do not expect it. By acknowledging our limitations this may further stimulate application of laboratory knowledge in coping with HSK which continues to present a major challenge in management.

HSV: CLINICAL TRIALS

C. Dawson

The Herpetic Eye Disease Study (HEDS) addresses problems in the management of ocular herpes simplex virus infections. The HEDS trials are randomized, masked and placebo controlled. They include three therapeutic and two preventive trials, and a study of factors triggering HSV ocular recurrences.

One completed HEDS therapeutic trial compared topical corticosteroid to placebo for patients with HSV stromal keratitis who also received prophylactic trifluridine drops. In this trial, the 10 week tapering course of topical corticosteroid drops was significantly better than placebo in reducing the progression or persistence of HSV stromal keratitis and shortening its duration. However, 22% of patients (11/49) on placebo also resolved during the 16 week course of the trial.

A second HEDS therapeutic trial compared 10 weeks of oral acyclovir (200 mg capsules) to placebo (2 capsules 5 times daily) for patients with herpetic stromal keratitis receiving a 10 week tapering course of corticosteroid and trifluridine drops. In this trial there was no beneficial effect of acyclovir.

Recruitment is still in progress for a trial of oral acyclovir or placebo (2 capsules twice daily) for one year to prevent HSV ocular recurrences. Patients in this trial may also enter a study on the risk factors for ocular HSV recurrences.

Other HEDS trials include a therapeutic study of oral acyclovir or placebo for steroidtrifluridine treated HSV iridocyclitis which is currently in press. Recruitment has also stopped in another HEDS trial comparing oral acyclovir to placebo capsules for trifluridine treated HSV epithelial keratitis to prevent subsequent stromal keratitis or iridocyclitis. Follow-up visits are still under way in this trial.

PREVENTION OF RECURRENT HSV KERATITIS

Herbert E Kaufman, Bryan M. Gebhardt, Emily D. Varnell, and James M. Hill

Louisiana State University Eye Center, New Orleans, Louisiana

In genital and labial herpes simplex virus, multiplication of the virus at the muco-cutaneous surface occurs and is necessary for viral pathology. Several studies have demonstrated that drugs such as acyclovir are effective in preventing recurrences of genital and labial HSV. The significant differences between infections at these sites and ocular HSV infection is that minimal to no viral replication is necessary for recrudescent disease on the ocular surface. Acyclovir is relatively ineffective in preventing ocular recurrences, probably because viral replication takes place in the distant nervous reservoir and infectious particles are transported to the ocular surface to set up the secondary infection. Recent studies in our laboratories have revealed that the beta adrenergic blocking agent, propranolol, can prevent viral reactivation in heat-stressed mice. We found that there was a statistically significant lower incidence of ocular shedding of virus in animals treated with propranolol as compared to those treated with placebo. In another series of experiments, we have also shown that recently identified inhibitors of viral thymidine kinase can also prevent viral reactivation in the trigeminal ganglion of heat-stressed mice. In a series of comparative experiments, we found that acyclovir is ineffective at preventing ganglionic viral reactivation in this mouse model. We believe that these results support our hypothesis that ganglionic reactivation is not prevented by acyclovir because the number of viral particles reaching the ocular surface are adequate to cause recurrent disease. On the other hand, it appears that pharmacologic intervention, such as with the use of beta adrenergic receptor blockers, may be an effective, new approach to preventing viral reactivation in the nervous system.

BRIDGING THE GAP BETWEEN THE BIOLOGY AND THE CLINICAL DISEASES OF VARICELLA ZOSTER VIRUS

Paul R. Kinchington

Department of Ophthalmology, University of Pittsburgh, Pittsburgh, Pennsylvania

Herpes Zoster Ophthalmicus (HZO) and most of the clinical manifestations caused by Varicella Zoster Virus (VZV) are well-documented and for the most part are readily recognizable in the clinic and are straightforward to diagnose. The diseases caused by this member of the herpesvirus family is largely seen in two phases of life; either as a consequence of a primary infection, which most often occurs during childhood, or as a result of virus which has reacted from a dormant or latent state within the host. Disease from this reactivated virus is usually seen in late adulthood and the retired population. The importance of Zoster and its complications have recently been highlighted by the AIDS epidemic and the increased use of immunosuppression, because zoster incidence increases dramatically in such individuals.

In contrast to a well characterized and comprehensive clinical picture of VZV disease, considerably less is understood about the biology of the virus itself. VZV has remained quite refractory to growth outside the human host, despite the effort of many researchers and virologists. In particular, very little is known of the virus in its dormant state, and current knowledge is conflicting and controversial. Only recently, largely through the application of the techniques of molecular biology, have we begun to understand in depth the fundamental events of the viral growth cycle during the acute, or active state of infection. This knowledge is a vital prerequisite for the design of new drugs to combat the diseases caused by this virus; it is also essential to understand how the virus can be combated in both the quiescent and active states of growth in the human.

In this short talk, I will highlight recent advances in specific areas of VZV biology which may impact upon the physician and the treatment and management of VZV disease.

EXTERNAL OCULAR EPSTEIN-BARR VIRUS (EBV) INFECTION

Stephen C. Pflugfelder

Bascom Palmer Eye Institute, University of Miami School of Medicine

Epstein-Ban virus (EBV) is a ubiquitous virus that infects the majority of humans by early adulthood. Similar to other herpesviruses, it has a lifecycle consisting of latent and replicative (lytic) phases. Two types of latent EBV infections have been identified: 1) active latent infection with transcription of EBV oncoproteins that transform (or immortalize) B cells into lymphoblasts, 2) passive latent infection that is typically utilized by the virus after infecting small resting B cells during which transcription of only one gene (EDNA-1) has been identified. Lytic infection occurs most commonly in mucosal epithelial cells that shed infectious virus. EBV was initially observed in biopsies of Burkitt's lymphoma, a neoplasia that occurs predominantly in children in certain tropical regions of Africa. EBV was subsequently found to be the agent responsible for infectious mononucleosis (IM), a common febrile illness. EBV has also been detected in other human neoplasias including nasopharyngeal carcinoma, thymic carcinoma, Hodgkin's disease, oral hairy leukoplakia, and B-cell lymphoproliferation in allograft recipients receiving immunosuppressive therapy.

There is increasing clinical and laboratory evidence suggesting that EBV is capable of infecting ocular surface epithelial cells. Expression of CD21, the putative EBV receptor, has been detected in conjunctival and corneal epithelial cells. EBV genomic sequences have been detected in normal human conjunctiva and corneal epithelium. Numerous cases of conjunctivitis and keratitis have been reported in patients with IM syndrome. EBV can cause dendritic epithelial keratitis, although stromal keratitis is the more common form observed clinically. Among the twelve reported cases of EBV stromal keratitis, there appears to be thee distinct morphologic patterns of the corneal lesions. Subepithelial infiltrates (type 1) most closely resemble those of adenovirus epidemic keratoconjunctivitis. Anterior-to-mid stromal opacities (type II) occur in two forms: small, granular, circular or ring-shaped opacities with minimal associated inflammation, or larger, blotchy, pleomorphic infiltrates with active inflammation. Full-thickness or deep stromal keratitis (type III) Is pleomorphic and blotchy, predominantly it involves the deep peripheral cornea, and may mimic luetic interstitial keratitis, or when unilateral, HSV stromal keratitis, direct and indirect evidence has been reported that EBV plays a pathogenic role in the lacrimal gland pathology of Sjögrens Syndrome. EBV may persist in a latent non-pathogenic form in a small percentage of normal lacrimal glands. EBV genomes, and antigens (both active latent and lytic) have been detected in residual glandular epithelial cells and the mononuclear cells infiltrating Sjögrens Syndrome lacrimal glands. EBV genomes have been detected in 80% of tear samples obtained from Sjögrens Syndrome patients suggesting that this virus may be shed from the diseased lacrimal glands onto the ocular surface. The efficacy of anti-viral therapy for ocular EBV infection has not been established. It is likely that some of the ocular inflammatory conditions observed in patients with acute EBV infection, such as stromal keratitis and uveitis, are due to inflammation insighted by the virus rather than active viral replication. Corticosteroid therapy either alone, or in combination with acyclovir. has been reported to be effective in these conditions, and may be considered for severe ocular inflammation.

RECENT ADVANCES IN THE PATHOGENESIS AND TREATMENT OF ADENOVIRUS OCULAR INFECTIONS

Jerold Gorden

University of Pittsburgh, Pittsburgh, Pennsylvania

Adenovirus ocular infections are the most common external ocular infections that occur worldwide. They are usually characterized by epidemics in the community and medical facilities. Although not blinding, ocular morbidity is significant for the affected individual and the broader economic ramifications in ophthalmology, business, education, and military preparedness are considerable. Recent advances in the molecular virology of adenoviridae will be presented. An understanding of the pathogenesis of adenovirus ocular infection has been advanced through the successful development on animal models that mimic human infection. The role of differences in adenovirus serotype and isolate virulence will be considered in terms of host specificity and clinical infections. Risk factors for the transmission of adenovirus within the ophthalmologist's office will be reviewed and appropriate recommendations made. Evaluation of current diagnostic tests including culture, enzyme immune assay, and PCR will be presented. Important advances in the development of specific antiviral agents for the treatment of adenovirus ocular infections (e.g., cidofovir) will be reviewed including the results of recent animal studies and the current status of clinical trials.

CORNEAL IMPRESSION TESTING FOR THE DIAGNOSIS OF RABIES

Andrew Billingsley and Gerald W. Zaidman

Department of Ophthalmology; Westchester County Medical Center New York Medical, College, Valhalla, New York

The antemortem diagnosis of rabies is very difficult. A confirmed diagnosis of rabies is usually obtained late in the disease or by post mortem brain biopsy. Once symptoms appear the disease is usually fatal. Therefore early diagnosis is important. Early diagnosis allows isolation of infected patients. Also post exposure treatment (with human rabies immune globulin and human diploid cell vaccine) has been effective in preventing the disease if applied very soon after exposure.

A 13 year old girl was admitted with signs of acute encephalitis of unknown etiology. Viral and bacterial cultures and fluorescent antibody testing of the blood, spinal fluid and saliva as well as testing for Lyme's disease and toxoplasmosis were negative. A skin biopsy from the nape of the neck was negative. Corneal impressions were taken four days after admission. Standard glass microscope slides were gently applied to the cornea until an impression was obtained. The slides were air dried and fixed with acetone. Fluorescent antibody testing of the smear (and two additional smears taken 2 days later) were positive for rabies. Subsequently the diagnosis was confirmed by serum serology and skin biopsy.

This case demonstrates that corneal smears can help in the diagnosis of acute rabies encephalitis. They should be part of the routine antemortem workup for presumptive rabies.

MAINTENANCE OF DNA FROM A REPLICATION-DEFICIENT HERPES SIMPLEX VIRUS IN CORNEAL KERATOCYTES

W.J. O'Brien and J.L. Taylor

Departments of Ophthalmology and Microbiology, Medical College of Wisconsin, Milwaukee, Wisconsin

The discovery of herpes simplex virus (HSV) DNA in corneal cells during asymptomatic periods, long after acute disease has resolved, suggests that replication deficient virus may be suitable as a vector for gene delivery to corneal cells and other cells of the eye. The aim of these studies was to determine the stability and configuration of viral DNA delivered to cells by the replication-deficient mutant of HSV-1 KOS strain, 5dl1.2. This virus possesses a deletion in the gene encoding infected cell protein 27 (ICP27), a gene of the immediate early class reported to be required for virus replication (McCarthy et al, J. Virol. 63: 18, 1989). In order to evaluate the stability and structure of the viral DNA, cultures of Vero cells, cornea stromal cells, and retinal pigment epithelia cells were infected at various multiplicities with HSV 5dl1.2. At various times after infection, cultures were observed and cells were harvested. Viral DNA was analyzed by embedding infected cells in agarose rods which were digested with proteinase K and detergents. Slices of the agarose containing embedded DNA were subjected to pulsed-field electrophoresis to separate linear DNA from circular and other replicative intermediate DNA forms. DNA structure was analyzed by the use of rare-cutting restriction endonucleases. Viral DNA was detected by *in situ* hybridization using HSV-specific probes and by amplification using the polymerase chain reaction (PCR). The synthesis of various classes of viral proteins was analyzed by immunoblots of infected cell lysates. In control cells, Vero 3.3, a cell line stably transformed to express HSV-1 ICP27, the replication-deficient virus replicated to titers of 10^7 pfu/ml, expressed a full compliment of viral proteins, and replicated DNA, generating mature, linear 150 kb genome as well as replicative intermediate forms. Based on digestion with the endonuclease, Spe I, the mature genome consisted of the usual four isoforms. In wild type Vero cells virus replication was reduced by $\geq 10^6$. Viral DNA persisted in the form of a replicative intermediate. In the absence of the production of detectable virus, viral DNA was detectable after 20 days and 5 passages by PCR. A dominate viral protein, ICP8, was detectable on immunoblots for 19 days. In corneal stromal cells the virus and viral DNA persisted in a manner similar to Vero cells. Viral DNA remained as a replicative intermediate after entering the cell. Surprisingly, a second eye-derived cell, the retinal pigment epithelium did support replication of the virus deletion mutant as evidenced by production of infectious progeny and production of viral proteins and unit length viral genome. These studies demonstrate several issues regarding gene delivery: (i) it cannot be assumed that the replication incompetence of a particular mutant virus is universal, (ii) viral DNA may persist in cells in the form of a replicative intermediate for extended periods, (iii) selected viral genes may be expressed despite the inability of virus to replicate, and (iv) HSV that is replication-deficient in corneal cells can deliver viral genes to corneal cells.

EFFECT OF GLYCOPROTEIN D₂ VACCINATION ON ACUTE AND RECURRENT OCULAR HSV-1 INFECTION

J.S. Pepose,[1] K.A. Laycock,[1] J.K. Miller,[1] K.K. Hook,[1] E.D. Fenoglio,[1] M. Francotte,[2] M. Slaoui,[2] P.M. Stuart,[1] and T.L. Keadle[1]

[1]Department of Ophthalmology and Visual Sciences, Washington University, St. Louis, MO and [2]SmithKline Beecham Biologicals, Rixensart Belgium

Purpose: To compare the prophylactic and therapeutic efficacy of herpes simpler virus type 2 (HSV-2) glycoprotein D (gD_2) vaccines in a mouse model of recurrent ocular HSV-1 infection. **Methods:** Vaccinations consisted of gD_2 in alum, gD_2 in alum/3DMPL, adjuvant or saline. In prophylactic studies, the corneas of vaccinated and control mice were inoculated with HSV-1 McKrae. In therapeutic studies, mice with preexisting latent ocular HSV-1 infection and mock infected controls were infected with gD_2 vaccines, adjuvant or saline. Corneal opacity, mortality, virus titers, latency, and reactivation rates were determined at time points before and after vaccination/infection and ultraviolet-B (UV-B)- induced recurrent ocular virus shedding. **Results:** Prophylactically, gD_2 alum and gD_2 alum/3DMPL vaccines decreased acute disease severity and mortality Only gD_2 alum/3DMPL vaccination resulted in significant reductions in latency, UV-B induced virus reactivation, and post reactivation disease. Therapeutically, gD_2 vaccination decreased the number of days recurrent viral shedding was detected. **Conclusions:** Whereas gD_2 vaccination was protective when administered prior to infection, its effects on reactivated latent ocular infections in mice was limited to reduced length of viral shedding, with no effect on subsequent ocular disease. These disparate findings underlie the need to evaluate herpes vaccines in models of both primary and recurrent ocular herpetic stromal keratitis, so that valid independent conclusions about their prophylactic and therapeutic value can be reached.

PENETRATING KERATOPLASTY FOR ACUTE PERFORATIONS IN HERPETIC KERATITIS

Ramón Naranjo-Tackman

Cornea Department, Asociación Para Evitar la Ceguera en México, México, D.F.

Purpose: The evaluation of clinical outcome of cases that underwent Penetrating Keratoplasty (PK) for recently perforated herpetic keratitis.

Methods: The retrospective evaluation of cases with active Herpetic Keratitis (HK), that evolved to corneal perforation, was done. Visual outcome, graft evolution as well as postoperative complications, were evaluated.

Results: The files of 13 cases: 13 eyes of 13 patients, were reviewed. Males were predominant in 62% of cases, with a mean age of 23.6 years of age (Range: 9 to 52 years). Right eyes were more affected than the left eye in 61% of cases. In 11 cases there was a history of recurrent herpetic keratitis, the average time of evolution of the herpetic disease since the first attack to the perforation, was 7.5 years, with a mean rate of recurrences of 3 episodes. Only 2 cases (15.38%) were reported as the initial episode, an both cases were associated with the use of topical steroids. In 11 cases (84.62%),perforation was central, for an average of 11 days before PK. Stains and cultures routinely practiced showed only saprophitic flora in all 13 cases.

In all cases a penetrating keratoplasty was performed, the size of grafts, varied from 6.5 to 9.0 mm in diameter. Only interrupted sutures were used. No associated surgical procedure other than anterior iris synechia liberation were performed. Postop treatment consisted in topical steroids and topical antiviral ointment (Ophthalmic acyclovir ointment), for a mean 11 months period. Post-op follow-up, ranged from 14 months to 4 years. Preop vision ranged from Light perception to count fingers, after surgery it improved In 10 eyes (BCVA:20/40 or better in 3 eyes)

Main complications were: Glaucoma 30.7%, Uncontrolled graft rejection: 23%, Cataract: 23%, Vascularization 38%. Recurrent herpetic ulcers in the graft: 2 eyes (15.38%).

Conclusions: Most of cases evolved after multiple recurrences. The main predisposing factor was topical steroids, specially in new cases. Main complications of the Grafts were the same as reported in other series, however results are encouraging, specially after long follow-up, with sustained combined steroid, antiviral therapy.

DE NOVO HERPES SIMPLEX VIRUS KERATITIS AFTER PENETRATING KERATOPLASTY

L. Remeijer, P. Doornenbal, A.J.M. Geerards, W.J. Rijneveld, and W.H. Beekhuis

Cornea and External Eye Disease Service; Eye Hospital Rotterdam; Rotterdam, The Netherlands

Background: In corneal transplantation for diagnoses not related to Herpes Simplex Virus(HSV) keratitis there is not always suspicion of an HSV infection in the case of nonspecific epithelial defects. The purpose of this study was to determine the incidence of "De Novo Herpetic Keratitis" after penetrating keratoplasty and to analyse possible factors contributing to this clinical entity.

Methods: We retrospectively studied the medical records of our group of patients transplanted in the period from January 1980 to January 1995.Factors related to the operation and possible reactivating stimuli were recorded.

Results: From 1980 to 1995 a group of 18 patients presented with epithelial herpetic keratitis in their corneal graft whereas the primary diagnosis was not related to HSV keratitis. The incidence of "De Novo Herpetic Keratitis" is 1,2 per 1000 person years. In most cases the infection occurs in the first two years after the operation and in the majority of cases known reactivating stimuli could have caused the HSV infection.

Conclusions: Herpes simplex virus keratitis can occur in penetrating keratoplasty even in the absence of a clinical history of HSV in the host. The high incidence of this clinical picture and the frequent occurrence of the infection in the first two years after the operation strongly indicates a relation between the corneal transplantation and the presentation of the infection.

DETECTION OF HERPES SIMPLEX VIRUS GENOMES IN TEARS FROM PATIENTS AFTER PENETRATING KERATOPLASTY USING POLYMERASE CHAIN REACTION

M. Tei, K. Nishida, T. Sasagawa, W. Adachi, and S. Kinoshita

Department of Ophthalmology; Kyoto Prefectural University of Medicine, Kyoto, Japan

Purpose: Diagnosis of recurrent herpetic epithelial keratitis after penetrating keratoplasty (PKP) is considered to be difficult, since many factors such as steroid administration, insufficient innervation in the graft modify ocular surface appearance. In diagnosing the herpetic epithelial keratitis mentioned above, polymerase chain reaction (PCR) method may be effective and swift, in comparison with viral culture, immunofluorescence, and serum antiboby. In the present study, we investigated the efficacy of PCR method in diagnosing HSV-suspected epithelial keratitis in patients after PKP for herpetic stromal keratitis.

Methods: Three eyes of 3 patients showed epithelial keratitis characteristic of large geographic-shaped ulcer located at host-graft border, weak ciliary injection and a little epithelial infiltration at the edge of the ulcer. Tears were collected by Schirmer's strips from these 3 patients and 3 eyes of 3 patients without recurrent HSV keratitis after PKP served as control. DNA was extracted and submitted to PCR. Subsequently, Southern blot hybridization was performed to determine herpes simplex genomes.

Results: Using PCR, we identified HSV DNA in 3 eyes (100%) of HSV-suspected epithelial keratitis, but not in control eyes.

Conclusions: The results indicate that PCR is an effective and swift method to diagnose possible herpetic epithelial keratitis after PKP, which is difficult to judge from clinical observation.

IMMUNOPATHOGENESIS OF HERPES SIMPLEX STROMAL KERATITIS

Corneal blindness secondary to scarring from recurrent herpes simplex keratitis (HSK) still occurs in epidemic proportions, despite 30 years of effective topical antiviral medication. Why some individuals are capable of an adequate immune response which clears the infection without producing excessive, tissue-damaging inflammation, while others are unable to do this is unclear. Our work in a defined murine model of necrotizing HSK has shown that discreet genetic differences produce profound immunologic and clinical differences following corneal encounter with HSV. Underregulation of an overly exuberant inflammatory response is only one of those differences responsible for the blinding keratopathy experienced by some individuals. We now know that in mice with a specific genotype, frank autoimmunity to corneal antigens develops, contributing to the necrotizing stromal keratitis seen in these mice. These data indicate even more profound reasons for major efforts at developing selective immunomodulatory strategies for treating The inflammatory response associated with HSK, with strategies that dissociate The anti-inflammatory effect from the wound healing impairment and infection enhancing effects of steroid therapy.

DIAGNOSTIC IMPRESSION CYTOLOGY FOR VIRAL DISEASES OF THE OUTER EYE

H. Araki, H. Nakagawa, N. Kimata, Y. Nakagawa, and M. Murata

Tokyo Women's Medical College, Tokyo, Japan

Purpose. To evaluate the efficacy of impression cytology (IC) for the diagnosis of viral diseases of the outer eye. **Materials and Methods.** Three common viral diseases of the oilier eye were studied. (1) Herpes simplex keratoconjunctivitis (n=20): Impression specimens were obtained from eyelid vesicles, bulbar an palpebral conjunctiva, and stellate, dendritic and geographic epithelial lesions of the cornea or conjunctiva. The specimens were stained for herpes simplex virus (HSV) antigens by peroxidase-antiperoxidase method using polyclonal anti-HSV antibodies. (2) Herpes zoster ophthalmicus (n=6): Specimens obtained from dendritic lesions were tested for varicella zoster virus (VZV) antigens by Immunofluorsecence with monoclonal anti-VZV antibodies. (3) Adenovirus (Adv) conjunctivitis: Eighty cases of acute follicular conjunctivitis, clinically suspected of Adv conjunctivitis were involved. Impression specimens from bulbar conjunctiva were stained for Adv antigens by modified avidin-biotin method using monoclonal anti-Ad antibodies. The patients were also examined for Adv antigens by using Adenoclone®. **Results.** (1) Twenty cases were all HSV isolation-positive. HSV antigens were identified in 100% of eyelid vesicle samples (9/9) and 91% of epithelial lesions(10/11) from the cornea and conjunctiva. In contrast, HSV antigens were rarely detected in bulbar (1/18) and palpebral (1/15) conjunctiva (2) antigens were detected from dendritic lesions in 3 cases (50%), including one case of zoster sine herpete. (3) Of 42 cases of Adv conjunctivitis proven by positive virus isolation, IC was positive in 36 cases, sensitivity 85.7% (36/42). In 38 adenovirus-negative cases, 35 cases showed negative in IC, specificity 92.1%

(35/38). Adenoclone® was 61.9% (26/42) sensitive and 100% (38/38) specific. **Conclusion.** We conclude that IC is an useful technique for the diagnosis of viral diseases of the outer eye because of its simple, rapid, noninvasive procedure and its ability to detect viral antigens even from minute lesions.

DETECTION AND TYPING OF HUMAN PAPILLOMAVIRUS (HPV) IN CORNEAL AND CONJUNCTIVAL TUMORS

S. Kumakura,[1,2] T. Iwasaki,[2] T. Sata,[2] R. Muramatsu,[1] T. Kurata,[2] and M. Usui[1]

Department of Ophthalmology, Tokyo Medical College[1]; Department of Pathology, NIH[2]; Tokyo, Japan

Purpose: Human papillomavirus (HPV) has been known to induce corneal and conjunctival tumors. Viral types reported in these tumors are HPV 6, 11 and, 16 which have been considered to be mucosal HPVs. In order to examine and characterize HPV present in corneal/ conjunctival tumors, we analyzed these tumors by polymerase chain reaction (PCR), and compared the sequences of amplified products to those of HPV reported in the literature. **Material and methods:** PCR using the Li consensus primers (MY1 1 and MY09, Manos MM and Y Ting, 1989) was performed on DNA extracted from formalin-fixed paraffin sections and frozen tissues of 10 cases of squamous cell papilloma, 4 cases of conjunctival dysplasia, and I case of carcinoma in situ. Sequencing of amplified fragments was analyzed on 3 recombinants clones from each specimen after TA ligation. **Results:** Amplified bands, about 450 bases in length, were found in 3 of 10 cases of squamous cell papilloma and in the 1 case of carcinoma *in situ*. No amplification was observed in any of the 4 cases of conjunctival dysplasia. Sequence analysis of DNA fragments in squamous cell papillomas showed the sequence of the HPV 11 genome, while the amplified fragment from the case of carcinoma in situ was of HPV16. Three conserved and 1 non-conserved point mutations and 1 insertional and 1 deletion triplets were found in amplified fragment of HPV 16 in carcinoma *in situ*, in comparison with the sequence of HPV 16 prototype cloned from invasive cervical carcinoma (Shwartz et al. 1982). In amplified fragments of HPV 11 in three squamous cell papilloma, only one conserved or non-conserved point mutations were found in comparison to that of HPV 11 prototype cloned from laryngeal papilloma, besides neither deletion or insertional changes were observed. B These results suggest that cornea and conjunctiva have a similar susceptibility to HPV that infects genital and laryngeal mucosa. In addition, in cases of squamous cell papilloma and carcinoma *in situ*, it appears that HPV causes similar histopathology to that seen in genital and laryngeal infections.

Session VIII

Keratoconus

40

THE CASE FOR EYE RUBBING AS THE MAJOR CAUSE OF KERATOCONUS

Jay H. Krachmer

Department of Ophthalmology
University of Minnesota
Minneapolis, Minnesota

ABSTRACT

Eye rubbing has been implicated as a cause of keratoconus for 35 years. Over that period of time there has been a growing body of information confirming that hypothesis. This paper presents examples and arguments supporting eye rubbing as an etiology for keratoconus.

EYE RUBBING AND KERATOCONUS

There are many cases documented in the literature which, short of absolute proof, establish that eye rubbing can cause keratoconus. Two cases are especially strong.

The first case is that of an 11-year-old boy.[1] He was born with an atrial ventricular septal defect and underwent open heart surgery at the age of two. Because of a conduction defect, he had paroxysmal atrial tachycardia and discovered at the age of five that he could regulate his heart rhythm by "vigorously" massaging his left eye. He had no sign of keratoconus at the age of seven, but when he was 11 years of age with blurred vision in the left eye, he was found to have keratoconus in that eye. He had 20/20 vision and no sign of keratoconus in the right eye. The left eye had a visual acuity of 20/200 with a 4 mm central cone and a curvature of 53.00x55.50 diopters. Keratometry was normal in the right eye. Computerized topography was not available at that time.

The second case occurred during the present era with the availability of photokeratoscopy performed by cornea specialists at the University of Southern California.[2] It even more powerfully establishes the fact that eye rubbing can cause keratoconus. A 31-year-old man had been "pressing vigorously" with his fists against his eyes to aid in daily ritual meditation. He had keratoconus with a visual acuity of 20/200 in the left eye and underwent successful penetrating keratoplasty. On initial examination, his right eye had absolutely no signs of keratoconus by methods of sophisticated examination including photokeratoscopy. He was warned against rubbing his eyes but eleven months later he was seen with decreased vision in his right eye. He had progressed from no corneal astigmatism or signs of keratoconus to nine diopters of astigmatism with stress lines and thinning and definite keratoconus. Even though he was warned against ocular massage, he admitted to continued vigorous massage with his fist against his right eye.

The opinion that eye rubbing can cause keratoconus has been repeatedly mentioned in the literature since the report of Ridley in 1961.[3] The lack of scientific proof and the anecdotal reporting have contributed to the failure of most to believe that eye rubbing can cause keratoconus. After all, all of us rub our eyes, why do only some of us have keratoconus? Eye rubbing is very difficult to qualitate and quantitate. An excellent attempt was made by Korb et al., in which they found, with a five year follow-up, that chronic, severe, forceful eye rubbing was strongly implicated in the evolution of keratoconus.[4]

Keratoconus is seen in a variety of clinical settings. Many of them are strongly associated with eye rubbing.[5] Keratoconus is much more frequently diagnosed in atopic patients than in the normal population. Because of itching, eye rubbing is a prominent activity in atopic patients with ocular involvement. Patients with Down's syndrome also have a higher frequency of keratoconus compared to the general population. Eye rubbing is a common characteristic in Down's patients. Leber's congenital amaurosis is frequently accompanied by keratoconus. These patients vigorously rub their eyes to stimulate the retina.

A subset of the controversy regarding eye rubbing in keratoconus surrounds the issue of whether or not contact lenses can cause keratoconus.[6] Eye rubbing in contact lens wearers occurs both by the mechanical rubbing of the plastic on the cornea, as well as the vigorous eye rubbing that takes place in many contact lens wearers after the lenses are removed. Contact lens wearers frequently admit to the joy of rubbing their eyes after the contacts are removed.

Floppy eyelid patients frequently have keratoconus.[7] Is it pure chance that floppy eyelid patients often also have keratoconus, and that if they have unilateral floppy eyelids the keratoconus is on the same side as the floppy eyelid? Without absolute proof, one could say that the patient would have developed keratoconus anyway and that it was just a coincidence that the keratoconus was related to the worse or only floppy eyelid eye.

Eye rubbing can cause keratoconus. The only question is the proportion of cases of keratoconus are caused by eye rubbing. It is possible that there are other factors that predispose the patient to corneal deformity, such as biochemically or anatomically abnormal corneal tissue.

All of us rub our eyes. Only some of us develop keratoconus. Millions smoke. Only some smokers suffer lung cancer. Everyone eats saturated fats. Fortunately, only some develop arteriosclerotic disease. Clearly, whether or not we have keratoconus, lung cancer, or arteriosclerotic disease depends to some degree on the magnitude of the eye rubbing, smoking, and saturated fat intake as well as biochemical, anatomical, and physiological predisposition to these conditions.

Genetic factors are being discovered which, when combined with smoking and saturated fat intake, can result in cancer and heart disease. Perhaps we will someday identify genetic factors which predispose some eye rubbers to developing keratoconus.

This discussion certainly does not prove that eye rubbing can cause keratoconus. It does not explain the cause of keratoconus in patients who definitely lack a history of eye rubbing. It is meant to emphasize the importance of eye rubbing in the etiology of keratoconus. Smoking is a causative factor in some patients with lung cancer. Eye rubbing is a causative factor in some patients with keratoconus.

REFERENCES

1. J.T. Coyle, Keratoconus and eye rubbing. *Am. J. Ophthalmol.* 97:527 (1984).
2. D.C. Gritz, and McDonnell, P.J., Keratoconus and ocular massage. *Am. J. Ophthalmol.* 106:747 (1988).
3. F. Ridley, Eye-rubbing and keratoconus. *Brit. J. Ophthalmol.* 45:631: (1961).
4. D.K. Korb, Greiner, J.V., and Leahy, C.D., Forceful eye rubbing as a causative factor in keratoconus. *Ophthalmology* 102(suppl.):152 (1995).
5. A.G. Karseras, and Ruben, M., Aetiology of keratoconus. *Brit. J. Ophthalmol.* 60:522 (1976).
6. M.S. Macsai, Varley, G.A., and Krachmer, J.H., Development of keratoconus after contact lens wear: patient characteristics. *Arch. Ophthalmol.* 108:534 (1990).
7. E.D. Donnenfeld, Perry, H.D., Gibralter, R.P., et al., Keratoconus associated with floppy eyelid syndrome. *Ophthalmology* 98:1574 (1991).

41

LONG-TERM FOLLOW-UP OF PENETRATING KERATOPLASTY FOR KERATOCONUS

Martin Filipec and Erik Letko

2nd Department of Ophthalmology
Charles University
Prague, Czech Republic

ABSTRACT

Long-term results of penetrating keratoplasty (PKP) for keratoconus in 104 grafts of 78 patients were evaluated in a retrospective study. Keratometry, visual acuity test, slit lamp examination, and specular microscopy of the grafts were performed and the charts of patients were reviewed. The mean follow-up time was 13.5 years. The mean astigmatism was 5.5 diopters. In 30 grafts followed for 12 years, the astigmatism was stable in 11 eyes (37%), increased in 10 eyes (33%), decreased in five eyes (17%), and fluctuated in four eyes (14%). Visual acuity better than 0.5 was achieved in 87.5% of eyes; graft was clear in 99% of eyes. The mean endothelial cell density in all grafts was 830 cells/mm^2 (range 550–1300 cell/mm^2). There was no statistically significant change in endothelial cell density within the time after surgery (p>0.05). In three eyes the endothelial cell density increased from 507 cells/mm^2 to 766 cells/mm^2. It was concluded that (1) the long-term results of PKP for keratoconus concerning visual acuity and graft clarity are excellent; (2) astigmatism is the most common complication and may change during the follow- up in any direction; and (3) endothelial cell density became stable after the fifth year post- keratoplasty and cell density may increase in some cases.

INTRODUCTION

Keratoconus is the leading indication for penetrating keratoplasty in patients younger than 60 years of age.[1,2] Results of penetrating keratoplasty for keratoconus are reported to be excellent, with graft survival ranging from 90% to 100%.[3–5] High astigmatism and, less often, loss of graft clarity, cataract and glaucoma are the most common complications impairing the visual acuity during long-term follow-up.[5,6] A slow decrease of endothelial cell density after penetrating keratoplasty in keratoconus was demonstrated previously,[6] whereas a second report failed to show any consistent changes in cell density.

Advances in Corneal Research, edited by Lass
Plenum Press, New York, 1997

during long-term follow-up.[7] There are only limited data on long-term results in penetrating keratoplasty for keratoconus with the longest mean follow-up time of 11.3 years.[3] Because the keratoconus patients indicated for surgery are usually young and their lifetime expectancy is the same as for the normal population,[8] it is extremely important to know more about the long–term results and expected graft lifetime after penetrating keratoplasty for keratoconus. The purpose of this retrospective study was to evaluate visual acuity, astigmatism, graft clarity, endothelial cell density, graft thickness and complications during long–term follow-up of post-keratoplasty patients.

MATERIALS AND METHODS

All available charts of patients who underwent penetrating keratoplasty for keratoconus between January 1, 1965 and December 31, 1990 in the 2nd Department of Ophthalmology in Prague were reviewed. Patients who had a minimum of six years' follow-up after their first graft were invited to return for a final clinical examination. Only those patients who agreed to this last examination were included in this study.

All patients were operated on using fresh donor tissue. The donor age ranged up to 65 years; harvested corneas were stored in a moist chamber at 4°C and used within six hours of enucleation. The technique of penetrating keratoplasty was evolving during the time period covered by this study. All penetrating keratoplasties performed before 1975 were performed without an operating microscope. Maltese cross and 8–0 silk as a suturing material were used in the years 1965 to 1969; 10–0 Nylon and continous or interrupted suture have been used since 1970. All donor and recipient corneas were trephined from the epithelial side; the sizes of trephines were the same for both.

The study included 104 eyes of 78 patients. The clinical examination included keratometry, final corrected Snellen visual acuity expressed in decimal scale, and slit lamp examination of the graft clarity and anterior segment. In a subset of 30 eyes, the postoperative astigmatism was measured in at least three examinations during a period of 12 years. Differences of more than 1.5 diopters of astigmatism were counted. Graft endothelial cell density and graft thickness were evaluated by specular microscopy (Keeler-Konan). Fixed frame analysis for cell counting was used. At least three cell counts in different locations, to minimize the error connected with this method, were performed per each photomicrograph. In a group of ten patients with a history of allograft rejection, the graft endothelial cell density was examined during an interval of 12 years. All patient clinical charts were reviewed and postoperative complications evaluated. For statistical analysis, ANOVA (analysis of variance) was used in this study.

RESULTS

One hundred four eyes of 78 patients were evaluated after penetrating keratoplasty. Twenty patients were female (26%) and 58 were male (74%). The female to male ratio was 1:3. The mean age at the time of surgery was 22 years (range 11–49 years). The mean follow-up time from the surgery to the last clinical examination was 13.5 years (range 6–30 years). The eyes were divided into five groups based upon the date of surgery (Table 1). The mean graft astigmatism in all 104 eyes was 5.5 cylindric diopters (range 0–21 diopters) (Table 1). There was a tendency for the postoperative astigmatism to be greater in patients grafted during the earlier years of the study period, but statistical significance

Table 1. Astigmatism, visual acuity, endothelial cell density and graft thickness

Groups of patients (date of PK)	No. of eyes	Astigmatism (diopters)	Visual acuity	Cell density (cell/mm^2)	Thickness (mm)
1966-70	5	10.7	0.58	812	0.61
1971-75	5	7.0	0.70	835	0.59
1976-80	7	6.8	0.64	837	0.59
1981-85	53	5.9	0.72	904	0.61
1986-90	34	4.0	0.74	850	0.61
	total = 104	mean 5.5	0.70	830	0.60

was seen only between the patient groups 1966–70 and 1986–90 (p=0.05) (Fig. 1). In 30 eyes, the evolution of astigmatism was measured during a mean follow-up time of 12 years (range 10 to 15 years). The astigmatism did not change in 11 eyes (37%), increased in 10 eyes (33%), decreased in five eyes (17%), and fluctuated in four eyes (14%).

The results of best corrected final visual acuity are shown in Tables 1 and 2. There was no statistically significant difference in the mean visual acuity among all five evaluated groups (p>0.05). The reasons for visual acuity lower than 0.5 in 13 eyes are listed in Table 3. Slit lamp examination revealed a clear graft in 103 eyes (99%); in one eye (1%) the graft was opaque. The reason for graft failure in this patient was infectious keratitis.

The most common complication of the keratoplasty was astigmatism higher than 5.0 diopters, seen in 45 eyes (43%) (Table 4). Allograft rejection occured in 26 eyes (25%). In eight eyes there were repeated episodes of graft rejection. The first rejection in this series was seen one month after the surgery, the latest 8 years after keratoplasty. The mean time of graft rejection was 15.8 months. The highest number of rejections developed within the first year after keratoplasty (Table 5). Of 78 unilateral keratoplasties, rejection occured after first keratoplasty in 19 eyes (24%). In 26 bilateral transplantations rejection occurred after second keratoplasty in seven eyes (27%). This difference was not statistically significant (p>0.05). Allograft rejection did not result in graft failure in any patient included in the study. In four patients cataract was diagnosed, and wide paretic pupil (Urrets-Zavalia syndrome) occured in one patient (Table 3).

The mean endothelial cell density in all examined grafts was 830 cells/mm^2 (range 550–1,300 cells/mm^2). Comparison of graft endothelial cell densities (Table 1) among the five groups examined did not demonstrate a statistically significant difference (p>0.05).

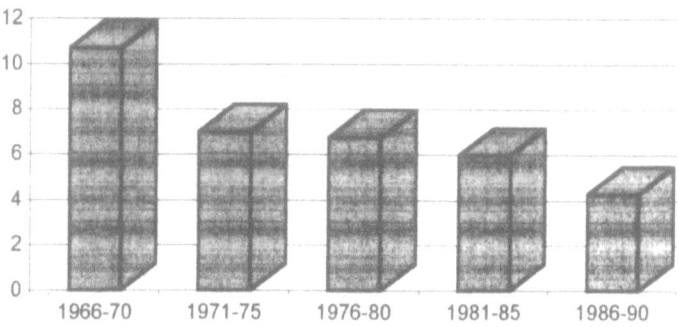

Figure 1. Mean astigmatism values (cylindric diopters) in five groups of patients based upon the date of surgery.

Table 2. Final visual acuity

Visual acuity	Eyes (%)
1.0–0.67	80 (77)
0.5–0.4	17 (16)
<0.4	7 (7)

Table 3. Reasons for visual acuity lower than
0.5 in 13 eyes

Reason	Eyes (%)
Cataract	4 eyes (30%)
High astigmatism	3 eyes (23%)
Amblyopia	3 eyes (23%)
Tapetoretinal degeneration	1 eye (8%)
Graft failure	1 eye (8%)
Urrets-Zavalia syndrome	1 eye (8%)

In a subset of 10 eyes, specular microscopy of graft endothelium was performed twice within an interval of 12 years after keratoplasty, as shown in Figure 2. All of these patients had a previous episode of endothelial graft rejection. The mean time of first examination was 1.5 year after keratoplasty (range 1 to 4 years); the mean endothelial cell density was 1,159 cells/mm^2 (range 283–2570 cells/mm^2). The mean time of second examination was 12 years (range 11 to 15 years) after keratoplasty, and the mean endothelial cell density was 778 cells/mm^2 (range 630–970 cells/mm^2). This cell density did not differ significantly (p>0.05) from the mean endothelial cell density seen in eyes without a history of allograft rejection examined at the same interval after surgery, 804 cells/mm^2 (range 550–1193 cells/mm^2). In three patients the graft endothelial cell density increased from a mean value of 507 cells/mm^2 at the first examination to 766 cell/mm^2 at the second examination, 12 years after the surgery (Figure 2). Corneal graft thickness, as measured

Table 4. Complications of keratoplasty
for keratoconus

Complication	Eyes (%)
High astigmatism (> 5.0 diopter)	45 (43)
Allograft rejection	26 (25)
Glaucoma	2 (2)

Table 5. Occurence of allograft
rejection within the time
after keratoplasty

Time after keratoplasty	Eyes (%)
1st year	17 (65)
2nd year	4 (15)
3rd year	3 (12)
4th-8th year	2 (8)

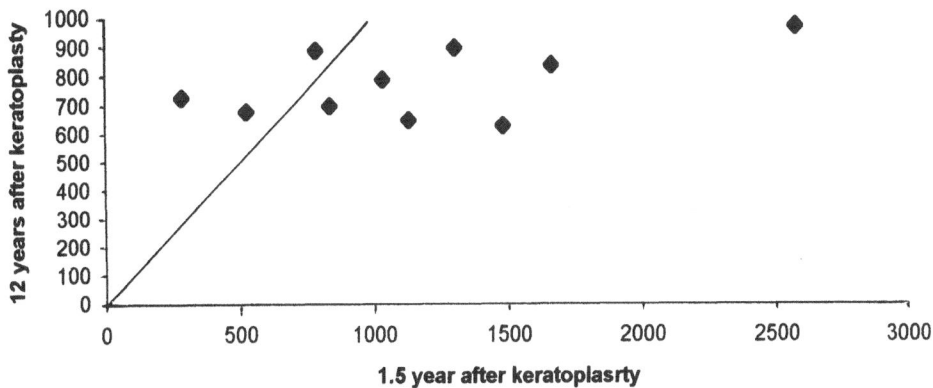

Figure 2. Graft endothelial cell density (cells/mm^2) 1.5 and 12 years after surgery in 10 eyes with a previous episode of rejection. In three eyes the graft endothelial cell density increased.

by means of specular microscopy (Table 1), was not statistically different among any examined groups ($p>0.05$).

Additional surgery was performed in 15 eyes (14.5%). Retransplantation was performed in two eyes, in one patient because of graft failure after infectious keratitis and in one patient because of high astigmatism. Refractive surgery was performed in 11 eyes and suggested after the last examination to 12 other patients. In two patients with glaucoma trabeculectomy was performed. Cataract surgery was suggested to four patients after the final clinical examination.

DISCUSSION

There is general agreement in the literature concerning the excellent results of penetrating keratoplasty for keratoconus.[3-7] This study confirms these excellent results during long-term follow-up; the mean follow-up time of 13.5 years is the longest among all published studies.

Mean astigmatism of 5.5 diopters in the last clinical examination is similar to the astigmatism seen by others.[9-12] Higher mean astigmatism in the group of patients operated on in the years 1965–1970 may be the result of slowly progressing disease. It is believed that the main reason is the surgical technique (Maltese cross suture, 6.0–7.0 mm graft diameter) used in that time. Recurrence of keratoconus as reported by some authors[13,14] was not observed in these patients. The studies concerning post-keratoplasty astigmatism generally consider the period of 12 to 24 months after suture extraction as sufficient for astigmatism to become stable. In this study, we observed changes in astigmatism greater than 1.5 diopters in 64% of these patients during the period of 10 to 15 years following surgery. This phenomenon may be the consequence of the presence and slow progression of keratoconus pathology in the periphery of the recipient cornea.

Visual acuity of 0.5 or better in 87.5% of eyes in this series is similar to that seen in other studies where this level of acuity was found in 73% to 91% of eyes.[3-7] The reasons for visual acuity worse than 0.5 in 13 eyes were directly related to the state of the graft only in four eyes. In three eyes the reason was high astigmatism, and in one eye this was due to graft failure following infectious keratitis. These findings are similar to those reported by other authors.[3-5] The rate of allograft rejection in our series of 104 keratoplasties is 25%; the reported rejection rate ranges from 10% to 39% after keratoplasty for keratoconus.[5,6,15] The role of second transplants in increasing the incidence of graft rejection is not definite. Both higher[16] and statistically not different[17] rates of rejection have been demonstrated. In this study, the occurence of graft rejection in unilateral keratoplasty is not statistically significantly different from that seen in bilateral keratoplasty (24% versus 27%).

Clear grafts as a result of penetrating keratoplasty for keratoconus are reported in more than 90% of eyes. Various studies with a mean follow-up time ranging from 3 to 11.3 years show 90% to 100% clear grafts.[3-6,18,19] In our series, corneal grafts were clear in 99% of eyes. In one eye the graft was opaque due to infectious keratitis in the early postoperative period. Incidence of permanent mydriasis (Urrets-Zavalia syndrome) is described by different authors in 0 to 17.7% of eyes.[20,21] In our series, paretic pupille was observed in one eye (1%). Graft endothelial cell densities in this study were not significantly different in any of the patient groups in relation to the time after the keratoplasty. Endothelial cell counts seem to become stable after the 5th year post- keratoplasty. In our series, the mean cell density was 830 cell/mm^2, and there was no tendency towards its decrease in the time after surgery. According to numerous studies, graft endothelial cell density dramatically decreases following penetrating keratoplasty by 18.3%-24% within the first three months and by 33.6 to 45% within the first year.[22-24] After 4.3 to 5.5 years of follow-up, endothelial cell density is decreased by 60 to 65%.[25,26] Ehlers and Olsen[6] demonstrated a slow decrease in endothelial cell density following penetrating keratoplasty in keratoconus (follow-up 3 to 12 years, mean 5.8 years). Linn[7] observed in 55 transplants for keratoconus a mean endothelial cell density of 941 cells/mm^2. Follow-up time in these grafts was 2.5 to 35 years. There was no decrease of cell density within the time after surgery. Current observations indicate that corneal grafts in keratoconus enter into a certain steady state period and the cell density does not change after that point after an initial period of 1 to 5 years of endothelial cell density decline. In a subset of 10 patients who suffered an episode of endothelial rejection, we were able to examine the graft endothelium during an interval of 12 years. A decrease in endothelial cell density after endothelial rejection has been described.[27,28] Twelve years after the rejection episode, no statistically significant differences in endothelial cell density were observed when compared with other grafts examined at the same time after keratoplasty. In three eyes, an increase of graft endothelial cell density from a mean of 507 to 766 cells/mm^2 was observed. In one of these grafts the difference between the two examinations was particularly prominent. This transplant, with a cell density of 283 cells/mm^2 after endothelial rejection, was edematous one year after penetrating keratoplasty. Giant endothelial cells with thickened cell walls were seen by specular microscopy only with difficulty. Twelve years later the graft was crystal clear, and endothelial cell density was 730 cells/mm^2. This observation, and also the fact that the endothelial cell density stabilized after the fifth year post-surgery among all patients studied, including those with up to 30 years follow-up, can be explained by two mechanisms. It has been postulated that corneal endothelial cells in primates and humans have no or very little capacity to proliferate.[29-31] Other authors[32,33] have demonstrated both migration and proliferation of corneal endothelial cells *in vitro* and also *ex vivo*. These observations suggest the possibility of slow endothelial cell proliferation and endothelial wound repair by this mechanism under certain conditions. Another possible mechanism of endothelial repair is the sliding of endothelial cells from the recipient cornea. It has been demonstrated following penetrating keratoplasty in rabbits[34] that endothelial cells have the ability to migrate from the donor to the host cornea. It is speculated that the same movement of healthy endothelial cells can occur in the opposite direction after keratoplasty in humans, that is from keratoconus recipient to donor cornea. The generally less favorable short and long-term follow-up results of penetrating keratoplasty in Fuchs dystrophy[35-37] also lend support to this idea.

We can further confirm very good results of penetrating keratoplasty for keratoconus with excellent prognosis concernig graft clarity, and low complications rate. Graft astigmatism is a limiting factor for even better results of visual acuity and may change during the long-term follow-up in any direction. High initial loss of endothelial cells after keratoplasty and even after correctly treated endothelial graft rejection in keratoconus are not critical for long-term graft survival in keratoconus patients. To explain mechanisms of partial graft repopulation by endothelial cells need further experimental and clinical studies.

REFERENCES

1. N. Mamalis, Craig, M.T., Coulter, V.L., et al., Penetrating keratoplasty 1981–1988: clinical indications and pathologic findings. *J. Cataract. Refract. Surg.* 17:163 (1991).
2. L. Hyman, Wittpenn, J., and Yang, C., Indications and techniques of penetrating keratoplasties. *Cornea* 11:573 (1991).
3. P.G. Paglen, Fine, M., Abbott, R.L., and Webster, R.G., Jr., The prognosis for keratoplasty in keratoconus. *Ophthalmology* 89:651 (1982).
4. F.W. Price, Jr., Whitson, W.E., and Marks, R.G., Graft survival in four common groups of patients undergoing penetrating keratoplasty. *Ophthalmology* 98:322 (1991).
5. K.S. Sharif, and Casey, T.A., Penetrating keratoplasty for keratoconus: complications and long-term success. *Br. J. Ophthalmol.* 75:142 (1991).
6. N. Ehlers, and Olsen, T., Long term results of corneal grafting in keratoconus. *Acta Ophthalmol.* 61:918 (1983).
7. L.G. Linn, Jr., Stuart, J.C., Warnicki, J.W.,et al., Endothelial morphology in long-term keratoconus corneal transplants. *Ophthalmology* 88:761 (1981).
8. R.H. Kennedy, Bourne, W.M., and Dyer, J.A., A 48-year clinical and epidemiologic study of keratoconus. *Am. J. Ophthalmol.* 101:267 (1986).
9. A. Anseth, Keratoplasty for keratoconus, a report of 50 operated eyes. *Acta Ophthalmol.* 45:684 (1967).
10. R.C. Troutman, and Meltzer, M., Astigmatism and myopia in keratoconus. *Trans. Am. Ophthalmol. Soc.* 70:265 (1972).
11. S.A. Boruchoff, Jensen, A.D., and Dohlman, C.H., Comparison of suturing techniques in keratoplasty for keratoconus. *Ann. Ophthalmol.* 7:433 (1975).
12. J.M. Richard, Paton, D., and Gasset, A.R., A comparison of penetrating keratoplasty and lamellar keratoplasty in the surgical management of keratoconus. *Am. J. Ophthalmol.* 86:807 (1978).
13. M.B. Abelson, Collin, H.B., Gillette, T.E., and Dohlman, C.H., Recurrent keratoconus after keratoplasty. *Am. J. Ophthalmol.* 90:672 (1980).
14. N. Bechrakis, Blom, M.L., Stark, W.J., and Green, R., Recurrent keratoconus. *Cornea* 13:73 (1994).
15. J.W. Chandler, Immune reaction and corneal graft rejection. *Trans. Pac. Coast. Oto.- Ophthalmol. Soc.* 55:209 (1974).
16. P.C. Donshik, Cavanagh, H.D., Boruchoff, S.A., and Dohlman,C.H., Effects of bilateral and unilateral grafts on the incidence of rejection in keratoconus. *Am. J. Ophthalmol.* 87:823 (1979).
17. J.N. Buxton, Schuman, M., and Pecego, J., Graft reactions after unilateral and bilateral keratoplasty for keratoconus. *Opthalmology* 88:771 (1981).
18. F.W. Price, Jr., Whitson, W.E., and Marks, R.G., Graft survival in four common groups of patients undergoing penetrating keratoplasty. *Ophthalmology* 98:322 (1991).
19. R.H. Keates, and Falkenstein, S., Keratoplasty in keratoconus. *Am. J. Ophthalmol.*;74:442 (1972).
20. J.H. Krachmer, Feder, R.S., and Belin, M.W., Keratoconus and related noninflammatory corneal thinning disorders. *Surv. Ophthalmol.* 28:293 (1984).
21. T. Bertelsen, and Seim, V., Irreversible mydriasis following keratoplasty in keratoconus. *Acta Ophthalmol. Suppl. (Copenhagen)* 125:45 (1975).
22. W.M. Bourne, and O'Fallon, W.M., Endothelial cell loss during penetrating keratoplasty. *Am. J. Ophthalmol.* 85:760 (1978).

23. W.M. Bourne, One-year observation of transplanted human corneal endothelium. *Ophthalmology* 87:673 (1980).

24. W.W. Culbertson, Abbott, R.L., and Forster, R.K., Endothelial cell loss in penetrating keratoplasty. *Ophthalmology* 89:600 (1982).

25. R.A. Laing, Sandström, M., Berrospi, A.R., and Leibowitz, H.M., Morphological changes in corneal endothelial cells after penetrating keratoplasty. *Am. J. Ophthalmol.* 82:459 (1976).

26. W.M. Bourne, and Kaufman, H.E., The endothelium of clear corneal transplants. *Arch. Ophthalmol.* 94:1730 (1976).

27. L.W. Hirst, and Stark, W.J., Clinical specular microscopy of corneal endothelial rejection. *Arch. Ophthalmol.* 101:1387 (1983).

28. M. Filipec, and Kraus, H., Specular microscopic study of endothelial rejection reaction after corneal transplantation. *Ces. Oftalmol.* 43:310 (1987).

29. D.L. Van Horn, and Hyndiuk, R.A., Endothelial wound repair in primate cornea. *Exp. Eye Res.* 21:113 (1975).

30. D.J. Doughman, Van Horn, D.L., and Rodman, W.P., Human corneal endothelial layer repair during organ culture. *Arch. Ophthalmol.* 94:1791 (1976).

31. J.A.Capella, Regeneration of endothelium in diseased and injured corneas. *Am. J. Ophthalmol.* 74:810 (1972).

32. W.F. Treffers, Human corneal endothelial wound repair. *Ophthalmology* 89:605 (1982).

33. K. Engelmann, and Friedl, P., Optimization of culture conditions for human corneal endothelial cells. *In Vitro Cell. Dev. Biol.* 25:1065 (1989).

34. R.J. Olson, and Levenson, J.E., Migration of donor endothelium in keratoplasty. *Am. J. Ophthalmol.* 84:7 (1977).

35. T. Olsen, Ehlers, N., and Favini, E., Long-term results of corneal grafting in Fuchs'endothelial dystrophy. *Acta Ophthalmol. (Copenhagen)* 62:445 (1984).

36. H.J. Völker-Dieben, Kok-Van Alphen, C.C., and DeLange, P., Corneal grafts for endothelial decompensation:the influence of intraocular lenses on cornealgraft survival. *Acta Ophthalmol.* 62:432 (1984).

37. F.W. Price, Whitson, W.E., and Marks, R.G., Graft survival in four groups of patients undergoing penetrating keratoplasty. *Ophthalmology* 98:322 (1991).

SECTION VIII: KERATOCONUS

Abstracts of Other Conference Presentations and Posters

FAMILIARITY IN KERATOCONUS AND RELATED TOPOGRAPHIC MEASURES

Yaron S. Rabinowitz,[1-5] Huiying Yang,[2-4] and Jerome I. Rotter[2-4]

[1] Cornea-Genetic Eye Medical Clinic and the [2] Medical Genetics Birth Defects Center Cedars-Sinai Medical Center [3]Departments of Pediatrics, [4]Medicine and [5]Ophthalmology U.C.L.A. School of Medicine, Los Angeles, California

Background: To date, there have been no formal studies to determine whether the underlying etiological factors in isolated keratoconus (KC) are environmental or genetic

Methods: We performed segregation analysis on 240 families ascertained through patients with a clinical diagnosis of KC using a computer program REGD (in the SAGE package) and tested for multiple potential inheritance models for KC.

Results: Using maximum likelihood statistics, we were able to reject a no major gene model, environmental effects, and sporadic occurrence (p<.05). The major gene model could not be rejected. Within this model, both autosomal dominant and additive models were rejected, but not autosomal recessive inheritance. This suggests that the distribution of KC in the families we studied is consistent with major gene effects which act in an autosomal recessive fashion.

Conclusions: Genetic factors are the main underlying etiological cause for KC. Our results, in combination with other reports of dominant inheritance in specific families, demonstrate that KC is likely to be a genetically heterogenous disorder. (Supported by NEI 09052)

POSSIBLE ROLE OF PROTEOLYTIC ENZYMES IN THE PATHOGENESIS OF KERATOCONUS

Joel Sugar and Beatrice Y.J.T. Yue

University of Illinois at Chicago

Keratoconus is a disorder of unknown etiology. Prior studies have shown decreased protein content in all keratoconus corneas along with reduced protein and collagen production in cultured stroma from some but not other keratoconus patients (PSEBM 1984; 175:336–341). In the face of reduced protein content and normal protein synthesis, at least in some keratoconus patients, the possibility that degradation processes play an etiologic role arises. Using histochemical techniques we have shown elevated levels of the lysosomal enzymes acid phosphatase, acid esterase, and acid lipase in the epithelium of keratoconus corneas when compared to normal control human corneas (Arch Ophthalmol 1989; 107; 1507–1510). Levels of matrix metalloproteinases MMP-2 and MMP-9 were not different between keratoconus and control corneas (Curr Eye Res 1992; 9:849–862). In addition levels of alpha-1-proteinase inhibitor were found to be reduced in the epithelium and stroma of keratoconus corneas (Exp Eye Res 1990; 50:549–554). Also levels of alpha-2-macroglobulin, another proteinase inhibitor, are reduced in both the epithelium and stroma of keratoconus corneas (Invest Ophthalmol Vis Sci 1994; 35:4008–4014). More recent studies of conjunctiva from keratoconus patients also shows elevated levels of epithelial acid esterase and acid phosphatase while conjunctiva from normal controls and patients with other corneal diseases does not (Arch Ophthalmol 1994; 112:1368–1374). Skin biopsies from keratoconus patients show normal enzyme levels.

These studies support a role of proteolytic enzymes in the loss of corneal tissue which occurs in keratoconus.

OF THE ROLE OF FIBROCYTES IN THE PATHOGENESIS OF KERATOCONUS

Yves Poulique

Goal: The precise molecular basis of keratoconus (KC) are still unknown. Alteration of the regulation of matrix metalloproteinase, with increased glucosaminoglycans content and dermatous keratan sulfates ratio in the extracellular matrix (ECM) was reported. Because of the frequent clinical association of keratoconus to atopy, we hypothesized that the synthesis and degradation of ECM may be modulated by cytokines involved in the immune or inflammatory responses.

Methods: Comparison is made of 9 strains of fibroblasts from KC to 12 strains from normal cornea maintained in culture from the 2nd to 10th passage (30 generations). We investigated the 111 receptors of IL-1, the kinetics of cyclooxygenase, the synthesis of PGE2, the components of the plasmin system (tPA, uPA, PAI) and the synthesis and effect of intrinsic TGF beta.

Results: As compared to normal corneal cells strains, fibroblasts from KC strains have a 4 folds more IL1 receptors, a 10 fold increase in cyclooxygenase's Vmax, a 10 fold increase in the basal production of PGE2, and stronger effect of t-PA and u-PA on the secretion of PGE2. t-PA/PAI ratio is reduced; a significant increase in the synthesis of TGF beta was observed in KC cells. These changes were consistently observed in subsequent passaged cells.

Conclusion: Modulation of ECM degradation may involve cytokines and enzymes from inflammatory pathways either as a primary or a secondary mechanism.

CONTACT LENSES, CORNEAL TOPOGRAPHY, AND KERATOCONUS

Penny Asbell

Mount Sinai Medical Center, New York, New York

Computerized corneal topography systems have been used to diagnose, analyze and map the progress of keratoconus. Spherical objects have been used as standards in evaluating computerized corneal topography systems. However, since it is well known that the human cornea is an aspheric surface, aspheric standards provide a better approximation of corneal contour and may be better to evaluate the accuracy and precision of these machines. Using two placido based photovideokeratoscopes, EyeSys and the TMS, radius of curvature readings at 4mm and 8mm diameters were obtained for four polymethylmethacrylate (PMMA) objects designed with micron accuracy by Computer Numeric Control (CNC) from Bausch & Lomb. Results indicate that EyeSys and TMS have available abilities to measure prolate (normal cornea) and oblate (changes noted after some surgeries—for example, radial keratotomy) corneas. In both systems, the error of measurement was found to increase from center to periphery and this may be due to spherically biased reconstruction algorithms employed in these systems. Aspheric standards should be developed to evaluate the accuracy of such corneal topography systems in the future and to check calibration machines in use.

Corneal images of 16 patients (22 eyes) clinically diagnosed with keratoconus were obtained by using EyeSys and PAR. Qualitative and quantitative analyses were performed for the following parameters: shape, location, apex of cone values, steepest and flattest points, cylindrical values, distance of apex to the line of sight, and the average of steepest and flattest points. Evaluating the qualitative measurements of shape and location we found differences in these parameters for both Systems.

Use of corneal topography to diagnose keratoconus and fit contact lenses is demonstrated, including use of an intermediate zone program to pick the initial base curve of a rigid gas permeable contact lens.

Future developments to aid in contact lens fitting of keratoconus will depend on the accuracy of measuring corneal topography and new development of useful criteria for contact lens fitting of the abnormal cornea.

THE COLLABORATIVE LONGITUDINAL EVALUATION OF KERATOCONUS (CLEK) STUDY

Karla Zadnik,[1] Joseph T. Barr,[2] Mae O. Gordon,[3] and Timothy B. Edrington[4]

[1]University of California, Berkeley, School of Optometry, [2]The Ohio State University College of Optometry, [3]Washington University, Department of Ophthalmology and Visual Sciences, [4]Southern California College of Optometry, and the CLEK Study Group

The Collaborative Longitudinal Evaluation of Keratoconus (CLEK) Study is a 16-center, observational investigation of keratoconus patients at all stages of the disease. Patients are eligible for the CLEK Study if they are at least 12 years old, have an irregular cornea in at least one eye, have Vogt's striae, Fleischer's ring, or scarring characteristic of keratoconus in at least one eye, do not have bilateral corneal transplants, and do not have bilateral macular disease, cataracts, intraocular lenses, or optic nerve disease (except glaucoma). As of February 16, 1996, 817 patients have been enrolled and have completed a CLEK Study Baseline Examination. They will be re-examined annually for three years. CLEK Study measures include quality of life assessment case history findings, contact lens wearing time, high and low contrast visual acuity with a variety of correction modes, slit lamp biomicroscopic findings, corneal scarring, corneal topography, contact lens fit, rigid contact lens base curve radius just clearing the corneal apex, corneal photography, and fluorescein pattern photography. From a database constructed of patients enrolled through January 8, 1996, the patients' baseline characteristics will be presented. The CLEK Study will evaluate changes with time in such critical parameters as corneal curvature, high and low contrast visual acuity, and photographically documented corneal scarring. Supported by National Eye Institute grants U10 EY10419, EY10069 and EY10077 and by Conforma Contact Lenses, Inc.

NONMECHANICAL TREPHINATION WITH THE EXCIMER LASER 193 MM IN PENETRATING KERATOPLASTY

G.O.H. Naumann, B. Seitz, A. Langenbucher, M.M. Kus, and M. Küchle

Department of Ophthalmology and University Eye Hospital, University Erlangen-Nürnberg, Erlangen, Germany

Background: Nonmechanical excimer laser trephination using open masks for penetrating keratoplasty (PK) was developed since 1986 in our institution and has been routinely used in over 165 eyes since 1989. The goal has been to avoid mechanical deformation, vertical tilt and horizontal torsion. We present results of a prospective study comparing keratoplasty with nonmechanical and mechanical trephination for Fuchs' dystrophy and keratoconus.

Methods: In this single surgeon prospective study, patients with keratoconus or Fuchs' corneal dystrophy undergoing PK were randomly assigned to either mechanical or nonmechanical trephination. Mechanical trephination was performed with a hand-held motor threphine (Geuder), whereas an excimer laser 193 mm (MEL 60, Aesculap-Meditec) with open metal masks and 8"Erlanger orientation teeth" was used for nonmechanical trephination. Graft diameter was 7.5/7.6 mm-in Fuchs' dystrophy and 8.0/8.1 mm in keratoconus. Double running sutures were used in all eyes. Regular examinations included keratometry, videokeratometry, best corrected visual acuity, determination of graft centration and noninvasive quantification of aqueous flare by laser tyndallometry.

Results: A total of 134 eyes (43 keratoconus nonmechanical; 42 keratoconus mechanical; 25 Fuchs' nonmechanical; 24 Fuchs' mechanical) were included in the study. Following removal of all sutures, mean astigmatism was 3.0 ± 2.1 D. following nonmechanical and 4.7 ± 5.1 D. following mechanical trephination ($p< 0.05$). Significant differences were observed for best corrected visual acuity (better following nonmechanical trephination, $p< 0.05$), graft centration (better in following nonmechanical trephination, $p<0.05$), regularity of astigmatism as determined by videokeratometry (higher following nonmechanical trephination, $p<0.05$), and postoperative blood-aqueous barrier breakdown as determined by laser tyndallometry (less extensive following nonmechanical trephination, p <0.05).

Conclusions: Nonmechanical trephination results in less astigmatism, better corrected visual acuity, better graft centration, higher regularity of astigmatism, and reduced blood-aqueous barrier breakdown. We recommend nonmechanical trephination for PK in nonvascularized corneas.

A RETROSPECTIVE ANALYSIS OF THE MANAGEMENT OF KERATOCONUS

William Drieke

We conducted a retrospective analysis of the management of 118 eyes of 66 new patients presenting with keratoconus at the University of Florida. Eyes were ultimately managed by one of three methods: glasses or no correction; contact lenses; or penetrating keratoplasty. The outcome of each management method was determined by evaluating initial and final vision and keratometry for each group. Twenty-one eyes received glasses or required no correction. Rigid gas permeable lenses, Dura-T style PMMA lenses, and specialty design gas permeable lenses were used to successfully fit 63 eyes. Twenty-eight eyes underwent penetrating keratoplasty (PK), and an additional six eyes were PK candidates. Factors associated with the need for PK included best corrected initial visual acuity of 20/40 or worse, average keratometry >55 D, and the presence of apical scarring (P<0.001).

ACCURACY OF THE PREDICTED VISUAL ACUITY IN THE HOLLADAY DIAGNOSTIC SUMMARY

Jayne S. Weiss and Nancy Oplinger

Kresge Eye Institute, Wayne State University, Detroit, Michigan

In the Holladay Diagnostic Summary Corneal Topography Program, the predicted corneal acuity (PCA) estimates the visual acuity if the cornea is the limiting factor in vision and posterior segment is normal.

We compared the PCA with the best corrected visual acuity (BVA) in order to determine the accuracy of the PCA measurement. We examined ten normal eyes and ten eyes with corneal abnormalities including prior penetrating keratoplasty, corneal scarring status post trauma, and keratoconus

The PCA was consistent with the BVA in all ten of the normal eyes. The PCA was less consistent with the BVA in all eyes with corneal abnormalities. The PCA was least accurate in patients with more than one diopter of astigmatism and less than or equal to sixty percent corneal uniformity index. In these cases, the PCA differed from the BVA by greater than three lines.

Therefore, the PCA appears to be less useful in predicting the BVA in patients with corneal abnormalities resulting in abnormal topography.

TRAUMATIC KERATOCONUS AFTER PROLONGED OBSESSIVE EYE COMPRESSION

M.F. Sartori, P.G. Manso, and M.C. Martins

Department of Ophthalmology, Jundiai School of Medicine, Brazil

Background: Keratoconus is usually a bilateral progressive pathology and is frequently associated with systemic diseases, especially atopy. **Purpose:** To report a probable prolonged trauma induced keratoconus. **Patients and Methods:** A 16 year old girl first reached our Ophthalmology Department complaining of blurred vision on the right eye. Personal history was unremarkable except for an obsessive habit to sleep with her thumb in mouth and the index finger compressing her right eye. Family history was also unremarkable for keratoconus or any other systemic syndromes neither any atopic disease. Ocular examination showed best corrected visual acuity of count-fingers , apparent ectasia of right cornea (positive Munson's sign), irregular reflex at retinoscopy, corneal thinning, vertical corneal stress lines and Fleischer's ring. UBM analysis confirmed biomicroscopic signs. Videokeratographic pattern of keratoconus was also present. Left eye examination was normal. Computer- assisted topographic analysis of some relatives were performed without any asymmetric corneal shape. The patient went on a psychological treatment and after one year of cutting off her old habit of compressing her eye, a penetrating keratoplasty was performed.

Pathologic changes of the graft showed fragmentation and fibrillation of Bowman's layer and basement membrane with fibroblastic activity of the affected area. At 3 months of follow-up, her uncorrected visual acuity is 20/40. **Conclusions:** Trauma should be concern in the pathogenesis of this reported keratoconus. Longer topographic follow-up of the fellow eye must not be missed.

TOPOGRAPHIC ANALYSIS OF 50 CASES OF EARLY KERATOCONUS

Ramón Naranjo-Tackman and Karla Uribe-Martínez

Cornea Department, Asociación Para Evitar la Ceguera en México, México, D.F.

Purpose: A topographic analysis of cases with suspicion of being incipient keratoconus, was made to identify the most important topographic characteristics of the initial stages of this ectasia.

Method: A prospective study of suspected cases of initial keratoconus, was made in patients with steep keratometric readings, slight distortion of keratomer mires, without clinical signs of keratoconus. In contact lens users, discontinuation of the lens was ordered for two weeks at least. The topographic study was made, using a TMS-1 corneal Topography System (Computed Anatomy, N.Y.). Several pictures were taken and analyzed using the absolute and adjustable scales. Simulated Keratometry (SimK) Surface Asymmetry Index (SAI), as well as localization, shape, maximal steep value, and distance to visual axis was evaluated in every case.

Results: 50 eyes of 28 patients were studied 6 patients only showed topographic evidence of the disease in one eye. The mean SimK values were: 47.16D.SAI values had a mean of 1.26. The most common pattern was a very asymmetric, angled Bowtie shape, that tended to take a "bean" shape, according to larger extent and steeper keratometric readings. The most frequent localization was the inferonasal quadrant. The steepest readings had a mean 52.10 D. Distance from visual axis was 1.63mm (mean value).

Conclusions: Corneal topography is the most reliable method to diagnose or confirm the diagnosis of an initial case of keratoconus, showing the limitations for a precise diagnosis that a keratomer has, in the absence of clinical data. This is specially important for refractive surgery, to avoid surgery on affected corneas.

THE ADAPTATION OF CONTACT LENSES IN KERATOCONUS

Remeto Leca

The adaptation of contact lenses was studied prospectively in 86 eyes of 50 patients with keratoconus between April 1991 and January 1993.

The patients' age varied from 11 thru 54 years with an average of 23,54 years. From this universe 60% was male and 10% was composed of white color individuals.

A proper adaptation observed in 6 eyes. During the period of time this study was done, from the remaining 80 eyes it was noticed an intolerance to the use of contact lenses in 2 other cases. It was recommended that a corneal transplantation was made in these 8 cases.

Among the 86 eyes studied most of the cases was of advanced keratoconus: 30 of these eyes showed that there was not least 1 cylindrical axis with more than 61 diopters.

A visual acuity equal or better than 20–50 was obtained in 79.06% of all cases. It clearly resulted from this study that a contact lenses adaptation must always be tried even in the most advanced cases of keratoconus, once the possibilities of getting good optical results are signficant.

REFRACIVE ASTIGMATISM AND VISUAL ACUITY FOLLOWING POST- KERATOPLASTY SUTURE REMOVAL IN KERATOCONUS

E. Graue, C. Trapatsas, Si De Ita Ji, T. Ramirez, R. Suarez, L. Moreno, and A. Climent

Instituto De Oftalmologia, Universidad Nacional Autonoma De Mexico, Mexico City

Purpose. To determine the refractive astigmatism and visual acuity following preadjustable post-keratoplasty suture removal in keratoconus with combination continuous interrupted sutures technique. **Methods.** In this retrospective study, 103 patients (105 eyes) diagnosed with keratoconus between 14 to 55 years-of-age undergoing penetrating keratoplasty, where evaluated from 1987 to 1995, comparing spherical and cylindrical factor, axis and visual acuity with combination continuous-8 interrupted sutures technique with Nylon 10–0 in two different groups between 6 to 12 months after surgery for both groups.

Group 1. Before suture removal. Group 2. First month post suture removal. **Results.** Removal of combination continuous interrupted sutures (mean time 9.01 months) caused an average decrease in astigmatism of 1.25 diopters ([)) from 5. 16+-3 .89 D to 3 .91+-2.77 D. However, the astigmatism in 59% of eyes changed 2 or more D and the range changed more than 20 degrees in 53% of the eyes. The spherical factor decreased 0.29 D. Both groups had AJV better than 20/60. 30.21% in Group 1 and 64.75% in Group 2 had A/V better than 20/30. There was an increase in the amount of astigmatism change with decreasing time between surgery and suture removal. **Conclusions.** Refractive astigmatism following preadjustable post-keratoplasty suture removal in keratoconus decreased with continuous interrupted sutures technique during the first 12 postoperative months, allowing a refined control, regarding that suture adjustment or removal of some interrupted suture during the first weeks postoperatively, reaching a faster visual recovery. Supported by Conacyt Grant F082I9110.

Session IX

Non-Microbial Keratitis and Immunology

SECTION IX: NON-MICROBIAL KERATITIS AND IMMUNOLOGY

Abstracts of Conference Presentations and Posters

SEASONAL ALLERGIC, VERNAL, AND ATOPIC CONJUNCTIVITIS

William J. Power

Departments of Cornea and Immunology
Massachusetts Eye and Ear Infirmary; Boston Massachusetts

Allergic disease is extremely common, with 15% of the world's population affected. The eye conditions associated with type I hypersensitivity as a major component are allergic conjunctivitis (both seasonal and perennial), vernal keratoconjunctivitis (VKC), atopic keratoconjunctivis (AKC) and giant papillary conjunctivitis. Corneal involvement occurs frequently in both VKC and AKC. Vernal keratoconjunctivitis is a rare allergic conjunctival inflammatory disorder which typically affects male children. Symptoms are usually worse in the spring but perennial disease also occurs. The predominant symptom of VKC is itching. Excessive tearing, mucus production, photophobia, and burning or foreign body sensation are common symptoms. Although VKC may be a self limiting disease, it is a debilitating and sight threatening condition. Mast cell-stabilizing agents form the mainstay of treatment on patients with VKC. These agents have no effect on blocking the effects of released mediators and to be effective they must be used prophylactically before exposure to antigen. Topical steroids may be used in the treatment of acute initial disease or to control breakthrough inflammation. A short pulse of prednisolone sodium 1%, used four times daily with a taper to stop over 7 to 10 days is usually sufficient.

Atopic keratoconjunctivitis (AKC) was defined by Hogan in 1952 as allergic keratoconjunctivitis occurring in association with atopic dermatitis (eczema). We recently reviewed the course of 20 patients with AKC who were followed for an average of 7.3 years (range 3–17 years). The mean age at presentation was 46 years. There was an associated personal history of eczema in 19 cases and asthma in 13 cases. Fifty per cent of patients had a positive family history of atopy. Significant keratopathy developed in 70% of patients, corneal neovascularization in 60%, fornix foreshortening in 25%, and symblepharon in 20% during the course of their disease. Eleven patients required penetrating keratoplasty (3 for tectonic purposes and 8 for visual rehabilitation). All patients were treated with systemic antihistamines and topical mast cell stabilizers. Eighty five per cent of patients required topical steroids at some point during the course of their disease. Psychoneurotic behavior, consisting of poor compliance with treatment and appointments and occasional self-destructive behavior necessitating psychotherapeutic counseling, was present in 6 patients (30%).

AKC is a potentially blinding disease which may result in a poor visual outcome as a result of corneal complications. Therapy requires a multidisciplinary approach. Patients should be made aware of the chronic nature of the disease and referral for counseling at an early stage may be appropriate for certain patients. Elective surgical intervention can be of benefit but should be performed only in those patients whose inflammation is controlled.

OCULAR CICATRICIAL PEMPHIGOID

C. Stephen Foster

Massachusetts Eye and Ear Infirmary, Boston, Massachusetts

Ocular cicatricial peiriphigoid is an autoimmune, progressive and blinding disease While immunosuppressive chemotherapy revolutionized the care of patients with this disorder, 10% of such individuals still have progressive disease despite all therapeutic attempts, and some patients are intolerant of chemotherapy. Additional insights into the relevant target antigen, the genetic susceptibility to the disease, triggering factors, and more selective treatment are greatly needed. At least one specific antigen in the lamina lucida in the conjunctival basal epithelial cell basement membrane zone has been identified as the target antigen for OCP; it is possible that others exist, since patients with OCP are diverse with respect to the class of antibody found at the BMZ and with respect to response to therapy. We are cloning the gene for the OCP antigen, and expect availability of large amounts of antigen to make possible the development of a sensitive serologic diagnostic test, and to lead to more selective immunomodulatory therapies, possessing less toxicity, for this blinding disease.

STEVENS-JOHNSON SYNDROME

Bartly J. Mondino

Jules Stein Eye Institute, University of California, Los Angeles, Los Angeles, California

Erythema multiforme is an acute, generally self-limited bullous inflammatory disease of the skin and mucous membranes. It develops as a reaction to a wide variety of exogenOus precipitating factors, such as infections and drugs. It has been reported following the use of topical ophthalmic scopolamine, tropicamide and sulfonamides. The minor form affects primarily the skin, whereas the major form (Stevens-Johnson syndrome) can have mucosal and skin involvement with associated toxemia, fever, prostration and even death. Immune complex formation may be important in the immunopathogenesis of the Stevens-Johnson syndrome.

Ocular involvement includes swollen, ulcerated, and crusted eyelids and conjunctivitis. In severe cases, pseudomembranous or membranous conjunctivitis may result in scarring, with associated complications of entropion and trichiasis, inability to fully close the eyelids, fibrosis of lacrimal puncta, dry eye and keratinization. As a result, corneal erosions, ulcers, opacification, and even perforation can occur.

Local treatment appears to have little influence on the severity of ophthalmic complications. The dry, scarred eye resulting from Stevens-Johnson syndrome may require artificial tears, closure of the lacrimal puncta, destruction of aberrant lashes, soft contact lenses to protect the cornea from drying and trichiasis, and lid scrubs followed by antibiotic ointment for the chronic blepharitis that may be found with this disease.

RHEUMATIC CORNEAL ULCERATION

Yuichi Ohashi, Shigeki Okamoto, and Masahiro Okamoto

Department of Ophthalmology, Ehime University School of Medicine, Ehime, Japan

Ocular complications associated with rheumatic arthritis (RA) include keratoconjunctivitis sicca, peripheral corneal infiltrate, sclerosing keratitis, scleritis and so on. Among these, corneal perforation has been increasingly encountered during the clinical course of RA patients and is one of the serious situations which require an immediate and proper management. The therapeutic strategies for corneal perforation should be modified according to the location and the size of the perforation.

Peripheral corneal perforation can be treated with the bandage use of soft contact lenses along with topical antibiotics and low doses of systemic corticosteroid. Peri-limbal conjunctival resection plus subconjunctival administration of corticosteroid is often helpful. To our experience, topical recombinant human epidermal growth factor has been of great benefit especially in cases with persistent aqueous leakage. When the perforation is too large to achieve anterior chamber reformation, off-axis, tectonic lamellar graft should be placed peripherally together with peri-limbal conjunctival resection and partial keratoepithelioplasty.

Central corneal perforation should be initially treated in a similar way to peripheral corneal perforation. When this maneuver fails, intracameral injection of viscoelastic materials should be considered as another option before penetrating keratoplasty is intended. Penetrating keratoplasty is the final choice and needs intensive postoperative care in order to avoid graft rejection as well as epithelial disturbances and subsequent stromal melting.

The exact pathogenesis of rheumatic corneal ulceration has remained unknown. We have recently disclosed an abnormal cytokine expression in the cornea of the mice with experimental rheumatic arthritis, which may partly explain the pathophysiology of acute keratolysis. The implication for future immunotherapy from our laboratory data will be presented.

MOOREN'S ULCERATION

Peter Watson

There has been a tendency among clinicians to call any peripheral corneal destructive change in the absence of any obvious systemic disease, Mooren's ulcer. This has led to considerable confusion in the literature, making it almost impossible to decide which of the many treatments suggested are likely to be effective in a particular case. With the advent of monoclonal antibody therapy it is now becoming vital that all the immune mediated diseases are fully characterised in order that the most appropriate therapy can be given.

The differential diagnoses of the various forms of Mooren's ulceration will be discussed together with recent pathological findings. A therapeutic regime will be suggested based on these findings.

VASCULITIC PERIPHERAL ULCERATIVE KERATITIS

Elisabeth M. Messmer[1] and C. Stephen Foster[2]

[1]University Eye Hospital, Munich, Germany; [2]Massachusetts Eye and Ear Infirmary, Harvard Medical School, Boston, Massachusetts

The onset of peripheral ulcerative keratitis in the course of a connective tissue disorder such as rheumatoid arthritis, relapsing polychondritis or systemic lupus erythematosus may reflect the presence of potentially lethal systemic vasculitis. Moreover, peripheral ulcerative keratitis may be the first presenting sign of systemic necrotizing vasculitis in polyarteritis nodosa or Wegener's granulomatosis and the ophthalmologist sometimes is the first contact with the health system. Although the exact pathogenesis of this severe corneal inflammation and destruction is not well understood, the body of evidence points to a dysfunction in immunoregulation. Immune complexes to autoantigens or some unknown antimicrobial antigen are deposited in scleral and limbal vessels and cause the activation of the complement cascade. Chemotaxis of neutrophils and macrophages, release of inflammatory mediators, proteolytic enzymes and kinins as well as the activation of the clotting cascade seem to be mainly responsible for the resulting tissue damage. Untreated conditions not only carry a grim prognosis for the eye, but are also lifethreatening for the patients. Aggressive immunosuppressive therapy with corticosteroids and cytotoxic agents is therefore mandatory in the treatment of these multisystem disorders associated with vasculitic peripheral ulceralive keratitis.

SCLEROKERATITIS

Maite Sainz de la Maza and C. Stephen Foster

Purpose: Inflammatory peripheral keratitis may accompany scleritis. Early recognition and treatment are essential to avoid corneal perforation. The authors analyze the characteristics of patients with sclerokeratitis to delineate the prognosis of the presence of keratitis in the course of scleritis.
Methods: Type of keratitis, type of scleritis, patient characteristics, ocular complications, previous ocular surgery, and specific disease association were evaluated in patients with sclerokeratitis; comparisons were made between patients with sclerokeratitis and patients with scleritis without keratitis, and between the different clinical types of keratitis in scleritis.
Results: Forty-seven of 172 patients with scleritis had keratitis (27%); they included 12 pa-

tients with peripheral corneal thinning, 11 patients with stromal keratitis, and 24 patients with peripheral ulcerative keratitis. Patients with sclerokeratitis had more necrotizing scleritis (57%, p=0.0001), decrease in vision (81%, p=0.0001), anterior uveitis (62%, p=0.0016), previous ocular surgery (38%, p=0.0001) and specific disease association (87%, p=0.0001) than did patients with scleritis without keratitis. Patients with peripheral ulcerative keratitis had more impending corneal perforation (100%, p=0.0001), previous ocular surgery (58%, p=0.0032), and specific disease association (100%, p=0.0066) than patients with the other types of keratitis in scleritis. **Conclusions:** The detection of inflammatory peripheral keratitis in a patient with scleritis connotes a poor ocular prognosis because it indicates extension of scleral inflammation to adjacent structures leading to ocular complications which may cause progressive visual loss. It also indicates a poor systemic prognosis because it is often associated with potentially lethal systemic diseases. Peripheral ulcerative keratitis entails the worst ocular prognosis because it is more often associated with impending corneal perforation than peripheral corneal thinning and stromal keratitis.

CORNEAL TRANSPLANT AND IMMUNOSUPPRESSANT

Atsushi Kanai

Department of Ophthalmology, Juntendo University School of Medicine, Tokyo, Japan

Despite the excellent anatomic and optical results obtained with keratoplasty, graft rejection remains a significant problem.

The incidence of graft rejection is variable, but in vascularized host cornea, prognosis of graft survival is not favourable. Corticosteroids are used for corneal transplantation to prevent graft rejection and are generally effective; however, side effects of steroid therapy are noticed. Immunosuppressive agents, such as azathioprine, cyclophosphamide, and antilymphocyte serum had been used in experimental setting as well as in a very limited series in humans. A significant improvement in the success rate of organ transplantation was achieved by the introduction of a new, powerful immunosuppressant, cyclosporin and FK-506. However, the systemic administration of these agents may be associated with side effects. Local administration of these drugs promises to be a new frontier for the prevention of corneal graft rejection.

MINOR H, RATHER THAN MHC, ALLOANTIGENS OFFER THE GREATER BARRIER TO SUCCESSFUL ORTHOTOPIC CORNEAL TRANSPLANTATION

Yoichiro Sano,[1,2] Bruce R. Ksander,[1] and J. W. Streilein[1]

[1]Schepens Eye Research Institute and Department of Ophthalmology Harvard Medical School, Boston, Massachusetts; [2]Department of Ophthalmology, Kyoto Prefectural University of Medicine, Kyoto Japan

Irrespective of HLA matching, a far higher proportion of human corneal allografts placed orthotopically in avascular corneal graft beds are accepted indefinitely, compared to other types of solid tissue allografts. However, many more corneal grafts are rejected if they are transplanted onto neovascularized recipient eyes. Using a murine model of orthotopic corneal transplantation in which grafts were placed in normal eyes, we have reported previously that grafts bearing minor H antigens alone are more likely to be rejected (approximately 50%) than are grafts displaying only MHC alloantigens (<20%). These studies have now been extended to include corneal grafts placed in neovascularized recipient eyes. Neovascularization was induced by placing sutures in the central cornea of one eye of recipient mice. Two weeks later, MHC class I only, class II only, minor H only, or MHC + minor H disparate corneal allografts were grafted into these eyes and their rejection rates were examined. While MHC + minor H disparate corneal allografts were uniformly rejected in neovascularized graft beds (10 out of 10), 66.7% (8 out of 12) of MHC class I only disparate grafts and 58.3% (7 out of 12) of MHC class II only disparate corneal allografts were rejected. Surprisingly, the rejection rate of minor H only disparate corneal allografts was 90.9% (10 out of 11). These findings indicate that, for orthotopic corneal allografts, minor H antigens offer a more formidable barrier to graft acceptance than do MHC-encoded antigens. We speculate that this unexpected outcome may reflect a reduced level of MHC expression on corneal tissue. Moreover since the cornea lacks bone marrow-derived dendritic cells, allorecognition by recipient T cells must occur via the *indirect* pathway, and in this situation minor H antigens may compete favorably with MHC antigens for processing and presentation by recipient APC.

$\delta\gamma$T CELLS IN MURINE CONJUNCTIVAL EPITHELIUM AND ITS MIGRATION TO CORNEAL EPITHELIUM

Y. Tagawa, A. Matsuda, and H. Matsuda

Department of Ophthalmology, Hokkaido University School of Medicine, Sapporo, Japan

Purpose: We have previously demonstrated that Langerhans cells and Thy-1 lymphocytes were major immunocompetent cells in murine conjunctival epithelium and a part of those Thy-1 cells expressed $\delta\gamma$T cell receptor in conjunctiva as same as those in epidermis(Thy-1 DEC). In this study we examined whether $\delta\gamma$T cells migrated to cornea by the stimuli to cornea. **Methods:** C3H/He mice were used throughout the experiments. 1)10–0 nylon suture were made in the center of the cornea. 2)OK-432, a group A streptococcal preparation of a potent immunostimulant were injected to the cornea. EDTA-separated epithelial sheets were immunostained by immunofluorescence after ten days in sutured eyes and five days in OK-432 injected eyes, respectively. The following monoclonal antibodies were used;1)anti-$\delta\gamma$T cell 2)anti-CD3. **Results:** In normal mice T cells and CD3 cells were observed in conjunctiva, but not in cornea. $\delta\gamma$T cells and CD3 cells were found in the center of the cornea in 10–0 nylon sutured eyes. In OK-432 injected eyes $\delta\gamma$T cells and CD3 cells were present in cornea and increased in number in conjunctiva. **Conclusions:** The above findings indicate that $\delta\gamma$T cells migrate to cornea and increase in number in conjunctiva responding to the stimuli to the cornea. Therefore, $\delta\gamma$T cells may play a role in the first line of defense in the ocular surface epithelium.

IMMUNOHISTOCHEMICAL STUDY OF THE CORNEA AND CONJUNCTIVA IN MOOREN'S ULCER AND THE TREATMENT WITH LAMELLAR KERATOPLASTY AND TOPICAL CYCLOSPORINE A

Zheng Wang, Jia-qi Chen, Long-shan Chen, Chnn-mao Feng, Yue-sheng Lin, and Bin Yang

Zhongshan Ophthalmic Center, Sun Yat-sen University of Medical Sciences, Guangzhou, China

Purpose: To investigate the local immunological changes in Mooren's ulcer and to determine whether postoperative topical cyclosporine A (CsA) would further improve the outcome of conventional lamellar keratoplasty for Mooren's ulcer. **Methods:** *Part I.* The corneal and conjunctival specimens from 14 patients with Mooren's ulcer who underwent lamellar keratoplasty and 6 cadaver eyes were stained immunohistologically for CD1, CD3, CD4, CD8, CD25 and HLA-DR. *Part II.* Forty-seven consecutive eyes in 44 patients with Mooren's ulcer were treated with lamellar keratoplasty. A crescent, annular, or a whole lamellar corneoscleral graft (with 2-mm scleral rim) was used, according to the extent of the ulceration. Sutures were not placed on the cornea so that to minimize suture induced nonspecific inflammations and corneal astigmatism. Postoperatively, cyclosporine A 1% eyedrops were given, 6 times a day for 2 months and then 4 times a day for 6 to 12 months. The patients were followed up for 18 months to 6 years. **Results:** *Part I.* The CD4+/CD8+ ratio was significantly higher than normal control. HLA-DR antigen was aberrantly expressed by the epithelial cells and keratocytes. *Part II.* Finally 45 eyes (95.7%) were cured. Thirty-seven eyes (78.7%) were cured after initial operation. Seven eyes (14.9%) were cured after 2 repeated procedures and 1 eye (2.1%) after 3 procedures. Recurrence occurred in 2 eyes even after 3 repeated procedures. Both the surgical outcome and the postoperative vision were improved compared with our results before topical CsA were used. **Conclusion.** The aberrant expression of MHC-II antigen by the resident cells and the raised local T_H/T_S ratio may play an important role in the pathogenesis of Mooren's ulcer. Lamellar keratoplasty is an effective treatment for Mooren's ulcer and postoperative topical CsA may further improve the result.

SUBCONJUNCTIVAL TREATMENT OF OCULAR CICATRICIAL PEMPHIGOID WITH MITOMYCIN C

Eric D. Donnenfeld,[1,2] Henry D. Perry,[1,3] Anastasios J. Kanellopoulos,[4] Gayle Grossman,[1] Stanley J. Berke,[1] and Richard T. Sturm[1]

[1]North Shore University Hospital, Manhasset, New York; [2]Manhattan Eye, Ear and Throat Hospital, New York; [3]New York Eye and Ear Infirmary, New York; [4]Massachusetts Eye and Ear Infirmary, Boston, Massachusetts

Purpose: Ocular cicatricial pemphigoid (OCP) is a potentially blinding disorder of autoimmune etiology, resulting in conjunctival cicatrization with subepithelial fibrosis. Treatment with systemic chemotherapy is not always successful, and may be associated with significant morbidity and on occasion, mortality. Mitomycin C interferes with fibroblast proliferation. We investigated the effect of localized treatment of OCP with Mitomycin C.

Methods: Three patients with undiagnosed OGP were treated by referring physicians for pseudopterygium (1 patient) and glaucoma (2 patients) with focal application of Mitomycin C to the bare sclera. This patient group stimulated us to evaluate the use of subconjunctival Mitomycin C for OCP. Four additional patients with known OCP received monocular subconjunctival injections of 0.5 ccs of .2 mg/ml Mitomycin C in the more affected eye. RESULTS. All 3 patients with topical applications of Mitomycin C showed focal quiescence of the disease with a mean follow-up of 2.1 years. Three of the 4 patients with subconjunctival Mitomycin C failed to show progression of the disease, while the untreated eye showed progression with a mean follow-up of 12 months. There were no significant side effects noted with the subconjunctival Mitomycin C injection. Histopathologic examination of 2 patients revealed a paucity of inflammatory cells and a lack of fibrosis in the areas treated with Mitomycin C, while control areas showed marked inflammatory changes, consistent with OCP.

Conclusion: Subconjunctival Mitomycin C requires further evaluation in the treatment of ocular cicatricial pemphigoid. (No proprietary interest.)

OCULAR SURFACE RECONSTRUCTION BY LIMBAL AUTOGRAFT TRANSPLANTATION WITH THE USE OF AMNIOTIC MEMBRANE

Jun Shimazaki and Kazuo Tsubota

Department of Ophthalmology, Tokyo Dental College, Chiba, Japan

Treatment of cicatricial ocular surface disorders such as chemical burn and recurrent pterygium is challenging. Limbal autograft transplantation has been shown to be effective for promoting corneal epithelialiation in some cases, but not in cases with severe conjunctival scarring. We treated such difficult cases by limbal autograft transplantation with the use of amniotic membrane, which has been used to supplement a thick basement membrane, decrease bacterial growth, and prevent tissue adhesion.

Three chemical burns and two recurrent pterygia with severe symblepharon were treated as follow: scar tissues were totally excised and a preserved amniotic membrane was placed on the exposed sclera. The amniotic membrane was obtained at a time of cesarean sections, and stored in -80C with DMSO. Limbal tissue was then excised either from contralateral eye in cases of chemical burn, or from ipsilateral eye in cases of pterygium. The graft was secured at limbal lesion where scar tissue invasion on the cornea was most prominent.

Postoperatively, ocular surface was promptly reconstructed in all cases, with a total lysis of symblepharon. No recurrence was noted in each patient with the mean follow-up of 7.6 months. Athough a long-term follow-up is necessary these results indicate that the procedure is useful for ocular surface reconstruction in cases of monocular conjunctival cicatricial disorders.

INTERSTITIAL KERATITIS IN SARCOIDOSIS

Janine A. Smith and Robert B. Nussenblatt

National Eye Institute; National Institutes of Health, Bethesda, Maryland

Interstitial keratitis (IK) is an exceedingly uncommon ophthalmic manifestation of sarcoidosis of symptomatic patients. Pulmonary involvement is most frequently encountered followed by ocular manifestations of disease such as uveitis, retinal phlebitis, choroidal granuloma formation and optic nerve edema. There are few reports of corneal changes seen in conjunction with sarcoidosis except for the well described association with calcific band keratopathy. Lennarson and Bamey recently reported a single case of childhood sarcoidosis with IK as the initial ocular manifestation of disease. Further review of the literature reveals only five cases of probable IK in patients with clear evidence of sarcoidosis; however, these are largely incompletely described.

Reported here are two cases of IK in adults with uveitis and pulmonary sarcoidosis. Case I: A 44 year old black woman with a history of skin lesions, shortness of breath and bilateral chronic, granulomatous anterior uveitis developed bilateral inferior, corneal stromal inflammation. Deep stromal vessels and scrolls of Descemet's membrane were also evident. Bilateral vitreous cells, inferior snowballs and sheathing of peripheral retinal vessels were noted. Although serum ACE, calcium and lysozyme were normal, chest x-ray showed bilateral interstitial disease but no hilar changes and CT revealed massive mediastinal lymphadenopathy consistent with sarcoidosis.

Case II: A 37 year old black woman with a history of bilateral chronic anterior uveitis was referred for evaluation and found to have bilateral corneal stromal scarring without vascularization. The inferior corneal opacification was triangular and symmetric reminiscent of the pattern of inflammation seen in the first patient and consistent with previous IK. Exam of the left eye further revealed vitreous cells and chorioretinal lesions of the inferior retinal periphery. Whereas serum calcium and lysozyme were normal, the ACE was elevated. Chest x-ray showed bilateral hilar and paratracheal lymphadenopathy and increased interstitial markings. Biopsy of a skin lesion showed noncaseating granuloma.

These two cases highlight an uncommon etiology of nonsuppurative corneal inflammation with vascularization. Sarcoidosis should be considered in the differential diagnosis of IK and further diagnostic work-up pursued as necessary.

IDENTIFICATION AND IMMUNOLOCALIZATION OF MACROPHAGE MIGRATION INHIBITORY FACTOR (MIF) IN HUMAN CORNEA

Akira Matsuda,[1] Jun Nishihira,[2] Yoshitsugu Tagawa,[1] and Hidehiko Matsuda[1]

[1]Department of Ophthalmology and [2]Central Reserch Institute Hokkaido University School of Medicine, Sapporo, Japan

We detected macrophage migration inhibitory factor (MIF) mRNA expression on human corneal epithelium and endothelium by reverse transcription-polymerase chain reaction, and demonstrated its immunolocalization using the polyclonal antibody prepared from immunizing a rabbit with human recombinant MIF. MIF mRNA was expressed in both the corneal epithelial cells and the endothelial cells. Immunohistochemical study showed that MIF was present basal cells of corneal epithelium and endothelial cells. Identification of MIF in differentiating corneal cells suggests that MIF plays an important role in corneal cell differentiation.

Session X

World Corneal Health

42

CHILDHOOD KERATITIS

Epidemiological and Microbiological Study

Anita Panda,[1] Namrata Sharma,[1] Rasik B. Vajpayee,[1] Geeta Satpathy,[1]
Surendra K. Angra,[1] and Madhu Vajpayee[2]

[1]Dr. Rajendra Prasad Centre for Ophthalmic Sciences
All India Institute of Medical Sciences
New Delhi, India
[2]Department of Microbiology
All India Institute of Medical Sciences
New Delhi, India

ABSTRACT

The objective of this study is to evaluate the demographic features, clinical profile, and microbiological agents in cases of microbial keratitis in children under 16 years of age over a period of 20 years. The study was designed as a retrospective analysis set in the Cornea Clinic of the Dr. Rajendra Prasad Center for Ophthalmic Sciences in New Delhi, a tertiary eye care referral centre. Culture-positive corneal ulcers in 1,118 consecutive eyes of 1,070 children were reviewed in this retrospective analysis. The study period was divided into Phase I (1975–1984) and Phase II (1985–1994). The most common predisposing factors identified were trauma (36.94%) and systemic illness (22.36%). Malnutrition, determined by body mass index was present in 87.85% of the children studied. Bacterial isolates were more common in Phase I and Phase II (77.2% and 35.4%, respectively) as compared to fungal (22.8% and 46.6%, respectively). A significantly higher incidence of fungal pathogens was noted in Phase II ($Z = 8.32$; $p < 0.001$). Additional highlights of Phase II included the emergence of *Staphylococcus albus* as a major Gram positive organism (43.5% vs. 26.5%) ($Z = 3.63$; $p < 0.001$), decrease in *Streptococcus pneumoniae* (30.6% vs. 8.7%) ($Z = 5.73$; $p < 0.001$), and no cases of *Neisseria gonorrhea*. *Pseudomonas aeruginosa* was the most common (49.1%) of the Gram negative organisms identified. Similarly, *Aspergillus* was the most common fungus isolated (49.4%), followed by *Fusarium* (11.7%). However, no significant variation in the isolation of Gram negative or fungal organisms was noted between the two phases. This study highlights the demographic features, risk factors, and changing etiological pattern of microbial keratitis in children. The causes of the changing microbial spectrum over the 20 years are also discussed. A prospective study evaluating the same is recommended.

Advances in Corneal Research, edited by Lass
Plenum Press, New York, 1997

INTRODUCTION

Microbial keratitis in adults has been described at great length in various reports.[1-3] However, not much information is available in pediatric patients.[4-6] Many age-related risk factors, including tear film dysfunction, lid abnormalities, blepharitis, neurotrophic keratitis, and exposure have a limited role in children.[5] The identification of principal risk factors predisposing to corneal infection has been emphasized in many series of microbial keratitis.[1-7] However, most of these studies included very few children. Lack of reliable history, delay in reporting the symptoms, inability to cooperate for biomicroscopic examination and subsequent corneal scraping often prolongs the interval to initial diagnosis and therapy of corneal ulceration in the pediatric age group.[6]

This retrospective study analyzed the demographic features, predisposing factors, clinical characteristics, and microbial pathogens responsible for childhood keratitis. Also studied were the microbial spectrum and the changing etiological agents over the 20 year study period.

PATIENTS AND METHODS

We undertook a retrospective analysis of culture-proven cases of microbial keratitis in children less than 16 years of age who presented to the Cornea Service at Dr. Rajendra Prasad Centre for Ophthalmic Sciences (New Delhi, India) between January 1, 1975 and December 31, 1994. Criteria for inclusion in the study were: (1) keratitis with clinical appearance consistent with infectious non-viral ulcer and (2) identification of pathogen on culture. The study period was divided into Phase I (1975–1984) and Phase II(1985–1994) to enable a review of the changing etiological pattern over the 20-year period.

The accumulated medical records were reviewed using a standardized protocol. A complete ophthalmic and related history was evaluated. Factors recorded included age, sex, predisposing factors, location, and size of the lesion and presence or absence of hypopyon or perforation. Body mass index (BMI), a determinant of malnutrition, was available in the last 370 cases (as a part of an ongoing prospective trial). This was calculated as follows:

$$\text{Body mass index (BMI)} = \text{Weight in kg} \div \text{Height in metres}^2$$

Clinical Evaluation

The location of the ulcer, whether central, paracentral, or peripheral was noted in each case. The size of the ulcer, as recorded in charts, was measure from its mid point and divided into small, medium, and large (Table 1).

Laboratory Diagnosis

The records showed that scraping specimens were obtained from the edge of the ulcer using standard technique either under topical anesthesia (with/without sedation) or under general anesthesia, depending upon the patient's cooperation (Table 1). Corneal scraping was done under general anesthesia, sedation, or topical anesthesia, depending on the level of a patient's cooperation. General anesthesia was required by 241 children (22.5%) (Table 2). In 77.5% of the children (829/1070), overall scraping and examination

Table 1. Location and size of keratitis

	No. of eyes (%)
I. Location	
Central	701 (62.7)
Paracentral	298 (26.7)
Peripheral	119 (10.6)
II. Size of ulcer	
Small (< 2 mm)	198 (17.7)
Medium (2-6 mm)	622 (55.6)
Large (> 6 mm)	298 (26.7)

was possible under topical anesthesia with or without sedation. Of the 482 patients who were less than five years of age, 290 required sedation with topical anesthesia. Sedation was achieved by chloral hydrate (100 mg/kg) and 4% xylocaine was used for topical anesthesia. All children older than 10 years of age cooperated for scraping under topical anesthesia, except one 12-year-old, mentally retarded child who required general anesthesia.

Scrapings were obtained with a platinum spatula and Gram stained smears prepared. KOH wet mount preparation for fungal organisms was also performed. The specimens obtained were inoculated onto blood agar, Sabouraud's agar plates supplemented with yeast extract and 50 ug/ml of gentamicin sulphate (without cycloheximide) at 20°C to enhance the growth of fungi, and 2% non-nutrient agar overlaid with *Escherichia coli* (which was available from 1989 onwards only).

A culture was considered positive when there was growth of 11 or more colonies of the same bacterial organism on two or more culture media or confluent growth on multiple "C" streaks on solid medium.[9] For fungi, growth of one or more colonies on two media or growth on one medium confirmed by a positive smear was considered a positive culture.[9]

Statistical Analysis

Statistical analysis to compare the proportion of organisms between two independent phases was done using Test of Proportion in two independent groups.

RESULTS

Out of a total of 4,863 cases of microbial keratitis seen at the tertiary center during the study period, 1,086 were children, i.e., overall incidence of childhood microbial keratitis was 22.3%. However, 16 cases were excluded from the study group for lack of com-

Table 2. Anaesthesia used for scrapping

Age in years	No. of children	General anaesthesia	Sedative + topical anaesthesia	Topical anaesthesia
0–5	482	192	290	–
6–10	396	48	297	51
11–15	192	1	–	191
		241	587	242

Table 3. Predisposing factors

Risk factors	No. of eyes (%)
Trauma	413 (37)
a) Home	40
b) Assault	101
c) Industrial	41
d) Bow and arrow	98
e) Rural/Vegetable matter	74
f) Others	59
Systemic illness	250 (22.4)
Previous ocular surgery	119 (10.6)
Exposure	101 (9)
Steroid use	48 (4.3)
Contact lens wear	84 (6.6)
Severe dry eye	65 (4.9)
Lid abnormality	38 (2.5)
Unidentified	30 (2.7)

plete data. Of 1,070 children enrolled for the study, 696 (65%) were males and 374 (35%) were females with a mean age of 6.5 ± 6 years (range 5 months to 15 years). Trauma was the most common predisposing factor (37%) (Table3). Bow and arrow injury was responsible for 24% of all trauma cases. The frequency of other identified factors is shown in Table 3. The BMI, available in only the last 370 cases, was calculated and severity of malnutrition correlated with the frequency of corneal ulceration in children (Fig. 1). Malnutrition was graded according to the BMI and was present in 87.85% of patients; of these 4.1% were labeled as suffering to a severe degree. Other systemic associations included bronchopneumonia, diarrhea, eruptive fevers, skin diseases, and neurological problems. Exposure keratopathy was seen in 9% of cases.

Clinical Characteristics

The right eye was involved in 677 cases (60.5%), the left eye in 441 cases (39.5%), and 48 (4.4%) children had bilateral corneal ulceration. The central location of the kerati-

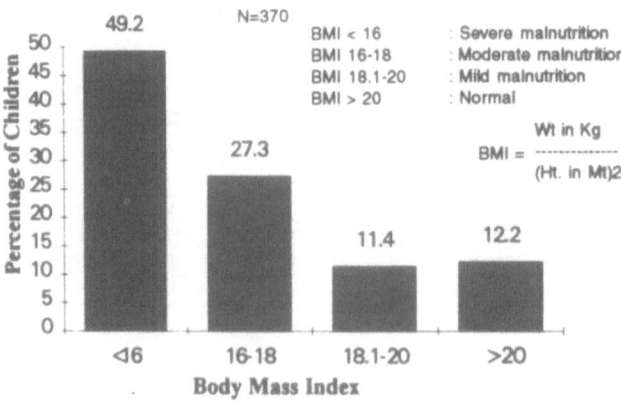

Figure 1. Body mass index (severity of malnutrition) of 370 children.

Table 4. Pathogens isolated

	No. of pathogens	No. of eyes
Bacteria alone	637	637
More than one bacteria	84	36
Fungus alone	415	415
Mixed (bacteria + fungus)	60	30
	1196	1118

tis was most common (62.7%), followed by paracentral and peripheral (Table 1). Most ulcers were of moderate size (55.6%) (Table 1). Hypopyon was present in 705 eyes (63.1%), while 192 (17.2%) eyes were associated with perforation.

Microbiological Evaluation

Of 1,196 pathogens isolated, 751 (62.8%) were bacterial and 445 (37.2%) were fungal. Of the 751 bacteria isolated, 657 were bacterial alone (single and polybacterial). Fungal isolates alone were seen in 37.1% of eyes (415). Mixed infection, with bacteria and fungus were seen in 30 eyes (Table 4). No *Acanthamoeba species* were cultured during the study period.

A retrospective analysis of Gram stained smear revealed a positivity of 77.2% in bacterial cases (580/751) and 27.2% in fungal cases (121/445). KOH wet mount preparation was positive in 92.4% (411/445).

A higher incidence of fungal pathogens (46.6%; 337/723) was seen in Phase II as compared to Phase I (22.8%; 108/473) as shown in Figure 2 (Z - 8.32; p < 0.001). Analysis of the bacterial isolates in two phases revealed a greater predominance of Gram positive bacteria (59.6%) over Gram negative (53.7%) in Phase II (Fig. 3). Significantly higher isolates of *Staphylococcus albus* (43.5%) were seen in Phase II, as compared to Phase I (26.5%; Z = 3.63; p < 0.001) (Table 5). *Staphylococcus aureus* did not show a sig-

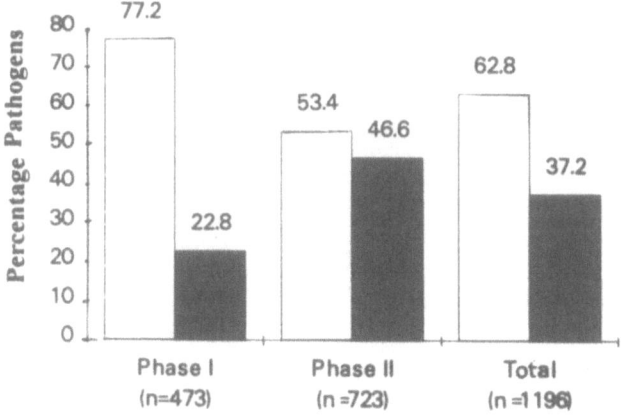

Figure 2. Pathogens isolated (bacteria and fungi) over the 2 phases.

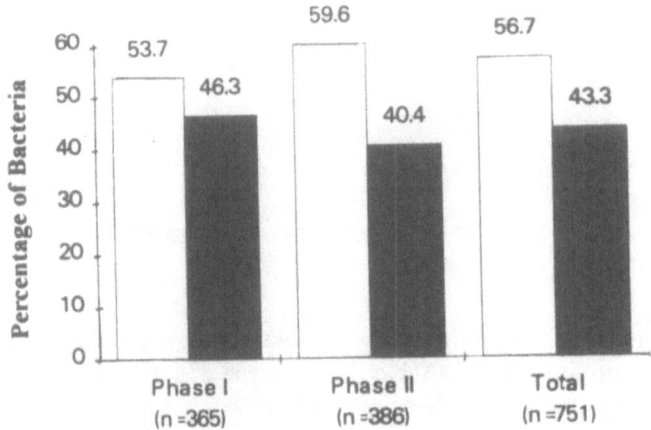

Figure 3. Bacteria isolated (Gram positive and Gram negative) over the 2 phases.

nificant change in its isolation in the two phases (29.6% vs. 31.3%; Z = 0.38; P > 0.05). *Streptococcus pneumoniae* was significantly decreased in the second phase (8.7 versus 30.6%; Z = 5.7; p < 0.001) (Table 5). Among the Gram negative organisms, *Pseudomonas aeruginosa* was the most common in Phase I (49.1%), the isolation of which significantly increased in the second phase (62.2%; Z - 2.36; p < 0.001), followed by *Neisseria gonorrhea* (10.7%). However, no case of the latter was noted in Phase II (Table 6). *Aspergillus* species was the leading fungus isolated, followed by *Fusarium* and no significant variation among the various fungal isolates was noted over the two phases (Table 7).

DISCUSSION

Microbial keratitis is a potentially blinding disorder in children. Very few studies are available highlighting the epidemiology, clinical features, and microbial spectrum of pediatric keratitis.[4-6] This is the first series reviewing the etiological factors, clinical features, and changes in microbial spectrum of childhood keratitis in a developing country over the 20 year study period. Various predisposing factors for adult microbial keratitis include trauma, use of contact lenses, systemic illness, previous ocular surgery, topical ster-

Table 5. Gram positive organisms isolated

Organism	Phase I (n = 196) *	Phase II (n = 230)*	Statistical analysis (Z value p value)	Total (%) (n = 426)*
Staphylococcus albus	52 (26.5)	100 (43.5)	-3.639 <0.001	152 (35.7)
Staphylococcus aureus	58 (29.6)	72 (31.3)	NS	130 (30.5)
Streptococcus pneumoniae	60 (30.6)	20 (8.7)	5.773 <0.001	80 (18.8)
Bacillus species	26 (13.3)	38 (16.5)	NS	64 (15.0)

NS: Not significant
*No. (%)

Table 6. Gram negative organisms

Organism	Phase I (n = 169)*	Phase II (n = 156)*	Statistical analysis (Z value p value)	Total (n = 325)*
Pseudomonas aeruginosa	82 (49.1)	97 (62.2)	-2.368 <0.01	180 (55.3)
Enterobacter sp.	17 (10.1)	15 (9.6)	NS	32 (9.8)
Klebsiella pneumoniae	11 (6.5)	9 (5.8)	NS	20 (6.3)
Proteus sp.	11 (6.5)	2 (1.3)	2.402 <0.01	13 (4.0)
Neisseria gonorrhea	18 (10.7)	0 (0)	4.194 <0.001	18 (5.5)
Haemophilus influenza	6 (3.6)	6 (3.9)	NS	12 (3.7)
Haemophilus aegypticus	9 (5.3)	8 (5.1)	NS	17 (5.3)
Acinetobacter sp.	12 (7.0)	16 (10.2)	NS	28 (8.6)
Moraxella sp.	2 (1.2)	3 (1.9)	NS	5 (1.5)

NS: Not significant
*No. (%)

oid medications, exposure keratitis, keratitis sicca, and recurrent erosions.[1-7] Although similar predisposing factors were found in children, a variation in the frequency of these risk factors has been noted.[4-6] Trauma was the most common local ocular predisposition regardless of age.[4-6] Ormerod et al. 91986) and Cruz et al. (1993) have noted trauma as the predisposing factor in 26% and 44% of cases, respectively.[4,5] The same was seen in 36.9% of cases in this series. Bow and arrow injury is more prevalent in this part of the world due to mythological and religious associations and was reported in 30% of all trauma cases in a previous study.[10] As a cause of microbial keratitis, this was responsible for 24% of all trauma cases. The introduction of the organism through an epithelial defect or gap in epithelial bridges is concurrent with penetrating or perforating corneal injury.[4] Although anterior segment surgery or previous corneal pathology is among the leading risk factors in

Table 7. Fungi isolated

Organism	Phase I (n = 108)*	Phase II (n = 337)*	Statistical analysis (Z value p value)	Total (n = 445)*
Aspergillus sp.	55 (50.9)	165 (49.0)	NS	220 (49.4)
Fusarium sp.	13 (12.0)	39 (11.6)	NS	52 (11.7)
Alternaria sp.	10 (9.3)	38 (11.2)	NS	48 (10.8)
Mucor sp.	2 (1.9)	16 (4.7)	NS	18 (4.0)
Penicillium sp.	5 (4.6)	20 (5.9)	NS	25 (5.6)
Rhizophus sp.	1 (0.9)	3 (0.9)	NS	4 (0.9)
Curvularia sp.	7 (6.5)	18 (5.3)	NS	25 (5.6)
Candida sp.	4 (3.7)	4 (1.2)	NS	8 (1.8)
Helminthosporium sp.	2 (1.9)	6 (1.8)	NS	8 (1.8)
Cladosporium sp.	2 (1.9)	5 (1.5)	NS	7 (1.6)
Unidentfied sp.	4 (3.7)	5 (1.5)	NS	9 (2.2)
Cephalosporium sp.	1 (0.9)	4 (1.2)	NS	5 (1.1)
Hermodendrum sp.	1 (0.9)	4 (1.2)	NS	5 (1.1)
Syncephalostrum sp.	–	6 (1.8)	NS	6 (1.3)
Phialophora sp.	1 (0.9)	4 (1.2)	NS	5 (1.1)

NS: Not Significant
*No. (%)

developed countries, this was not so in our study.[4-6] Systemic illness was responsible for a substantial number of cases (22.4%) in this series). This was possibly due to greater predominance of diarrhea, bronchopneumonia, eruptive fevers, and skin diseases associated with malnutrition. These are the major contributing factors for occurrence of corneal infections in tropical climates and developing countries. This was further substantiated by assessment of BMI, a determinant of malnutrition, which was available for 370 patients and revealed the presence of malnutrition in 87.9% of them.

The incidence of fungal keratitis demonstrated a significant increase in Phase II as compared to Phase I (46.6% vs. 22.8%; $Z = 8.32$; $p < 0.001$). Fungal infections are particularly common in hot and humid tropical countries; any corneal injury contaminated with soil or vegetable matter is a potential site for mycotic infection.[11] The increased frequency and distribution of corneal mycotic infection in recent years (Phase II) is probably due to the indiscriminate use of topical steroids and antibiotics.[11] However, the possibility of a referral bias cannot be ruled out in such cases, i.e., only ulcers not responsive to antibiotics were referred to our tertiary center. Due to lack of facilities for optimal microbiological investigations, particularly in peripheral health care centers, there is an increase in the number of children who receive therapy before specimens for culture are made.[6] Also, there is a tendency on the part of the ophthalmologist to start maximal medication prior to microbiological evaluation.

Indigenous bacteria, such as *Staphylococcus albus*, are being isolated with increasing frequency in corneal ulcers, more so in polymicrobial infections.[3] An overwhelming increase (26.5% vs. 43.5%; $Z = -3.6$) in these organisms was noted during the last ten years of our study. *Bacillus* species infections were seen in 15.02% of cases. Since many of the children's injuries involved playing with sticks, bow and arrow, or exposure to vegetable debris, these types of unusual virulent organisms can be expected to invade the cornea. A significant association with *Streptococcus pneumonia* in the 0–19 year old age group is well known.[4,13] However, once a common cause of corneal ulceration prior to the advent of modern lacrimal surgery, this has decreased in frequency in recent times.[13] Therefore, fewer cases of *Streptococcus pneumoniae* were encountered in the second phase.

Pseudomonas aeruginosa was the most common Gram negative organism isolated in our study. However, no case of *Neisseria gonorrhea* was noted in the last 10 years of the study, which has been attributed to improved antenatal, natal, and postnatal care, as well as to better prophylaxis available against these organisms.[6]

Similar to findings in adult keratitis, the *Aspergillus* species was the most common fungal pathogen isolated in the pediatric patients in the present study, as has been noted worldwide and in India, alike.[14,15]

The major thrust of this study was to identify the predisposing factors of childhood keratitis, as well as to review the changing patterns in isolation of various pathogens over the last two decades.[1] Judicious collection of samples from the ulcer is mandatory for proper isolation of the organism and hence, prompt and appropriate medication. This series represents the first review of microbial keratitis in children in developing countries, where this disease entity is very frequently encountered. However, a prospective trial evaluating the demographic features, clinical profile, microbial spectrum, treatment modalities, and visual outcome data in children with microbial keratitis would enable a better understanding of this clinical challenge.

REFERENCES

1. D. Locatcher-Khorazo, Seegal, C., and Gutierrez, E.H., Bacterial infections of the eye. In, *Microbiology of the Eye*, D. Locatcher and Seegal, B.C., eds. St. Louis, C.V. Mosby (1972).

2. D. Ormerod, Hertzmark, E., Gomez, D.S., et al., Epidemiology of microbial keratitis in southern California: a multivariate analysis. *Ophthalmology* 94:1322 (1987).

3. T.J. Liesegang, and Forster, R.K., Spectrum of microbial keratitis in South Florida. *Am. J. Ophthalmol.* 90:38 (1980).

4. L.D. Ormerod, Murphree, A.L., Gomez, D.S., et al., Microbial keratitis in children. *Ophthalmology* 94:449 (1986).

5. O.A. Cruz, Sabir, S.M., Capo, H., and Alfonso, E.C., Microbial keratitis in childhood. *Ophthalmology* 100(2):192 (1993).

6. T.E. Clinch, F.E. Palmon, F.E., Robinson, M.J., et al. Microbial keratitis in children. *Am. J. Ophthalmol.* 117:65 (1994).

7. D.B. Jones, Initial therapy of suspected microbial ulcers. II. Specific antibiotic therapy based on corneal smears. *Surv. Ophthalmol.* 24:97 (1979).

8. F.S. King, and Burgess, A., Anthropometric Reference Values in Nutrition for Developing Countries. Second Edition. New York, Oxford University Press (1993).

9. J.A. Washington, Initial processing for cultures of specimens. In, *Laboratory Procedures in Clinical Microbiology*, Second Edition, Chapter 3. New York, Springer Verlag.

10. A. Panda, Bhatia I.M., and Dayal, Y., Ocular injury. *Afro Asian J. Ophthalmol.* III:163 (1985).

11. F.M. Polack, Kaufman, H.E., and Newmark, E., Keratomycosis. *Arch. Ophthalmol.* 85:410 (1971).

12. C.S. Foster, Fungal Keratitis. *Infect. Dis. Clin. North Am.* 6(4):851 (1992).

13. M. Okumoto and Smolin, G., Pneumococcal infections of the eye. *Am. J. Ophthalmol.* 79:719 (1975).

14. B.R. Jones, Principles in management of oculomyocosis. *Am. J. Ophthalmol.* 79:719 (1975).

15. O.P. Kulshreshtha, Bhargava, S., and Dube, M.K., Keratomycosis: a report of 23 cases. *Indian J. Ophthalmol.* 21:51 (1973).

43

EOSINOPHILS IN OCULAR INFLAMMATION

Histological and Ultrastructural Characteristics of Onchercercal Keratitis

Eric Pearlman,[1,2,3] David S. Bardenstein,[1,3] James W. Kazura,[2] and Jonathan H. Lass[1]

[1]Center for Vision Research
Department of Ophthalmology
[2]Department of Medicine
[3]Department of Pathology
Case Western Reserve University
Cleveland, Ohio

ABSTRACT

Eosinophils are implicated in allergen-mediated keratitis and conjunctivitis, including hay fever conjunctivitis and vernal keratoconjunctivitis. Eosinophils are also associated with sclerosing keratitis caused by the parasitic helminth *Onchocerca volvulus*, which causes River blindness. These studies use a murine model to investigate the role of eosinophils in onchocercal keratitis.

PATHOGENESIS OF ONCHOCERCIASIS

Onchocerciasis remains the third leading cause of infections blindness world-wide. Sclerosing keratitis, which is the major cause of visual impairment in infected individuals, develops as a result of the host immune response to degenerating parasites in the corneal stroma. The impact of this disease is outlined in two reports from the World Health Organization, which estimates that at least 270,000 people are blinded by onchocerciasis and 500,000 are severely visually impaired, mostly due to sclerosing keratitis.[1,2] In some villages in hyperendemic areas of Africa, up to 10% of inhabitants have serious visual impairment as a result of onchocerciasis, causing severe socioeconomic strains on the community. Adult worms reside subcutaneously in host-derived nodules and release numerous first stage larvae (microfilariae, Mf) which migrate through the skin, often causing a severe eosinophil-mediated dermatitis.[3,4] Ocular pathology occurs when *O. volvulus* Mf enter the cornea after migrating through the periorbital skin and conjunctiva. So long as they remain alive, Mf elicit little or no inflammatory response, and motile worms can be detected in the cornea by routine slit lamp examination. When the Mf die, parasite antigens are released into the micro environment of the corneal stroma and trigger a local inflammatory response. In individuals who have been sensitized by chronic exposure to the parasites, the immediate inflammatory response is characterized by discrete areas of corneal inflammation termed punctate keratitis.[5] These lesions, which comprise local edema with infiltrating lymphocytes and eosinophils, resolve spontaneously with minimal visual impairment.[6] In contrast, in heavily infected individuals where there is prolonged invasion of the cornea by large numbers of Mf, the inflammatory response results in sclerosing keratitis, which is characterized by scarring and severe visual impairment.[7]

As human corneas are difficult to obtain, understanding of the immunopathology of human keratitis comes from studies on: a) adjacent conjunctival tissue of infected individuals; b) dermal tissue from infected individuals; and c) animal models of onchocercal keratitis, as described below.

Reports of the immune mechanisms associated with ocular onchocerciasis are limited to adjacent conjunctival tissue in which abscesses comprising dead microfilariae with eosinophils and lymphocytes have been reported.[7] T cells were also found to infiltrate the conjunctiva of patients, and resident cells were in a state of activation as measured by elevated major histocompatibility complex (MHC) class II expression.[8] Chan et al., detected IL4-mRNA in conjunctival biopsies from seven out of ten of these patients, but found no correlation with disease status.[9]

Skin punch biopsies are routinely performed to monitor the effect of mass chemotherapy and onchocerciasis control.[2] Treatment with diethylcarbamazine (DEC) rapidly kills Mf in the tissue, and the acute response to DEC accelerates the chronic inflammatory response that normally occurs in infected individuals[10] and supports the notion that the inflammatory response is directed at antigens released from dead and degenerating Mf. Conclusions from studies on onchocercal dermatitis may thus be cautiously extrapolated to mechanisms underlying sclerosing keratitis. In this regard, the most consistent finding in DEC-treated individuals relates to eosinophils. Blood eosinophilia and serum IL-5 (which stimulates eosinophil production) increases dramatically after DEC treatment, coincident with a decline in skin Mf counts.[11] In addition, Eosinophil Major Basic Protein (MBP) and Eosinophil Derived Neurotoxin (EDN) in blood plasma are significantly elevated.[10] DEC treatment also results in a pronounced inflammatory response in the skin of chronically infected individuals. This phenomenon, known as the Mazzotti reaction, causes severe pruritis and exacerbated keratitis and correlates with increased eosinophil degranulation and deposition of granule proteins in the skin.[10]

EXPERIMENTAL ONCHOCERCAL KERATITIS

As human corneas are difficult to obtain, animal models have been used to investigate the immune mechanisms underlying onchocercal keratitis (for a recent review, see Pearlman[12]). Eosinophils are prominent cells in the corneal stroma of rabbits inoculated subconjunctivally with *O. volvulus* microfilariae (Mf),[13] guinea pigs inoculated subconjunctivally or intrastromally with the cattle parasite *O. lionalis*,[14,15] and mice injected intrastromally with soluble. *O. volvulus* antigens.[16] Prior immunization was shown to exacerbate keratitis.[14,15] As there is no rodent model for *O. volvulus* infection, guinea pigs and mice are sensitized by subcutaneous immunization, and Mf degeneration and release

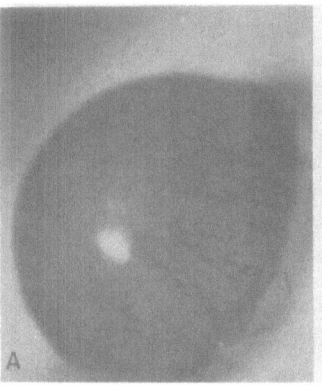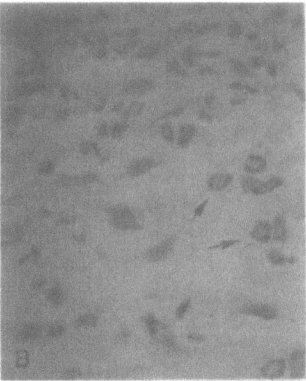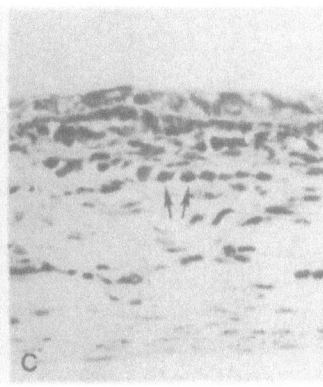

Figure 1. Clinical and histological features of experimental onchocercal keratitis. BALB/c mice were immunized subcutaneously and injected intrastromally with soluble antigens from the parasitic helminth *Onchocerca volvulus*, which causes River Blindness. (A) Clinical appearance of the cornea 7 days after intrastromal injection. Note the corneal opacification and neovascularization typical of human disease. (B) Corneal stroma stained with hematoxylin and eosin demonstrating a pronounced cellular infiltrate. Arrowheads indicate cells with nuclear morphology and eosin staining typical of murine eosinophils. (C) Corneal stroma immunostained with antibody to eosinophil major basic protein. Arrowheads indicate two positively stained cells.

of parasite antigens in infected individuals are reproduced by instrastromal injection of soluble *O. volvulus* antigens. Using this experimental approach, murine corneas develop the same clinical response as reported for human disease, i.e., corneal opacification and neovascularization.[16–19] Corneal opacification develops rapidly and peaks at 4–7 days after injection, whereas neovascularization progresses more gradually.[16] Figure 1A shows a mouse cornea Day 7 after intrastromal injection, with severe opacification and numerous corneal vessels.

Cells comprising the inflammatory infiltrate are detected after staining 5 μm corneal sections with hematoxylin and eosin. Corneal sections show a pronounced cellular infiltrate comprised of granulocytes, histiocytes and lymphocytes (Figure 1B). Many of the granulocytes have horseshoe-shaped nuclei, typical of murine eosinophils. However, to determine more definitively the identity of these cells, sections were immunostained with serum to murine eosinophil major basic protein (MBP; kindly provided by Dr. Gerry Gleich of the Mayo Clinic; Rochester, MN). Numerous cells were identified as eosinophils using these antibodies (Figure 1C). This approach not only provides a more reliable method for quantitation of these cells, but extracellular staining is suggestive of degranulation and release of MBP in the stromal matrix. These studies are currently underway.

Eosinophils contain unique and highly characteristic cytoplasmic granules in which there is a central electron-dense core and a more electron-lucent granule matrix.[20] Ultrastructural characteristics of eosinophils in the corneal stroma are showing in Figure 2. The normal rounded appearance of these cells is distorted, presumably as a result of distension from the tightly packed collagen lamellae. Pleomorphism in this model has been more extensively characterized in a recent publication.[21] Furthermore, examination of the corneal stroma by ultrastructural analysis identified eosinophils that would otherwise be difficult to discern, and supports the concept that these cells are quantitatively the most important cell in this model.[21]

Cytokine modulation of onchocercal keratitis has demonstrated that the presence of eosinophils correlates with the severity of the clinical response—in the absence of inter-

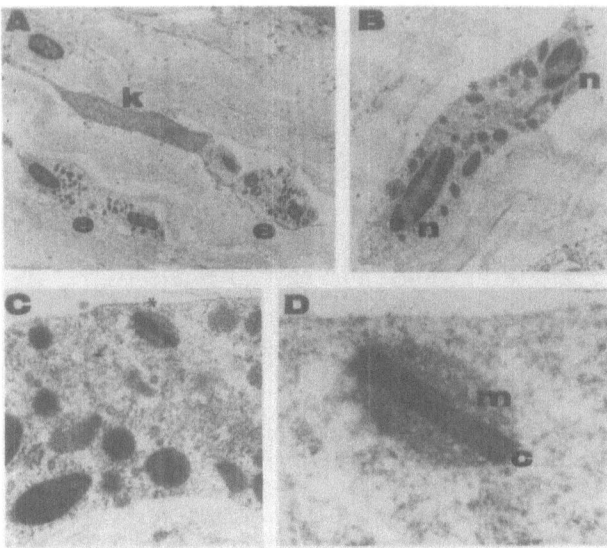

Figure 2. Corneal stroma from mouse described in Figure 1. (A) Eosinophils (e) in the corneal stroma in the same field as a keratocyte (k) (x 3,300). (B) A single distended eosinophil showing bilobed nucleus (n) and characteristic granules (indicated by *) (x 13,000). Same granule at higher magnification (x 24,000 panel C, and x 130,000 Panel D). The granule core (c) and matrix (m) are indicated.

leukin (IL)-4, keratitis is less severe, with fewer eosinophils present in the corneal stroma.[16,22] Conversely, mice given recombinant murine Il-12 have an exacerbated response associated with increased numbers of eosinophils in the corneal stroma.[23] In addition, it was found that the β-chemokine eotaxin is important in recruitment of eosinophils to the corneal stroma.[24] Based on these studies, a series of events leading to the clinical signs of onchocercal keratitis has been proposed (Table 1), providing the basis for the cur-

Table 1. Predicted sequence of events in onchocercal keratitis (from [12])

Repeated subcutaneous immunization with parasite antigen (as a model for chronic infection) selectively induces IL-4 and IL-5 secretion which stimulate production IgE and eosinophils, respectively (16).

Injection of parasite antigen into the corneal stroma (as a model for parasite invasion into the cornea, followed by death and release of helminth antigens) triggers release of eotaxin and other chemokines (12) and also elevates expression of vascular adhesion molecules ICAM-1, ICAM-2, and VCAM-1 on limbal vessels.

Circulating eosinophils expressing the counter-receptors LFA-1 and VLA-4 bind to vascular endothelial cells and migrate into the corneal stroma and towards the site of injury via a chemokine gradient.

Eosinophils in the cornea bind antigen by surface-bound IgE. Cross-linking of IgE receptors mediates eosinophil degranulation and release of Major Basic Protein (MBP) and other granule proteins.

Eosinophil MBP released into the stromal matrix has a cytotoxic effect on resident corneal epithelial cells, keratocytes, and endothelial cells.

Dysfunction of resident cells results in abnormal regulation of corneal hydration, causing stromal edema and subsequent corneal opacification. (Neovascularization likely results from angiogenic factors released from inflammatory cells and from collagen breakdown products.)

rent studies on molecular mechanisms for eosinophil recruitment to the corneal stroma and subsequent eosinophil degranulation.

As eosinophils and MBP are also important in vernal keratoconjunctivitis,[25] and eosinophils are implicated in ocular allergies such as hay fever conjunctivitis (review[26]) findings from the current studies may be more broadly applicable and indicate possible strategies for immune intervention.

ACKNOWLEDGMENTS

The authors gratefully acknowledge the technical assistance of Eugenia Diaconu, Alan W. Higgins, Fred E. Hazlett, and Jamie Albright. These studies were supported by National Institutes of Health grant EY 10320 and Al 35938, by the Research to Prevent Blindness Foundation, and by the Ohio Lions Foundation.

REFERENCES

1. World Health Organization Expert Committee on Onchocerciasis. Third Report. *WHO Tech. Rep. Series 752* Geneva (1987).
2. World Health Organization Expert Committee on Onchocerciasis. *Onchocerciasis and Its Control. WHO Tech Rep. Ser. 852* Geneva (1995).
3. E. Ottesen, Immune responsiveness and the pathogenesis of human onchocerciasis. *J. Infect. Dis.* 171:659 (1995).
4. E. Pearlman, Immunopathology of onchocerciasis: a role for eosinophils on onchocercal dermatitis and keratitis. *Chem. Immunol.* In press. (1997).
5. A. Garner, Pathology of ocular onchocerciasis: human and experimental. *Trans. Roy. Soc. Tropical. Med. Hyg.* 70:374 (1976).
6. F. Rodger, Pathogenesis and pathology of ocular onchocerciasis. *Am. J. Ophthalmol.* 49:560 (1960).
7. C.D. Mackenzie, Williams, J.F., Sisley, B.M., et al., Variations in host response and the pathogenesis of human onchocerciasis. *Rev. Infect. Dis.* 6:802 (1985).
8. C.C. Chan, Ottesen, E.A., Awadzi, K., et al., Immunopathology of ocular onchocerciasis. I. Inflammatory cells infiltrating the anterior segment. *Clin. Exp. Immunol.* 77:367 (1989).
9. C.C. Chan, Li, Q., Brezin, A.P., et al., Immunopathology of ocular onchocerciasis. III: Th-2 helper cells in the conjunctiva. *Ocular Immunol. Inf.* 1:71 (1993).
10. S.J. Ackerman, Kephart, G.M., Francis, H., et al., Eosinophil degranulation. An immunologic determinant in the pathogenesis of the Mazzotti reaction in human onchocerciasis. *J. Immunol.* 144:3961 (1990).
11. A.P. Limaye, Abrams, J.S., Silver, J.E., et al., Interleukin-5 and the posttreatment eosinophilia in patients with onchocerciasis. *J. Clin. Invest.* 88:1418 (1991).
12. E. Pearlman, Experimental onchocercal keratitis. *Parasitol Today* 12: 261 (1996).
13. A. Garner, Duke, B.O., and Anderson, J., A comparison of the lesions produced in the cornea of the rabbit eye by microfilariae of the forest and Sudan-savanna strains of *Onchocerca volvusus* from Cameroon. II. The pathology. *Z. Topenmed. Parasitol.* 24:385 (1973).
14. J.J. Donnelly, Rockey, J.H., Bianco, A.E., and Soulsby, E.J.L. Ocular immunopathologic findings of experimental onchocerciasis. *Arch. Ophthalmol.* 102:628 (1984).
15. A.A. Sakla, Donnelly, J.J., Lok, J.B., et al., Punctate keratitis induced by subconjunctivally injected microfilariae of *Onchocerca lienalis*. *Arch. Ophthalmol.* 104:894 (1986).
16. E. Pearlman, Lass, J.H., Bardenstein, D.S., et al., Interleukin 4 and T helper type 2 cells are required for development of experimental onchocercal keratitis (river blindness). *J. Exp. Med.* 182:931 (1995).
17. B. Chakravarti, Lass, J.H., Diaconu, D.S., et al., Immune-mediated *Onchocerca volvulus* sclerosing keratitis in the mouse. *Exp. Eye Res.* 57:21 (1993).
18. B. Chakravarti, Herring, T.A., Lass, J.H., et al., Infiltration of CD$+ T cells into corneal during development of *Onchocerca volvulus*-induced experimental sclerosing keratitis in mice. *Cell. Immunol.* 159:306 (1994).

19. M.Y. Gallin, Murray, D., Lass, J.H., et al., Experimental interstitial keratitis induced by *Onchocerca volvulus* antigens. *Arch. Ophthalmol.* 106:1447 (1988).

20. G. Gleich, and Loegering, D., Immunobiology of eosinophils. *Annu. Rev. Immunol.*2:429 (1984).

21. D.S. Bardenstein, Lass, J.H., Kazura, J.W., and Pearlman, E., Pleomorphism of stromal eosinophils in murine experimental onchocerciasis. *Ocular Immun. Inf.* In press. (1997).

22. E. Pearlman, Lass, J.H., Bardenstein, J., et al., *Onchocerca volvulus* mediated keratitis: cytokine production by IL-4 deficient mice. *Exptl. Parasit.* 84:274 (1996).

23. E. Pearlman, Lass, J.H., Bardenstein, D.S., et al., IL-12 exacerbates helminth-mediated corneal pathology by augmenting cell recruitment and chemokine expression. *J. Immunol.* 158:867 (1997).

24. M.E. Rothenberg, MacLeaon, J., Pearlman, E., and Leder, P., Targeted disruption of the chemokine eotaxin reduces peripheral blood and antigen induced tissue eosinophillia. *J. Exp. Med* In Press (1997).

25. S.D. Trocme, Gleich, G.M., Kephart, G.M., and Zieske, J.D., Eosinophil granule major basic protein inhibition of corneal epithelial wound healing. *Invest. Ophthalmol. Vis. Sci.* 35:3051 (1994).

26. S.D. Trocme, and Aldave, A.J., The eye and the eosinophil. *Surv. Ophthalmol.* 39:241 (1994).

44

MICROBIAL CONTAMINATION OF DONOR EYES

Anita Panda, Namrata Sharma, S. K. Angra, and A. Kumbar

Dr. Rajendra Prasad Centre for Ophthalmic Sciences
All India Institute of Medical Sciences
New Delhi, India

ABSTRACT

A total of 2,150 consecutive eyes enucleated from the deceased between 1 and 18 hours after death were obtained from various sources. Microbiological evaluation of the donor tissues before and after antiobiotic therapy was undertaken in all eyes. Positive cultures were obtained in 44.88% of the donor eyes; bacterial growth was seen in 41.06% of the eyes; and fungus noted in 3.81%. The number of pathogens isolated correlated directly with the death enucleation time. *Staphylococcus albus* was the most frequent bacterial isolate (37.03%), followed by *Pseudomonas aeruginosa* (14.72%). Antibiotics effective against most pathogens were Chloramphenicol and Framycetin. Polymyxin B was effective against *Pseudomonas* and cloxacillin against *Staphylococcus*. Thus, pre-enucleation instillation of framycetin (soframycin) eye drops in the donor eye followed by treatment of the donor eye ball with a 20 ml solution of normal saline containing 0.3 mg/ml of chloramphenicol for 10 minutes in the Eye Bank was recommended.

INTRODUCTION

Although the incidence of graft infection due to donor eye contamination is infrequent, it does jeopardize an otherwise successful penetrating keratoplasty.[1] Donor rim culture and sensitivity reports are especially valuable in institution of prompt treatment of post-surgical endophthalmitis.[2-4] The donor eyes are obtained from the deceased at various sites, including home, mortuary, and ward, which are not strictly sterile areas. Positive donor rim culture has been correlated with septic conditions at the time of death, prolonged corneal storage time, technique of removing the eye or cornea, prolonged death enucleation time, and antibiotic used in the storage media.[1,2] This study reviewed the cultures of donor eye balls used for penetrating keratoplasties, performed from June 1992 to July 1995 at the national Eye Bank. The incidence of microbial contamination, efficacy of the

Advances in Corneal Research, edited by Lass
Plenum Press, New York, 1997

antimicrobial drugs, and the effect of death enucleation time to obtain sterile donor corneas were also studied.

MATERIALS AND METHODS

In this study, 2,150 consecutive donor eyes received from various sources were reviewed. In all eyes, the cause of death, death enucleation time, and place of enucleation were noted.

After all the eye balls were received at the Eye Bank in moist chamber, two limbal swabs were obtained from each eye ball (Ia and Ib). None of the eyes received either normal saline irrigation or antibiotic drops in the conjunctival cul de sac prior to enucleation. Each eye ball was treated with a 20 ml solution of normal saline containing 0.4 mg/ml of gentamicin, for 10 minutes in a sterile bottle. After the antibiotic treatment, repeat limbal swabs (IIa and IIb) were taken from all eye balls.

Both Ia and IIa labeled swabs were sent for microbiological evaluation in glucose broth, while Ib and IIb were sent in Sabouraud's medium.

Identification of the pathogens was achieved by using standard bacteriological techniques. If there was any growth of bacteria, the antibiotic sensitivity was tested by the disc diffusion method on Muller Hinton agar media. However, no antifungal sensitivity was done in positive fungal culture.

RESULTS

Donor age varied from 5 months to 80 years. The cause of death was attributed to road traffic accidents in two-thirds of patients, and to cardiac or respiratory failure in one-third of patients.

Of the 2,150 donor eyes, 965 (44.88%) showed a positive culture. Pathogenic bacteria was grown in 883 eyes (41.06%), while fungal growth was seen in 82 eyes (3.81%) (Table 1).

Death enucleation time varied from 1 hour to 18 hours. The same was less than or equal to 6 hours in 358 donor (33.09%), while the rest (724; 66.91%) were subjected to enucleation 6 hours or more after death (Table 2). Longer death enucleation period was associated with increased number of pathogens accounting for 20.66% in less than 3 hours, 22.08% in 3–6 hours, 53.92% in 6 to 10 hours, and 67.66% in more than 10 hours (Fig. 1). By far the most prevalent bacteria cultured was *Staphylococcus albus* (37.03%), followed by *Pseudomonas* (14.72%), and *Acinetobacter* (14.38%) (Table 3). The incidence of other pathogenic bacteria varied from 1.82% to 10.3%. The post-treatment growth of bacteria was reduced from 41% to 36% (Table 3).

Table 1. Frequency of microbial contamination

Donor eyes tested	2150
Positive cultures	965 (44.88%)
Positive bacterial growth	883 (41.06%)
Positive fungal growth	82 (3.81%)

Table 2. Death enucleation time (DET)

In hours	No. of donors	No. of eyes
< 3	150 (13.86%)	300 (13.94%)
3 to ≤ 6	208 (19.23%)	412 (19.16%)
> 6 to 10	588 (54.34%)	1172 (54.52%)
> 10	136 (12.57%)	266 (12.38%)
Total	1082 (100%)	2150 (100%)

The isolated pathogens were tested for sensitivity to 10 antibiotics (Table 4). The most effective antibiotics for *Pseudomonas aeruginosa* were polymyxin B (95.3%) and Framycetin (80%). Similarly the most effective antibiotics for *Staphylococcus aureus* and *albus* were chloramphenicol and cloxacillin (56.6%, and 51.98%), respectively. Framycetin and chloramphenicol were more sensitive than other antibiotics in all isolated pathogens (Table 4). Gentamicin, a commonly-used drug for donor eye treatment was resistant to the isolated pathogens, the frequency varied from 50% to 86.66% (Table 5).

DISCUSSION

Positive bacterial cultures from donor eyes have been reported in 4.2 and 100% of cases (Table 6).[1,2,5–11] The low incidence of pathogens in the series reported earlier was

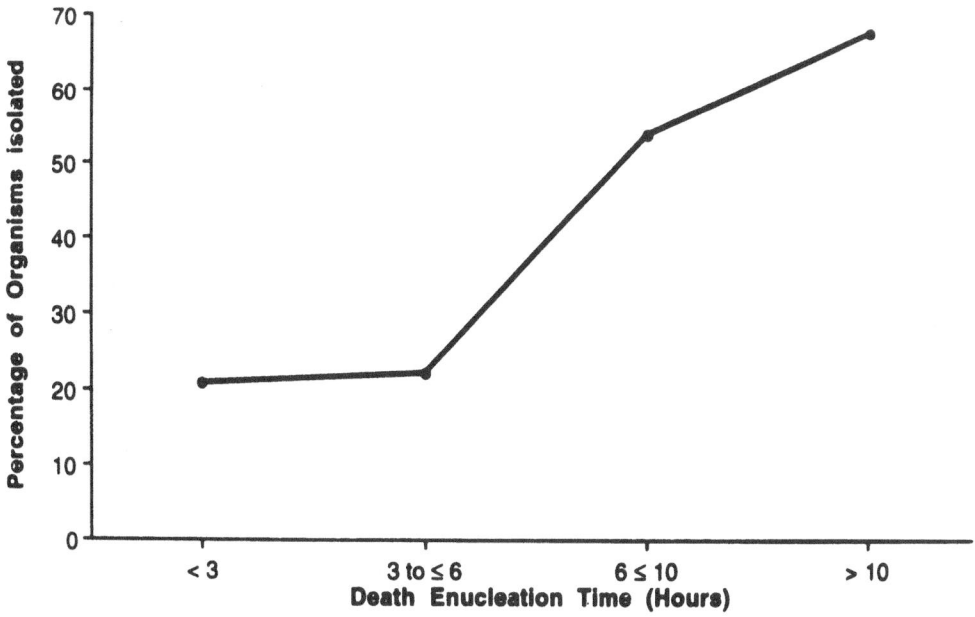

Figure 1. Death enucleation time vs. pathogens.

Table 3. Bacteria isolated

Bacteria	I (Pre-treatment) n = 883 (41.1%)	II (Post-treatment) n = 786 (36%)
Staph. albus	327 (37.03%)	303 (38.55%)
Staph. aureus	53 (6.02%)	50 (6.36%)
Pseudomonas aeruginosa	130 (14.72%)	105 (13.36%)
Enterobacter aerogenes	91 (10.30%)	88 (11.20%)
Klebsiella sp.	42 (4.75%)	39 (4.96%)
Moraxella sp.	16 (1.82%)	12 (1.53%)
Alkaligens faecalis	30 (3.39%)	25 (3.18%)
E. Coli	45 (5.09%)	42 (5.34%)
Acinobacter sp.	126 (14.38%)	102 (12.98%)
Alpha Streptococcus	23 (2.50%)	20 (2.54%)

due to pre-enucleation instillation of antibiotics in conjunctival cul de sac and irrigation of the same with normal saline.[9] In the present series, neither irrigation nor antibiotic instillation was done in the conjunctival cul de sac. This could be the reason for isolation of a higher percentage of pathogens in comparison to a previous study[9] where routine use of antibiotic drops was followed. The other reason for the higher percentage could be due to prolonged death enucleation time. In the previous study, the death enucleation time was within 6 hours in all enuclateions,[9] while in the present study over two-thirds of enucleations were carried out 6 hours or more following death. As the majority of the eyes in this series were obtained from medico-legal cases, the time of enucleation was delayed because of completion of legal formalities. The site of the enucleation of eyes was the mortuary in most cases where the maintenance of asepsis is not strictly assured.

Gentamicin was earlier thought to be an ideal drug and therefore recommended for the use in M.K. media and also for pretreatment of donor eyes at many Eye Banks.[10] However, the survival of many pathogenic organisms is known in gentamicin supplemented M.K. media.[11] In the present series, the resistance of the pathogens to gentamicin varied from 50–86%. This could probably explain a low rate of disinfection in the donor eyes following gentamicin therapy. In 1984, Poole et al., followed by Jose, et al. (1995) reported resistance to gentamicin in about 50% of all organisms isolated and *Stapylococcus epidermidis*, respectively.[8,12] Although polymyxin B was highly effective against *Pseudomonas aeruginosa* (95.3%) and *E. coli* (53%) in the present series, the sensitivity rates to other organisms such as *Enterobacter, Acinetobacter,* and *Klebsiella* were poor (14–35%). Jose et al. highlighted the efficacy of gentamicin and streptomycin for the decontamination of donor eyes.[12] Streptomycin sensitivity was not evaluated in the present study, as the results of the same were not very encouraging in a previous series.[9] Framycetin was found to be the most sensitive antibacterial agent against all pathogens (40–80%). Similarly,

Table 4. Sensitivity pattern

Organisms	No. of Strains	C	T	F	G	CL	P	S	A	CP	CF
Staph. albus	327	170 (51.98)	162 (49.54)	166 (50.76)	119 (36.39)	178 (54.43)	NT	94 (28.74)	NT	NT	NT
Pseudomonas aeruginosa	130	32 (24.61)	28 (21.53)	104 (80.0)	21 (16.15)	10 (7.6)	124 (95.3)	21 (16.15)	–	21 (16.15)	10 (7.6)
Acinobacter sp.	126	65 (51.58)	60 (47.61)	85 (67.46)	25 (19.84)	NT	30 (23.80)	15 (11.90)	5 (3.96)	15 (11.90)	15 (11.90)
Enterobacter aerogenes	91	28 (30.76)	24 (26.37)	52 (57.14)	8 (8.79)	NT	32 (35.16)	4 (4.39)	–	16 (17.58)	–
Staph. aureus	53	30 (56.60)	20 (37.73)	25 (47.16)	15 (28.30)	25 (47.16)	NT	15 (28.30)	NT	NT	NT
E. Coli	45	6 (13.3)	6 (13.3)	36 (79.0)	6 (13.3)	–	24 (53.0)	9 (20.0)	9 (20.0)	–	–
Klebsiella sp.	42	21 (50.0)	15 (35.71)	30 (71.0)	21 (50.0)	–	6 (14.28)	3 (7.0)	3 (7.0)	–	3 (7.0)
Alkaligens faecalis	30	–	6 (20.0)	12 (40.0)	6 (20.0)						
Alpha Streptococcus	23	8 (34.78)									
Moraxella sp.	16	16 (100.0)									

C = Chloramphenicol; G = Gentamycin; S = Sisomycin; CP = Ciprofloxacin; T = Tetracycline; CL = Cloxacillin; A = Amikacin; CF = Cefazolidine; F = Framycetin; P = Polymyxin B

Table 5. Response of pathogens to gentamycin

	No. of Strains	Sensitive	Resistant	N.T.
1. *Staph. albus*	327	219 (66.97)	74 (22.62)	34 (10.39)
2. *Pseudomonas aeruginosa*	130	21 (16.15)	109 (83.84)	–
3. *Acinobacter sp.*	126	25 (19.84)	90 (71.42)	11 (8.73)
4. *Enterobacter aerogenes*	91	8 (8.79)	75 (82.41)	8 (8.79)
5. *Staph. aureus*	53	15 (28.30)	35 (66.03)	3 (5.66)
6. *E. coli*	45	6 (13.3)	39 (86.66)	–
7. *Klebsiella sp.*	42	21 (50.00)	21 (50.00)	–
8. *Alkaligens faecalis*	30	6 (20.00)	24 (80.00)	–

chloramphenicol sensitivity varied from 13.3–100%. Moreover, it was the only drug found to be sensitive against *Moraxella*.

Cloxacillin gives better results only in cases of the *Staphylococcal* group of organisms. However, polymyxin B and cloxacillin were effective against a limited group of organisms. As the new generation antibiotics were not widely tested for all pathogens in our laboratory, their use cannot be recommended for the routine treatment of donor eyes. Thus, the two most effective drugs for prevention of microbial contamination in this series were chloramphenicol and framycetin.

Fungal contamination of donor corneas, though not common, is a serious problem, especially with regard to post-surgical outcome.[13-15] In 1983, Nelson et al. reported 5.2% growth of fungi on organ-cultured corneas.[13] The report from our center revealed fungal isolation in 2.3% and 3.6% of donor eyes in two successive studies.[9,10] Although antibacterial therapy is routinely given to prevent microbial contaminations, antifungals to prevent fungal endophthalmitis, though advocated, are not routinely used.[13]

Thus, the pre-enucleation instillation of framycetin (soframycin) drops into the decased eye every 5 minutes while the surgeon is getting ready for the eye removal procedure is recommended. Similarly, the donor eye balls should be treated with a 20 ml solution of normal saline containing 0.3 mg/ml of chloramphenicol, for 10 minutes. However, the sensitivity patterns of newer antibiotics should be tested routinely to assess their efficacy.

Table 6. Reports on bacterial growth (comparative study)

Authors and years	No. of eyes studied	Percent + VE culture
Rollins et al. (1964)[5]	100	61
Polack FM et al. (1967)[6]	240	100
Rycroft BW (1956)[1]	107	43
Bobergans et al. (1962)[2]	63	87.3
Pardos GJ et al. (1982)[7]	4167	12.4
Poole TG et al. (1984)[8]	70	20.00
Panda et al. (1988)[9]	1516	21.8
Satpathy et al. (1993)[10]	1557	42.77
Jose et al. (1995)[11]	1097	4.2
Present study (1996)	2150	44.88

REFERENCES

1. B.W. Rycroft, The donor corneal graft. *I Curso International de Oftalmologica* 2:711 (1956).
2. J. Bobergans, Badsberg, E., and Rasmussen, J., Frequency of infection in donor eyes. *Br. J. Ophthalmol.* 46:365 (1962).
3. P.L. Farell, Fan, J.T., Smith, R.E., and Trousdale, M.D., Donor cornea bacterial contamination. *Cornea* 10:381 (1991).
4. A.S. Leveille, McMullian, F.D., and Cavanagh, H.D., Endophthalmitis following penetrating keratoplasty. *Ophthalmology* 90:38 (1983).
5. H.J. Rollins, and Stocker, F.W., Bacterial flora and preoperative treatment of donor corneas. *Am. J. Ophthalmol.* 59:247 (1965).
6. F.W. Polack, Khorazo, D.L., and Elizabeth G., Bacteriologic study of donor eyes. *Arch Ophthalmol.* 78:219 (1967).
7. G.J. Pardos, and Gallagher, M.A., Microbial contamination of donor eyes. *Arch Ophthalmol.* 100;1611 (1982).
8. T.G. Poole, and Michael S., Donor eyes contamination. *Am. J. Ophthalmol.* 97:560 (1984).
9. A. Panda, Angra, S.K., Venkateshwarlu, K., et al., Microbial contamination of donor eyes. *Jpn. J. Ophthalmol.* 32:264 (1988).
10. G. Satpathy, and Angra, S.K., Changing pattern of microbial contamination and antimicrobial sensitivity in donor eyes. *Ann. Ophthalmol.* 25:44 (1993).
11. J.C. Baer, Nirankari, V.S., and Glaros, D.S., Survival of *Streptococcus viridans* in gentamicin supplemented McCarey-Kaufman medium. *Cornea* 8:131 (1989).
12. A.P.G. Jose, Mohamad, R.D., Dua, H.S., et al., Positive donor rim culture in penetrating keratoplasty. *Cornea* 14:457 (1995).
13. J.D. Nelson, Mindrup, E.A., et al., and Ching, C.K., Fungal contamination in organ culture. *Arch. Ophthalmol.* 101:280 (1983).
14. M.S. Insler, and Urso, L.F., *Candida albicans* endophthalmitis after penetrating keratoplasty. *Am. J. Ophthalmol.* 104:57 (1987).
15. W. Behrens-Baumann, Ruechel, R., Zimmermann, O., and Vogel, M., *Candida tropicalis* endophthalmitis following penetrating keratoplasty. *Br. J. Ophthalmol.* 75:565 (1991).

45

SEVERE CORNEAL ULCERATIONS AND VITAMIN A DEFICIENCY

A Case Series

Tomy Starck

Department of Ophthalmology
University of Texas
Health Science Center at San Antonio

ABSTRACT

This paper reports a case series of patients with corneal complications associated with vitamin A deficiency (keratomalacia) in a developed country. Entry criteria for this series include presence of unilateral or bilateral sterile or infectious corneal ulceration after the patient had been found to have low serum vitamin A levels. Patients were prospectively identified from November 1, 1991 to October 30, 1995. Additional findings such as xerophthalmia, Bitot's spots, decreased serum retinol binding protein (RBP), and abnormal electroretinogram and dark adaptation tests were included to support the diagnosis but were not essential.

Seven patients and nine eyes with hypovitaminosis A-related corneal ulcers were identified. Five of the seven patients were of Hispanic background and all had a history of alcoholism and poor nutrition. One patient admitted concomitant drug abuse. Serum vitamin A level was <30 mcg/dl in all patients and four patients were below 10 mcg/dl. In three patients with cornea superinfection only bacteria were isolated. Despite immediate restitution of vitamin A levels, most patients required repeated cyanoacrylate glue or emergent corneal transplant. Two patients who were treated early in the process of corneal ulceration retained good vision (>20/40). Nonetheless, the results were poor in patients in whom consultation was performed late in the disease.

From this study, it was concluded that severe simultaneous or sequential bilateral corneal ulceration in the presence of chronic alcoholism or drug abuse should raise clinical suspicion for vitamin A deficiency. Any corneal ulcer in this setting should be considered a consequence of such deficiency until proven otherwise. Failure to recognize this entity may undermine the visual prognosis already compromised by delayed corneal wound healing, increased susceptibility to bacterial infection, frequently debilitated general health, and lack of compliance.

Advances in Corneal Research, edited by Lass
Plenum Press, New York, 1997

INTRODUCTION

Keratomalacia (KM) or severe corneal ulceration occurs as a result of vitamin A deficiency, usually associated with prolonged starvation among impoverished populations.[1] Adults on adequate diets are rarely affected in developed countries. However, vitamin A deficiency and xerophthalmia still occur in affluent Western societies, especially as a result of chronic alcoholism, drug abuse, and subsequent malnutrition. A case series of seven patients with severe unilateral or bilateral corneal ulcerations associated with alcoholism and drug abuse-related vitamin A deficiency in a developed country is presented in this paper.

METHODS

Seven patients and nine eyes with corneal complications associated with serum vitamin A deficiency were seen at the affiliated hospitals of the University of Texas Health Science Center at San Antonio from November 1, 1991 to October 30, 1995. To be included in this series, the patient needed to have any corneal ulceration with associated serum hypovitaminosis A. Additional clinical findings such as conjunctival and corneal xerosis, night blindness, Bitot's spots, decreased total retinol binding protein (BRP), and abnormal electroretinogram (ERG) and dark adaptation also were included to support the diagnosis.

A complete eye examination was performed at the initial visit and in all seven patients corneal scrapings obtained with a platinum spatula were directly inoculated on sheep blood agar, chocolate agar, Sabouraud's dextrose agar, and thioglycolate broth. Additional scraped material was sent for viral cultures and Gram staining. Systemic and autoimmune etiologies were excluded based on thorough review of systems and a blood work-up that included SMA-20, Rheumatoid factor (RF), ESR, Complement (C3,C4), ANA, MHATP, RPR, SSA, SSB, cANCA, and pANCA.

A blood sample (5 cc) for vitamin A levels was obtained in fasting conditions and after 24 hours of alcohol abstinence. The specimens were protected from light exposure and preserved at room temperature or refrigeration at 4°C. The blood samples were processed promptly by the high pressure liquid chromatography (HPLC) method. A value of 30–95 mcg/dl was considered normal. Additional frozen serum samples were obtained in some patients for total RBP. These were also protected from light and processed by HPLC. A range of 2.2–6.4 mcg/dl was considered normal.

Electroretinogram and dark adaptation tests were performed in patients in which placement of the electrodes would not further jeopardize the integrity of the eye.

Initial treatment of the corneal ulcer included topical fortified tobramycin sulfate solution (14 mg/ml) and fortified cafazolin sodium solution (100 mg/ml) every hour for the first 48 hours. Cycloplegic agents were administered for patient comfort. If the index of suspicion for hypovitaminosis A was high, empiric vitamin A replacement was started at a dose of 200,000 IU of retinyl palmitate orally on two successive days after blood samples had been obtained.

All patients were seen on an outpatient basis at the initial visit, and were subsequently hospitalized to ensure compliance with the prescribed treatment regimen.

When impending corneal perforation was suspected, cyanoacrylate glue and a bandage contact lens were applied. If this therapy proved to be insufficient to restore the integrity of the eye, tectonic or penetrating corneal graft was performed.

SELECTED CASE REPORTS

Case #1

A 27-year-old, white woman with a history of alcohol, methadone, and cocaine abuse, along with poor nutrition complained of severe photophobia, nyctalopia, diffuse conjunctival injection, and progressive visual loss OU over the previous month.

On ocular examination the best corrected visual acuity was finger counting at 2 feet OD and 20/70 OS. Slit-lamp biomicroscopy revealed positive diffuse rose bengal staining and bilateral corneal perforations with positive Seidel's test (Fig. 1). Both ulcers were located inferiorly with infiltration only present at the base. Corneal cultures were negative, a was the work-up for immunologic-vasculitic processes. Pretreatment serum vitamin A level was 10 mcg/dl. Despite intensive nutritional supplementation, vitamin A replacement, and application of cyanoacrylate glue twice to both eyes, the patient finally required an emergency penetrating keratoplasty OD and a tectonic corneal graft covered by a conjunctival flap OS. Subsequent cataract extraction and posterior chamber intraocular lens placement were also required in the right eye. After two years of follow-up, both anterior segments remain stable with visual acuity of 20/40 OD and 20/70 OS. Her nutritional status and vitamin A levels continued to be normal without any further diet supplementation.

Case #4

A 37-year-old, well-nourished Hispanic man presented with a 5-day history of right eye redness, blurred vision, and photophobia. A history of chronic pancreatitis and alcohol abuse was obtained.

On ocular examination the best corrected visual acuity was 20/400 OD and 20/30 OS. Slit-lamp examination revealed Bitot's spots OU and an inferonasal corneal ulcer with 70% thinning OD (Fig. 2). Dense infiltration around the ulcer and hypopyon were also present. Basal tear secretion was 8 mm OD and 4 mm OS. Corneal cultures were positive for *Klebsiella oxytoca*. Serum vitamin A level was < 10 mcg/dl. The patient was treated with fortified antibiotics and vitamin A replacement. One month later, the cornea had healed completely with visual acuity improved to 20/30 and 80 mcg/dl of serum vitamin A levels.

Case #5

A 63-year-old, Hispanic man was brought to the emergency room by neighbors because he "seemed to be lost" during the week prior to admission. A history of night blindness, chronic alcoholism, and severe malnutrition was obtained.

On ocular examination, the best corrected visual acuity was hand motions OD and NLP OS. On slit-lamp examination, both conjunctivas showed multiple areas of severe keratinization and xerosis. His right eye had an 8 x 7 mm central corneal perforation with iris entrapment and flat anterior chamber. His left eye showed evidence of previous perforation with a vascularized healed corneal scar (Fig 1). Corneal cultures were negative. Serum vitamin A level was < 10 mcg/dl. Retinol binding protein (RBP) serum level was 1.0 (N: 2.2–6.4). ERG and dark adaptation were not performed due to corneal perforation. Emergency penetrating keratoplasty and cataract extraction OD were performed with subsequent early rejection and persistent epithelial defects which eventually closed. Three months postoperatively, his vision remained hand motions at 1 foot OD and he is currently scheduled for a second transplant. Since his admission, his nutritional status and vitamin A levels have improved to normal levels.

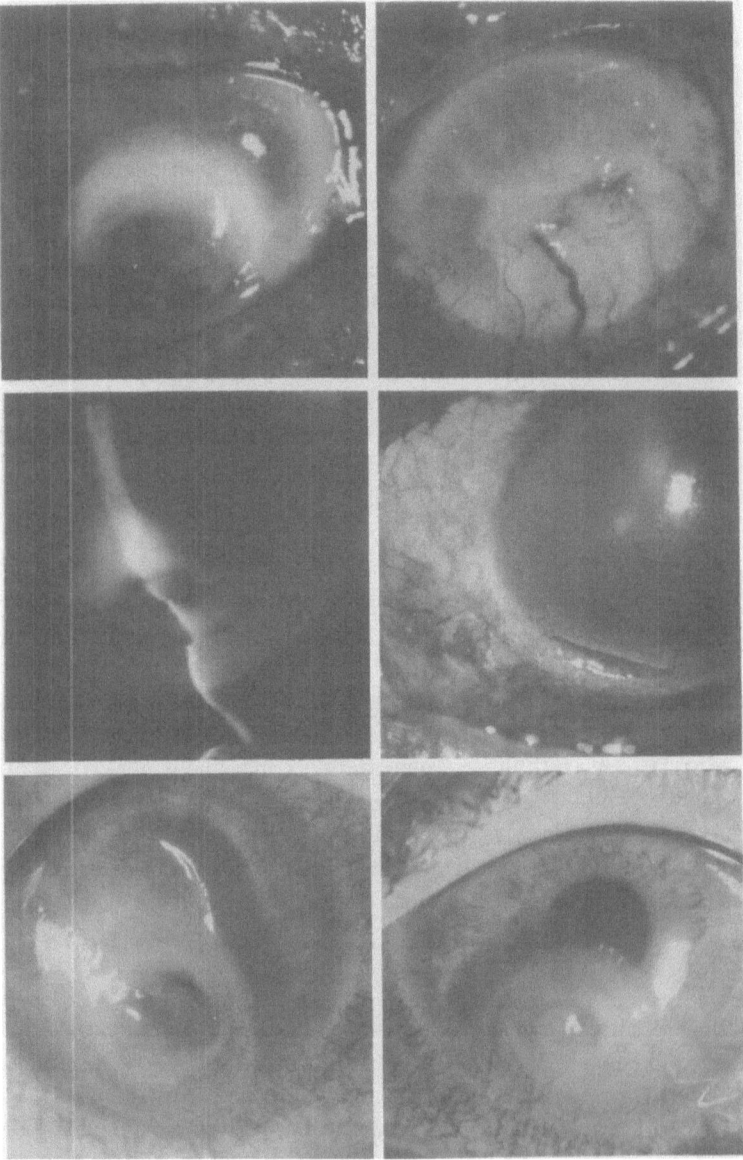

Figure 1. Top left: (Case 5) Severe corneal perforation and necrosis in a 63-year-old chronic alcoholic. **Top right:** Fellow eye of the same patient discloses evidence of previous perforation with a vascularized healed corneal scar. **Middle left:** (Case 7) Right eye of a 59-year-old cachectic alcoholic male who complained of nyctalopia one year prior to admission. Severe inferior corneal ulceration and necrosis developed, which eventually required a corneal patch graft. **Middle right:** Left eye of the same patient with inferior ulceration and positive rose Bengal staining. **Bottom right & left:** (Case 1) Bilateral perforated inferior corneal ulcers in an alcoholic and drug abuser with vitamin A deficiency.

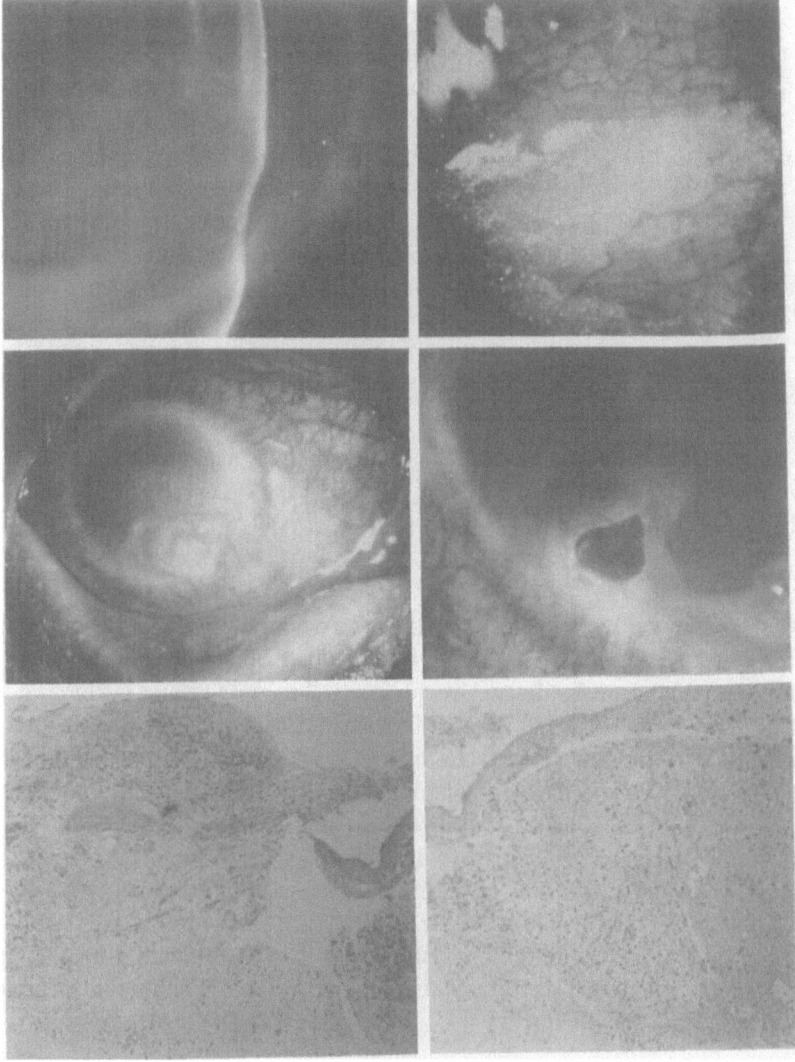

Figure 2. Top left & right: (Case 4) Conjunctival xerosis and Bitot's spots in a 37-year-old male with history of alcohol abuse and pancreatitis. Right eye reveals inferonasal corneal ulceration with dense stromal infiltration and thinning. Note the presence of hypopyon. **Middle left:** Severe corneal perforation with necrosis in a 73-year-old cachectic chronic alcoholic with hypovitaminosis A. **Middle right:** (Case 6) Left corneal ulceration of a 45-year-old male with hyctalopia, alcoholism, and poor nutrition. **Bottom left & right:** Corneal specimen of case #5, shows loss of corneal epithelium and keratinization, severe necrosis with neutrophyl inflammatory reaction and intense fibrinoid deposition.

Case #6

A 45-year-old male presented with a three-week history of red, scratchy, painful eyes. History of consumption of three to four quarts of beer daily, poor nutrition, and nyctalopia was elicited. Additionally, high hyperopia and amblyopia OS were reported by the patient.

On initial examination, visual acuity was 20/30 OD and 20/200 OS. The bulbar and palpebral conjunctiva was dry and without luster OU with significantly decreased tear break-up time. Paralimbal Bitot's spots and diffuse conjunctival rose bengal staining were evident OU. The left cornea revealed a sharply demarcated, 50% thinned corneal ulcer with minimal surrounding inflammatory reaction (Fig. 2). On dilated fundus examination, multiple peripheral yellow-white dots were found at the level of the RPE OU. Vitamin A level was < 10 mcg/dl and RBP 1.2 mcg/dl. Corneal cultures were negative. An ERG and dark adaptation tests revealed widespread pathology affecting cones and, more severely, rods. After vitamin A supplementation, the ocular surface progressively improved within 2–4 weeks with arrest of the corneal thinning OS. Subjectively, the patient reported improvement of night vision within one week. Visual acuity was unchanged due to amblyopia OS. Post-treatment vitamin A levels remain normal.

Case #7

A 59-year-old, black male complained of decreased visual acuity, photophobia, and red, painful eyes for several weeks. History revealed that one year prior to admission, the patient had been seen at the emergency room by a physician for difficulties with night vision despite 20/20 vision OU Additionally, a history of alcohol abuse, poor nutrition, and cirrhosis was elicited.

On examination, his visual acuity was light perception OD and hand motions at 1 foot OS. Slit-lamp examination showed a right eye perforated inferior peripheral corneal ulcer that was Seidel positive despite iris plugging (Fig. 1). Stromal infiltration at the superior edge was evident. The left cornea showed an arcuate inferior peripheral ulcer with approximately 90% thinning (Fig. 1). Conjunctival and corneal xerosis with positive rose bengal staining OU was found. His vitamin A level was <10 mcg/dl and RBP of <1.0 mcg/dl. Corneal cultures showed light growth of *Xanthomonas maltophilia* OD. The patient was immediately started on fortified antibiotics, and vitamin A supplementation. ERG and dark adaptation test showed severe depression of mostly rods OU. Two attempts at corneal gluing OD failed, and he finally underwent a patch graft with anatomical restoration of the eye. After sealing the corneal ulcer in the left eye with glue, the ocular surface and progressive corneal melting were arrested. At three months follow-up his visual acuity was 20/50 OD and 20/20 OS.

RESULTS

During the four-year study period, seven patients were identified as having hypovitaminosis A-related corneal ulcerations (Table 1). Patient ages ranged from 27 to 63 years of age. There were six men and one woman. All patients, but two were Hispanic. All patients had significant history of chronic alcohol abuse and, in addition, one patient was addicted to methadone and cocaine. All patients showed serum vitamin A levels below 30 mcg/dl with four of them with <10 mcg/dl. Three patients in whom RBP was obtained (cases 5, 6, and 7) had levels reported to be abnormally low. Three of seven patients in whom ERG/dark adaptation studies were able to be performed showed widespread depressed cone and rod function, mostly affecting rods. Two of these patients improved dramatically after 1–2 weeks of vitamin A replacement.

On initial presentation, all patients had corneal ulcerations. Two of seven had simultaneous bilateral ulceration and three of seven showed evidence of sequential bilateral cor-

Table 1. Corneal ulcers associated with vitamin A deficiency

Patient	Risk factors	Exam	Visual acuity	Vitamin A/RBP	Cultures	Procedures	Final VA
27 y/o WF	Alcohol, Methadone & Cocaine abuse Poor Nutrition	Bilateral corneal perf. Nyctalopia Conj. xerosis	CF OF 20/70 OS	10 mcg/dl	Neg.	Glue x (2) PK OD Tectonic graft OS ECCE OD	20/40 OD 20/70 OS
63 y/o HM	Chronic alcohol. Poor nutrition	Corneal perf. OD Old scar OS	HM OD 20/200 E @ 1 foot OS	22 mcg/dl	Staph. ureus	Glue	Lost F/U
42 y/o HM	Chronic alcohol. Cirrhosis Hepatic encephalop.	Conj. Xerosis OD C. Perf. OS	20/30 OD NLP OS	13 mcg/dl	Strep. viridans Diphth.	Gue x (2) Enucle.	No change
37 y/o WM	Chronic alcohol. Chronic pancreat.	Keratitis OD Bitot's spots OU	20/400 OD 20/30 OS	<10 mcg/dl	Klebsiella oxytoca	Medical Rx	20/30 20/30
63 y/o HM	Chronic alcohol. Severe malnutr.	Nyctalopia Corneal perf. OD Corneal scar OS	HM OD NLP OS	<10 mcg/dl 1.0 mcg/dl	Neg.	PK + ECCE + PCIOL OD	HM OD NLP OS
45 y/o HM	Chronic alcohol. Malnutrition	Nyctalopia Corneal ulcer OS Bitot's spots OU Retinopathy OU Amblyopia OS	20/30 OD 20/200 OS	<10 mcg/dl 1.2 mcg/dl	Neg.	Medical Rx	20/30 OD 20/200 OS
64 y/o BM	Chronic alcohol. Poor nutrition Cirrhosis	Nyctalopia Corneal ulcers OU Corneal Perf. OD Conj/Corneal xerosis	LP OD HM OS	<10 mcg/dl 1.0 mcg/dl	Xanthamonas Malthophilia	Patch graft OD Glue (x2) OS	20/50 20/50

OU: Both eyes; OD: Right eye; OS: Left eye; NLP: No light percep¬tion; LP: Light percepion; PK: Penetrating keratoplasty; ECCE: Extracapsular cataract extraction; PCIOL: Posterior chamber intraocular lens; RBP: Retinol Binding Protein; VA: Visual acuity; HM: Hispanic male; WF: White female; WM: White male; BM: Black male.

neal involvement. All but one patient showed clinical signs of generalized malnutrition but none were hospitalized at the time of the initial visit.

Two of nine eyes cultured positive for Gram-positive organisms (*Staphylococcus aureus*, *Diphteroids*, and *Streptococcus viridans*) and of nine were Gram-negative (*Klebsiella oxytoca* and *Xanthomonas maltophilia*). All patients with positive cultures had active ulceration. Five of nine eyes were found to be sterile despite severe corneal ulcerations and necrosis. All viral cultures were negative.

Despite the fact that all patients received aggressive medical treatment, four of seven patients required application of cyanacrylate glue for impending or actual corneal perforations. Three of them required treatment twice. Two patients received emergent penetrating keratoplasty or corneal patch graft. All but one were preserved anatomically. Visual acuity improved in five of nine eyes and remained unchanged in four eyes. One eye required enucleation and one patient was lost to follow up.

DISCUSSION

Vitamin A deficiency is considered to be a problem of developing countries with estimates of more than 5 million new cases of xerophthalmia annually, and one-quarter million resulting in blindness every year.[2,3] When encountered in developed countries, xerophthalmia, and specifically keratomalacia, often occur in conjunction with cystic fibrosis or other forms of malabsorption or dietary restriction.[4-13] As keratomalacia is uncommon, it is frequently overlooked, and results are tragic. In recent years, an increased prevalence of alcoholism and drug abuse has raised the number of patients with insufficient dietary intake or inadequate intestinal absorption with subsequent vitamin A deficiency and corneal complications.[14,15]

The mechanism(s) by which vitamin A deficiency causes corneal ulceration and necrosis remains controversial.[16] Vitamin A is necessary for the normal production of mucin by conjunctival goblet cells.[17,18] Absence of mucin in the tear film leads to increased surface tension and very rapid preocular tear film break-up time. The formation of keratinized plaques may contribute to epithelial loss either by traumatic sloughing of cornified epithelium or by inducing an irregular wetting of the corneal surface with a delle-like lesion. All of these factors may act upon an already compromised epithelial basement membrane. In fact, morphometric analysis of vitamin A deficient rats has revealed significant reduction in the frequency and size of hemidesmosomes.[19] These changes were reversed with adequate vitamin A supplementation. Once epithelial cell loss has occurred, stromal melting and subsequent perforation may result, but stromal necrosis also can occur despite intact epithelium.

It appears that vitamin A deficiency can also induce alterations of the corneal metabolism, leaving the stroma more susceptible to necrosis.[20] Independent of the vitamin A status, corneal ulceration and stromal necrosis may develop in patients with drug abuse, such as crack cocaine.[21] It is believed that a drug-induced neurotrophic cornea plays a significant role in the pathogenesis of the disease of these patients. Another factor that may play a role is possible exposure keratopathy of the lower third of the cornea during the drug- or alcohol-related stupor. Patient #1 could have had multiple mechanisms for epithelial breakdown and corneal perforation.

Individuals deficient in vitamin A are often protein deficient, which affects the transport of vitamin A into cells. Nevertheless, it seems unnecessary to have both in order to develop corneal complications as illustrated in Patient #4. Moreover, Sommer et al.,[22] elegantly demonstrated that even the most severe corneal alterations were compatible with normal indices of protein and anthropometric status, but not with normal serum vitamin A levels.

Yet another unresolved question is the role of infection in corneal perforation. Bacterial infection has long been suspected as a contributing factor in the causation of blindness.[23] DeCarlo et al.,[24] found that vitamin A deficient rabbits were more susceptible than control animals to infection, even with similar levels of protein-calorie malnutrition. Other studies have shown that with vitamin A deficiency there is an increased adherence of bacteria to the keratinized surface, the plasma antiproteases are decreased, and glycoprotein synthesis is altered.[25,26] One study found a direct correlation between the severity of corneal involvement and the frequency with which pathogenic bacteria were cultured from the conjunctival sac.[20] In this series, four of the seven patients were culture positive (Table 1). No susceptibility to any specific microorganism was found. The clinical appearance of the corneal ulcer was not a reliable guide to diagnosis and prognosis was demonstrated by the wide variation between Patients #4 and #5. Only one patient had developed hypopyon during the course of the disease, but its significance cannot be determined. It is still uncertain whether infection is just a contributing factor or an actual initiator of stromal necrosis.

Histopathologic changes in the ocular surface epithelium of vitamin A deficient patients include keratinization, squamous metaplasia, and loss of conjunctival goblet cells.[4] Pathological review of corneal specimens from patients #1, #5, and #6 revealed thinned corneal epithelium that had totally disappeared from the site of perforation. Corneal epithelial keratinization was observed in some areas. Inflammatory reaction, mostly composed of neutrophils, was present with severe necrosis and formation of fibrinoid material at the wound site (Fig. 2). Despite presence of severe necrosis, a Brown-Hopp stain did not reveal any bacterial colonies.

The diagnosis of keratomalacia should be based on clinical observation. The sudden onset of bilateral, rapidly deepening corneal ulcers, with or without inflammation, seen in this group of patients suggested this diagnosis. As pointed out by Sommer,[1] corneal ulceration unresponsive to antimicrobial therapy in an alcoholic should be considered a consequence of vitamin A deficiency until proven otherwise. Rapid diagnosis and appropriate therapy may restore corneal integrity and prevent visual loss. Failure to diagnose this condition invariably leads to corneal perforation and often blindness. Tests such as electroretinography (ERG) and dark adaptation may help to confirm the diagnosis. Nonetheless, because of the severe bilateral nature of the disease, it is not always possible to obtain these tests. In addition, if the electrodes are placed outside of the cornea, there are no electrophysiologic guidelines to compare the results. Conjunctival impression cytology, total serum retinol binding protein (RBP) and holo-RBP may be useful adjunctive tests to add into the work-up of these patients.

If the index of suspicion is high, empiric vitamin A replacement should not be delayed. Replacement of vitamin A as recommended by the World Health Organization should be followed. A dose of 200,000 IU of retinyl palmitate orally on two successive days, and a third dose 1 to 4 weeks later, should be given. Appropriate corneal cultures should be obtained and bacterial coverage provided. Another possible treatment is the use of topical retinoid, which can speed the corneal healing, but does not have any significant impact on the overall clinical outcome.[27] Any protein deficiency should be corrected. If diagnosis is made early in the process of corneal ulceration, the prospects for obtaining clear cornea and good vision are high, as demonstrated by some of our patients. Unfortunately, some of our patients sought attention with late involvement in the only remaining eye. In such cases, tissue adhesive with an overlying soft contact lens may not seal a large perforation and a patch graft or penetrating keratoplasty is warranted in order to preserve the anatomy.

Although corneal perforations secondary to vitamin A deficiency are considered rare in the United States, this series reports a subset of patients in whom the ophthalmologist must maintain a high index of suspicion of vitamin A deficiency in the differential diagnosis of corneal melting and perforation.

ACKNOWLEDGMENTS

Supported in part by an unrestricted grant from Research to Prevent Blindness.

REFERENCES

1. A. Sommer, Vitamin A deficiency and xerophthalmia. *Arch. Ophthalmol.* 108:343 (1990).
2. A. Sommer, *Nutritional Blindness: Xerophthalmia and Keratomalacia* Oxford University Press, New York (1981).
3. A. Sommer, Tarwotjo, I., and Hussaini, G., Incidence, prevalence, and scale of blinding malnutrition. *Lancet* 1:1407 (1981).
4. P. Fells, and Bors, F., Ocular complications of self induced vitamin A deficiency. *Eye* 89:221 (1969).
5. G.M. Gombos, Hornblass, A., and Vendeland, J., Ocular manifestations of vitamin A deficiency. *Ann. Ophthalmol.* 2:680 (1970).
6. R.S. Smith, Farrel, T., and Bailey T., Keratomalacia. *Surv. Ophthalmol* 20:213, 1975.
7. J. Oliver, Keratomalacia on a "healthy diet". *Br. J. Ophthalmol.* 70:357 (1986).
8. A.N.H. Main, Mills, P.R., Russell, R.I., et al., Vitamin A deficiency in Crohn's disease. *Gut* 24:1169 (1983).
9. G.C. Brown, Felton, S.C., and Benson, W.E., Reversible night blindness with intestinal bypass surgery. *Am. J. Ophthalmol.* 89:776 (1980).
10. D.B. Sloan, Wood, W.J., and Iserhagen, R.D., Short-term night blindness associated with colon resection and hypovitaminosis. *Arch. Ophthalmol.* 112: 162 (1994).
11. P. Gouras, Carr, R.E., and Gunkel, R.D. Retinitis pigmentosa in abetallipoproteinemia: effects of vitamin A. *Invest. Ophthalmol. Vis. Sci.* 10:784 (1971).
12. R.A. Petersen, Petersen, V.S., and Robb, R.M. Vitamin A deficiency with xerophthalmia and night blindness in cystic fibrosis. *Am. J. Dis. Child.* 116:662 (1968).
13. M.A. Sperling, Hiles, D.A., and Kennerdell, J.S., Electroretinographic responses following vitamin A therapy in abetalipoproteinemia. *Am. J. Ophthalmol.* 73:342 (1972).
14. E.P. Suan, Bedrossian, E.H., Eagle, R.C., et al. Corneal perforation in patients with vitamin A deficiency in the United States. *Arch. Ophthalmol.* 108:350 (1990).
15. R.M. Russell, Morrison, S.A., Smith, F.R., et al., Vitamin A reversal of abnormal dark adaptation in cirrhosis: study of effects on the plasma retinol transport system. *Ann. Intern. Med.* 88:622 (1978).
16. P.B. Donzis, and Mondino B.J., Management of noninfectious corneal ulcers. *Surv. Ophthalmol.* 32:94 (1987).
17. A. Sommer, and Green, W.R., Goblet cell response to vitamin A treatment for ocular xerophthalmia. *Am. J. Ophthalmol.* 94:213 (1983).
18. V. Rao, Friend, J., Thoft, R.A., et al. Conjunctival goblet cells and mitotic rate in children with retinol deficiency and measles. *Arch. Ophthalmol.* 105:378 (1987).
19. N.B.K. Shams, Hanninen, L.A., and Chaves, H.V., Effect of vitamin A deficiency on the adhesion of rat corneal epithelium and basement membrane complex. *Invest. Ophthalmol. Vis. Sci.* 34:2646 (1993).
20. A. Sommer, Green, W.R., and Kenyon, K.R., Clinicohistopathologic correlations in xerophthalmic ulceration and necrosis. *Arch. Ophthalmol.* 100:953 (1982).
21. R. Sachs, Zagelbaum, B.M., and Hersh, P.S., Corneal complications associated with the use of crack cocaine. *Ophthalmology* 100:187 (1993).
22. A. Sommer, et al. Nutritional factors in corneal xerophthalmia and keratomalacia. *Arch. Ophthalmol.* 100:399 (1982).

23. M.J. Valenton, and Tan, R.V., Secondary ocular bacterial infection in hypovitaminosis A xerophthalmia. *Am. J. Ophthalmol.* 80:673 (1975).

24. J.D. DeCarlo, Van Horn, D.L., Hyndium, R.A., et al., Increased susceptibility to infection in experimental xerophthalmia. *Arch. Ophthalmol.* 99:1614 (1981).

25. T.C. Kiorpes, Molica S.J., and Wolf, G., A plasma glycoprotein depressed in vitamin A deficiency in the rat: Alphamacroglobulin. *J. Nutr.* 104:1659 (1976).

26. J.Y. Kim, and Wolf, G., Vitamin A deficiency and the glycoproteins of rat corneal epithelium. *J. Nutr.* 1104:710 (1974).

27. A. Sommer. Treatment of corneal xerophthalmia with topical retinoic acid. *Am. J. Ophthalmol.* 95:349 (1983).

46

CORNEAL AND CONJUNCTIVAL INTRAEPITHELIAL NEOPLASIA

A Clinical and Histopathological Analysis

Francisco Barraquer[1] and Luis F. Mejía[2]

[1]Instituto Barraquer de América
 Santafé de Bogotá, Columbia
[2]Instituto de Ciencias de la Salud -CES
 Medellín, Columbia

ABSTRACT

A retrospective study identifying 306 patients (326 pathology samples; 59.74% of whom were males) with a corneal and conjunctival intraepithelial neoplasia (CIN) was performed. The neoplasia was conjunctival in 213 (69.6%) and corneal in 94 (30.7%) of the cases studied. Mean age in the conjunctival group was 48.2 ± 16.2 years, while in the corneal group it was 59.2 ± 14.8 years ($p = 0.0001$). There was a predominance for the CINs to locate on exposed interpalpebral areas.

Mean follow-up time was 21.9 months. Among the mild-moderate dysplasias, 2.9% recurred, compared to 8.06% of the severe-ca in situ dysplasias. The resection border was more frequently involved in the 18 cases that recurred (61%) than in the 308 that did not recur (37.9%).

Overall, there were 18 recurrences (5.52%) in a mean time of 20 months. This group was statistically different regarding male sex, prolonged sun exposure, more advanced dysplastic stage, and resection border involvement. Thus, a complete resection and appropriate anatomical reconstruction are considered essential for the proper management of this entity.

INTRODUCTION

Corneal and conjunctival intraepithelial neoplasia (CIN) is being increasingly recognized in ophthalmology because of its oncological as well as its functional implications. The term CIN was first employed during the 70s in gynecology referring to cervical interaepithelial neoplasia. Its main objective was to include all intraepithelial dysplastic le-

Advances in Corneal Research, edited by Lass
Plenum Press, New York, 1997

sions in one group with similar risk factors, management, and prognosis.[1] In 1978 Jakobiec and Pizarello used such a denomination for the first time in ophthalmology referring to conjunctival intraepithelial neoplasia.[2] Later on, Waring, Roth, and Elkins used it to describe corneal intraepithelial neoplasia,[3] so that nowadays the term CIN in ophthalmology means essentially dysplasia at the limbal junctional zone.

CIN usually appears in the 5th to 6th decades, more frequently in caucasian males,[2,4–7] unilaterally, and predominantly in the interpalpebral zone.[8–11] An actinic[2,4,10,12–17] as well as a traumatic influence[2,18] has been proposed. A viral etiology has also been suggested (HPV type 16),[19–23] like that of uterine cervix CIN, in which this etiology is more firmly established.[24]

Considering that monoclonality is a fundamental neoplastic characteristic, cellular genome alterations will perpetuate only when taking place in stem cells, since these are the only ones capable of self renewal. The stem cells of the ocular surface are located at the basal cell layer on the limbus. This explains why the CINs are connected to the limbus, comprising the corneal and conjunctiva simultaneously, although asymmetrically.

MATERIALS AND METHODS

This was a retrospective study done through the Pathology Laboratory at the Instituto Barraquer de America in Bogota. The study checked on all cornea and/or conjunctiva specimens previously classified as squamous cell carcinoma, CIN, papilloma, keratotic plaque, solar keratosis, and pseudoepitheliomatous hyperplasia, either clinically or histologically, between 1964 and 1994. The clinical records were reviewed regarding patient's age, sex, job, symptoms, previous treatments, physical examination findings, result of the anterior segment angiography, treatment, and follow-up.

Semiological analysis was based on slit-lamp pictures taken preoperatively, looking for:

- Growth pattern:

  - Gelatinous: Gray-whitish, somewhat raised outgrowth, less brilliant than the normal epithelial surface (Fig. 1).
  - Leucoplastic: White, dry, or creamy outgrowth with an irregular surface (Fig. 2).

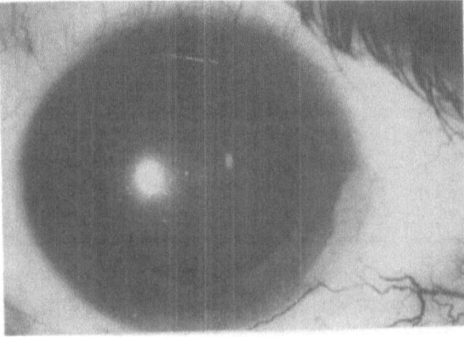

Figure 1. Gelatinous growth pattern.

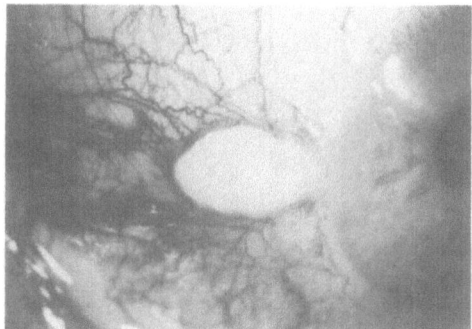

Figure 2. Leucoplastic growth pattern.

- Velvety: Pink-reddish convex outgrowth with a delicate vascular supply (Fig. 3).
- Papillomatous: Pink-whitish, vaulted, multinodular outgrowth (Fig. 4).

- CIN Location: Corneal or conjunctival, according to which side comprised a grater percentage of the lesion, by ocular surface quadrants.

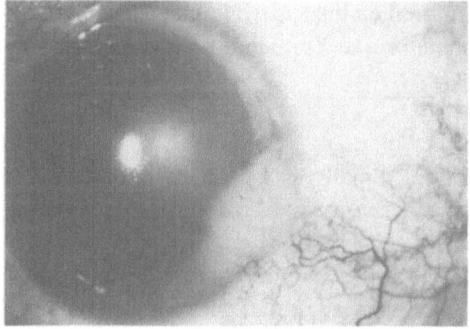

Figure 3. Velvety growth pattern.

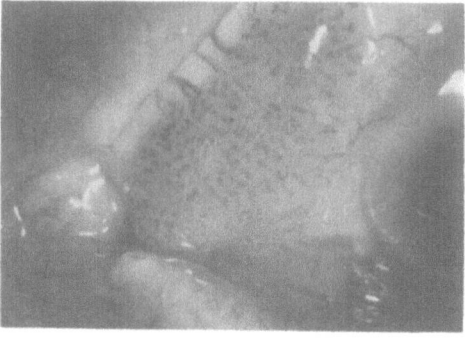

Figure 4. Papillomatous growth pattern.

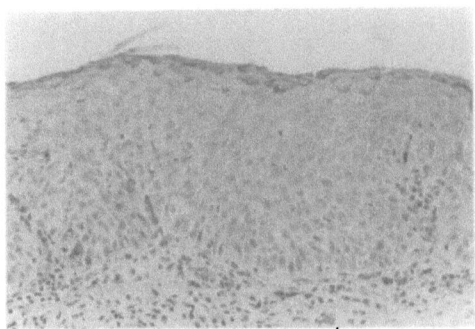

Figure 5. Mild–moderate dysplasia. Epidermoid fusiform cellularity. Magnification 63x.

- Advance Border: Convex or fimbriated
- Vascularity: Avascular, slight pannus, fibrovascular pannus, vertical vessels and vertically branching vessels.

Hematoxilin and eosin (HE) and periodic acid of Schiff (PAS) stained slides were reviewed, considering:

- Dysplasia Stage

  - Mild-moderate: Involvement of up to 2/3 of epithelial thickness. There is appropriate maturation on the superficial layers (Fig. 5).
  - Severe carcinoma *in situ*: Epithelial involvement grater than 2/3 of its thickness (Fig. 6).

- Cellularity:

  - Fusiform Basaloid: Small fusiform cells oriented perpendicularly to the basement membrane; delicate and eosinophilic cytoplasm; ellipsoid, moderately chromatic nuclei.
  - Epidermoid Fusiform: Medium-sized cells; more copious, eosinophilic cytoplasm; nore vesicle-shaped, although elongated nuclei.

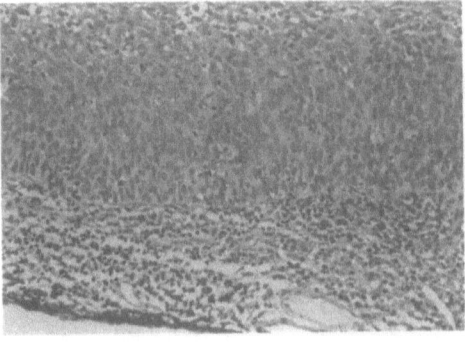

Figure 6. Severe–Ca "*in situ*" dysplasia. Epidermoid fusiform cellularity. Note basal mononuclear cell infiltration. Magnification 63x.

Table 1. CIN related consultation causes (n= 188)

Sign/symptom	Number	Percentage
Pterygium/Pinguecula/mass	142	75.53
Red eye	66	35.10
Ocular burning sensation	59	31.38
Foreign body sensation	30	15.95
Poor visu al acuity	18	9.57

- Epidermoid: Epithelioid cells, pleomorphic and bizarre with an eosinophilic and extensive cytoplasm; large nuclei and prominent nucleoli.

- Presence of suprabasal mitosis (≥ per 100x field), basal mononuclear cell infiltration, hyper- and parakeratosis, vascularization type, and resection border status.

RESULTS

This study identified 326 samples corresponding to CIN, pertaining to 306 patients. The mean patient age was 51.7 ± 16.5 years (range 10–88 years) and 59.74% were males. Daily activities were related to a prolonged sun exposure in 18.25% of the cases. The initial consultation complaint was CIN-related in 188 patients (61.43%), as illustrated in Table 1. Frequently the patient had more than one of the signs/symptoms. Symptoms had been present for a mean of 8.3 ± 12.4 months, and in most cases (75.16%) patients had received no treatment at all. Among the 76 patients (28.84%) who had received some treatment, 20 had been operated on—most with a diagnosis of pterygium—the remaining 56 patients had received multiple medical treatments without improvement.

The CIN was conjunctival in 213 (69.6%) and corneal in 94 (37.7%) patients; in one patient it was symmetrically corneal and conjunctival. Mean age of the patients in the conjunctival group was 48.2 ± 16.2 years, while in the cornel group it was 59.2 ± 14.8 years (p = 0.0001). The initial clinical diagnosis was corrected in 71.5% of cases. The most frequent misdiagnoses (undiagnosed CIN) were pterygium, pinguecula, and papilloma. Quadrant distribution of the CINs on the ocular surface evidences an exposed area predominance; often a lesion comprised more than one quadrant (Table 2).

When the quadrant distribution was analyzed according to patient age it was evident that the younger group had a nasal zone predominance while the older one has a superior quadrant predominance (Table 3). This pattern was statistically significant in the conjunctival group (p = 0.0001).

In the conjunctiva, the most frequent growth pattern was leucoplastic (43.19%), followed by gelatinous (22%), papillomatous (20.9%), and velvety (14%). In the cornea, the most frequent type was gelatinous (64.13%), followed by leucoplastic (15.5%), papillomatous (11.8%), and velvety (8.5%). These differences probably correspond to the variable

Table 2. Quadrant distribution

CIN	Nasal	Temporal	Superior	Inferior
Conjunctival	64.3%	29.5%	5.1%	11.2%
Corneal	61.9%	39.1%	16.3%	38.0%

Table 3. Age (yrs)–CIN location relationship

CIN	Nasal	Temporal	Superior	Inferior
Conjunctival	46.0	52.7	65.0	54.1
Corneal	56.5	61.9	57.4	57.2

difficulty with which the lesion is perceived against its background. The most frequent advancing border found, both in conjunctiva and in cornea, was the fimbriated one (80.1% and 92.4%, respectively).

One of the most characteristic semiological images of the CINs was the presence of blood vessels not reaching the lesion's advancing border. In early stages, when still avascular, 16.4% of the conjunctival and 10.6% of the corneal CINs were identified. This was probably due to the nutrition of the conjunctival neoplasia from the lamina propria, which lets them grow larger while still avascular. In addition, it was harder to identify early fine blood vessels against the white scleral background. The presence of a slight pannus and fibrovascular pannus was recognized slightly more frequently in the cornea than in the conjunctiva. However, when the vertical vessels began to appear — reflecting a greater volume — these percentages grew closer (11.7% in the cornea and 8.9% in the conjunctiva) and in the case of vertically branching vessels, it was greater in the conjunctiva (19.2%) than in the cornea (17%).

A similar operative technique was used for all patients: the CIN was dissected with Westcott scissors from bulbar conjunctiva up to the limbus, and intraepithelially from the cornea towards the limbus with a fine flat spatula. Once both slopes had been dissected, the CIN was sectioned with curved Vannas scissors at the limbus. When the limbus was irregular it was leveled with an aerotor; a free conjunctival graft or limbal-conjunctival graft (if the resection border was greater than 120°) was used to obtain an adequate anatomical reconstruction.[25] Postoperatively, patients were given antibiotic/steroid drops t.i.d. for 10 days, at which time the sutures were removed.

Mean follow-up time was 21.9 months. Mean visual acuity at first follow-up visit was 0.72 ± 0.37, and at the last one it was 0.81 ± 0.29 (p = 0.0001). The were 18 recurrences (5.52%) at a mean time of 20 months. This group was statistically different regarding sex (83.3% males), sun exposure (44.4% had prolonged sun exposure) and poorer final visual acuity (0.57 ± 0.32; p = 0.04).

Histopathological Analysis

A total of 326 samples were processed at the pathology laboratory. Conjunctival CINs were associated to a pterygium or pinguecula in 54% of cases. There was a slightly greater percentage of lesions showing an earlier stage in the corneal group, as was expected due to its easier clinical detection. Hence, the incidence of mild-moderate dysplasia was 46.1% in the cornea and 42.2% in the conjunctiva; the incidence of severe CA *in situ* dysplasia was 54.9% in the corneal and 60.4% in the conjunctiva. Sometimes there was more than one dysplastic pattern in the sample. No relationship between age and dysplastic stage was found. The more advanced the dysplasia, the greater the probability of recurrence. Thus, only 2.9% of the mild-moderate dysplasias recurred compared to 8.06% of the severe CA *in situ* dysplasias. The cellularity type was similar in the corneal and conjunctival groups, as follows: epidermoid fusiform in 83.6%, epidermoid in 22.1%, and

Table 4. Dysplasia stage-cellularity type relationship

Dysplasia	Fusif. Basaloid	Epiderm. Fusif	Epidermoid
Cornea			
Mild-moderate	100%	44.28%	36.36%
Severe-"in situ"	0%	55.72%	63.63%
Conjunctiva			
Mild-moderate	42.85%	23.37%	42.22%
Severe-"in situ"	57.15%	76.62%	57.77%

fusiform basaloid in 2.6% of cases (mean corneal and conjunctival values). The marked predominance of the epidermoid fusiform cellularity is sound, as it represents an intermediate stage in the benign morphological alteration sequence that begins with the more benign fusiform basaloid type and is most advanced with the epidermoid one.

When analyzing the association between a specific type of cellularity and the dysplastic stage, there was a trend towards a more severe corneal dysplasia associated with the epidermoid cellularity while in the conjunctiva this was associated with epidermoid-fusiform cellularity as shown in Table 4. The resection border was involved in 124 samples (38.03%); this number was significant when discriminating between the incidence of border involvement among the 18 cases that recurred (61%) and in the 308 that did not recur.

CONCLUSIONS

CIN has a multifactorial etiology, with different external influences partly depending on the age group. Hence, the predilelction for exposed areas in young people and for the superior one in older groups suggests two different etiologies. It is likely that in younger patients there is a grater relation to the actinic factor, while in the older group it corresponds to the mutagenicity directly related to aging.

Although some groups have suggested the use of conjunctival[26-30] and exfoliative[27,31,32] cytology for the diagnosis of these lesions, a good physical examination complemented with an anterior segment angiography when deemed necessary should be enough to correctly diagnose most CIN.

Classifying the CINs in different dysplastic stages is useful from both the pathological and prognostic standpoint. The dysplastic stage initially found is an important prognostic factor as 2.9% of the mild-moderate dysplasias recurred, while 8.06% of the severe-CA *in situ* dysplasias recurred.

A clear relationship was found between the resection borders status and the recurrence rate; so, 61% of recurring cases showed resection border involvement in the initial surgical sample, while 37.9% of those who did not recur showed it. Most of these recurrences appeared during the first two years, which denotes the necessity of a strict control of these patients for at least such a period.

No clinical sign that might allow prediction of the dysplastic stage of the lesion was found. Therefore, a careful follow-up and the verification of growth will determine the appropriate moment for resection. The basis for the surgical management of this entity is the complete resection of the anomalous tissue[33] with a subsequent adequate reconstruction of the ocular surface. Thus, a superficial keratectomy is not considered necessary in the management of this entity. Likewise, the use of adjunctive procedures or drugs such as cryotherapy,[5,34–36] radiotherapy,[37–39] Thiotepa,[4] or 5-Fuorouracil[40] are not considered necessary when employing a sound surgical technique.

While relatively low in virulence, the CIN has shown a tendency to recur. In this series, the recurrence rate was 5.52%, but in other series it varied between 10% and 40%,[5,7,13,33,41,42] usually being around 20%. Several studies have shown the mean age of patients with *in situ* squamous cell carcinoma to be 5 to 9 years less than that of patients with invasive squamous cell carcinoma,[4,7] which suggests a temporal relation between these two entities. However, their course should not be considered analogous to that of cervical intraepithelial neoplasia where 50% of cases progress to invasive carcinoma in 6 to 9 years,[43] compared to only 4.8% of the conjunctival CINs[2] and an even small number of the corneal CINs (0.3%-0.6%).[3,33]

REFERENCES

1. R.M. Richart, Cervical intraepithelial neoplasia. *Pathol. Annu.* 8:301 (1973).
2. L.D. Pizzarello, and Jakobiec, F.A., Bowen's disease of the conjunctiva: a misnomer. In *Ocular and Adnexal Tumors*, F.A. Jakobiec, ed., Aesculapius, Birmingham (1978).
3. G.O. Waring, Roth, A.M., and Ekins, M.B., Clinical and pathologic description of 17 cases of corneal intraepithelial neoplasia. *Am. J. Ophthalmol.* 97:547 (1984).
4. J.C. Erie, Campbell, R.J., and Liesegang, J., Conjunctival and corneal intraepithelial and invasive neoplasia. *Ophthalmology* 93:176 (1986).
5. F.T. Fraunfelder, and Wingfield, D., Management of intraepithelial conjunctival tumors and squamous cell carcinomas. *Am. J. Ophthalmol.* 95: 359 (1983).
6. M. Harrison, and Glasson, W., Conjunctival and limbal tumours. *Aust. N.Z. J. Ophthalmol.* 13: 193 (1985).
7. C. Ni, Searl, S.S., Kriegstein, H.J., and Wu, B.F., Epibulbar carcinoma. *Int. Ophthalmol. Clin.* 22:1 (1982).
8. Napora A., et al., Factors associated with conjunctival intraepithetial neoplasia: a case control study. *Ophthalmic Surgery* 21:27 (1990).
9. R.J. Campbell, and Bourne, W.M., Unilateral central corneal epithelial ophthalmology 88:1231 (1981).
10. C. Ni, et al., Epibulbar carcinoma. *Int. Ophthalmol. Clin.* 22:1 (1982).
11. F.C. Blodi, Squamous cell carcinoma of the conjunctiva. *Doc. Ophthalmol.* 34:93 (1973).
12. A.F. Cruess, Wasan, S.M., and Willis, W.E., Corneal epithelial dysplasia and carcinoma in situ. *Can. J. Ophthalmol.* 16:171 (1981).
13. A.R. Irvine., Dyskeratotic epibulbar tumors. *Trans. Am. Ophthal. Soc.* 61:243 (1963).
14. A.R. Irvine., Epibulbar squamous cell carcinoma and related lesions. *Int. Ophthalmol. Clin.* 12:71 (1972).
15. A.S. Clear, Chirambo, M.C., and Hut, M.S.R., Solar keratosis, pterygium, and squamous cell carcinoma of the conjunctiva in Malawi. *Br. J. Ophthalmol.* 63:102 (1979).
16. G.A. Lee, Williams, G., Hirst, L.W., and Green, A.C., Risk factors in the development of ocular surface epithelial dysplasia. *Ophthalmology* 101:360 (1994).
17. K.F. Tabbara, Kersten, R., Dauk, N., and Blodi, F.C., Metastatic squamous cell carcinoma of the conjunctiva. *Ophthalmology* 95:318 (1988).
18. F.C. Blodi., Squamous cell carcinoma of the conjunctiva. *Doc. Ophthalmol.* 34:93 (1973).
19. M.G. Odrich, Jakobiec, F.A., et al., A spectrum of bilateral squamous conjunctival tumors associated with Human Papillomavirus Type 16. *Ophthalmology* 98:628 (1991).
20. J.M. McDonnell, McDonnell, P.J., Mounts, P., et. al., Demonstration of papillomavirus capsid antigen in human conjunctival neoplasia. *Arch. Ophthalmol.* 104:1801 (1986).
21. J.M. McDonnell, Mayr, A.J., and Martin, W.J., DNA of human papillomavirus type 16 in dysplastic and malignant lesions of the conjunctiva and cornea. *N. Engl. J. Med.* 320:1442 (1989).
22. J.M. McDonnell, McDonnell, P.J., and Sun, Y.Y., Human papillomavirus DNA in tissues and ocular surface swabs of patients with conjunctival epithelial neoplasia. *J. Invest. Ophthalmol. Vis. Sci.* 33:184 (1992).
23. J.M. McDonnell, Wagner, D., Ng, S.T., et al., Human papillomavirus type 16 DNA in ocular and cervical swabs of women with genital tract condylomata. *Am. J. Ophthalmol.* 112:61 (1991).
24. L. Gissmann, Linking FIPV to cancer. *Clinical Obstetrics and Gynecology* 32:1 (1989).
25. J.I. Barraquer, et. al., In, *The First Cornea World Congress.* J.H. King, Jr, and McTigue J.W. eds., Butterworths, Washington (1965).

26. H. Gelender, and Forster, R., Papanicolau cytology in the diagnosis and management of external ocular tumors. *Arch. Ophthalmol.* 98:909 (1980).

27. P. Dykstra, and Dykstra, B.A., The cytologic diagnosis of carcinoma and related lesions of the ocular conjunctiva and cornea. *Trans. Amer. Acad. Ophthal. Otolaryng.* 73:979 (1968).

28. G.R. Nolan, Hirst, L.W., Wright, R.G., and Bancroft, B.J., The application of impression cytology to the diagnosis of conjunctival neoplasms. *Diagn. Cytopathol.* 11:246 (1994).

29. M. Muscara, Guiffre, G., Trombetta, C.J., et al., Nucleolar organizer regions (NORs) in dysplastic and neoplastic epithelial lesions of the conjunctiva. *Pathologica* 83:281 (1991).

30. S.S. Weissman, Char, D.H., Herbort, C.P., et al., Alteration of human conjunctival epithelial proliferation. *Arch. Ophthalmol.* 110:357 (1992).

31. M. Spinak, and Friedman, A.H., Squamous cell carcinoma of the conjunctiva. Value of exfoliative cytology in diagnosis. *Surv. Ophthalmol.* 21:351 (1977).

32. H. Gelender, and Forster, R.K., Papanicolau cytology in the diagnosis and management of external ocular tumors. *Arch. Ophthalmol.* 98:909 (1980).

33. J.C. Erie, Campbell, R.J., and Liesegang, T.J., Conjunctival and corneal intraepithelial and invasive neoplasia. *Ophthalmology* 93:176 (1986).

34. F.T. Fraunfelder, and Wingfield, D., Management of intraepithelial conjunctival tumors and squamous cell carcinomas. *Am. J. Ophthalmol.* 95:359 (1983).

35. R.D. Divine, and Anderson, R.L., Nitrous oxide cryotherapy for intraepithelial epithelioma of the conjunctiva. *Arch. Ophthalmol.* 101:782 (1983).

36. F.T. Fraunfelder, and Wingfield, D., Therapy of intraepithelial epitheliomas and squamous cell carcinoma of the limbus. *Trans. Am. Ophthalmol. Soc.* 79:290 (1980).

37. J. Francois, Kluyskens, J., and Rabaey, M., Intraepithelial epithelioma of the conjunctiva and cornea (Bowen's disease) healed by contact radiotherapy. *Brit. J. Ophthalmol.* 34:360 (1950).

38. P. Lommatsch, Beta-ray treatment of malignant epithelial tumors of the conjunctiva. *Am. J. Ophthalmol.* 81:198 (1976).

39. L. Cerezo, Otero, J., Aragon, G., et al., Conjunctival intraepithelial and invasive squamous cell carcinomas treated with Strontium-90. *Radiother. Oncol.* 17:191 (1990).

40. R.P. Yeatts, Ford, J.G., Stanton, C.A., and Reed, J.W., Topical 5-fluorouracil in treating epithelial neoplasia of the conjunctiva and cornea. *Ophthalmology* 102:1338 (1995).

41. J. Carroll, and Kuwabara, T., A classification of limbal epitheliomas. *Arch. Ophthalmol.* 73:545 (1965).

42. G.A. Lee, and Hirst, L.W., Ocular surface squamous neoplasia. *Surv. Ophthalmol.* 39:429 (1995).

43. R.M. Richart, and Barron, B.A., A follow-up study of patients with cervical dysplasia. *Am. J. Obstet. Gynecol.* 105:386 (1969).

SECTION X: WORLD CORNEAL HEALTH

Abstracts of Other Conference Presentations and Posters

BACTERIAL CORNEAL ULCERS

In the developing countries of the world, corneal ulceration is a major cause of blindness. This situation is especially true in areas where trachoma, onchocerciasis, leprosy, and other infectious causes of ocular disease are endemic. As a result, corneal opacification is second only to cataract as the most important cause of visual disability in the world today. Studies from several developing countries have reported the incidence of bacterial and fungal pathogens isolated from ulcerated corneas. Comprehensive epidemiologic surveys investigating the predisposing and demographic factors contributing to corneal ulceration, however, are rare. Since the epidemiologic pattern of corneal ulceration varies significantly from region to region, an understanding of the epidemiologic pattern in different parts of the world is essential for the development of a global strategy for prevention of blindness caused by corneal ulceration.

Patients with corneal ulceration were examined at Tribhuvan University Teaching Hospital in Kathmandu, Nepal, and Aravind Eye Hospital Madurai, India. The results of our studies will be reported.

PROGRESS IN TRACHOMA PATHOGENESIS AND CONTROL PATHOGENESIS

The histopathology of trachoma, the lack of known chlamydial toxins, and the absence of viable organisms in a high proportion of cases of inflammatory, and most cases of scarring disease suggest that it is an immunopathological disorder. It has been assumed for many years that the inflammatory response was due to cell-mediated delayed hypersensitivity to chlamydial antigens. Recent studies in humans have cast doubt on this hypothesis. Cell-mediated immune responses to whole organisms, to recombinant major outer membrane protein and to the chlamydial heat shock protein hsp-60 were depressed in subjects with persistent inflammatory, or with scarring disease, whereas anti-chlamydial antibody levels in both tears and serum were increased in these subjects. This suggests that, as for other intracellular pathogens, aT-helper I type cell-mediated immune response is associated with protection from disease. A case-control study of scarring trachoma in the Gambia has recently shown that the class I HLA allele A*6802 is significantly associated with severe scarring. An association has also been shown with polymorphisms in the promoter region of the TNF alpha gene.

Control

Recent studies have evaluated health education and oral azithromycin in the control of trachoma. In Tanzania an intensive education campaign increased the prevalence of clean faces and reduced the prevalence of severe inflammatory trachoma among children over a 1 year period. In the Gambia, a single dose of azithromycin (20 mg/kg) was equivalent to 6 weeks of topical tetracycline in the treatment of active disease. Reinfection was however rapid in both groups. A multicentre study to evaluate mass treatment with 3 oral doses of azithromycin in trachoma control is currently being conducted.

MITOMYCIN C IN PTERYGIUM SURGERY

M. Srinivasan and P. Sathyan

Purpose: To evaluate the safety and efficacy of single intraoperative application of 0.02% mitomycin-C in pterygium surgery.

Methods: 469 eyes of 410 patients in the age group ranging from 20 years to 80 years had 0.02% intraoperative mitomycin for one minute in pterygium surgery performed by single surgeon in the same institute between April 1993 to June 1995. Consecutive patients with advanced pterygium were operated. Follow-up period ranges from 6 months to 26 months.

Results: 445 eyes had primary pterygia and 24 had recurrent pterygia. 232 were males and 178 were females. 399 eyes had only nasal pterygium. 2% of these eyes had recurrence of pterygium following this technique. 4% had tenons granuloma. No other adverse reactions was noticed.

Conclusion: We find single application of 0.02% mitomycin-C for one minute intraoperatively in pterygium surgery is safe and effective in preventing recurrence of pterygium.

EYE BANKING IN DEVELOPING COUNTRIES

Gullapalli N. Rao

L.V. Prasad Eye Institute, Hyderabad, India

Corneal blindness is a major problem in developing countries and consequently effective eye banking is a great necessity in these countries. Lack of public awareness, religious superstition, governmental negligence, lack of infrastructure and trained manpower are major stumbling blocks to progress. Several models that have improved the situation now exist in some countries.

In India, with the support of several international organisations such as International Federation of Eye Banks several new concepts are being developed. Eye Bank Association of India was formed with permanent headquarters coordinating the activities throughout the country. Models of high quality eye banking in all aspects were also created along with manpower training. Efforts are being made to get appropriate legislative measures enacted by the government.

All these can be replicated in other parts of the developing world.

CHALLENGES OF INTERNATIONAL EYE BANKING

Frederick N. Griffith

International Federation of Eye Banks, Baltimore, Maryland

While eye banking in most developed countries has evolved to a high level of efficiency, varying cultures, customs and conditions pose continuing challenges, especially in developing countries. The areas of concern are several, including: (1) understanding and sensitivity to religious, traditional & cultural differences; (2) encouragement of tissue retrieval laws; (3) upgrading of existing eye banking facilities & personnel; (4) provision of adequate equipment, space and supply availability; (5) organization of full-time, around-the-clock staffing; (6) establishment of uniform quality control standards and monitoring; (7) management of tissue in tropical climates; (8) develop equitable tissue distribution systems; (9) elevate the perception of the eye bank as a community resource with an active and supportive advisory board; (10) network communications through fax and E-mail. During the past decade, the methodology of the IFEB has evolved to include site visits involving Ministries of Health, ophthalmic faculties, hospitals and legislators to determine feasibility, and to ultimately ensure an appropriate organizational basis as well as financial resources plus staff, supplies and dedicated supporters. Since 1988, the IFEB has established 15 eye banks outside the U.S. and is working to upgrade four existing facilities, while seven new eye banks are currently under development. IFEB centers in Cairo and Prague also serve as training sites for technical personnel. Corneal preservation media is being distributed from IFEB-established facilities in Egypt and India. Although the challenges are ongoing, these experiences and accomplishments suggest that locally appropriate adaptations of current methodology and technology can prove rewarding in advancing the cause of international eye banking.

KERATOEPITHELIOPLASTY FOR SEVERE, RECURRENT PTERYGIUM

Tatsuo Yamaguchi

St. Luke's International Hospital; Tokyo, Japan

Since Thoft first described keratoepithelioplasty in 1984, this procedure has been used to treat eyes with chemical burns, Mooren's ulcer, and Stevens-Johnson syndrome, with good results. We have examined the results of using this procedure in eyes with severe, recurring pterygium.

Keratoepithelioplasty was performed in seven patients, ages 39 to 72 years, who had undergone pterygium surgery from one to four times previously. There were five men and two women. The grafts were prepared from fresh donor cornea, cut to a depth of 2/3 to 3/4 of the full thickness using a Graefe blade. One edge of the grafts was cut straight. After removal of the pterygium, three grafts were sutured together side to side and then sutured tightly to the limbus with 10–0 nylon, with the straight edge facing the conjunctiva. Finally, the conjunctiva was sutured to the bare sclera.

With a mean follow-up of 68 months (range, 53–63 months), six of the seven cases have had no recurrence; one case developed a recurrence 2 months after surgery after the graft was rejected. Postoperatively, astigmatism decreased an average of 0.25 D (range, increase of 1.25 D - decrease of 2.52 D).

The efficacy of this procedure may be the result of contact inhibition between the epithelial cells in the graft and in the conjunctiva and between the keratocytes in the graft stroma and the fibroblasts in the conjunctival stroma. We believe that this procedure is useful in the treatment of severe, recurring pterygium.

CORNEAL AND CONJUNCTIVAL INTRAEPITHELIAL NEOPLASIA: A Clinical and Histopathological Analysis

Louis Mejia

Corneal and Conjunctival Intraepithelial Neoplasia (CIN) is being increasingly recognized in ophthalmology as the importance of an early diagnosis is realized both from the oncological and functional point of view.

We performed a retrospective study through the archive of the Pathology Laboratory of Instituto Barraquer de América, finding 374 specimens (306 patients) corresponding to ICN, which had a clinical, photographic and angiographic follow up of at least 6 months. Males (59.74%) were affected slightly more often than females, with a mean age of 51.7±16.5 yrs. The main cause of consultation was a pterygium, pinguecula or ocular surface mass (57.44%). Conjunctival CIN's comprised 69.6% of the lesions while corneal accounted for 30.7%. Overall, the most common location of the lesions were in the interpalpebral fissure. Younger patients had a predominance for nasal areas while older patients had a predominance for the superior quadrant of the ocular surface. Recurrence rate was 5.6%, at an average of 20 months.

Histopathologically, there was a predominance for "Slight to Moderate Dysplasia" in the Corneal group (46.1%), and "Severe to Ca 'in Situ' dysplasia" in the Conjunctival one (60.4%). Recurrent cases had a greater proportion of Severe-Ca "in Situ" Dysplasia (79%) on the material obtained in the first surgery. Overall, the resection border was involved in 39.2% of cases: it was involved in 61 % of the recurrent cases and in 37.9% of those who did not recur.

SURGICAL MANAGEMENT OF AN ADVANCED PTERYGIUM INVOLVING THE ENTIRE CORNEA

Li Lim and Donald T.H. Tan

Singapore National Eye Centre

Introduction: Conjunctival autografting for pterygium is an effective surgical modality which has been shown to reduce the incidence of recurrence. We present a unusual case of a primary pterygium which involved tile entire surface of the cornea, and which therefore posed a significant surgical challenge to visually rehabilitate the eye.

Case Report: A 63 year old farmer presented with primary pterygia in both eyes. The right cornea was totally replaced by fibrovascular pterygium tissue, resulting in a visual acuity of light perception. The pterygium in the left eye also encroached on the visual axis and visual acuity was 6/60.

A surgical procedure was planned in which excision of the the total pterygium in the right eye was performed in conjunction with procurement of an annular-shaped conjunctival graft obtained from the superior bulbar conjunctiva. Postoperatively there was no recurrence of the pterygium (at 5 months) and the cornea remained non-vascularised. Visual acuity remained at counting fingers due to the presence of deep stromal scarring.

Five months after conjunctival autograft surgery, a penetrating keratoplasty cataract extraction and intraocular lens implantation was performed. Five months postoperatively, visual acuity was 6115 with a refraction of plano/-2.00 x 75 deg. The graft has remained clear and there has been no recurrence of the pterygium.

Summary: Surgery to visually rehabilitate a severe pterygium affecting the entire cornea can be successful. The technique of annular conjunctival grafting is a useful surgical procedure for cases in which conjunctival grafts are required for large, subtotal limbal conjunctival defects.

SURVIVAL OF CORNEAL GRAFTS IN INDIA

Gullapalli N. Rao, Lalit Dandona, Krishman Ragu, M. Janarthanan, and Thomas J. Naduvilath

L.V. Prasad Eye Institute; Hyderabad, India

The purpose of this study was to evaluate the survival of corneal grafts after penetrating keratoplasty (PK) at a premier eye care institution in India. All 13964 PKs done during 1987–95 at the L.V. Prasad Eye Institution, Hyderabad, India, a tertiary referral institution, were reviewed. Kaplan-Meier survival analysis was used to evaluate graft survival for the various categories of indications for PK. Multiple logistic regression was used to study the effect of age, sex and socioeconomic status on graft survival.

Survival analysis was done for the 1,725 optical PKs performed. The 239 therapeutic PKs for active infectious keratitis were not included in this analysis. The overall survival of all 1,387 first optical PKs at 1, 2 & 5 yrs was 79.6%, 68.7% & 46.5%, respectively. The highest 5 year graft survival of 95.1% was for keratoconus. Corneal dystrophies had survival rates of 87%, 75.5% & 56% at 1, 2 & 5 yrs These survival rates were 80.1%, 72.3% & 52.2% for corneal scars excluding adherent leukomas, and 75%, 58.5% & 31.5% for adherent leukomas. The 1, 2 & 4 yrs survival for pseudophakic and aphakic bullous keratopathy were 80.1%, 67.5% & 52.9%, and 74.4%, 60.9% & 39.5%, respectively. The lowest survival was for regrafts, 53.1% at 1 yr and 23% at 4 yrs Patients with lower socioeconomic status had significantly lower graft survival for all categories of indications for PK than those with Irigher socioeconomic status (P < 0.0001). The major reasons for graft failure were allograft rejection in 29.2%, high IOP in 16.9%, graft infection in 15.4%, and surface problems in 12.7%.

Keratoconus, having excellent graft survival, made up only 6.8% of the optical PKs. The indications for PK having poor graft survival made up almost half of the total cases of optical PKs in our series: regrafts 19.5%, aphakic bullous keratopathy 13.4%, adherent leukomas 8.5%, and the miscellaneous category including congenital conditions 6.7%. Comparison of graft survival rates between India and the developed world is influenced by the higher proportion in India of those indications known to have poor survival prognosis and by the significantly lower graft survival in patients with lower socioeconomic status.

CORALLINE HYDROOXYAPATITE KERATOPROSTHESIS

Carlos R. Leon, Jose I. Barraquer, Jr., and Jlse I. Barraquer

Instituto Barraquer de America

Purpose: The ideal prosthesis will let the tissue grow into the supporting material and have a similar curvature as the recipient cornea. Hydroxyapatite (HA) is highly biocompatible, causes minimal tissue inflammation, is not resorbed, and allows rapid host tissue ingrowth. **Materials and Methods:** We developed a new support for keratoprosthesis (Kpro), made of porous hA with a similar curvature as normal cornea, diameter of 10 mm, 1 to 1.5 mm thick and a 3 mm central opening into which the optic cylinder was fitted and fixed with a cement that did not affect the vitality of HA. They were implanted unilaterally in eyes of 12 New Zealand rabbits intralamellarly and between a homologous episclerokeratoplasty. **Results:** We observed good vascularization (the pores are filled with fibrovascular tissue throughout and some osteoblasts line the HA material), no signs of infection or extrusion, no epithelial downgrowth, nor detection of any adverse tissue reaction. **Conclusion:** This type of biocompatible HAKPro with a biointegrable, nonbiodegradable, and colonizable haptic has been accepted by the rabbit cornea (for 11 months) and a clinical trial in selected patients could be justified.

WORLD TREND OF CONTACT LENS PRACTICE

Dorothy Leason,[1] Chris O. Imafidon,[2] Bernice K. Glover,[3] Joe E. Imafidon,[4] Khan Briggs,[5] and Emmanuel Mukoro[6]

[1]London, UK; [2]Cambridge, UK; [3]New Jersey; [4]Nigeria; [5]Nigeria; [6]Nigeria

Abstract: A questionnaire was distributed from Munich, Germany to all countries in Europe, Latin America, the Middle East, Far East and Africa on the database of the WCO. An analysis of the returned forms showed a new trend in world contact lens. Singapore emerged as the country with the highest percentage of lens wearer in the population. The United States of America and Luxembourg were the next in the chart of high lens usage. The most commonly fitted lens type was sofi lens but Columbia showed a huge preference for rigid lenses (60% of the lenses were RGP). Austria and India had no preference at all (50% RGP, and 50% soft).

Countries with the biggest optometric involvement with lens fitting were Sweden and Norway (98%). India and Belgium showed 50% optometric interest while France and Greece had the least optometric interest. Results of this survey on regulation of practice, and training of practitioners will also be presented. (Acknowledgment: VDC, WCO, and the International body of Contact Lens Practitioners.)

(Acknowledgements: Wolfgang Cangolati).

LONG TERM RESULTS OF THE FALCINELLI OSTEO-ODONTO KERATOPROSTHESIS (OOKP)

Christopher Liu[1] and Sergio Pagliarini[2]

[1]Sussex Eye Hospital, Brighton, England and Moorfields Eye Hospital, London, England
[2]"La Sapienza" University, Rome, Italy

There is a need for keratoprosthesis surgery for cases of corneal blindness not amenable to conventional corneal grafting. Excellent results of OOKP surgery have been reported by Falcinelli using his modified technique whereas early followers of the original Strampelli technique were met with poor results. The purpose of the present study was to validate Falcinelli's results by independent assessment.

Of 153 patients who had OOKP surgery recalled, 45 patients (56 eyes) participated in a structured interview arid examination in a 3 week period in July 1994. During the same period and at subsequent visits, the authors observed OOKP surgery to learn and to gain insight into the surgical procedure.

The mean follow up time was 5.11 years (range 0.2 - 16) with chemical burn (26 eyes) and ocular pemphigoid (13 eyes) making up the major indications. All eyes had either perception of light (PL) or band movement (HM) vision pre-operatively. 41 eyes (77.4%) saw 6/12 (20/40) or better post-operatively. There were three cases of non-improvement of visual acuity: PL to PL due to glaucoma (1 case); PL to NPL due to endophthalmitis (2 cases). The reasons for poor corrected visual acuity in other cases were either retinal or glaucomatous and not due to the formation of retroprosthetic membrane. Glare in bright light was a universal problem.

Retention results: 1 eye was enucleated (infection) and 3 eyes were awaiting repeat insertion of osteo-odonto block. Pre-existing city eye state was not a prognostic factor. The state of the buccal mucosal graft was invariably good but may require maintenance surgery.

Despite the excellent results reported above, the technique is not without problems in that the surgery is complex, multi-staged and is traumatic; it involves the loss of a tooth All patients experienced glare and a limited visual field (40° with the new 4 mm optic). The diagnosis and management of glaucoma and retinal detachment is difficult in the presence of an OOKP, although it is possible to do so. Despite the above problems, all the patients examined bar two were satisfied with the results and would go through the same procedure again if they were asked again.

We conclude that modem OOKP surgery, when performed adequately, is a valid technique for select cases of corneal blindness not amenable to conventional corneal graft surgery. Indeed, for many desperate cases, the Falcinelli OOKP provides the only hope for long term restoration of vision. The first author of this report is pleased to offer an OOKP.

MAST CELL STABILIZERS VS STEROIDS IN THE TREATMENT OF PERENNIAL VERNAL KERATOCONJUNCTIVITIS (VKS) – A WEST AFRICAN EXPERIENCE

K. Glover,[1] K. Kponyo,[2] Chris O. Imafidon,[3] Joe B. Imafidon,[4] Khan Briggs,[4] and Emmanuel Mukoro[4]

[1]New Jersey; [2]Legon, Ghana; [3]Cambridge, UK; [4]Ile-Ile, Nigeria

ABSTRACT: In tropical West African sub-region, vernal keratoconjunctivitis (VKC) is a perennial cause of ocular allergy. Treatment modalities include steroids and mast cell stabilizers. This study involves the use of both modalities in the treatments of VKC in Ghana and Nigeria, West Africa. Seventy-five per cent of the patients using (Lodaxamide) reported improvement in symptoms within 48 hours compared to 50% of the patients on steroids. Five per cent of the patients using steroids developed corneal ulcers compared with 0% of the patients oil Alomide. This study underscores the fact that in tropical countries where VKC is perennial and not seasonal, physicians should endeavour to use mast cell stabilizers because they are efficacious and with fewer side effects.

INDICATIONS FOR CORNEAL TRANSPLANTATION IN INDIA

Gullapalli N. Rao, Lalit Dandona, Krishnan Ragu, M. Janarthanan, Raviridranath Shenoy, and Thomas J. Naduvilath

L.V. Prasad Eye Institute, Hyderabad, India

The purpose of this study was to evaluate the indications for penetrating keratoplasty (PK) at a premier tertiary eye care institution in India. The records for all PKS done at the L.V. Prasad Eye Institution, Hyderabad, India, a tertiary referral institution, during 1987–95 were reviewed retrospectively. The indications for PK were studied. The effect of age, sex and socioeconomic status on the indications was evaluated by multiple logistic regression. A total of 1,964 PKs were done on 1,632 patients, 1,128 (69.1%) males and 504 (30.9%) females, in the age range of 7 days to 90 years and a median of 40 years. For the 1,964 PKs the indications were corneal scarring in 551 (28.1%) cases including adherent leukoma in 147 (7.5%), regrafts in 336 (17.1%), active infectious keratitis in 239 (12.2%), aphakic bullous keratopathy in 231 (11.8%), pseudophakic bullous keratopathy in 209 (10.6%), corneal dystrophies in 165 (8.4%) including Fuchs' dystrophy in 23 (1.2%), keratoconus in 118 (6%), and miscellaneous in 115 (5.9%). Out of the 1,218 PKs done on patients < 50 years of age, the most common indication was corneal scarring in 426 (35%) cases. Out of the 746 PKs done on patients ~ 50 years of age, the two most common indications were aphakic and pseudophakic bullous keratopathy in 188 (25.2%) and 171(22.9%) cases, respectively. The proportion of PKs done in patients with lower socioeconomic status was significantly higher for corneal scarring ($P < 0.0001$), active infectious keratitis ($P < 0.0001$) and regrafts ($P = 0.0009$) than in the higher socioeconomic status. Corneal scarring, including adherent leukoma, and active infectious keratitis are relatively more common indications whereas keratoconus, pseudophakic bullous keratopathy and Fuchs' dystrophy are less common indications for PK in India than reported from the developed world. Indications for PK which carry a better prognosis for graft survival are relatively less common in India than in the developed world.

ENDOPHTHALMITIS FOLLOWING PENETRATING KERATOPLASTY

Satish Gupta, Murali Krishnamachary, Nibaran Gangopadhyay, and Pranab Kumar Sen

L.V. Prasad Eye Institute, Hyderabad, India

PURPOSE: To evaluate the incidence and etiopathogenesis of endophthalmitis following penetrating keratoplasty (PK).

METHODS : Incidence of endophthalmitis was retrospectively studied in 1725 corneal transplants, performed for optical reasons, between 1987 & 1995. We analysed the clinical presentation, risk factors, mode of management and outcome.

RESULTS: Nineteen (1.08%) patients developed endophthalmitis. Clinical diagnosis of endophthalmitis was substantiated by ultrasonic evaluation in four patients and vitreous aspirate in 16 patients. Seven vitreous specimens demonstrated microorganisms, six of which were bacterial and one fungal. Average duration, following surgery, for onset of endophthalmitis was 22.5 days. Preoperative aphakia (n=10;) pseudophakia (n=2) and performance of intraoperative vitrectomy (n=7), were the most common risk factors. Moist chamber was used as a mode of transport for 12 donor eyes. 8 donor rims grew micro-organisms on culture, three of which had the same organism as was obtained from the vitreous. All patients were on topical steroids at presentation. Twelve patients underwent vitrectomy and ten required regrafts. Four grafts remained clear, 4 eyes went into phthisis, five had to be eviscerated and in the rest the grafts failed.

CONCLUSIONS: Post-PK endophthalmitis can result from host-related (aphakia), donor-related (contaminated donor rims), intra-operative (vitrectomy) and/or post-operative (steroids) factors. Despite aggressive management visual results continue to be poor.

CORNEAL TOPOGRAPHIC CHANGES FOLLOWING RETINAL AND VITREOUS SURGERY

H. Lichter, N. Loya, D. Weinberger, R. Axer-Siegel, L. Mutzmacher, and Y. Yassur

Department of Ophthalmology; Beilinson Medical Center, Petah; Tiqva, Israel

Purpose: To evaluate the corneal topographic changes following retinal and vitreous surgery. **Methods:** A total of 46 patients who underwent various vitreoretinal surgery was divided into 3 groups: (1) Encircling buckle - 25 patients; (2) Pneumatic retinopexy - 11 patients; (3) Vitrectomy - 10 patients. Corneal topography was performed before and after surgery by video-keratography. **Results:** Encircling buckle may cause an increase of "with the rule astigmatism." Local buckle elements affect the quadrant involved. There was no significant corneal topographic changes following pneumatic retinopexy. Vitrectomy increases the steepness of the cornea toward the scleral sutures.

Conclusions: Of the various retinal and vitreous surgery procedures, the buckle induces the majority of corneal changes. Pneumatic retinopexy does not induce any significant topographic changes. Videokeratography is a valuable tool for evaluating these changes.

Session XI

Microbial Keratitis–Non-Viral

47

MEDICAL AND SURGICAL TREATMENT OF FUNGAL KERATITIS

M. Srinivasan

Aravind Eye Hospital
Madurai, India

ABSTRACT

Fungal ulcer represents a significant ophthalmologic entity in developing countries like India, where some centers find that more than 50% of the total suppurative keratitis that presents is due to this cause. Unfortunately, no antifungal antibiotics are available in countries where fungal ulcers are common. Thus, a large proportion of severe fungal ulcers perforate, resulting in unilateral corneal blindness. This paper examines the treatments available for fungal ulcer.

INTRODUCTION

Fungal ulcer is emerging as the most common cause of suppurative keratitis in developing countries, particularly in India. About 1,100 fungal corneal ulcers are being treated annually at Aravind Eye Hospital and Post Graduate Institute of Ophthalmology (Madurai, India), a tertiary care center. It constitutes more than 50% of total suppurative keratitis and it is possible that even this huge number is statistically underestimated since many patients with suppurative keratitis seek traditional therapy and do not consult an ophthalmologist. In addition, most ophthalmologists lack diagnostic laboratory facilities.

Other locations show similarly high incidences of fungal keratitis. In south Florida, for example, fungi account for 35% of the isolates in microbial keratitis. In Bangladesh the proportion is between 36% and 40%, while the proportion is 30% in south India and 17% in Nepal. In temperate climates it ranges between 2% and 2.5%.[1] In general, no appropriate antifungal antibiotics are available in countries where fungal ulcers are common. Seventy percent of the fungal ulcers in India are due to filamentous fungi and most common among them are *Fusarium* and *Aspergillus*.[2] *Candida* is very rare. Management of fungal keratitis would improve if broad spectrum antifungal agents with specific effectiveness against the common fungi mentioned earlier were readily available. However, in spite of adequate appropriate antifungal therapy, 50% of severe fungal ulcers perforate, re-

Advances in Corneal Research, edited by Lass
Plenum Press, New York, 1997

sulting in unilateral corneal blindness. The majority of these perforations are not grafted due to lack of donor material in Asian countries. Perhaps early diagnosis and highly potent dugs could reduce corneal blindness due to fungal keratitis.

MEDICAL TREATMENT OF FUNGAL KERATITIS

There are many agents available for treatment of fungal keratitis. These agents are listed in Table 1 and more detailed descriptions of their use and effectiveness follow.

Polyenes

Amphotericin B. Amphotericin is not available as an ophthalmic preparation. This agent is unstable, thermolabile toxic, and is considered to be the most effective against yeasts, with some action against filamentous fungi like *Aspergillus*. Systemic use may produce chills, rigors, nausea, vomiting, and phlebitis, and higher doses will cause renal damage. Amphotericin B is supplied in powder form in 50 mg vials with desoxycholate as a buffer and should be dissolved in distilled water or with 5% dextrose since saline causes it to precipitate. Once dissolved, this agent can be used for a week; it must be kept in an amber-colored bottle and protected from heat and light. Most often patients complain of burning sensation. This author has had the experience of pseudomonas contaminating the prepared amphotericin-B solution, resulting in perforation of two eyes. In these cases, pseudomonas was cultured from both the eye and the solution. Since it has no preservative, one should be careful and look for contamination if the fungal ulcer suddenly worsens.

Table 1. Classification of antifungal agents

Polyenes:
 Amphotericin-B
 Natamycin
 Nystatin
Azoles:
 Imidazole
  Miconazole
  Ketaconazole
  Clotrimazole
  Econazole
 Triazole
  Itraconazole
  Fluconazole
Pyrimidine:
 Flucytosine
Other agents:
 Silver sulfadiazine
 Povidone-iodine
 Chlorhexidine

Dosage: Topical: 0.15 to 0.5% instilled as frequently as possible, as in any other suppurative keratitis. *Subconjunctival:* 1–2 mg—toxic, produces conjunctival necrosis. *Systemic:* Intravenous route—begin with 0.1 mg to 0.25 mg per kilogram of body weight; can be increased gradually up to 1 mg/kg/day. This mode of treatment is usually recommended in systemic necrosis.

Natamycin. This is the only antifungal agent approved by the FDA. Found to be effective against *Fusarium* and *Aspergillus*, it is supplied as 5% suspension and does not produce any serious adverse reaction when applied topically. The suspension sometimes accumulates over the base of the ulcer as a yellowish-white exudate. Natamycin is supplied as a 15 ml vial in the USA and in a 3 ml vial in India. Since it is not cost effective, many patients in developing countries cannot afford Natamycin. Although it has been reported to cure 16 out of 18 eyes with *Fusarium keratitis* by Jones and colleagues,[3] Natamycin is not an effective agent against deep filamentous fungal ulcers.

Nystatin. Nystatin is not a broad spectrum antifungal agent. It is reported to be effective against *Candida* and *Aspergillus* and is marketed in India as an ophthalmic ointment as 100,000 units/gm. Nystatin does not penetrate well when used systemically and produces contact dermatitis when used topically. It is applied 5 times day until a response is achieved. Unfortunately it is poorly absorbed orally and is quite toxic when administered parenterally.

Azoles

Imidazole. Miconazole. In addition to its antifungal activity, Miconazole also exhibits mild activity against Gram positive bacteria. It is prepared as 1% or 2% solution in arachis oil or 0.7% methyl cellulose. The commercially available intravenous preparation (Monistat) can be administered topically as such. A dosage of 200–400 mg of miconazole given orally has been found to be effective against keratomycosis. Since the course of treatment is prolonged, this drug ends up being too costly. It is also hepatotoxic. Topical and subconjunctival miconazole have been effective in human keratitis caused by *Aspergillus*, *Fusarium*, *Candida*, and other genera in limited uncontrolled trials.[3] The primary mechanism of action of azole compounds is inhibition of fungal cytochrome P-450 enzymes, which are required in the demethylation of lanosterol in the synthesis of ergosterol, the major sterol of most of the fungal cell membranes.

Keratoconazole. This agent is available as 200 mg tablets, prepared as a topical solution as mentioned earlier for miconazole. Oral ketoconazole is given in a dose of 200–400 mg per day. This agent is reported to be effective against *Aspergillus, Fusarium,* and *curvularia* infections in humans.[4] Side effects include hepatitis, and rare, but lethal jaundice develops in 1 in 10,000 patients.

Clotrimazole. A 1% or 2% topical preparation of clotrimazole can be made with arachis oil, although nausea, vomiting, and hepatotoxicity have been reported. Clotrimazole is said to have greatest value in the treatment of *Aspergillus* infections *in vivo.*

Econazole. A 1% topical preparation of econazole in arachis oil can be applied topically for several days without any corneal toxicity, and the pharmacy at Moorfields Eye Hospital in London routinely makes econazole available to the patients attending the cornea service. This agent has a wide spectrum of activity against filamentous fungi *in vitro.*

Triazole. Flucanazole is hydrophilic and penetrates well into body fluids and tissues. Available since 1988, this agent represents a major advance in antifungal treatment.

Fluconazole is water soluble at neutral pH and is available as intravenous preparation and tablets. At a dosage of 100 to 200 mg orally per day, it is found effective against *Candida sp.* This agent has not been widely used against filamentous ocular fungi *in vivo*, but it does appear to be highly effective against candida.

Itraconazole is available as a 200 mg capsule to be taken with meals.

*Pyrimidine. **Flucytosine*** is not a broad spectrum antifungal, but is effective against *Candida*. It possesses synergism when combined with amphotericin-B. Given orally as 150 mg/kg/day, this agent is very expensive and can be applied as a 1% solution.

*Other Antifungal Agents. **Silver sulfadiazine*** was tried as an antifungal agent in Delhi, India and was reported to be highly effective against fusarium.[5] These authors claim 80% success rate using silver sulfadiazine in 20 cases of smear positive fungal ulcers and effective against 85% of *fusarium keratitis*. In the late 1980s, this treatment was projected as a wonder drug against fungal ulcers in India, but now it is not routinely tried. It is available as 1% suspension and as ointment.

Povidone iodine. *In vitro* study of this agent claims very good results at 5% concentration, but the results are disappointing *in vivo*. If other antifungals are not available, one can start with povidone iodine.

Chlorhexidine gluconate. A double-masked randomized study using chlorhexidine gluconate in different concentrations (0.05%, 0.1%, and 0.2%) in 60 culture-proved fungal ulcers was performed recently. Better results were obtained with the 0.2% solution when compared with the lower concentrations and with the natamycin group of agents. The corneal toxicity found with this agent was mild and reversible.

SURGICAL TREATMENT OF FUNGAL KERATITIS

If corneal infection progresses in spite of maximum antifungal therapy, consideration must be given to surgical intervention. There are several surgical methods available to arrest and eliminate corneal suppuration. Any one or a combination of these methods could be adopted according to the nature and extent of severity of corneal infection. Surgical methods available are (1) tissue adhesive; (2) conjunctival flap; (3) tectonic graft; (4) penetrating graft; and (5) evisceration.

Tissue Adhesive

Small corneal perforations (less than 1.5 mm) occurring early in the course of medical therapy can be managed with the tissue adhesive n-butyl-2-cyanoacrylate and bandage contact lens. Even though n-butyl cyanoacrylate glue is not approved by the FDA it is used with the patient's consent when indicated. Apart from helping as a mechanical support, it also has some antibacterial effect. Because many patients in India cannot afford to pay for bandage lenses and because there is often poor lens hygiene, it is often preferable not to fit a bandage contact lens after application of glue. Although the adhesive is an irritant, patients tolerate it well without the lens. In some patients severe vascularization is observed a few days after the application of the glue; this observation disappears once the adhesive is removed or falls out spontaneously.

Conjunctival Flap

This procedure, which may take any of three forms, is recommended before the ulcer perforates and can be performed under local or general anesthesia as indicated by the age and general condition of the patient. Pedicle flap or raquet flap is easy to perform and promotes healing in peripheral small ulcer. Total conjunctival flap is not done frequently as before due to improved medical therapy and availability of corneal tissue for grafting. Although conjunctival flap (Gunderson flap) hastens healing of the ulcer, it is technically difficult to perform the procedure due to severe inflammation and chemosis of the conjunctiva. The tissue bleeds profusely and is easily friable. If properly done under operating microscope better results can be obtained. The disadvantages of the procedure are that it obscures the view of the ulcer and precludes monitoring of its progress. Sometimes nonresponding ulcers perforate along with the flap and resurgery is not possible. Moreover, a conjunctival flap procedure does not remove the infected material and prevents penetration of antifungal agents. Mobilization of adequate flap may not be possible in eyes that had prior antiglaucoma surgery and cataract surgery.

Full Thickness Corneal Grafting

Indications for full thickness corneal grafting include impending perforation; perforation more than 2 mm; failed medical therapy; elimination of infection; or diagnostic. Unless there is marked perforation, this procedure can be performed under routine retrobulbar and facial block anesthesia. For perforation with lens extrusion, eyes with larger perforation, and in children general anesthesia is recommended. Local anesthesia makes the eye white, minimizing intraoperative bleeding. The grafting is planned according to the location of the ulcer. For peripheral ulcers, eccentric graft rather than a larger graft involving a segment of healthy cornea may be performed. A 0.5 mm oversized button is used and interrupted sutures are preferred. As far as possible, the lens should be left undisturbed to prevent spreading of infection to the posterior segment. To minimize the problem during trephination, it is convenient for the surgeon to use vacuum trephines in the host. During surgery, as in most perforations, the chamber is flat without aqueous, and technically it is very difficult to feel the penetration into the anterior chamber, which is usually noticed by aqueous leak in optical grafts. Hence, chances of injury to the lens and iris are high if new disposable, unguarded trephines are used. If there is severe hypotony one can make the recipient bed through freehand cut. Viscoelastics or glue on the table may make the globe tense, facilitating smooth recipient cut. Bleeding occurs when the inflammatory membranes and exudates are peeled off from the iris surface and it could be stopped by washing with BSS for a few minutes or by using viscoelastics. On rare occasions, parsplana vitreous aspiration may be required to make the eye soft for proper apposition of the graft host junction. Frequent breaking of the sutures indicates marked positive pressure within the globe, which is managed by vitreous aspiration. In large perforation where the lens is exposed preoperatively, it is better to remove it as extracapsular extraction through the trephined area. In most cases the etiology cannot be confirmed by culturing the recipient cornea because the ulcer becomes sterile once it perforates.

Tectonic and Lamellar Grafts

These grafts can be performed in eyes with small perforations like a fistula. A partial thickness (4 or 5 mm) donor cornea could be placed as a patch graft over the defect after debriding with a weckcel and anchored with interrupted or star shaped suturing using 10–0 nylon. This technique only helps as structural support and doesn't eliminate the sepsis or infected material. Tectonic graft is used in eyes with larger perforation in which glue is contraindicated and in places where trained corneal surgeons are not available.

Evisceration

This is an ancient ocular surgical procedure performed in an eye with gross sepsis. This author prefers evisceration to enucleation as it is technically easy to perform in a proptotic eye with severe conjunctival chemosis. Usually performed under local infiltration in all four quadrants with a fine, sharp, short needle. Prosthesis is not recommended at this stage. Rarely, it is performed as an emergency procedure for spontaneous explusive hemorrhage due to sudden perforation of the ulcer. In undiagnosed cases, the contents can be sent for microbiological investigations.

Postoperative Management of Fungal Keratitis

After surgery, the preoperative antifungal agents are continued and topical steroids can be started even from the first postoperative day in a minimal dosage (administered twice a day). Later the frequency is increased depending upon the condition of the graft. Antiglaucoma medications are begun if the intraocular pressure remains high. During 1995, this author performed full thickness therapeutic graft on 76 eyes of 76 patients with suppurative keratitis. Among them, 51% had fungal ulcer, 20% had bacterial, and the rest sterile. Of these patients, 62% were males and 60% of them were between 20 and 50 years of age. In 75% of these patients presentation to this service occurred one week after onset of ulcer. Of the grafts performed, 75% were for ulcers of more than 3 weeks duration. At two months follow-up 55% of the grafts remained clear. Of the 76 grafts performed only two eyes developed reinfection 3 weeks after surgery and both belong to fungal keratitis (*Fusarium*). Results showed that 39% of these eyes had visual acuity better than 3/60 to 6/60 and 13%, 6/36 to 6/6. The outcome would have been better if fresh good donor tissue had been used.

CONCLUSION

Fungal ulcer is emerging as one of the leading causes of uniocular corneal blindness in developing countries, especially in India. Non-availability of broad spectrum antifungal agents and delayed diagnosis are the two main reasons for this preventable corneal blindness.

REFERENCES

1. M Hegen, Wright E, Newman M, et al., Causes of suppurative keratitis in Ghana. *Br. J. Ophthalmol.* 79:1024 (1995).
2. M. S. Srinivasan and George C., The current status of fusarium species in mycotic keratitis in south India. *Indian J. Med. Microbiol.* 11(2):140 (1993).
3. D.B. Jones, Forster, R.K., and Rebell, G., Fusarium solani keratitis treated with natamycin. *Arch. Ophthalmol.* 88:147 (1972).
4. K.J. Johns, and O'day, D.M., Pharmacologic management of keratomycosis. *Surv. Ophthalmol.* 33:178, 1988.
5. M. Mohan, Gupta, S.K., and Kaira, V.K., Topical silver sulphadiazine: a new drug for ocular keratomycosis. *Br. J. Ophthalmol.* 72:192 (1988).

48

AXIAL MYOPIA IN KERATITIS PHLYCTAENULOSA CAUSED BY FORM DEPRIVATION MYOPIA

C. Meyer,[1] G. Duncker,[2] and H.-J. Meyer[3]

[1]Klinik für Augenheilkuride Medizinische
Universität zu Lübeck
Germany
[2]Klinik für Ophthalmologie
Christian-Albrechts-Universität
Kiel, Germany
[3]Augenklinik Marienhospital
Osnabrueck, Germany

ABSTRACT

Animal experiments carried out by Chew, Norton, Schaeffel or Wallmann[1-10] revealed that translucent occluders or concave lenses can induce axial eye elongation a so-called form deprivation myopia (FDM).

In order to find a clinical correlate, this retrospective multicenter study examined 156 cases of keratitis phlyctaenulosa peracta. The majority of cases were corneal transplant patients. The pre-operative refraction of this group showed -4.44 dpt on average whereas it is +0.5 dpt in the general population. In patients with an early onset of the corneal disease, i.e., prior to the age of five, myopia was higher than in cases where the onset was late. It was possible to establish biometrically the axial length in 62 patients which was on average 26.58 mm, thus being approximately 3 mm above Rohen's mean norm. These results confirm that form deprivation controls the linear growth of the eye, not only in animal experiments, but also in clinical cases.

INTRODUCTION

The distribution of refractions in various populations is well documented from major epidemiologic studies in the 1940's and 1950's.[11-14] There are more recent studies by Norton,[2-4] Seko,[16] Chew,[1] and Wallmann[8-10,15] into causes and etiology of axial myopia. Experimental studies by Schaeffel[6,7] are particularly interesting. They were able to induce axial eye elongation in chickens by using translucent occluders or concave lenses[5,18] and called it form deprivation myopia (FDM). Apart from individual reports, [19–22] there is not yet any clinical confirmation of these experiments, especially none involving major groups of patients. Due to the great number of cases with corneal transplants at the "Augenklinik Osnabrück," the "Augenklinik of Lübeck University," and the "Klinik für Ophthalmologie of Kiel University" many cases of keratitis phlyctaenulosa peracta with simultaneous high myopia became apparent. By the beginning of the century for the same keratitis many synonyms like keratitis scrophulosa, phlyctenulosa, lymphatica or superficialis were introduced. Keratitis phlyctaenulosa usually produces stromatous, extensive, prominent infiltration starting from the limbus and spreading towards the center. Infants and school children aged between 6 and 10 years with asthenic or pasty constitution are affected especially in spring and summer[23] when living under adverse hygienic conditions and being subject to a poor diet. More often a non lymphatic-exudative diathesis is present. Duke-Elder described the behavior of these children: "During the day the child hides away in a dark corner, blurring his face in his hands; and during the night he curls up under the blankets."[24] And Goldmann remembers: "In our pediatric ward we had two main diseases; the keratitis scrophulosa (phlyctenulosa) and the conatal keratitis parenchymatosa."[25] Girls are affected much more frequently than boys. In a study of 4,635 Eskimos with keratitis phlyctaenulosa Philip et al. found a characteristic distribution of corneal opacities and severity according to age. Opacity was infrequently seen in children under the age of 5. But 53% of school-age children and 45% of adults showed corneal scarring. The opacity was more frequently among females then males.[26] Over 80% of the children with keratitis phlyctaenulosa show a positive tuberculin reaction and an increased IgE-immunoglobulin level in the blood plasma. This can be interpreted as hyperergic reaction to microbial allergens.[27–29]

Phlyctaenulosa changes of the cornea occur more often in times of war and distress. An increased number of cases has been registered recently by us, mainly in patients from former eastern block countries or the Middle East. Many of these patients had undergone a corneal transplant - mainly in the 1980. Because of the early onset of the disease and the nebulous image caused by corneal scars at an early age, the conditions could be comparable to those found in animal experiments previously mentioned. The authors designed a retrospective multi center study involving 156 patients suffering from keratitis phlyctaenulosa peracta—mainly corneal transplant patients—to establish age of onset, refraction and ultrasound biometry.

METHODS

Total Test Group

Over the last three decades, several hundred patients suffering from keratitis phlyctaenulosa peracta had been referred to the three centers in question, 156 of those patients underwent follow-up checks and were entered into the study 135 of these patients had undergone a penetrating keratoplasty in one or both eyes. In 78 patients this was combined either with a cataract operation (n=45), or a triple procedure (n=34) had been carried out.

Exclusion criteria were: inaccurate diagnosis as keratitis of other origin (e.g., herpes), inaccurate anamnesis or suspected keratoconus. In each case the clinical diagnosis was confirmed by a histologic examination of the trepanations which was carried out at the ophthalmic clinics of the University of Erlangen, Kiel and Heidelberg. Of the 156 phlyctaenulosa patients 43 (27.6%) were male and 113 (72.4%) were female. The high proportion of two thirds of female patients corresponds to bibliographical references.[23,26]

Some patients suffered from such pronounced corneal clouding that no pre-operative refractions could be established. In 125 cases pre-operative refraction data were available. Cylindrical refraction was converted into spherical equivalents. The study always first analyzed the more affected eye for the refraction—more often this was the eye with the initial onset. In cases of keratoplasty of both eyes the eye that had been operated upon first was included in the study. In cases of postoperative aphakia the established refraction was reduced by 12 diopters.

As biometry was first established as a clinical routine about 10 years ago, researchers were only able to establish objective data concerning axial length from medical records of more recent years. However, since the beginning of this study they have carried out biometry in further patients suffering from keratitis phlyctaenulosa According to the patients the onset of keratitis phlyctaenulosa was between their first and 30th birthdays. The average age was 5.6 years. From literature two distinct phases in eye growth are recognized: a rapid infantile phase and a slow juvenile phase.[14,18,20,28,29] Because early onset of the disease is often early and there is danger of amblyopia being involved, special care with the anamnesis was taken prior to the corneal transplant. In particular, all patients were asked whether the corneal disease had started before they had completed their 4th year of age. More specific information about the age of onset was not available because many patients could not exactly recall their early childhood which. 29 patients did not remember exactly when they started to suffer from the corneal disease because it was either, when they were very young or the disease started intermittently, which is characteristic. However, data about the age of onset was more reliable, when it had started after the age of five. That is why patients were separated into two different groups: Group I onset up to the completed 4th year of age (n=93): Group II onset from the age of five years (n=63)(Fig. 1).

RESULTS

Refraction

First of all the refraction data were compared with the epidemiological normal distribution (dark checkered columns in the diagram) according to Stenstroem.[32] He examined the refraction of 10,000 patients and came up with data ranging from -15.25 dpt to +8.0 dpt and a statistical average of +0.5 dpt.

Refractions of patients in the current study ranged between -20.5 dpt and +8.75 dpt, the average being -4.44 dpt, meaning a standard deviation of 5.70 (gray dotted columns). 22% of patients suffered low myopia of down to -3.0 dpt. In one third of the cases medium myopia of between -3 .0 dpt and -9.0 dpt were found. A further 20% of cases showed extremely high myopia of down to -20.5 dpt And in another 20% of cases results revealed hypertropia. A comparison of both groups revealed a marked shift towards myopia of almost 5 dpt in phlyctaenulosa patients. The distinction between the two groups in the t-test was highly significant (p < 0.001). In addition, it was found that in patients suffering from phlyctaenulosa corneal scars the distribution of refractions is scattered over a much wider range (Fig. 2).

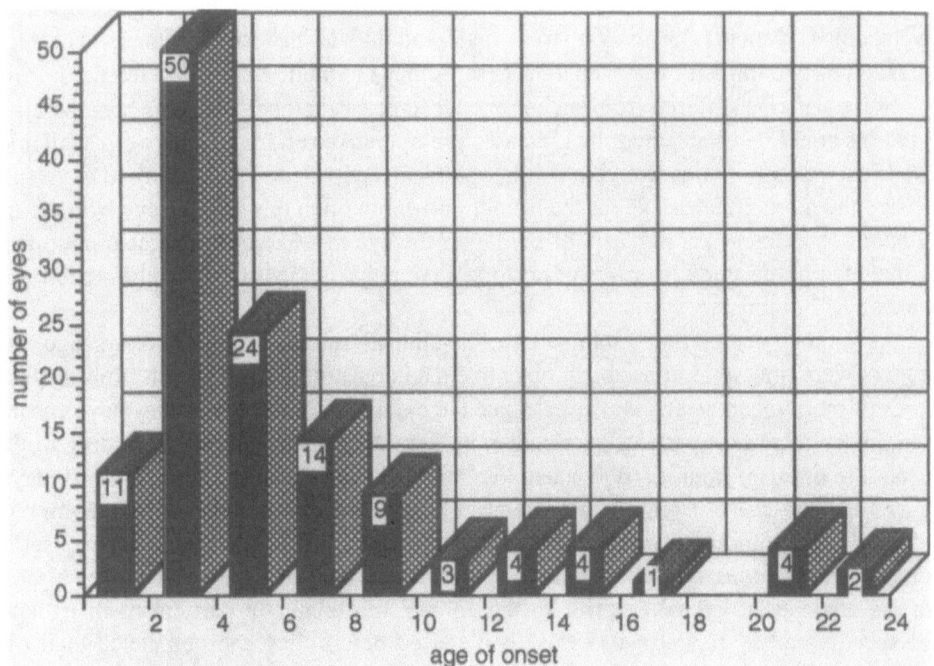

Figure 1. Onset of disease in 156 patients suffering from keratitis phlyctaenulosa.

Refraction and Age of Onset

Patients in this study were separated into the two groups mentioned above. The results for these groups are as follows

Group I. Onset up to the completed 4th year of age (n=93). In 70 patients of this group refractions could be worked out. They ranged between +8.75 dpt and -20.5 dpt. An average of -6.2l dpt was worked out, standard deviation: 5.67. Approximately 16% of patients suffered from lower myopia of down to -3.O dpt, more then 40% revealed data ranging between -3.0 dpt and -9.0 dpt. It was most striking that nearly a third of these patients showed very high myopia of over -9.0 dpt. It must be said that around 12% of patients were hyperopic (Fig. 3).

Group II. Onset from the age of five years (n=63). Refractions of 55 patients were known. They ranged between -19 dpt and +8.5 dpt. The average was -2.11 dpt, standard deviation 4.88, thus being considerably lower than of group I. Cases of low and medium myopia amounted to one third each. The number of patients suffering from very high myopia was around 7.0%, thus being considerably lower. Around 20% of patients suffered from hypertropia (Fig. 4).

Both groups are normally distributed and show a significant difference in the unpaired t-test (p< 0.01).

Axial Length

Biometry was carried in 62 patients. Axial lengths ranging between 21.35 mm and 30.43 mm were revealed (black columns with white dots). The average was 26.58 mm,

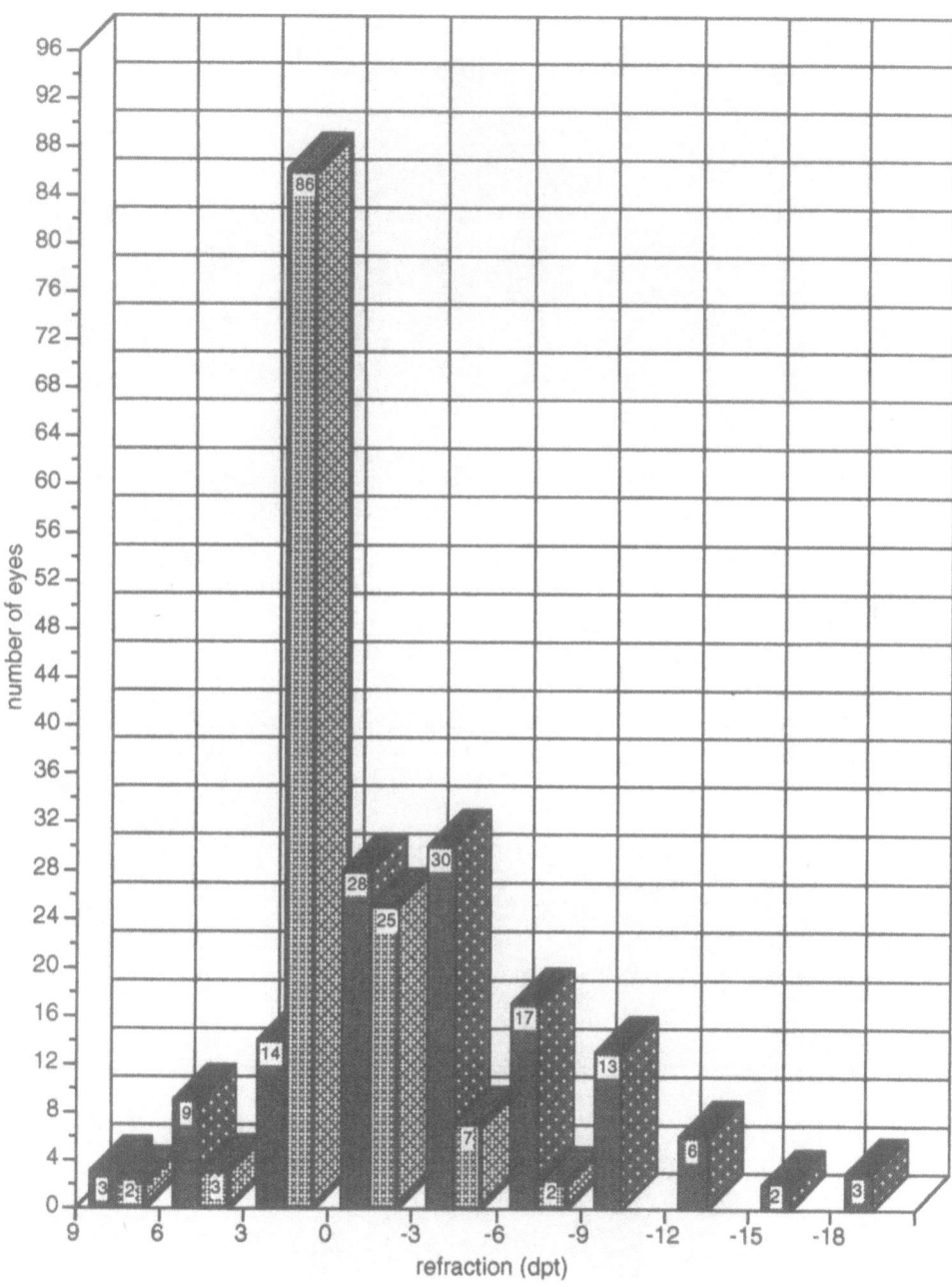

Figure 2. Refraction: comparison of all keratitis phlyctaenulosa patients (light gray, dotted columns) with normal distribution according to Stenström (dark checkered columns).

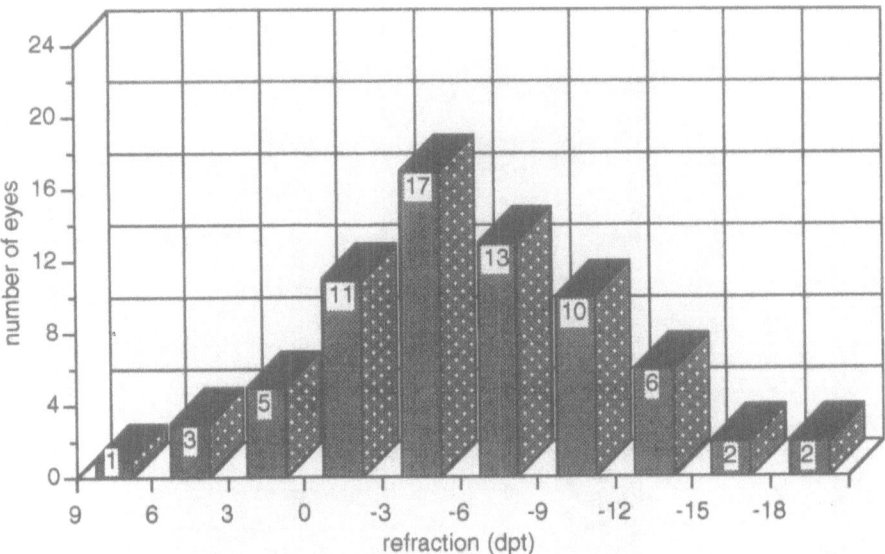

Figure 3. Refractions: 70 patients in group I; onset of disease prior to completion of 4th year of age.

and thus considerably higher than results from measurements in the general population. Hoffer[33] found the mean axial length measurement for 7,500 eyes to be 23.65 mm. Only 4.4% of his population had measurements more than 26.00 mm.

Latest biometric examinations carried out by Haiges[34] in 15,072 patients revealed an average axial length of even 23.48 mm, standard deviation 1.67; 11% of his cases were over 25 mm, another 11% under 22 mm.

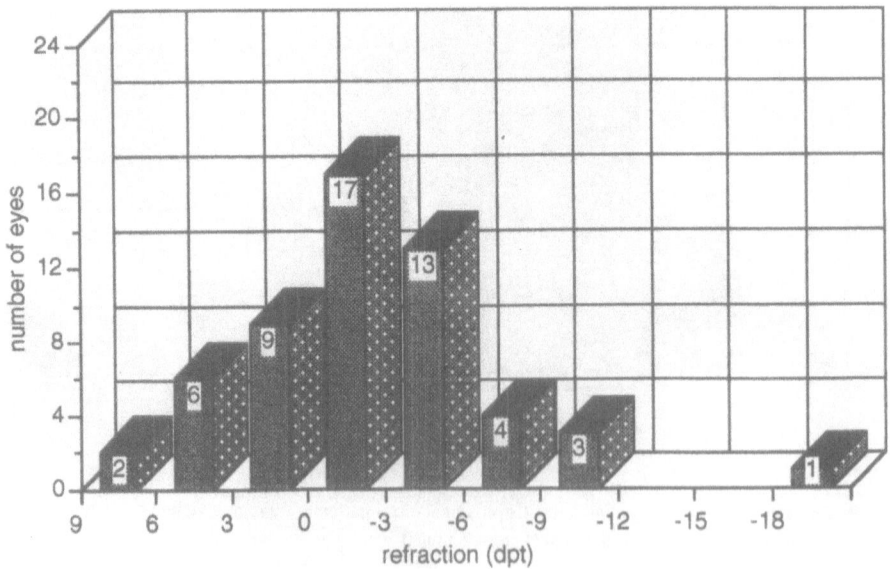

Figure 4. Refractions: 55 patients in group II; onset of disease after the age of 5 years.

In contrast Stenstroem[32] observed axial lengths ranging between 21.26 mm and 32.00 mm. His average is 24.00 mm, standard deviation 1.09. Rohen[35] also defines 24.00 mm as the normal axial length.

The study compared Stenstroem's figures with those of the current phlyctaenulosa patients. Both groups showed a significant difference of p < 0.001 in the t test (Fig. 5).

A more accurate breakdown on the age of onset into groups revealed the following.

Group I. In this group researchers carried out 38 biometries and came up with measurements ranging between 23.72 mm and 30.43 mm. The statistical average was 27.28 mm

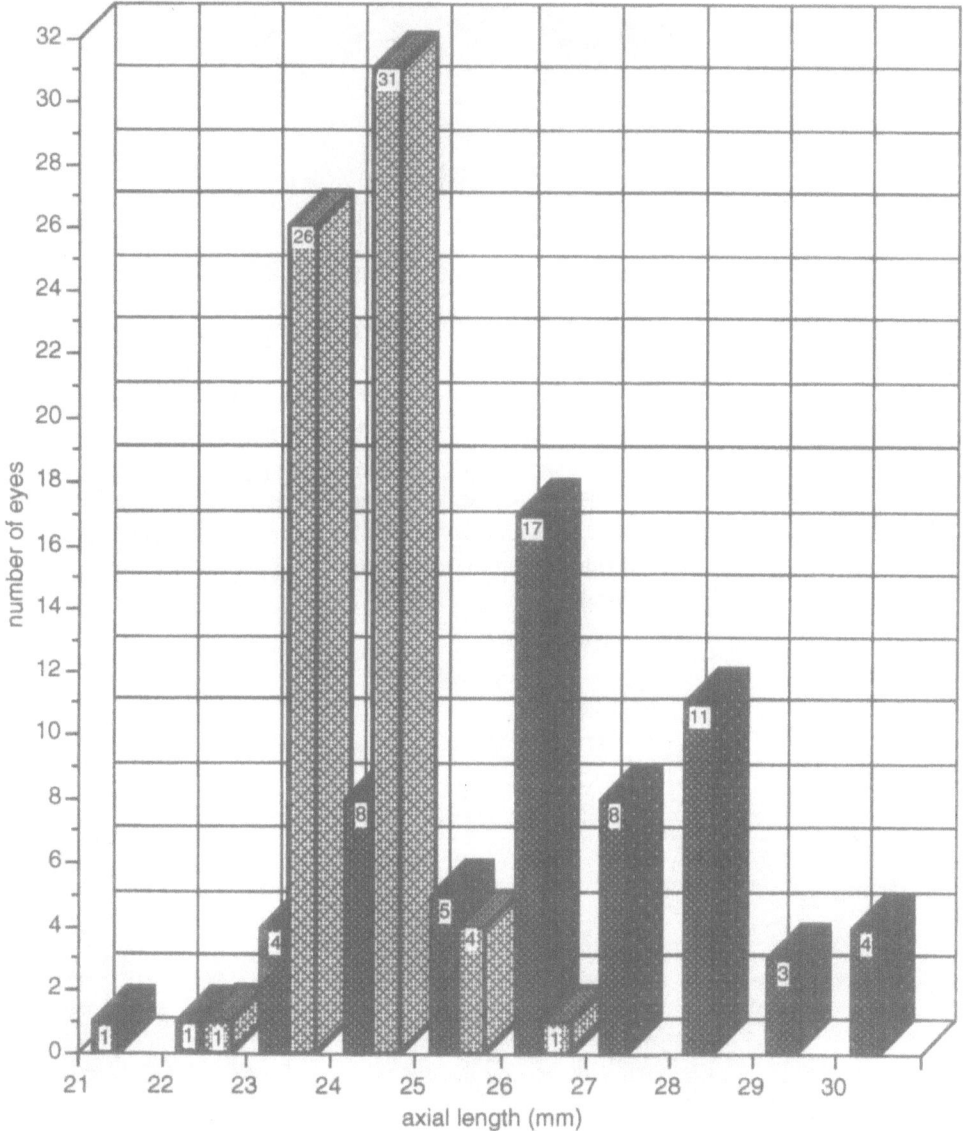

Figure 5. Axial lengths: comparison of all keratitis phlyctaenulosa patients (black columns with white dots) with normal distribution according to Stenström (lightly checkered columns).

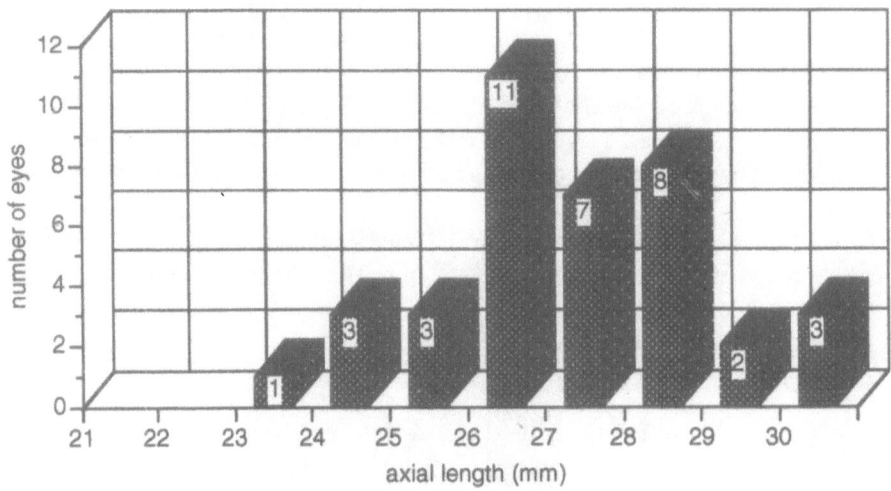

Figure 6. Axial length: 38 patients in group I.

and the standard deviation at 2.03. In almost 80% of the cases we found axial lengths over 26 mm (high myopia). One patient had axial length below the mean of 24.00 mm (Fig. 6).

Group II. There were 24 biometries in group II. The average was 25.5 mm, standard deviation

2.40. Age of onset varied considerably in this group, data ranged between 21.35 mm and 30.28 mm. In almost half of cases the axial lengths exceeded more than 26 mm. Results also revealed 5 patients with shorter bulbi, i.e., below 24 mm (Fig. 7).

There was no significant difference between the two groups.

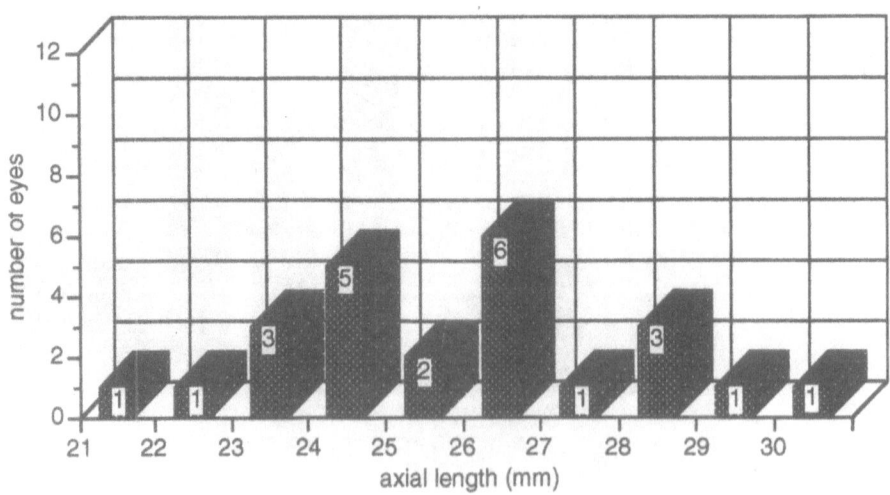

Figure 7. Axial length: 24 patients in group II.

DISCUSSION

In cases of keratitis phlyctaenulosa with onset in early childhood axial myopia were frequently noticed. Zrenner and Schaeffel, who induced axial eye elongation in chickens by using translucent occluders or concave lenses, explain it as form deprivation myopia (FDM) and discuss various mechanisms.[6,18]

One is based on the feedback mechanism theory, meaning that several instances follow the optical image and judge the image quality. This image analysis defines the actual value of the image definition. After comparison with the desired value, the control element is operated until the optimum image definition is found. Thus the photoreceptors are adjusted to the image level throughout the entire visual field locally in the eye. Troilo et al.[15] showed that occluders depriving only one half of the retina from vision had only a restricted elongation in the deprived area. On the other hand chicks with optic nerve section but without occluders have smaller eyes than normal. These results suggest that two different mechanisms may control eye growth. One within the eye and the other in the brain.

For both mechanisms the following evidence was found: Central electronic physiology experiments demonstrated that deprived animals have 15% smaller cells of the geniculate nuclei. Within the striate cortex binocular neurons are reduced to a third and abnormal distribution of cytochrome oxidase and other metabolic enzymes are found.[36–38]

Liang et al.[39] found in deprived eyes a thickening of the rod photoreceptors in the outer segment. Their distal tips apposed the basal lamina of the pigment epithelium or indented the cell nuclei and may contribute to axial elongation. Wallman's results[8] also argue for a local regulation of ocular growth that is depending on vision. To explain the epidemiological association of myopia in humans with large reading, he postulated: most nonfoveal retinal neurons have large receptive fields, they can not resolve the individual letters on the page, this may lead to being less activated and induce myopia. Seko et al.[16] found after two weeks occlusion a significant lower level of basic fibroblast growth factor (bFGF) and a significant higher level of transforming growth factor (TGF beta 2) in the treated eyes and concluded a regulative response for ocular enlargement for these and other proteins. Schaeffel et al.[7] reported that 6-hydroxy dopamine of retinal amacrine cells can suppress induced form deprivation and exaggerate axial growth up to a certain amount.

It is also discussed whether accommodation effort is of any significance for the optimum growth of the eye. It goes without saying that results from animal experiments with tree shew, chickens and monkeys can only to a limited extent be applied to humans.[40,41] One thing, however, seems to be certain: the growth of young human eyes is also being controlled by visual impressions.

The earlier the deprivation is initiated and the longer it is maintained, the greater the degree of the relative myopia in the deprived eye.[38]

Clinical studies on FDM are few and only involving small groups.[42] Research by O'Leary[21] is particularly interesting, as it depicts a longitudinal study. He followed the progress of 18 young patients suffering from ptosis and found, the younger the patients, the stronger was the progression of myopia. In one case myopia rose to -12.5 dpt within 4 years.

Thirteen patients with unilateral infantile traumatic cataract developed in all cases significantly greater axial length in the affected eye. The difference ranged from 0.1 to 11.5 mm.[19] Sinskey et al.[43] operated a child at the age of 7 with bilateral developmental cataract. Only one eye received an IOL. Within the next 11 years the other eye, which was corrected by contact lens, showed an increased axial elongation. Huber[44] implanted in infantile unilateral cataracts overcorrecting IOL's so that the eyes were slightly short-sighted afterwards. He found in all cases a further increasing myopisation of up to -6.0 dpt set in within six years. Biometries confirmed linear growth of these eyes. Similar findings on eyes with juvenile cataract are reported by Kora et al.[45] Another interesting ultrasound study from Moorfields on 10 patients with congenital hereditary endothelial dystrophy (CHED) showed by ultrasound examinations axial myopia in all patients. There was an inverse relationship between axial length and visual results following penetrating keratoplasty.[16]

All clinical reports concerning FDM refer to single or just very few cases. For the first time researchers could prove in a multicenter study involving large groups of patients that corneal clouding at a young age can quite regularly induce FDM. The current study's keratitis phlyctaenulosa patients showed an average myopia of -4.44 dpt. The wider range of refractions of between +8.75 dpt and -20.5 dpt in comparison to normal distribution can also be explained. A feedback mechanism which is disturbed by deprivation is unable to accurately recognize the image quality and cannot adjust the desired value for an optimum image definition. Another interesting feature is how myopia depends on the age of onset. Patients who suffered the corneal disease prior to the age of five years, showed considerably higher myopia and fewer cases of hypertropia than patients with a later onset. One can imagine that especially very young eyes react particularly strongly to disturbances in the feedback mechanism caused by deprivation. In order to counter the objection that cases of short-sightedness do not represent axial myopia, but could be caused by the lens' increased power of refraction or a steeper corneal radius, researchers referred to biometries in 62 patients. They confirmed that these patients suffered a genuine axial myopia and came up with basically the same results on average as the refraction determination. The average axial length in phlyctaenulosa patients was 26.58 mm, thus being almost 2.58 mm above the average norm of 24.00 MM from Stenstroem or Rohen[32,35] and more then 3 mm above the average axial length after Haiges[34] and Hoffer.[33] In conclusion patients with an early onset had longer eyes than those who suffered the disease later on in life. Altogether the findings of this study confirm that foim deprivation can also induce axial myopia in human eyes.

REFERENCES

1. S.J. Chew, and Beuerman, R.W., Visual form deprivation induces myopia in the infant rabbit, which is reduced by muscarinic antagonists applied directly to the sclera (abstract). *Proc. 5th. Int. Conf. Myopia, MIRF* (1995).
2. T.T. Norton, Experimental myopia in tree shrewes. In *Myopia and the Control of Eye Growth. (CIBA Symposium #155)* R.G. Bock and Widdows, K., ed., Wiley, Chichester (1990).
3. T.T. Norton, and Siegwart, J.T., Local myopia produced by partial visual-field deprivation in tree shrew. *Soc. Neurosci.* 17:558 (1991).
4. T.T. Norton, and Rada, J.A., Reduced extracellular matrix in maximmalian sclera with induced myopia. *Vision Res.* 35:1271 (1995).
5. F. Schaeffel, Experimentelle Ergebnisse zur Entstehung von Refraktionsfehlern. *Zbl. Prakt. Augenheilkd.* 13:221 (1992).
6. F. Schaeffel, Wilhelm, H., and Zrenner, E., Inter-individual variability in the dynamics of natural accommodation in humans: relation to age and refractive errors. *J. Physiol.* 461:301 (1993).
7. F. Schaeffel, Hagel, G., Bartmann, M., et al., 6-hydroxy dopamine does not affect lens-induced refractive errors but suppresses deprivation myopia. *Vision Res.* 34:143 (1994).
8. J. Wallman, Turkel, J., and Trachtmann, J., Extreme myopia produced by modest changes in early visual experience. *Science* 201:1249 (1978).
9. J. Wallman, Gottlieb M.D., Rajaram, V., and Fugate-Wentzek, L.A., Local retinal regions control local eye growth and myopia. *Science* 237:73 (1987).

10. J. Wallman, Nature and nurture of myopia. *Nature* 37:201 (1994).

11. A. Betsch, Über die menschliche Refraktionskurve. *Klin. Monatsbl. Augenheilkd.* 82:365 (1929).

12. B.J. Curtin, *The Myopias: Basic Science and Clinical Management.* Harper & Rowe, Philadelphia (1985).

13. H.G. Krumpaszky, und Klauß V., Epidemiologie der Refraktionsfehler. In, *Jhrbuch der Augenheilkunde 1995* A. Kampik, ed., Optik und Refraktion (1995).

14. K.J. Saunders, Early refractive development in humans. *Survey of Ophthalmology* 40:207 (1995).

15. S. Troilo, Gottlieb, M.D., and Wallman, J., Visual deprivation causes myopia in chicks with optic nerve section. *Curr. Eye Res.* 6:993 (1987).

16. Y. Seko, Shimokawa, H., and Tokoro, T., Expression of bTGF and TGF beta 2 in experimental myopia in chicks. *Invest. Ophthalmol. Vis. Sci.* 36:1183 (1995).

17. W. Wesemann and Schaeffel, F., Beeinflußt die Seherfahrung den Refraktionszustand? Ein Bericht über neue tierexperimentelle Untersuchungen zur Emmetropisierung des Auges in der Wachstumsphase. *Augen. Fortbildung.* 15:40 (1992).

18. E. Zrenner, and Schaeffel F., Myopie: Augenwachstum und Ursachen der Fehlsteuerung sowie experimen-telle Engriffsmglichkeiten (abstract). *Ophthalmolog.* 89(Suppl.):R35 (1992).

19. A. Calossi, Increase of ocular axial length in infantile traumatic cataract. *Optom. Vis. Sci.* 71:386 (1994).

20. D.A. Goss, Cox, V.D., Herrin-Lawson, G.A., et al. Refractive error, axial length and height as a function of age in young myopes. *Optom. Vis. Sci.* 67:332 (1990).

21. D.J. O'Leary, and Millodot, M., Eyelid closure causes myopia in humans. *Experientia* 35:1478 (1979).

22. I.C.J. Wood, and Hodi, S., Refractive findings of a longitudinal study of infants from birth to one year of age (abstract). *Invest. Ophthalmol. Vis. Sci.* 32:971 (1992).

23. A. Sorsby, The aetiology of phlyctenular ophthalmia. *Br. J. Ophthalmol.* 26:159 (1942).

24. FS. Duke-Elder, *System of Ophthalmology, Volume 8.* C.V. Mosby, St. Louis (1965).

25. H. Goldmann, Der Weg der Augenheilkunde in den letzten 50 Jahren. *Schweiz Med. Wochenschr.* 98:809 (1968).

26. R.N. Philip, Comstock, G.W., and Shelton, J.H., Phlyctenular keratokonjunctivitis among Eskimos in southern Alaska - epidemiologic characteristic. *Am. Rev. Resir. Dis.* 9:171 (1965).

27. M. Cremer, Klinik und Behandlung der Augentuberkulose. *Tub Artz.* 5:406 (1951).

28. R. Marquardt. Cronisch-enzuendliche Konjunktivitis. In, *Die Cronisch-Entzuendlichen Erkrankungen des Auges. Buecherei des Augenarztes, Vol., 101* Lund O-E Waubke, T.N., ed., Enke, Stuttgart (1984).

29. R. Sachsenweger, and Friedberg, D., Refraktionsanomalien. In, *Lehrbuch der Augenheilkunde, Vol. 13* H. Pau, ed., Fischer, Stuttgart (1992).

30. A.J. Adams, Axial length elongation, not corneal curvature, as a basis of adult onset myopia. *Am. J. Optom. Physiol. Opt.* 64:150 (1987).

31. A. Sorsby, Leary, G.A., and Richards, M.J., Correlation ametropia and component ametropia. *Vision Res.* 2:309 (1962).

32. S. Stenstroem, Untersuchungen über die Variation und Kovariation der optischen Element des menschlichen Auges, trans. D. Woolf, *Am. J. Optom.* 25:218 (1948).

33. K.J. Hoffer, Biometry of 7500 cataractous eyes. *Am. J. Ophthalmol.* 90:360 (1980).

34. W. Haigis. Biometrie bei komplizierten Ausgangssituationen. In, *9. Kogress der DGII*, R. Rochels, et al., eds., Springer, Berlin, Heidelberg (1995).

35. J.W. Rohen. Anatomie und Embryologie. In, *Augenheilkunde in Klinik und Praxis.* F.J. Hollwich, ed., Thieme, Stuttgart (1977).

36. M.L.Crawford, deFaber, J.T., Harwerth R.S., et al., The effect of reverse monocular deprivation in mon-keys. *Exp. Brain Res.* 74:338 (1989).

37. M.L. Crawford, Pesch, T.W., von Noorden, G.K., et al., Bilateral form deprivation in monkeys. Electro-physiologic and anatomic consequences. *Invest. Ophthalmol. Vis. Sci.* 32:2328 (1991).

38. E.L. Smith, Harwerth, R.S., Crawford, M.L., and von Noorden, G.K., Observation on the effects of form deprivation on the refractive status of the monkey. *Invest. Ophthalmol. Vis. Sci.* 28:1236 (1987).

39. H. Liang, Crewther, D.P., Crewther, S.G., and Barila, A.M., A role for photoreceptor outer segments in the induction of deprivation myopia. *Vision Res.* 35:1217 (1995).

40. K.M. Chung, Critical review: effects of optical defocus on refractive development and ocular growth and relation to the accommodation. *Optom. Vis. Sci.* 70:228 (1993).

41. K. Zadnik, and D.O. Mutti, How applicable are animal myopia models to human juvenile onset myopia? *Vision Res.* 35:1283 (1995).

42. C.S. Hoyt, Stone, R.D., Fromer, C., and Billson, F.A., Monocular axial myopia associated with neonatal eyelid closure in human infants. *Am. J. Ophthalmol.* 91:197 (1981).

43. R.M. Sinskey, Stoppel, J.O., and Amin, P.A., Ocular axial length changes in a pediatric patient with aphakia and pseudophakia. *J. Cataract Refract. Surg.* 19:787 (1993).

44. C. Huber., Myopische ÀÛnderungen der Refraktion bei Kindern mit einseitiger Linsenimplantation. *Augenspiegel* 24:48 (1994).
45. Y. Kora, Shimizu, K., Inatomi, M., et al., Eye growth after cataract extraction and intraocular lens implantation in children. *Ophthalmic Surg.* 24:467 (1993).

SECTION XI: MICROBIAL KERATITIS–NON-VIRAL

Abstracts of Other Conference Presentations and Posters

RAPID DIAGNOSIS OF OCULAR SURFACE INFLAMMATION

The traditional diagnosis of ocular surface inflammation relies upon analysis of scrapings and culture of ihe surface discharge or exfoliated cells. Both time consuming and of variable accuracy, such an approach is not likely to define rapid specific treatment nor prove cost-effective office management. This overview of office techniques capable of providing rapid and accurate diagnosis of ocular surface inflammation, especially of allergic or infectious etiologies, will identify those modalities that are practical and reliable for the clinician. Comparative cost analysis and regulatory aspects will be reviewed.

THE PATHOPHYSIOLOGY OF BACTERIAL KERATITIS

George A. Stern

Dept. of Ophthalmology, University of Florida College of Medicine, Gainesville, Florida

The pathogenesis of bacterial infections of the cornea shares a series of events in common with infections of other tissues, including 1) localization of micro-organisms to the site of infection, 2) adherence of organisms to the tissue, 3) invasion and induction of an inflammatory response, 4) tissue necrosis, and 5) repair.

A number of factors, especially contact lens wear and trauma, are known to predispose to corneal infection. These risk factors bring organisms to the site of infection and compromise the epithelial surface, setting the stage for adherence. Contact lenses are frequently contaminated by adherent bacteria which cause the infection. In addition, lenses, especially when worn on an extended wear (overnight) basis, cause superficial epithelial sloughing and subepithelial edema, which potentiate bacterial attachment.

Once the epithelium has been breached, bacteria adhere to injured cells by an adhesion-receptor interaction. In most cases, adhesions are components of bacterial cell wall appendages, and receptors are epithelial cell membrane glycoproteins which have been exposed by injury. Contact lenses potentiate adherence by shielding the cornea from the flow of tears and blinking. Once bacterial adhere, they begin to replicate, colonize the tissue, and invade the underlying stroma.

Once bacteria reach the stroma, they rapidly spread both radially and deeply. This spread is probably the result of two bacteria-derived matrix metalloproteinases (MMPs), elastase and alkaline protease, which act on corneal ground substances. An inflammatory response, characterized by the influx of PMNs, quickly ensues. PMNs are chemotactically attracted to the cornea by the secretion of exotoxin A, which causes keratocyte death, and activation of the alternate pathway of the complement system by bacterial endotoxins. PMNs principally reach the cornea by exudation from the limbal vessels into the tear film, followed by migration through the epithelial defect. Contact lenses delay PMNs reaching the stroma, prolonging the period of unchecked bacterial replication. Additional proteolytic enzymes, both MMPs and serine proteases, are produced by PMNs, and are responsible for true collagenolysis which leads to corneal destruction.

If the inflammatory process proceeds unchecked, the cornea will become destroyed and perforate. If the effects of inflammatory process, supplemented by antibiotics, succeed at arresting the spread and replication of bacteria, the cornea will undergo a phase of repair characterized by neovascularization, collagen resynthesis (scarring), and re-epithelialization.

A CENTRAL ROLE FOR HYPOXIA IN THE PATHOGENESIS OF CONTACT LENS-RELATED KERATITIS IN ANIMALS AND MAN

H.D. Cavanagh, H. Ren, W.M. Petroll, and J.V. Jester

Department of Opthalmology, University of Texas Southwestem Medical Center at Dallas, Dallas, Texas

Contact lens-related keratitis is the most serious clinical complication of lens use in 20–30 million wearers in the United States. While risk of extended wear (EW) is well documented, not all ulcers are explained by EW; if EW were eliminated. ulcers would still occur in significant numbers (CLAO J 22 30 (1996). We have proposed the testable hypothesis that lens use produces hypoxia to the epithelial surface inversely determined by lens O_2 transmissibility, and that this hypoxia results in graded changes in the corneal surface correlated with increasing bacterial binding. We recognize the possibility that for hydrogel lenses, a separate contribution may be made to this process by concurrent hypercapnia. Currently, we have established and validated a rabbit test animal model, and have begun a clinical trial in human subjects. Effects of rigid and hydrogel lens wear are quantitated non-invasively by confocal microscopy and by measurements of Pseudomonas aeruginosa (PA) binding to corneal epithelial cells shed from controls vs wearers, obtained by irrigation cytology. Pilot results reveal the novel finding that short-term effects of human lens wear produce striking retention of surface cells with decreased shedding, but increased bacterial binding in both EW and daily wear. Importantly, use of both ultra-high O_2 transmissible rigid and hydrogel test lenses do not appear to produce increasing PA biding; thus, it may be possible in future to increase significantly patient safety by preventing lens-related keratitis. (Supported by NEI EY10738, Bausch & Lomb, Inc., The

Pearle Vision Foundation, and Senior Scientist Awards (HDC, JW) and an unrestricted grant from Research to Prevent Blindness, Inc., New York, New York.)

MEDICAL AND SURGICAL THERAPY OF BACTERIAL KERATITIS

Joseph Frucht-Pery

Department of Ophthalmology, Hadassah University Hospital, Jerusalem, Israel

Staphylococcal and pseudomonas species are the most commonly isolated bacterial organisms from corneal ulcers.

Staphylococcal corneal ulcers causing less severe infections while pseudomonas corneal ulcers may perforate the cornea in a short period of time.

The diagnosis of the specific bacteria requires microbiologic evaluation. Once the cultures are taken, empiric broad spectrum antibiotics are initiated. Fortified aminoglicosides; gentamicin or tobramycin 1 .4%-2%, and cefazolin or vancomycin 5% are applied to cover gram negative and gram positive bacterial infections. Topical quinilone: ciprofloxacine 0.3% ophthalmic solution is as well an effective treatment, but increasing resistance of gram positive bacteria strains suggest extra caution and requires additional antibiotic to cover the gram negative strains. When bacteria is identified, treatment can be changed according to the specific sensitivity of this bacteria. When clinical improvement occurs, treatment change is riot required. However if clinical deterioration occurs, treatment should be stopped, the cause of infection should be reinvestigated, and treatment should be modified.

In case of major corneal tissue loss and perforation of the cornea, tissue glue [cyanoacrylate] may seal the perforation. When perforation is large, keratoplasty is required for tectonic or therapeutic reasons. The outcome of surgery in acute stage of infection is less favorable and postoperative complications such as glaucoma and graft rejections may compromise the final outcome of visual acuity.

PATHOPHYSIOLOGY OF FUNGAL KERATITIS

E.C. Alfonso

Bascom Palmer Eye Institute, University of Miami, Miami, Florida

Fungal keratitis is difficult to diagnose clinically, laboratory confirmation is important, and pharmacotherapy is not always effective. The organisms most commonly associated with corneal invasion are *Fusarium*, *Candida*, *Aspergillus*, and *Cephalosporium*. They can be found in soil, air, and organic waste. *Candida* has been isolated from the conjunctiva of normal adults and from in-use topical medications. The source of *Fusarium*, *Aspergillus* and *Cephalosporium* is usually organic material. The organisms do not penetrate an intact epithelium. For *Candida*, the organisms have been shown to attach to diseased epithelium and injured stroma. Invasion is secondary to trauma for filamentous fungi and due to a combination of trauma and impaired host defenses for yeasts. Trauma usually occurs in an agricultural setting, gardening or the outdoors. Host defenses may be impaired due to a defective host surface, or the use of topical corticosteroids Fifteen percent of patients developing fungal keratitis also have diabetes mellitus. Once in the stroma, an inflammatory response develops. Clinically, the eye develops conjunctival hyperemia and an inflammatory reaction in the stroma and anterior chamber. In *Candida* keratitis, the infiltrate is round with smooth edges, may be deep, and contains organisms and inflammatory cells. The corneal stromal appearance of feathery edges and satellite lesions in *Fusarium* keratitis is related to invasion of the organism and an inflammatory cell reaction. The infiltrate in the stroma may be covered by intact epithelium. The organisms may invade deep in the stroma, and with filamentous fungi penetration through an intact Descemet's membrane has been documented. The organisms produce toxins and enzymes. Soluble antigens also enhance the inflammatory response of the host. Once the organisms gain access into the anterior chamber, they are difficult to eradicate.

POST KERATOPLASTY *CANDIDA ALBICANS* KERATITIS

William Reinhart

Case Western Reserve University, Cleveland, Ohio

Three patients from the author's corneal transplant practice, one each in 1982, 1989 and 1995, were first diagnosed with deep corneal stromal infiltrates 59–77 days post keratoplasty. Specimen cultures from each patient grew out Candida. All visible deep stromal infiltrates were closely associated with nylon sutures, although two of the three infiltrates appeared to originate at the deep corneal transplant wound interface with projection of the inflammatory mass into the anterior chamber. The single patient with a deep stromal suture related abscess was cured with topical antifungal medication, whereas the two patients with anterior chamber involvement required intra-ocular surgery and either systemic and/or intra-ocular as well as topical antifungal medication for resolution. None of the three preservation media used: MK plus organ culture, Optisol with gentamycin, and Optisol with gentamycin and streptomycin, contained an antifungal.

THE PATHOPHYSIOLOGY OF PARASITIC KERATITIS

Colin M. Kirkness

Tennent Institute of Ophthalmology University of Glasgow, Scotland

Parasitic infections of the cornea involve mainly protozoans of which *Acanthamoebae* are the commonest organisms encountered, although more recently *Microsporidia*, *Vahlkampfia* and *Hartmanella* have also been described. First reported over 20 years ago, amoebic keratitis proved to be a devastating corneal infection with a prolonged morbidity and frequently resulted in loss of vision or even the eye.

Recent years have seen increased numbers of cases being identified. "Soft" contact lenses are tile most commonly reported vector for transference of tile organisms from contaminated water to the ocular surface. The organisms are ubiquitous and tile cysts may be resistant to the disinfection systems of most urban water supplies. Poor contact lens hygiene and ineffective disinfection routines allows growth of the *Acanthamoebae* in the biofilm of the storage case.

Once on the ocular surface, the organisms appear capable of invading intact epithelium producing first a diffuse epitheliopathy followed by ulceration in a dendritifiorm pattern. Bowman's membrane is penetrated leading to rapid invasion of the stroma, first centrally then spreading deeper and more peripherally. The corneal nerves may aid the penetration of Bowman's membrane and keratoneuritis is pathognomonic of this disease. Keratocyte death occurs, possibly as a result of the digestion of the nuclei by the amoebae. Polymorphonuclear leucocytes are only then recruited and a ring abscess appears. Failure to treat by this stage may lead to severe corneal disruption, scleritis, perforation and even retinal infarction.

Early diagnosis and treatment with the newer antiarnoebic drugs can now prevent serious corneal damage and permit restoration of normal vision.

THE INFLUENCE OF RISK FACTORS ON THE MANAGEMENT AND OUTCOME OF TREATMENT FOR SUSPECTED BACTERIAL KERATITIS

N. Morlet,[1] C. Pavesio,[1] D. Minassian,[1] A. Tullo,[2] J. Dart,[1] and the Ofloxacin Study Group

Moorfields Eye Hospital, London, Manchester Royal Eye Hospital, UK

It is well recognised that a number of conditions predispose people to bacterial keratitis; however, little is known about how these factors may influence the outcome of this condition.

We prospectively evaluated patients presenting with suspected bacterial keratitis over a period of 12 months and recorded their clinical outcomes. We looked for known risk factors at presentation as well as documenting the clinical features. All patients were treated with either topical ofloxacin 0.3% alone or cefuroxime 5% and gentamicin 1.2%. At each visit the clinical features were recorded along with evidence of therapeutic response or treatment toxicity.

Of the 106 patients observed, 18 required a change in management - 9 were considered treatment failures, 5 possible treatment failures (2 had possible HSV keratitis) and 3 had frank drug toxicity (in addition to 4 others in the previous 2 groups). Another 15 had failed to reepithelialise 2 weeks after commencement of treatment.

Compared with the other 73 patients treated, this group were older (69.7% vs 11.3% >60 yrs) presented later (54.5% vs 19.8% >4 days) and had larger ulcers (72.7% vs 6.6% >5 mm^2) They were more likely to have previous corneal disease (60.6% vs 14.2%) and few had no previous ophthalmic problem (77.9% vs 58.5%). Fewer had associated contact lens use (18.2% vs 33%). Many were on current topical treatment (72.7% vs 51%) in particular topical steroids (42.4% vs 2.8%).

Not only do recognised factors put the patient at risk for bacterial keratitis, they are related to management difficulties and prolonged morbidity.

MANAGEMENT OF CULTURE NEGATIVE CORNEAL ULCERS

Murali Krishnamachary, Tinwin, M.S, Satish Gupta

L.V. Prasad Eye Institute, Hyderabad, India

Purpose: To study the clinical and management course of culture negative corneal ulcers (CNCU).

Methods: In a retrospective study of 1141 corneal ulcers seen between 1991 and 1994, 105 (9.20%) were diagnosed as CNCU's. Diagnosis of CNCU was made when organisms could not be isolated on culture from clinically diagnosed patients of infectious keratitis. Predisposing factors, clinical presentation, management and outcome were analysed.

Results: Mean age was 29.3 years (M:F, 2.3:1) with a average follow-up of 67.8 days. CNCU's were classified as small (<2.0 mm; n=42), medium (2–5 mm; n=39), and large (>5.0 mm; n=24). Majority (n=80) of the patients received broad-spectrum antibiotics. Eighty four ulcers healed, 12 were lost to follow-up, three underwent penetrating keratoplasty, and the rest were showing improvement when last seen. The healing rate was 57.9, 19 and 17.9 per 100 person months and mean time to heal was 1.7 ± 2, 5.2 ± 6.7, and 5.4 ± 5:9 months for small, medium and large CNCU's respectively (p=0.01 04, ANOVA).

Conclusion: Successful management of CNCU's depends on clinical judgement, size of ulcer, past clinico-microbiological experience and meticulous follow-up.

ANTIBIOTIC RESISTANCE—NEW HOPE FOR OPTIMISM

Jules Baum

Boston Eye Associates; Chestnut Hill, Massachusetts

With the recent emergence of vancomycin-resistant enterococci (VRE) and the potential transmission of such resistance to staphylococci, especially methicillin-resistant *S. aureus* (MRSA), pressure for the development of new antibiotics and mechanisms to deal with the threat has resulted in the engineering of new molecules and reason for cautious optimism.

Several synthesized agents of a new class of compounds with a new chemical structure, the oxazolidinones, have been found to be highly effective against VRE and MRSA in experimental studies because they lack recognition by the pathogen and because they inhibit protein synthesis at a stage earlier than other antibiotics that act similarly. Preliminary studies in humans disclose no adverse effects.

Two other newly engineered antibiotics, one a variant of vancomycin, the other derived originally from the fungus, streptogramins, also appear to be very effective against both VRE and MRSA. The latter also kills penicillin-resistant pneumococcus.

Some pathogens are resistant to certain antibiotics because of their ability to pump out the antibiotic by turning on cell membrane proteins known as "efflux pumps", thus maintaining a subcidal or substatic intrabacterial drug level. Newly synthesized congeners of tetracycline, known as tetracycline resistance blocking agents, effectively block several different efflux pumps and, when given in combination with a tetracycline, kill resistant species of staphylococci and enterococci as well as resistant strains of E. coli.

Whereas pessimism has prevailed regarding our future ability to eradicate bacterial pathogens associated with vision-destroying infections, there is new cause to believe that several new agents, some undergoing preliminary experimental investigation, one currently in stage 3 clinical trials, may be available for our use within the next decade.

A POPULATION-BASED STUDY OF MICROBIAL KERATITIS IN CHILDREN: 1983–1989

C.W. Flowers, Jr., R.S. Baker, and R. Casey

Charles R. Drew University of Medicine, Los Angeles, California, Jules Stein Eye Institute, UCLA School of Medicine, Los Angeles, California

Background: Microbial keratitis in children poses a significant diagnostic and therapeutic challenge. Given the devastating visual consequences this condition can have among the pediatric population, and the limitations of existing data, we set out to perform a population-based study of microbial keratitis in children to characterize the distribution of disease, determine the age, race, and sex specific incidence rates, identify key etiologic determinants, and estimate the cost of care.

Methods: Using the California Discharge Database, a statewide population-based survey of microbial keratitis in children was performed. Hospital discharge data was derived from all inpatient admissions to nonfederal, acute care hospital facilities within the state of California for the years 1983 through 1989. Study eligibility was limited to inpatient admissions in which the age at admission was less than 15 years of age and ulcerative keratitis was the principal diagnosis or within the first 10 reported diagnoses. Population denominators were obtained from the 1990 census data for the state of California.

Results: During the period of observation, 312 pediatric patients were admitted with a diagnosis of corneal ulcer, with 207 (66%) being admitted with this condition as the principal diagnosis. Five years of age was the median age of admission, and patients less than one year of age had the highest frequency of admission for corneal ulcer. The mean overall annual incidence rate for pediatric corneal ulcer was 0.71 per 100,000 per year (95% CI, 0.57 to 0.85). The incidence was highest among individuals in the 0–4 year age group, and patients belonging to the African-American and Hispanic racial groups (0.81(95% CI, 0.56 to 1.06), 0.98 (95% CI, 0.54 to I .42), and 0.90 (95% CI, 0.72 to 1.08) per 100,000 per year respectively). Gender specific rates showed no sexual predilection, although male patients had a slightly higher mean overall annual incidence rate. The predominant risk factors for the development of microbial keratitis in children were congenital anomalies (ocular and non-ocular), trauma (ocular and non-ocular), iatrogenic complications, perinatal conditions, and CNS disorders. Over one-quarter of the patients underwent an ocular procedure, with corneal reparative procedures and penetrating keratoplasty being the most common. The estimated mean cost per patient, based on hospital charges alone, was $4,840.11 for patients with a principal diagnosis of corneal ulcer and $44,790.88 for patients with corneal ulcer as a secondary diagnosis.

Conclusions: Children in the 04 year age group, children of black and hispanic race, children with congenital anomalies, perinatal conditions, CNS disorders, and children who are victims of trauma appear to be at highest risk for the development of microbial keratitis. Therefore, preventative strategies and early intervention programs must be targeted toward these high risk groups.

PATHOGENESIS OF ACANTHAMOEBA KERATITIS: ROLE OF DOMESTIC WATER CONTAMINATION

Trevor Gray*, Simon Kilvington, Nigel Morlet, and John Dart

Moorfields Eye Hospital; CityRoad London

Aim: DNA typing techniques are used to establish the link between culture-proven cases of Acanthamoeba keratitis and amoebic contamination of domestic water sources.

Methods: Nineteen consecutive, traceable patients with culture-proven Acanthamoeba keratitis diagnosed between August 1994 and March 1995 were included. Each patient was supplied with a domestic water sample kit and questionnaire. Domestic water samples were collected from all bathroom, bedroom and kitchen taps and cultured for free living amoebae (FLA) only. Water sample collection occurred from June to October 1995. Mitochondrial DNA RFIP typing was performed on all Acanthamoeba isolates to determine the genetic similarity between corneal and domestic isolates.

Results: *Acanthamoeba spp.* contamination of domestic water sources was found in 4/19 sample sets. Two of these patients were found to have identical Acanthamoeba species growing from their corneas and domestic water samples. FLA were isolated from 16/19 respondents' domestic samples. FLA growth varied significantly with the tap temperature and location: 32 isolates from 36 cold taps compared with 5 isolates from 36 hot taps and 17 isolates from 19 mixer taps. All *Acanthamoeba spp.* were grown from bathroom(3)/ bedroom(1) cold taps. In this patient community, only the kitchen cold tap is supplied with fresh mains water, all other taps are fed from ceiling holding tanks. The number of isolates and amount of FLA grown from these two sources differed significantly: 10 isolates from kitchen cold taps (including 7 mixers) vs 23 isolates from bathroom cold taps (including 2 mixers).

Conclusions: The role of domestic storage tank fed water as a probable source of pathogenic *Acanthamoeba spp.* is confirmed in two of the nineteen cases. This further supports the advice to avoid using tank fed tap water in contact lens care routines. The significantly lower FLA growth from hot taps appears to support the thermal sensitivity or environmental preference of these amoebae. Unfortunately, the domestic water source with the highest potential for Acanthamoeba and other FLA contamination, is the bathroom basin cold tap.

ACRIDINE ORANGE STAINING IN RAPID DIAGNOSIS OF ACANTHAMOEBA KERATITIS

Tae-Won Hahn, Woo-Jin Sah, Man-Soo Kim, and Jae Ho Kim

Department of Ophthalmology; Catholic University Medical College; Seoul, Korea

Acanthamoeba keratitis is an uncommon but one of the most severe infectious disease of the cornea. Delayed diagnosis or misdiagnosis as herpes simplex virus keratitis leads to extensive corneal inflammation and profound visual loss. Therefore, rapid diagnosis of acanthamoeba keratitis is essential for an appropriate treatment and a favorable prognosis. We evaluated the value of acridine orange staining in two cases of acanthamoeba keratitis for rapid diagnosis from corneal scrapings and contact lens solution. Gram stain and culture were also made.

Corneal scrapings stained with acridine orange revealed green to yellowish polygonal, cystic or nonstaining cystic structures consistent with the appearance of acanthamoeba among inflammatory cells and the corneal epithelial cells. Contact lens solution in one patient's contact lens case also showed variably stained polygonal cystic structures. *Acanthamoeba castellani* was identified by growth in culture in one case, and the other amoeba is being studied for species identification.

Although we evaluated the usefulness of acridine orange staining on only two cases of acanthamoeba keratitis, we think that this staining is simple, rapid and reliable in the rapid diagnosis of acanthamoeba keratitis.

POST CATARACT SURGERY OCULOMYCOSIS

Madhukar K. Reddy, Savita Rawal, Taraprasad Das, Usha Gopinathan, and Gullapalli N. Rao

L.V. Prasad Eye Institute, Hyderabad, India

Purpose: To study the clinical profile of fungal infections following cataract surgery.

Methods: A retrospective review of medical records over a 3.5 year period (February 1992 - June 1995) of patients presenting as fungal keratitis or endophthalmitis within six months of cataract surgery at a referral eye hospital was performed.

Results: A total of 19 patients (13 males, 6 females) were seen; 8 presented initially with keratitis, 8 with endophthalmitis along with keratitis and three as endophthalmitis only. The mean time of presentation was 48 days after surgery. Topical corticosteroids were used definitely by 11 patients (63%) and 8 patients (42%) had diabetes mellitus. Corneal suppurative infiltration along the surgical wound was present in 16 patients (84%) and anterior vitreous exudates in 3 patients (16%). *Aspergillus sps.* were isolated on culture from 84% of corneal scrapings or vitreous biopsy. Infection by yeasts was not encountered.

3/8 (38%) eyes presenting with keratitis and 7/11 eyes (64%) presenting with endophthalmitis were eviscerated or advised evisceration. Resolution of infection occurred in the remaining patients with medical and or surgical management.

Conclusion: In the tropics, post cataract surgical fungal infection, presents commonly as infiltration at the surgical wound and is associated with poor visual prognosis. *Aspergillus sps.* are the commonest causative organisms. The infection initiated in the anterior segment probably spreads to the posterior segment at a later stage.

FLUORESCENT GRAM STAIN: A NEW METHOD IN THE DIAGNOSIS OF BACTERIAL KERATITIS

Savitri Sharma,[1] Bhaskar Roychoudhruy,[2] Madhukar K. Reddy,[2] and Gullapalli N. Rao[2]

Devchand Nagardas Jhaveri Microbiology Centre[1] and Sight Savers' Cornea training Centre. L.V. Prasad Eye Institute, Hyderabad, India

Purpose: To evaluate the efficacy of a new method of gram stain (BacLight) in the diagnosis of infectious keratitis and compare the results to conventional gram stain (CGS).

Methods: In a prospective study on 39 corneal ulcer patients, corneal scrapings were stained using BacLight (according to manufacturer's instructions) and examined by fluorescent microscopy. The scrapings were also stained with CGS as well as subjected to culture. Smears stained by both procedures were read by an observer masked to the results of culture. **Results:** The observations of gram reaction and morphology of bacteria, using BacLight and CGS, were compared against culture to determine the sensitivity, specificity and predictive values of the tests (Pig). The positive predictive value of CGS was significantly higher than BacLight though the difference in sensitivitv and specificity was not significant. Bacterial morphology was detected with equal accuracy by both methods. **Conclusions:** The efficacy of fluorescent gram staining is lower than CGS and needs improvement before it can be used as a diagnostic tool in infectious keratitis.

SENSITIVITY OF POTASSIUM HYDROXIDE PREPARATION AND CALCOFLUOR WHITE STAIN IN THE DIAGNOSIS OF MYCOTIC AND ACANTHAMOEBA KERATITIS

Savitri Sharma,[1] Usha Gopinathan,[1] Jeevan Jyothi,[1] Madhukar K. Reddy,[2] and Gullapalli N. Rao[2]

Devchand Nagardas Jhaveri Microbiology Centre[1] and Sight Savers' Cornea Training Centre[2], L.V. Prasad Eye Institute; Hyperabad, India

Purpose: To compare the sensitivity of potassium hydroxide (KOH) mount and calcofluor white (CFW) stain in the detection of fungal elements and Acanthamoeba cysts in corneal scrapings from infectious keratitis patients. **Methods:** Eight nine subjects with culture proven infectious keratitis (Mycotic-67, Acanthamoeba-22) were included in the study. All subjects had undergone microbiological evaluation consisting of microscopic examination of corneal scrapings and culture for bacteria, fungus, and Acanthamoeba. Smears were examined by staining with Gram, giemsa, and CFW with KOH. KOH and CFW were added on the same sample to obviate sample variation and readings were recorded separately using fluorescence (CFW) and light (KOH) microscopy. **Results:** The findings of KOH and CFW were compared in culture proven cases of fungal and Acanthamoeba keratitis. The sensitivity of KOH vs CFW was 77.6% vs. 80.5% (p - 0.3398) for detection of fungal elements and 54.5% vs. 59.0% (p = 0.3817) for Acanthamoeba cysts. **Conclusions:** While KOH is comparable to CFW in the diagnosis of mycotic and Acanthamoeba keratitis, both modalities are significantly more efficacious (p = 0.0181, 0.0212) in the detection of fungal elements than Acanthamoeba cysts in corneal scrapings.

CHARACTERISATION OF CORNEAL LESIONS CAUSED BY ACTIVE PROTEINASE AND BY CONIDIA OF ASPERGILLUS FLAVUS

Philip A. Thomas and P. Geraldine*

Joseph Eye Hospital, Tiruchirapalli 62000, India *Bharathidasan University,Tiruehirapalli 620024, India

AIM: Although Aspergillus species are important causes of keratitis in many countries, the role of Aspergillus proteinases in pathogenesis of Aspergillus keratitis is unclear.

We sought to characterise, in an experimental animal model, the corneal lesions caused by viable conidia and by an active proteinase from a corneal isolate of Aspergillus flavus. **METHODS:** A metalloproteinase was recovered from a 10-day growth of A.flavus in a defined liquid medium; 20 uL of this was inoculated intrastromally into one cornea of each of 10 rabbits. Viable conidia from a 48 hr growth of the fungus were suspended in 8 saline(5 x 10 CFU/ml); 20 uL of this was injected into steroid pretreated corneas of another 10 rabbits. **RESULTS:** Rapidly-evolving but localised damage was seen in corneas injected with active proteinase. Slowly evolving, spreading lesions were seen in corneas injected with viable conidia. Tissue sections revealed marked damage to stromal collagen fibrils and keratocytes in corneas, irrespective of whether proteinase or conidia had been injected. **CONCLUSIONS:** These data indicate that proteinase and conidia of A. flavus can cause lesions in corneal tissue. Such proteinases may contribute greatly to corneal damage in clinical A.flavus keratitis. Hence, proteinase-neutralising agents may have to be used as adjuncts in treating such patients.

NOCARDIA ASTEROIDES KERATITIS AFTER RADIAL KERATOTOMY

Elcio H. Sato, Denise Freitas, Edson Mori, and Claudio Macedo

São Paulo Federal University - Paulista School of Medicine, São Paulo, Brazil

Purpose: To present two cases of *Nocardia asteroides* keratitis after radial keratotomy. In our knowledge they are the two first of such cases. **Methods:** Two patients that had been operated by the same surgeon presented with suspected infectious keratitis that not responded to antibacterial and antifungal therapy. Due to the worsening of the infection the patients were referred to us. **Results:** Microbiological exams were positive to Nocardia asteroides, therefore treatment with topical and oral sulfadiazine was started. The keratitis in both patients slowly responded to the therapy. **Conclusions:** Although infrequent, *Nocardia asteroides* keratitis it is important to consider in the differential diagnosis of infectious keratitis after radial keratotomy, even more when the keratitis do not respond to traditional antibacterial and antifungal therapy.

KERATITIS SCROPHULOSA CAN CAUSE FORM DEPRIVATION MYOPIA

C. Meyer[1,2] and G. Dunker [3]

[1]Augenklinik Marienhospitel, Johannisfreiheit 2–4, 49078 Osnabrück, Germany
[2]Augenklinit der Medizinischen Universität 2tl Lübeck, Ratzeburger Allee 160, 23538 Lübeck, Germany [3]Christian-Albrechts-Universität, Klinik für Ophthalmologie, Hegewischstraße 2, 24105 Kiel, Germany

Introduction: In the past a lot of experimental studies on the causes of myopia have been published. Zrenner and Schaeffel reported that translucent occluders may induce axial eye elongation in animals. This axial growth is also called form deprivation myopia

(FDM). From clinical experience it is well known, that patients with keratitis scrophulosa frequently have high myopia.

Study: Searching for a clinical correlate, we designed a retrospective multi center study. 150 patients with keratitis scrophulosa peracta—mainly corneal transplant patients—were preoperatively reviewed concerning the following features:

1. age of onset
2. refraction
3. biometry

Results: Our results showed, a refraction of -4.27dpt on the average: The age of onset was form 1 year to the age of 21 with a mean of 5.3 years. If the onset of keratitis scrofulosa was before the age of 5, the myopia was found to be higher (-5.68dpt) than in patients with later age of onset (-2.54dpt). In epidemiologic studies Stenström found +0.5dpt as the mean refraction in the general population. The ultrasound results revealed a mean axial length of 26:89mm, the average is 23.50mm—nearly 3.5mm above the mean.

POSTOPERATIVE ENDOPHTHALMITIS: INCIDENCE, PREDISPOSING SURGERY, CLINICAL SPECTRUM AND OUTCOME

Solel Somani, Aaron Grinbaum, and Allan R. Slomovic

Purpose: To describe predisposing surgery, clinical course and final visual outcome of culture-proven and culture-negative post-surgical endophthalmitis. **Method:** The medical records of 144 patients with culture-proven (n=91) and culture-negative (n=53) post-surgical endophthalmitis from January 1989 to March 1995 were retrospectively reviewed. **Results:** An infectious agent was identified in 91 cases (63.2%). The most common organism isolated was coagulase-negative Staphylococci in 48 cases (53%). In the culture-proven group, cataract surgery was the most common predisposing procedure account for 85% (77/91) of the cases, 62 following extracapsular cataract extraction and 15 following phacoemulsification, with an incidence of 0.28% following both these techniques. While 95% of the culture positive cases received intra-ocular antibiotics following diagnosis, 51 cases (56%) also underwent a vitrectomy. Of the culture-proven cases, 24 (31%) achieved a visual acuity of 20/50 or better while 16 cases (21%) had a vision of no light perception (including 5 eyes that underwent enucleation). 21 cases (40%) infected with low virulence organisms (coagulase-negative Staphylococci or Proprionebacterium acne) were associated with a visual acuity 20/50 or better in comparison to 3 cases (13%) infected with other more virulent organisms (P<0.05). **Conclusions:** While endophthalmitis is most common after cataract surgery, there appears to be no significant difference in the incidence following extracapsular cataract extraction and phacoemulsification. Post-surgical endophthalmitis caused by organisms other than coagulase-negative Staphylococci or P. acne have a poor visual outcome.

INDEX